Integrative Geriatric Medicine

Integrative Medicine Library

Published and Forthcoming Volumes

SERIES EDITOR

Andrew Weil, MD

Donald I. Abrams and Andrew Weil: *Integrative Oncology*

Robert Bonakdar and Andrew W. Sukiennik: *Integrative Pain Management*

Timothy P. Culbert and Karen Olness: *Integrative Pediatrics*

Stephen DeVries and James Dalen: *Integrative Cardiology*

Randy Horwitz and Daniel Muller: *Integrative Rheumatology, Allergy, and Immunology*

Mary Jo Kreitzer and Mary Koithan: *Integrative Nursing*

Daniel A. Monti and Bernard D. Beitman: *Integrative Psychiatry*

Gerard Mullin: *Integrative Gastroenterology*

Robert Norman, Philip D. Shenefelt, and Reena N. Rupani: *Integrative Dermatology*

Myles D. Spar and George E. Munoz: *Integrative Men's Health*

Victoria Maizes and Tieraona Low Dog: *Integrative Women's Health*

Aly Cohen and Frederick S. vom Saal: *Integrative Environmental Medicine*

Richard Carmona and Mark Liponis: *Integrative Preventive Medicine*

Barbara Bartlik, Geovanni Espinosa, and Janet Mindes: *Integrative Sexual Health*

Integrative Geriatric Medicine

EDITED BY

Mikhail Kogan, MD, ABOIM, RCST

Medical Director, GW Center for Integrative Medical Center (www.gwcim.com)
Associate Director, Geriatric, Palliative, and Integrative Medicine Fellowships
Director, Integrative Medicine Track Program
Faculty, GW Center on Aging, Health, and Humanities
Assistant Professor of Medicine
George Washington University
Washington, DC
Founder and Chair of the Board, AIM Health Institute, Washington, DC-based nonprofit
organization delivering free integrative health services to underserved communities
(www.healthaim.org)

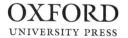

OXFORD
UNIVERSITY PRESS

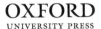

OXFORD
UNIVERSITY PRESS

Oxford University Press is a department of the University of Oxford. It furthers the University's objective of excellence in research, scholarship, and education by publishing worldwide. Oxford is a registered trade mark of Oxford University Press in the UK and certain other countries.

Published in the United States of America by Oxford University Press
198 Madison Avenue, New York, NY 10016, United States of America.

CIP data is on file at the Library of Congress
ISBN 978-0-19-046626-8

1 3 5 7 9 8 6 4 2

Printed by Webcom Inc., Canada

CONTENTS

FOREWORD

ANDREW WEIL, MD

Series Editor

An unprecedented demographic change is occurring in our society. Never before has there been such a high proportion of old people. What's more, the oldest old—those 85 and above—are now the fastest-growing segment of the population. Japan is a bit ahead of the United States in the graying of society, and the change there has greatly impacted the economy and many social institutions, including the national health care system.

Old people tend to be sicker than young people. Many of the most serious forms of chronic illness become much more frequent after age 60, cardiovascular and neurodegenerative disease and cancer especially. We often refer to these as the diseases of aging, but they are not inevitable consequences of living longer. Research shows that the aging process is independent of age-related disease, meaning that it is possible to live long and well, enjoying relatively good health until an inevitable period of disability and decline at the end of life. The goal of healthy aging is to reduce the risk and delay the onset of age-related disease and experience "compression of morbidity"—that is, a rapid and brief decline before death.

To achieve that goal people must attend to all the factors under their control that influence health and risks of disease: diet, physical activity, rest and sleep, mental and emotional wellness, for example. They must also avoid harmful habits and behavior, make appropriate use of preventive medical services, and practice self-care. It is very much in society's interest to teach people about healthy lifestyle choices and incentivize people to make them. Conventional medicine is not very effective at managing age-related diseases once they are established, and the effort to do so is a major drain on the resources of our failing health care system. We have yet to feel the impact of the demographic bulge of baby boomers now approaching old age; the more sick seniors we have to care for, the greater the economic burden we will have to bear.

Physicians and allied health professionals have a major responsibility to promote health, prevent illness, and help aging people increase their chances of compressing end-of-life morbidity. Given our rapidly growing older population, it is disappointing how few geriatricians we have: about 7,000 for the whole country. Worse, geriatrics is one of the few medical specialties that is shrinking, a less and less popular choice for young doctors to make when they finish residency training in internal medicine. Additionally, like conventional medicine in general, geriatrics has been limited by narrowly focusing on the physical body, paying insufficient attention to the influence of lifestyle factors on health and to the human organism's capacity for healing, and ignoring the potentially valuable concepts and practices of other medical systems, such as traditional Chinese medicine.

Integrative medicine has a much broader perspective. It addresses the whole person (body, mind, spirit, community member), includes lifestyle medicine, and draws on the best complementary and alternative practices as well as conventional ones. A new integrative model is needed to revitalize the field of geriatrics, attract more health care professionals to it, and provide for the needs of our graying society.

My friend and colleague, Dr. Mikhail Kogan, has compiled this volume with that new model in mind. It offers a wealth of useful, evidence-based information to help practitioners better care for older patients and is a valuable addition to the Weil Integrative Medicine Library series of Oxford University Press.

CONTRIBUTORS

Alyssa Adams, PsyD
Washington DC VA Medical Center
Washington, DC

Tania Alchalabi, MD
Assistant Professor in Geriatrics and
    Palliative Medicine
George Washington University
Washington, DC

Alice Berg
George Washington University
Washington, DC

Patricia A. Bloom, MD, FACP, AGSF
Clinical Associate Professor
Brookdale Department of Geriatrics
    and Palliative Medicine
Icahn School of Medicine at Mount
    Sinai
New York, NY

Ryan Bradley, ND, MPH
Assistant Professor
Division of Preventive Medicine
University of California, San Diego
La Jolla, CA

Marc Brodsky, MD
Assistant Clinical Professor of
    Medicine
Department of Medicine
Columbia University College of
    Physicians and Surgeons
New York, NY

Meredith Bull, ND, NS4
Bastyr University
Seattle, WA

Mara Caroline, MD
Temple University School of Medicine
Philadelphia, PA

Stephanie Cheng, MD
Assistant Professor of Medicine
University of California, San Francisco

Joseph P. Cleaver, MD, ABAARM
Paradigm Wellness Medical Group
San Francisco, CA

Elizabeth L. Cobbs, MD
Professor, Medicine, Geriatrics and
  Palliative Medicine
George Washington University
Chief, Geriatrics, Extended Care,
  Palliative Care
Washington DC VA Medical Center
Washington, DC

Aaron A. Davis, DO
Holy Cross Hospital
Taos, NM

Dimple Desai, MD
Department of Family Medicine
The University of Texas Medical
  Branch at Galveston
Galveston, TX

Anca Dinescu, MD
Assistant Professor, Internal Medicine
George Washington University
Washington, DC

Aviva Ellenstein, MD, PhD
Assistant Professor of Neurology
Medical Faculty Associates
George Washington University
Washington, DC

Yael Flusberg, E-RYT 500, RMT, MS
Yoga Therapist
GW Center for Integative Medicine
Washington, DC

Angela Gabriel, MSOM, L.Ac.
Acupuncturist
GW Center for Integative Medicine
Washington, DC

Marie Anne Gebara, MD
Neuropsychiatry Fellow
Department of Psychiatry
University of Pittsburgh School of
  Medicine
Pittsburgh, PA

Ronald Glick, MD
Assistant Professor of Psychiatry
  and Physical Medicine and
  Rehabilitation
University of Pittsburgh School of
  Medicine
Pittsburgh, PA

Mimi Guarneri, MD
Founder and Medical Director
Scripps Center for Integrative
  Medicine
Attending Physician, Cardiovascular
  Disease
Scripps Clinic
La Jolla, CA

Ann E. Hansen, DVM, MD
Acting Instructor of Medicine
Department of Medicine
Division of General Internal Medicine
University of Washington School of
  Medicine
Boise Veterans Affairs Medical Center
Boise, ID

Tiffany C. Hoyt M.Ac., Dipl. O.M., L.Ac.
Acupuncturist
GW Center for Integative Medicine
Washington, DC

Amanda Hull, PhD
Field Implementation Lead
VHA Office of Patient Centered Care
  & Cultural Transformation
Portland, OR

Luann Jacobs, MA-CCC/SLP, RMT
Reiki Master Teacher
Director of Reiki Program
GW Center for Integative Medicine
Washington, DC

Robert L. Jayes, MD
Associate Professor of Medicine
George Washington University
    Medical Faculty Associates
Washington, DC

**Robert M. Kaiser, MD, MHSc, FACP,
AGSF**
Attending Physician, Geriatrics and
    Extended Care
Medical Director, Home Based
    Primary Care Program
Washington DC VA Medical Center
Associate Professor of Medicine,
    Division of Geriatrics and Palliative
    Medicine
The George Washignton University
    School of Medicine
Washington, DC

Mary Kendell, MS, WHNP-BCV
Nursing Practitioner
Washington, DC

**Mikhail Kogan, MD, ABOIM, RCST
Associate Professor of Medicine**
Medical Director GW Center for
    Integrative Medicine
Associate Director Geriatrics,
    Palliative Care, Integrative Medicine
    Fellowship Programs
George Washington University
Washington, DC

Mariatu Koroma-Nelson, MD, MPH
Virginia Hospital Center
Geriatrician
Palliative/Hospice and Integrative
    Medicine
Arlington, VA

Angela Lee, MD, MPH
Associate Clinical Professor
Palliative Medicine
George Washington University
Washington, DC

Eric Lenze, MD
Professor of Psychiatry
Washington University School of
    Medicine in St. Louis
St. Louis, MO

**Amy Littlefield ND, MSOM,
LAc, FABNO**
Naturopathic Physician,
    Accupuncturist
Owner
Vermont Wellness Medicine and
    Integrative Oncology
Middlebury, VT

Tahira I. Lodhi, MD
Assistant Clinical Professor of Medicine
Division of Geriatrics and Palliative
    Medicine
George Washington University
Washington, DC

Beverly Lunsford, PhD, RN
Assistant Professor, George
    Washington School of Nursing;
    Director, Center for Aging,
    Health and Humanities; Director,
    Washington D.C. Area Geriatric
    Education Center Consortium
Washington, DC

Dale Lupu, MPH, PhD
Associate Research Professor
Center for Aging, Health and
    Humanities
School of Nursing
Professional Lecturer in Health Policy
School of Public Health
George Washington University
Washington, DC

Elizabeth R. Mackenzie, PhD
Adjunct Associate Professor
University of Pennsylvania
Graduate School of Education
Human Development & Quantitative
    Methods
Philadelphia, PA

**Nisha J. Manek, MD, FACP, FRCP
(U.K.) Chair**
Kingman Rheumatology, Kingman
    Regional Medical Center, Member,
    Mayo Clinic Network
Kingman, AZ

Anne McDonald, MFA, OTR/L
AmSAT certified Alexander Teacher
Guild certified Feldenkrais
    Practitioner
Occupational Therapist
Feldenkrais Guild© of North America
    (FGNA)
American Society for the Alexander
    Technique (AmSAT)
American Occupational Therapy
    Association (AOTA)
Washington, DC

Juliet M. Mckee, MD
Associate Professor, Family Medicine
Assistant Dean of Student Affairs
University of Texis Medical Branch
Galveston, TX

Kyle Meehan, MD
Department of Family & Community
    Medicine
College of Medicine Tucson
The University of Arizona
Tucson, AZ

Ronak Mehta, MD
Complementary and Integrative
    Medicine Physician
Washington, DC

Terry A. Mikovich, RN, BSN, MPS
Home-Based Primary Care Program
    Director
Department of Veterans Affairs
Washington DC VA Medical Center
Washington, DC

George Muñoz, MD
Oasis Institute and Arthritis Osteoporosis
    Treatment and Research Center
Aventura, FL

Maryclaire O'Neill, DO, DABFM, IFMCP
Family Medicine Physician
Integrative Primary Care
Chinle, AZ

Deirdre Orceyre ND, MSOM, LAc
GW Center for Integrative Medicine,
    Naturopathic Medical Director, GW
    Comprehensive Breast Center, GW
    University Hospital; Georgetown
    University, Dept. of Biochemistry
    and Cellular and Molecular Biology
Washington, DC

Christina Prather, MD
Associate Professor of Geriatric
    and Palliative Medicine, George
    Washington University
Washington, DC

Christina M. Puchalski, MD, FACP, FAAHPM
Professor of Medicine and Health
  Science
Director, The George Washington
  University Institute for Spirituality
  and Health (GWish)
Co-Director, MFA-GWU Supportive
  and Palliative Outpatient Clinic
The George Washington University
  School of Medicine and Health
  Sciences
Washington, DC

Birgit Rakel, MD
Assistant Professor
Director of Integrative Women's
  Health
Myrna Brind Center for Integrative
  Medicine at the Marcus Institute
Thomas Jefferson University
Philadelphia, PA

Seema Rao, MD, ABOIM
Geriatrician
Scripps Clinical Medical Group Inc
San Diego, CA

Eric J. Roseen, DC, MS
Research Fellow
Department of Family Medicine
Program for Integrative Medicine &
  Health Disparities
Boston University
Boston Medical Center
Boston, MA

Katalin Roth, JD, MD
Professor
Division of Geriatrics and Palliative
  Medicine
Department of Internal Medicine
Medical Faculty Associates
The George Washington University
  School of Medicine and Health
  Sciences
Washington, DC

Anna Rotkiewicz, MD
Assistant Professor
Department of Internal Medicine
Division of Geriatrics
University of Texas Medical Branch
Galveston, TX

Alice Schmidt Kehaya, MS4
George Washington University
Washington, DC

Ilana Seidel, MD
American Board of Integrative
  Medicine
San Francisco, CA

Angela J. Shepherd, MD
Professor Family Medicine
University of Texas Medical Branch
Galveston, TX

Justin Sevier, NREMT-P
George Washington University
Washington, DC

Michelle Sierpina, PhD, MS
Founding Director, Osher Lifelong
  Learning Institute, OLLI at UTMB
  Health; University of Texas
  Distinguished Teaching Professor
Galveston, TX

Victor Sierpina, MD
WD and Laura Nell Nicholson
   Professor of Integrative Medicine
Professor, Family Medicine
University of Texas Distinguished
   Teaching Professor
Department of Family Medicine
UTMB—Health
Galveston, TX

Mary Starich, PhD
Certified Advanced Rolfer™
GW Center for Integrative Medicine
Washington, DC

Karen Welch, MD, ABFM
Fellow in Integrative Medicine and
   Behavioral Health
University of Texas Medical Branch at
   Galveston
Galveston, TX

Julie Wendt, MS, CNS
Nutritionist and Health Coach, GW
   Center for Integative Medicine
Washington, DC

Margie Wentzel, MS, WHNP-BC, CNM
Gynecologist (OBGYN)
Shady Grove Facility
Alexandria, VA

James Yang, MD, MPH
Faculty Member, Instructor
Integrative and Metabolic Medicine
   Program
Department of Health Sciences
George Washington University
Washington, DC

1

Introduction

MIKHAIL KOGAN AND KYLE MEEHAN

Yesterday I was clever, so I wanted to change the world. Today I am wise, so I am changing myself.

Rumi, 13th-century Sufi poet

Dedication (from the book editor, Dr. Mikhail Kogan)

To my parents and grandparents, who raised me to respect the elders and be proactive about my health. Specifically, to my father, Rudolf, whose example influenced my lifelong interest in exercise and a healthy diet, and my mother, Zina, father, and grandparents, Shura and Yakov, who taught me the value of being close to nature and using nature-given products to assist with healing our body and mind. To my wife, Angela, who taught me how to integrate diverse concepts across different fields of medicine, such as allopathic and Chinese medicine, and who showed me how to see the importance in the shades of gray in times when I only saw things as black and white. To all my mentors, patients, and Sufi community friends, who nurtured the sense of a sacred respect for our elders.

Preface

Over the past century, the world has seen a steady increase in the life expectancy of humans. This positive trend is multifactorial due to a better quality of life, better medical care, and dramatic improvements in public health.

Unfortunately, in the last few years the life expectancy in the United States has stalled for all demographics and in the case of white women has actually decreased (http://www.cdc.gov/nchs). There are a number of explanations as to why this is happening, but we believe that in part this phenomenon is driven by over-medicalization of our health and lifestyles. Many people are now born into the world by cesarean section deliveries. We are fed processed and synthetic foods throughout our lives. Instead of traveling by foot and working manually, we move from place to place by automated transportation and our work is made easier by machines. Many medical ailments are now addressed first by different medications rather than by lifestyle changes. The over-medicalization of lives and health care is even more pronounced in the field of geriatrics, the health care for the aging population. This book does not try to answer why this over-medicalization is happening or attempt to solve any politicoeconomic reasons for this trend. Instead, this book demonstrates to health care providers and care partners of the elders that there are other ways of helping them to maintain and even improve their health, while minimizing the amount of medical interventions. This book will discuss lifestyle interventions such as dietary and exercise changes, as well as the introduction of evidence-based complementary modalities such as acupuncture, mind–body therapies and practices, and the use of natural supplements and products to enhance the health of the older patient.

Traditional use of the words "geriatric" and "elderly" implies the process of frailty and disease. We will try to use the word "elder" as much as possible, keeping with the international movement to reframe health care for the aging population away from disease and illness and toward health and wellness. Similarly, we will attempt to use "care partners" instead of "caregivers." Using term "elder," we aim to align readers with the traditional use of this word in cultures where elders were carriers of knowledge, wisdom, and traditions.

Case Study

Mr. R, an 80-year-old Jewish Russian man, was told in his late 20s that he had only a few years to live due to "severe incurable asthma." Being strong-minded and intellectually driven, he ignored this prognosis and took up the hobby of long-distance running. In just a few years, Mr. R completely recovered from his asthma and finished his first marathon in his mid-30s. In addition, Mr. R took up a comprehensive hybrid calisthenics and weight-training program that he still maintains at the age of 80. In the last few years he developed elevated blood pressure, for which he takes two medications, and he has suffered from nonspecific back pain, which he addresses by "running more." In addition to robust exercise and a healthy diet, Mr. R formed a habit of spending regular time in nature kayaking, hiking, and cross-country skiing with friends and family members. Mr. R's early life experience of being given a grim prognosis, which he avoided by a drastic lifestyle modification and the introduction of regular exercise into his life, made him a very smart health care consumer. Despite consulting with his doctors on all health problems, he preferred to first try lifestyle changes and natural approaches for his health care and ailments such as allergies and prostate enlargement.

This case demonstrates a few key issues that this book addresses. Severe illness early in life allowed Mr. R to channel his energy into discovering his own path to wellness. He created ongoing effective exercise and diet routines that not only cured his asthma but also maintained his health. Mr. R also credited his exercise program as his main stress management tool. An unforeseen benefit of his self-reliance was that he needed to access medical services only for routine checkups and acute emergencies, thus minimizing his risk of iatrogenic medical interventions and side effects and of medications. By the time this book was finished, Mr. R completed another Philadelphia marathon at the age of 80, taking fourth place in the 75+ age group and first place in the 80+ group. It should come as no surprise to the reader that this patient is Dr. Kogan's father, who became his role model for living and advocating for healthy lifestyle changes for himself, his family, and his patients.

A question that medical professionals, researchers, and lay people alike have continued to ask and study is why individual humans look so dramatically different both externally and internally when compared to one another in old age. Why do some people age quickly and become diseased, while others age slowly and stay productive and healthy into the dusk of their lives? From the study of individuals, families, communities, and populations at large many factors that drive the healthy aging process have become clear, and yet these factors have largely been ignored by the Western medical system.

It seems that developed Western countries have traded the innate healing presence within all of us, which allows for healthy aging but requires daily attention and a commitment to health care maintenance and a balanced lifestyle, for convenience, instant gratification, and the "quick fix" in medicine and health. Because of this trade, developed Western countries now consider healthy aging to be a rarity rather than an accessible reality for most. If we continue to allow people to believe that healthy aging is unattainable, the reality of achieving optimal health for the aging will become less and less possible for the majority. A philosophical shift in how we view aging and the possibility of healthy aging within our society is essential to change the reality of aging for our population.

As we grow older, our health care needs become biologically more and more unique, and yet our current health care system does not accommodate this diversity and often treats patients of the same age similarly or compartmentalizes care of patients by their disease only. For each medical problem and diagnosis there exists a set of general protocols accepted by health care practitioners as standard practice. However, these protocols almost never take into account what individuals are eating, how they are exercising, what their support system or community looks like, how they manage stress, and how they spend their leisure time. This book will present information that would suggest attention to such aspects of an individual's life is essential when recommending interventions for health promotion and disease treatment.

The scientific community agrees that only 20% of our longevity is based on genetics,[1] although many chronic illnesses have much higher heredity rates—for example, early Alzheimer's disease is hereditarily linked in over 50% of cases.[2] With genetics playing a significant role in determining our longevity, but not ultimately determining our lifespan, we would expect a continuous rise in life expectancy as modern medicine improves.

The books *The Blue Zones* and *Healthy at 100* describe places in the world where people routinely live until the age of 100 or longer while remaining highly functional, with a high quality of life and health well into the ninth or even tenth decade of life. These areas are now called "blue zones" after the bestselling book with the same name.[3] The healthy aging phenomena of the populations described within the books raise the question as to why, in industrialized countries, health drastically declines with age, despite the knowledge of which lifestyle factors can lead to a longer lifespan and healthier living. In industrialized countries, elderly people have more chronic illnesses and disability, which leads to a steady increase in health care spending as the populations age.[4] There is a drastic difference among the older nursing home residents in developed countries compared to the healthy elderly individuals who are able to continue to perform hard physical labor into their 90s, as found in the blue zones.

Dan Buettner, the author of *The Blue Zones*, described the following areas as having the highest prevalence of centenarians: Sardinia, Italy; Okinawa, Japan; Nicoya Peninsula, Costa Rica; Loma Linda, California (where a large number of Seventh Day Adventists live); and Ikaria, a small island off Greece. In his book, Buettner explores what is unique about the lifestyle in these parts of the world, where many centenarians are still active and free of chronic diseases, as compared to other developed parts of the world, where their contemporaries are plagued by disease and decreased functionality and quality of life.[3]

All the blue zones have a number of lifestyle similarities (and a number of differences as well). Residents' diets consist of whole foods. Food processing is limited to drying and fermenting. Simple carbohydrates and sugars are either completely absent or present in very small amounts. All blue zone cultures have adopted the philosophy that food is medicine. In terms of exercise, most of the inhabitants tend to move a lot throughout the day, in many instances walking or tending to gardens or farms for hours each day. In some communities, people walk upwards of marathon distance to perform their activities of daily living. The third and fourth essential shared qualities of these cultures are that these people live in community and strongly value rest and sleep. As a result of their diet, exercise, and community living, these populations share meaningful life engagement and positive attitudes, all contributing to extended life expectancy and sustained health and function into their late years of life.

While no single answer exists as a key to the fountain of youth, the overarching answer to how to live a longer, healthier life is simple and obvious. Western societies have lost the structure of healthy lifestyles as the pillar of health and disease prevention and treatment and no longer rely on regular exercise, a healthy diet, living in community, and fostering social connections as the key to health and disease-free living. Instead, Western societies rely on the medicalization of health. When the field of medicine became a for-profit industry, medical treatments and interventions that generate the most capital and are easiest to incorporate into practice flourish, while cheap but time-intensive lifestyle optimization interventions that need to be done throughout one's life have been largely ignored. With aging, the difference between an individual who takes healthy living as his or her personal responsibility and commits to lifestyle optimization versus an individual who relies on the medical community to solve his or her health care needs becomes more and more obvious. We must ask ourselves, as health care providers, how we can learn to guide our patients into their older age while staying healthy. The authors believe it is our duty as health care professionals to take an active role in teaching patients how to maintain a healthy lifestyle for optimal aging. We cannot wait for our governments or any other organizations to lead the culture shift toward healthier lifestyles for ourselves and our patients. Throughout this book, especially in the first section, we describe lifestyle methods that people who live in the blue zones of the world use in their daily life, and we offer recommendations of how to incorporate these methods into the lives of our patients in the industrialized world and in the care of the elderly to ensure healthier aging of our population.

While many theories of aging exist, none explains the process completely. We will not explore these theories in detail in this book and instead will concentrate on the practical approaches on how to maintain health and treat medical problems with lifestyle changes. However, a basic list of these theories is important to introduce to the readers in order to create a more robust picture on aging as a process.[5] The most common theories of aging can be divided into two major categories: programmed aging and damage- or error-based aging. In the programmed theories of aging, a number of genes turn on or off with time, which leads to programmed hormonal and immunological shifts, which lead to aging. The damage- or error-based theories of aging encompass multiple related yet unique theories, detailed in Box 1.1.

Aging is an undeniable, unavoidable reality for all of us, but becoming chronically ill is not a certainty. We believe that we can dramatically reduce the amount of chronic illness by radically modifying our nation's lifestyle. We also know that this shift is necessary to avoid dramatic financial and overall national health consequences for our society in the upcoming decades. The health care providers taking care of the geriatric population are the ones who see the end product of unhealthy living in the United States, but health care providers are not adequately taught how to reverse and prevent chronic illness during their training. Unfortunately, the idea of preventing a disease like cancer or Alzheimer's disease through lifestyle optimization and changes is often met with strong skepticism inside medical academia. This book serves as a guide for those health care providers who want to learn how to optimize and

---

Box 1.1. Damage- or Error-Based Aging Theories

1. Free radical accumulation/antioxidant system failure—leads to accumulation of toxins and gradual organ failure
2. Mitochondrial deterioration—leads to a decline in energy production of the organism
3. Social isolation/disengagement and decrease in activity (the "use it or lose it" theory)
4. Neuroendocrine theory—gradual decline in hormonal production leads to dysregulation of multiple hormonally controlled pathways.
5. Membrane theory of aging—encompasses and uniquely combines a number of earlier-described theories such as free radical, mitochondrial dysfunction, and neuroendocrine dysregulation
6. Glycosylation or cross-linking theory—the oxidation of sugars, specifically glucose, leads to the cross-linking of glucose to other molecules, which are then harmfully deposited in the body and trigger inflammation and free radical formation
7. Chronic inflammation—not usually listed as one of the aging theories, but recent research demonstrates that it is a strong contributor to multiple chronic illnesses and leads to premature aging and early demise of organisms. Therefore, much of this book attempts to provide working approaches on how to curb chronic inflammation to prevent disease and dysfunctional aging.

maintain health in elderly patients using evidence-based tools and avoiding over-reliance on the medical-industrial complex.

Unfortunately, the field of geriatrics is not one in which medical students are often interested due to many factors, some of which include the lack of exposure to the field in their medical training, the lack of perceived prestige of the field, and the lack of financial incentive, as it is one of the lowest-paying specialties. In April 2008, the Institute of Medicine published a grim report entitled "Retooling for an Aging America." The detailed report summarized data showing that not only is there a dramatic shortage of geriatricians in the United States currently, but also that all health care providers lack basic training in geriatrics even though a large percentage of their patient population is in this age range.[6] The field of geriatrics does not employ a lot of new technology or pharmacology, which is seen as "successful" and "cutting edge," and therefore is often considered a less glamorous or exciting field of medicine to those in training. Care for the elders requires (1) patience; (2) being able to see the "forest" of health and functional reserve beyond the "trees" of symptoms and illnesses; (3) being an outstanding and compassionate communicator and educator; and (4) what is one of the most challenging things in medicine, the capacity to be able to confront one's own mortality every day, using this reality and reflection as a tool for professional and personal growth rather than letting it cause despair. Despite all of these challenges, geriatricians as a group are often cited as the most satisfied with their choice of specialty, with lower rates of burnout and depression compared to individuals in other specialties.[7,8]

The Outline of the Book

The task of incorporating old wisdom of the key aspects to staying healthy into an increasingly complex health care system is not an easy one, and it must start with understanding the categories that make up a healthy lifestyle. The first section of this book describes the largest and most important lifestyle categories and how they apply to the field of geriatrics and the health of the older patient. These categories are (1) nutrition, (2) exercise, and (3) mind–body and spirituality. The environmental and genetic factors affecting health are described in different chapters throughout the book. In the chapter on exercise, we will cover the important concept of functional reserve and how to maintain or even improve it throughout one's life.

In the sections that follow, we will describe alternative methods to maintaining and promoting health while aging. Some of these alternative modalities have not been rigorously studied in the current scientific environment of randomized controlled trials, but have been used by people for hundreds if not thousands of years, are generally highly individualized, and have high safety profiles as compared to Western medical interventions such as medications and surgery. While we believe that every provider interested in treating older patients must have a good working understanding of nutrition, exercise, and mind–body/spirituality, using alternative modalities such as acupuncture or herbs may be outside of the scope of one's practice. In these cases, understanding when it is appropriate or useful to refer your patient to an alternative or complementary provider for coordination of care and interdisciplinary management of a patient's health is essential. Each chapter in the second section of this book will help the readers to become familiar with (1) the basics of each described modality; (2) what health promotion, disease prevention, or disease treatment it can be effectively used for; (3) common pitfalls, such as side effects, cost, lack of insurance coverage, or lack of licensing for the practitioners; and (4) how to utilize each method despite these issues. We do apologize in advance that for those readers who are highly trained in any given modality(s), the corresponding chapter(s) may appear overly basic. The intent of this book and these chapters is to provide basic knowledge for effective treatments and a guide for when it is appropriate and beneficial to make referrals into these modalities, as well as how to advocate for your patients within these modalities and our current health care system. Each chapter in this section has detailed descriptions of the required licensing and regulations of these modalities and describes additional references and training opportunities for such practices.

The third section of the book concentrates on addressing the most common geriatric conditions and is organized in an organ-based approach. In the practice of integrative health we usually try to stay away from the reductionist organ-based approach by focusing on the whole body, mind, and spirit, but for the sake of the standard geriatric texts and organization of the ideas in the book it is divided into organ systems. Again, we apologize in advance that some seemingly important topics are either totally missing (renal section) or represented only superficially (dermatology or otorhinolaryngology). This is due to number of factors, including (1) the lack of clearly evidenced integrative approaches outside of the common lifestyle interventions covered in the first section of the book, (2) the need to concentrate on areas that are more readily optimized by integrative approaches, and (3) the need to cover in greater detail areas where significant gaps exist in current medical model (chronic pain). Unfortunately, with the strict limits on the size of the book, many sacrifices had to be made.

The final section of this book addresses specific scenarios and professional environments in which many practitioners work while providing services to the aging patient.

While recognizing that this book is not a complete integrative geriatrics textbook, we hope that it will be a useful reference for a variety of health care providers who work with an aging population. We also hope that this book will add to the body of knowledge that may be used to advocate for the importance of high-quality care for our elders.

REFERENCES

1. Murabito JM, Yuan R, Lunetta KL. The search for longevity and healthy aging genes: Insights from epidemiological studies and samples of long-lived individuals. *J Gerontol Ser A Biol Sci Med Sci.* 2012;67A(5):470–479. doi:10.1093/gerona/gls089.

2. Gatz M, Reynolds CA, Fratiglioni L, et al. Role of genes and environments for explaining Alzheimer disease. *Arch Gen Psychiatry.* 2006;63(2):168–174. doi:10.1001/archpsyc.63.2.168.

3. Buettner D. *The Blue Zones: Lessons for Living Longer From the People Who've Lived the Longest.* 9th ed. Washington, DC: National Geographic; 2012.

4. Parker MG, Thorslund M. Health trends in the elderly population: Getting better and getting worse. *Gerontologist.* 2007;47(2):150–158. doi:10.1093/geront/47.2.150.

5. Jin K. Modern biological theories of aging. *Aging Dis.* 2010;1(2):72–74. doi:10.1016/j.bbi.2008.05.010.

6. Drootin M. Retooling for an aging America: Building the healthcare workforce. *J Am Geriatr Soc.* 2011;59(8):1537–1539. doi:10.1111/j.1532-5415.2011.03503.x.

7. Aronson L. Why geriatrics? *Ann Intern Med.* 2010;152:61.

8. Leigh JP, Tancredi DJ, Kravitz RL. Physician career satisfaction within specialties. *BMC Health Serv Res.* 2009;9:166. doi:10.1186/1472-6963-9-166.

2

Geriatric Nutrition

JULIE WENDT, ANNA ROTKIEWICZ, AND ALICE BERG

Food is our first medicine. In the elderly over the age of 65, nutritional risk factors such as vitamin deficiency, malabsorption, and inadequate food intake contribute to four of the ten major causes of death: diabetes, stroke, cancer, and heart disease.[1] As almost half of all deaths in the United States in 2010 were due to cancer and heart disease, proper nutrition appears essential for the prevention of disease-related morbidity and mortality.[1] The practice of integrative nutrition therapy aims to use food therapeutically in order to stimulate the body's innate healing mechanisms and optimize health.

Studies exploring the link between longevity and diet have reinforced the idea that health-promoting lifestyle habits delay the onset of age-related illness and death.[1] As inflammatory processes drive chronic disease, any dietary intervention should aim to mitigate inflammation and promote the anti-inflammatory cascade.[2,3] For example, the role of inflammation in the pathophysiology of symptomatic Alzheimer's disease (AD) is underscored by a phenomena called "resilient brain aging." Patients with resilient brain aging lack neuroinflammation, a finding that may contribute to their functionally asymptomatic status despite later autopsy evidence consistent with AD histopathology.[4] One of the key interventions in integrative neurological care includes an anti-inflammatory diet optimized to include key therapeutic foods for brain health (Table 2.1).

The anti-inflammatory diet should include a variety of plant foods that represent the full spectrum of colors as well as contain high amounts of vitamins and mineral antioxidants.[7] Dietary interventions that include antioxidants and phytonutrients may help to reverse the oxidative damage

Table 2.1. Inflammatory and Anti-inflammatory Foods

Food Category		Examples
Foods to minimize that *cause* inflammation[5,6]	Refined sugar and artificial sweetener	White, brown, maple syrup, corn syrup, agave nectar, rice syrup, sucralose, saccharin, aspartame, acesulfame potassium K and neotame
	Processed foods containing:	Refined carbohydrates, trans fats, rancid vegetable oils high in oxidized omega-6 fatty acids, and synthetic folic acid
	Food additives and chemicals	Artificial colors, chemical preservatives, and additives such as carrageenan
	Foods known to frequently cause sensitivity reactions: gluten-containing grains, dairy, eggs, corn, soy	
	Alcohol in excess	
Foods to emphasize that *reduce* inflammation[7,8]	Clean protein	100% grass-fed animal products, wild-caught seafood, nuts and seeds, legumes and pulses
	Fresh or frozen fruits and vegetables	Organic produce where possible, prioritizing those foods that are the heaviest in pesticide residue as outlined in the Environmental Working Group's Dirty Dozen list[9]; a wide range of color and variety of produce, striving for 8–10 servings per day
	Healthy fats	Nuts, seeds, avocados, olives, grass-fed butter and ghee, coconut oil, olive oil, flax oil, medium-chain triglyceride (MCT) oil, red palm oil, rendered grass-fed animal fat
	Balanced glycemic load	Certain combinations of macronutrients can help regulate glucose homeostasis. Namely, combining a food high in fat and a food high in protein with each meal and snack may prevent spikes in blood sugar by modulating insulin release and by mitigating the glucolipotoxic impact of high sugar intake.[10]

(continued)

Table 2.1. Continued

Food Category	Examples
Nutrient dense[11]	Includes foods that are: – Rich in all of the vitamins, minerals, micronutrients, and phytonutrients required to support biochemical processes at the cellular level – Combined to provide an appropriate macronutrient balance of protein, fat, and carbohydrates – Focused on dietary fiber and preferentially feeding the commensal microbiota that reside within the gut and that: – Provide systemic benefits via anti-inflammatory metabolites such as butyrate, acetate, propionate, niacin, long-chain fatty acids such as omega-3, succinate, kynurenic acid[12] – Endogenously produce nutrients such as vitamin K and B vitamins such as riboflavin, folate, cobalamin[13] – Are rich in resistant starch, which supports endogenous production of short-chain fatty acids such as jicama, garlic, Jerusalem artichoke, tiger nut, plantain, dandelion, chicory, and cooked and cooled beans, potatoes, or grains

associated with aging. With advancing age, an accumulation of reactive oxygen species from cellular metabolism can lead to degradation of cell membranes and an increase in toxins, which build up and cause pathology at the cellular level before spreading and causing disease in tissue and organ systems.[1,14] In 2014, Centers for Disease Control & Prevention researcher Jennifer Di Noia, PhD, identified 41 "Powerhouse Fruits and Vegetables" based on the percentage of key vitamins and minerals within these foods.[15] These foods include watercress, Chinese cabbage, chard, beet greens, spinach, chicory, leaf lettuce, parsley, romaine lettuce, collard greens, turnip greens, mustard greens, endive, chive, kale, dandelion, red pepper, arugula, broccoli, pumpkin, Brussels sprouts, scallion, kohlrabi, cauliflower, cabbage, carrots, tomatoes, lemons, iceberg lettuce, strawberries, radishes, winter squash, oranges, limes, grapefruits, rutabagas, turnips, blackberries, leeks, and sweet potatoes.

Nutritional Themes in the Aging Population

Even with an optimal lifestyle, the aging process inherently creates changes within the body that require careful clinical consideration in order to prevent age-related diseases from reducing a patient's quality of life. The following are some common age- and nutrition-related changes:[16]

- Inflammation and oxidation
- Malnutrition and malabsorption
- Decreased metabolism and corresponding weight gain
- Anorexia, weight loss, and resulting frailty

The natural aging process predisposes patients to nutritional deficiencies that must be monitored even in the healthiest of patients. Often, functional requirements for vitamins increase at the same time that appetite and physical capacities decrease, putting the geriatric patient in a vulnerable state of reduced nutrient stores.[17] Deficiencies in B vitamins, hydrochloric acid (HCl), vitamin D, iron, zinc, selenium, and magnesium can have a significant impact on health (Table 2.2).[18,19] Hence, foods high in these vitamins should be included in all dietary recommendations (Table 2.3).

Table 2.2. Key Nutritional Deficiencies Associated with Aging

Nutrient/Substance[20]	Food Sources	Function	Notes
Thiamine (vitamin B1)	Pork, trout, black beans, mussels, tuna, acorn squash, brown rice, sunflower seeds	Energy metabolism, growth of cells	Measured indirectly via transketolase
Pyridoxine (vitamin B6)	Chickpeas, beef liver, tuna, salmon, chicken, potatoes, turkey, banana	Neurotransmitter synthesis, involved in >100 enzyme reactions, amino acid metabolism, immune function	Can be conditionally deficient when B9 and B12 are deficient; functional marker is homocysteine (as well as B12)
Folate (vitamin B9)	Beef liver, spinach, black-eyed peas, asparagus, Brussels sprouts, romaine lettuce, avocado, broccoli, mustard greens	Amino acid metabolism, synthesis of nucleotides	Folic acid is a synthetic form of B9 found in all processed foods that can interfere with absorption of methylated folate in patients with MTHFR SNP.
Cobalamin (vitamin B12)	Clams, liver, trout, salmon, beef, nutritional yeast	Red blood cells, nerve function, DNA synthesis	Blood markers of functional deficiency are elevated Methylmalonic acid and homocysteine (as well as B6).
Calciferol (vitamin D)	Cod-liver oil, swordfish, tuna, sardines, liver, egg	Bone homeostasis, calcium (Ca) absorption, immune function, anti-inflammatory pathway	Interplay between serum Ca homeostasis, parathyroid hormone, and $1,25(OH)2D$
Hydrochloric acid (HCl)	Apple cider vinegar	Denatures proteins, increases absorption of minerals, kills pathogens	GERD is usually a function of low stomach acid and an insufficient lower esophageal sphincter feedback loop.

Iron	Oysters, white beans, dark chocolate, beef liver, lentils, spinach, tofu	Hemoglobin, connective tissue, energy cycle	Iron from food comes in heme (animal) and non-heme (plant) forms. Heme iron is more bioavailable.
Zinc	Oysters, beef, crab, lobster, pork, beans	Immune function, protein synthesis, wound healing, DNA synthesis	Three ounces of oysters contain nearly 500% of the RDA for zinc. Functional deficiency symptoms include poor wound healing, decreased taste or smell, skin disorders, and depressed immune function.
Selenium	Brazil nuts, yellowfin tuna, halibut, sardines, ham, shrimp	Antioxidant, DNA repair, thyroid function, immune function	No more than two Brazil nuts should be consumed per day to avoid risk of selenosis.
Magnesium (Mg)	Almonds, cashews, peanuts, spinach, wheat, soy milk, black beans, edamame, peanuts, avocado, potato, brown rice	Protein synthesis, muscle and nerve function, blood pressure and blood glucose control, involved in >300 enzymatic reactions	Difficult to measure Mg status as most is in bones and blood; best test is Mg RBC, which still misses some patients with functional deficiency. Key signs of deficiency are muscle twitches and cramps, nervous tension, and difficulty sleeping.

Table 2.3. Food Sources of Accessory Nutrients and Phytochemicals

Nutrient[21,22]	Food Sources (in order of highest levels per serving)
Selenium	Wheat germ, Brazil nuts, wheat, tuna, wheat bran, beef liver, Swiss chard, oats
Vitamin E	Wheat germ oil, sunflower seeds, almonds, safflower and sunflower oil
Vitamin C	Acerola, chili peppers, guava, red peppers, kale, parsley, collard greens, turnip greens, green peppers, broccoli, Brussels sprouts, mustard greens, watercress, cauliflower
Beta-carotene	Green plants, carrots, sweet potatoes, squash, spinach, apricots, green peppers, mangoes, yams
Lycopene	Tomatoes, carrots, green peppers, apricots, pink grapefruit, red cabbage, berries, plums
Flavonoids 1. Anthocyanidins 2. Flavones 3. Citrus bioflavonoids 4. Isoflavones	1. Blueberries, red grapes, purple cabbage 2. Onions, parsley, sage, tomatoes, strawberries, black currant, orange 3. Orange, lemon, lime, grapefruit 4. Soy, red clover
Lutein	Green plants, corn, potatoes, spinach, carrots, tomatoes, most fruit
Zeaxanthin	Spinach, paprika, corn, fruit
Resveratrol	Grapes, red wine, peanuts, cocoa, blueberry, bilberry, cranberry
Zinc	Oysters, seeds, nuts, legumes, whole grains
Glutathione	Asparagus, avocado, walnuts, tomatoes, spinach, carrots, grapefruit, apples (raw highest amounts)

Malnutrition and Malabsorption

MALNUTRITION

The decline of appetite with increasing vitamin and mineral needs leaves the elderly population especially vulnerable to malnutrition. The National Institutes of Health has developed a checklist as part of the Nutrition Screening Initiative (NSI) to guide clinicians in the review of clinical symptoms that predict a nutritional intake below the advised Recommended Dietary Allowance (RDA):[18]

Warning Signs of Malnutrition (DETERMINE):
D Disease
E Eating poorly
T Tooth loss, mouth pain, chewing difficulty

E Economic hardship

R Reduced social contact and eating meals alone

M Multiple medicines (three or more prescribed and/or over-the-counter medications)

I   Involuntary weight loss or gain (10 pounds in 6 months) (This is a red flag)

N Needs assistance with self-care

E Older than 80 years of age with increasing fragility

Addressing each of these social and physical impairments will ensure that the elderly patient receives optimal nutrition. For example, practitioners using the NSI screening can connect a patient who has tooth loss, mouth pain, and/ or chewing difficulty with a nutritionist who can suggest alternatives such as nutrient-dense soups and smoothies.

Malabsorption

Digestion and assimilation require three basic biological processes: mastication, digestion, and absorption. Pathology in any aspect of this cascade will likely result in maldigestion and malabsorption syndromes in the geriatric population due to age-related physical and biochemical decline.[17] Therapeutic dietary approaches to mitigate malabsorption include the following:

- *Bitter greens and apple cider vinegar* prior to meals in order to support HCl production for protein denaturation and mineral absorption.[23] Many elderly individuals have gastroesophageal reflux disease (GERD) due to a decline in lower esophageal sphincter integrity and low HCl levels, the latter of which can result from *Helicobacter pylori* infection-related chronic gastritis.[19]
- *Medium-chain triglyceride (MCT) oil,* which is absorbed directly into cells, bypassing the need for the carnitine shuttle and for bile salt emulsification required for longer chain fatty acids.[24] Coconut oil contains 60% MCTs.[25]
- *Traditionally fermented vegetables and beverages* inoculate the digestive tract with beneficial microbes that support digestion and offer a rich source of easily absorbed nutrients.[26] Examples include sauerkraut, kimchi, kefir, yogurt, and kombucha.
- *Traditionally prepared broth* from animal bones and cartilage that are high in glutamate, a nonessential amino acid that can heal the endothelial lining of the intestinal tract and improve absorptive capacity.[27]

Metabolism and Corresponding Weight Gain

Research has correlated metabolic syndrome–involving obesity with a con-stellation of disease states, such as cardiovascular disease, diabetes, arthritis, urinary incontinence, depression, pulmonary abnormalities, cataracts, cancer, and sarcopenia.[28-30] Rather than simply a function of the height to weight ratio (Body Mass Index [BMI]), obesity in the geriatric population requires con-sideration of the normal physiological increase in fat content and decrease in lean muscle mass that occurs with age. Moreover, as the BMI calculation can be misleading in the elderly due to loss of height from kyphosis and other factors, tools such as bioimpedance analysis and dual x-ray absorptiometry (DEXA) provide a useful window into body composition and therefore health risk in this population.[29,30] Basic caloric restriction without consideration of fat and lean muscle mass can lead to sarcopenia and malnutrition, which in turn increase weakness and fall risk in the elderly.[31] Successful weight loss in the elderly is therefore contingent on the ability to skillfully guide diet and exer-cise regimens such that fat mass decreases while bone mass, muscle mass, and adequate nutritional status are maintained.[30]

Anorexia of Aging

I am grateful to old age because it has increased my desire for good conver-sation and decreased my desire for good food.
M. Tullius Cicero, *Cato Maior de Senectute, 43* B.C.

Anorexia of aging is a multifactorial syndrome defined by decreased appe-tite and food intake with advancing age. While the mechanisms underlying this condition are not completely understood, the consequences are serious and may lead to under-nutrition, weight loss, frailty, sarcopenia, disability, and poor health outcomes.[32,33] In particular, protein energy malnutrition (PEM) can lead to thymus dysfunction, along with associated immune dysfunction, a decreased response to immunization, a decrease in T-cell production, infec-tions, as well as cognitive abnormalities, edema, anemia, dehydration, fatigue, weakness, falls complicated by hip fracture, pressure ulcers, impaired wound healing, and even death.[34]

Although anorexia of aging may affect up to 30% of all elderly individu-als, it often goes undiagnosed or inappropriately categorized as a normal con-sequence of aging.[33] All too often clinicians fail to evaluate whether elderly patients are receiving adequate food intake to meet their energy and nutri-ent requirements.[32] Complicating diagnosis, disease presentation tends to be atypical in the elderly as symptoms can be nonspecific, poorly described, and difficult to assess. In addition to the normal decline in physiological reserves with age, patients may have multiple organ system failure, chronic illnesses, nutritional deficiencies, functional impairments, iatrogenic effects from polypharmacy, and social and environmental factors that contribute to and underlie anorexia of aging (Fig. 2.1).[35]

For instance, the function and number of olfactory and taste receptors degenerate with age and with certain diseases, medications, and environmental exposures, in effect contributing to diminished interest and pleasure in eating.[36,33] If elderly persons also suffer from missing or damaged teeth or ill-fitting dentures, they can have difficulty masticating, further leading to nutritional deficiencies through decreased or less varied food intake. Worsening the situation, the inherent stress of aging, coupled with that caused by deteriorating functional status, loss of independence, loss of loved ones, social isolation, disease, dysbiosis (an imbalance of gut flora), and food allergies, can lead to higher cortisol and catecholamine hormone release, which in turn promote increased secretion of pro-inflammatory cytokines like interleukins and tumor necrosis factor-alpha (TNF-α). These pro-inflammatory cytokines are correlated with increased catabolism, cachexia, and decreased appetite through dysregulation of hormones that influence gastric emptying and satiety, or the feeling of fullness after eating.[32,33,37,38]

Proton-pump inhibitor treatment of GERD likewise delays the gastric emptying rate and increases antral stretch time by decreasing gastric HCl production, thereby slowing the digestion rate, prolonging the feeling of fullness, and reducing food intake.[39] In addition to diminished stomach HCl production due to medications and age, the elderly can have a diminished output of pancreatic enzymes and bile salts, leading to food intolerances, further inflammation, and a stressed immune system. Dysbiosis can cause additional intestinal inflammation and fat malabsorption, which can result in cachexia. Small intestine bacterial overgrowth in particular damages the intestinal barrier, causing increased permeability and possible bacterial translocation.[40]

Age-related medical factors such as gastrointestinal diseases, malabsorption, congestive heart failure, chronic obstructive pulmonary disease, and hyperthyroid disease are also associated with increased energy requirements, anorexia, and malnutrition.[32] Beyond physiological causes, elderly people may have trouble accessing and preparing food and feeding themselves due to sensory hearing and vision deficits, in addition to financial constraints, mobility impairments, lack of caregiver support, poor cognition, and institutionalized living. Finally, mood changes such as grief, anxiety, and depression are highly correlated with appetite reduction in the elderly and represent key targets for evaluation and treatment.[33]

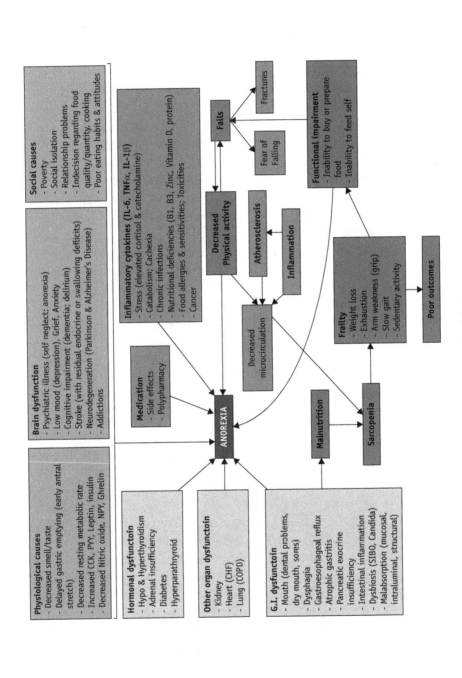

FIGURE 2.1. Preventive and therapeutic interventions for anorexia in the elderly.

SCREENING

Identification of risk factors for anorexia of aging can help with early diagnosis, improved quality of life, and improved clinical outcomes, which are likewise enhanced by multipronged cognitive, behavioral, nutritional, pharmacological, and social interventions that can help avoid complications such as infections, falls, hospitalizations, nursing home placement, and all-cause mortality.[32] Validated tools like the Simplified Nutritional Assessment Questionnaire (SNAQ) for detecting a greater than 5% weight loss and the Mini Nutritional Assessment (MNA) for detecting malnutrition are quick and reliable screening tools for anorexia of aging. Additionally, the FRAIL-NH scale for frailty incurred through reduced food intake and weight loss, and the Geriatric Depression Scale (GDS), may also be helpful indicators of this condition (see Table 2.3).[33]

NUTRITIONAL ASSESSMENT TOOLS

Many physical and biochemical markers are used to assess the nutritional status of the elderly patient (Table 2.4). A comprehensive case history including detailed dietary intake, precursor and triggering events, and lifestyle choices such as sleep, stress management, and exercise should be taken into consideration when interpreting laboratory values and physical signs and symptoms. Key considerations in nutritional assessment include evaluating inflammation and oxidation, malnutrition and malabsorption, decreased metabolism and corresponding weight gain, and anorexia, weight loss, and resulting frailty.

TREATMENT

Along with exercise to bolster strength, reduce depression, lower pro-inflammatory cytokines, stimulate metabolism and appetite, and stimulate microcirculation for delivery of nutrients to muscle cells, protein supplementation of at least 1.0 to 1.2 grams per kilogram of body weight per day has been shown to increase lean muscle mass and strength, thus protecting against the progression of frailty.[32,33] As elderly patients have a diminished anabolic response to increased protein compared to younger individuals, they may also require leucine-enriched essential amino acid supplementation for adequate protein synthesis.[33] Small yet frequent meals, along with additional behavioral and environmental alterations, may also enhance food intake and nutritional status (Table 2.5).

Table 2.4. Nutritional Assessment Tools for the Geriatric Population

Region/ Subject	Indications	Assessment	Clinical Notes	Therapeutic Foods[21]
Physical Assessment*	*Tongue* – Red, inflamed – Coated – Bald, slick, red	– Niacin deficiency – Digestive enzymes, probiotics, fiber – B vitamins, cobalamin, iron		Brewer's yeast, rice and wheat bran, liver, peanuts, sesame and sunflower seeds, oysters, white beans, dark chocolate, lentils
	Mouth – Cheilosis	– Riboflavin, iron		Oysters, white beans, dark chocolate, beef liver, lentils, spinach, tofu, brewer's yeast, almonds, wheat germ, rice
	Ears – Hard ear wax – Vertical lobe crease – Sound sensitivity – Tinnitus	– Omega 3 – Magnesium, B complex, omega 3, CoQ10 – Mg, zinc – Niacinamide, pyridoxine	– Allergies – Cardiovascular risk – Allergies, Temporomandibular joint disorders	Fatty fish, leafy greens, oysters, nuts, pumpkin seeds, ginger, kelp, molasses, buckwheat, wheat
	Eyes – Burning, itching, bloodshot – Dry, soft cornea, xerosis – Eyelid pallor – Iris: copper ring – Vision dysfunction	– Riboflavin – Vitamin A, zinc – Iron – Zinc – Vitamin A, zinc, omega 3, thiamine	– Excess copper, Wilson's disease – Hypoadrenalism	– Prioritize foods with high zinc content and limit foods with high copper. – Liver, chili peppers, dandelion root, carrots, dried apricots, leafy greens

	Hair – Lackluster – Thinning/loss	Biotin, essential fatty acids, protein, zinc	Screen for hypothyroid and excess vitamin A.	Brewer's yeast, liver, soy, rice, peanuts, nuts, fatty fish, oysters
	Nails – White spots – Pale nail beds	– Zinc – Iron deficiency		Oysters, pumpkin seeds, ginger, pecans, split peas, brazil nuts, wheat, rye, oats
	Skin – Acne, eczema, dermatitis, psoriasis – Peeling hands/feet – Rosacea	– Zinc; vitamins A, D, and B; niacin – Omega 3; vitamins A and D; zinc – Riboflavin + B complex	Dairy sensitivity?	Oysters, mushrooms, fatty fish, red palm oil, nuts and seeds, leafy greens
	Sinusitis	Vitamins C, A, B5; zinc; quercetin; β-carotene	Allergies, especially dairy.	Acerola, chili peppers, guavas, sweet peppers, leafy greens, onions, apples, pomegranate
Subjective Testing	Decreased taste and/or smell	Use Zinc Tally test to assess zinc sufficiency.	– RA related to zinc deficiency – Medications influence zinc status. – Toxins block zinc.	
	Metallic taste		Excess zinc, toxic metals	

(continued)

Table 2.4. Continued

Region/ Subject	Indications	Assessment	Clinical Notes	Therapeutic Foods[21]
Objective Testing	Mini Nutritional Assessment—Short Form (MNA-SF)		In a 2012 prospective cohort study, MNA-SF scores of 11 or below correlated with nutritional malnutrition that was confirmed with biochemical workup of albumin, cholesterol, vitamins A and D.[41]	
	SNAQ (Simplified Nutritional Assessment Questionnaire)	Anorexics at risk of weight loss over the next 6 months		
	All patients	Genetic testing (www.23andme.com)	Use full genetic code in various interpretive online applications to assess SNPs that respond well to directed nutritional interventions such as COMT, MTHFR, CBS, MAO, and DAO.	
	Urinary 8-OHdG	Increase food-based antioxidants	Oxidative stress marker that is adversely involved in aging process	

Uric acid elevation	Essential fatty acid deficiency	Associated with antioxidant deficiency and high-sugar diet or diabetes
Bioimpedance analysis		Inexpensive and noninvasive technology to estimate body composition (fat, water, bone)[42]
Complete blood count	– Transferrin (half-life 8 days) – Prealbumin (half-life 17–21 days) – Albumin (half-life 17–21 days) – Hypocholesterolemia – Iron – Iron binding capacity – Total lymph count[17,43]	

* Modified with permission from Dana Laake, RDH, LDN, MS.

Table 2.5. Screening and Therapeutic Interventions for Anorexia in the Elderly

	Screening/Therapeutic Interventions[32, 33, 36, 44–46]	Notes
1	Evaluate for the ability to follow up with a plan; assess:	– Comprehension – Motivation and emotional resilience – Psychological and psychiatric issues (depression, grief) – Medications*/treatments that may dampen appetite (e.g., certain psychiatric, cardiovascular, and anti-rheumatic drugs) or cause dry mouth (e.g., atropine) or sores (e.g., chemotherapy and radiation)
2	Evaluate:	– Ability to chew (dental evaluation) – Ability to swallow (speech evaluation) – Gastrointestinal function (for detailed information, see functional laboratory studies chapter 25) – Other organ dysfunction (laboratory, workup studies) – Evaluation of nutritional deficiencies (e.g., SpectraCell, NutraEval) – Subjective Global Assessment (nutritionally focused physical exam)
3	Treatment of the underlying problem as found above	Many times a multifactorial issue
4	Promote food intake by modifying environment and implementing behavioral interventions:	– *Social interaction*: touch, verbal cueing, dining with others – *Physical alterations*: daily 15-minute sun exposure; increase physical activity – *Food alterations*: Enhance taste, enhance appearance and presentation, adjust texture (smoothness); several food choices to give a sense of control; provide maximal amount of patient-preferred food; serve favorite food late in the day when satiety is decreased – *Environmental alterations*: Dining location decorated with art, warm colors, a fish tank, good lighting, music for increased relaxation; adequate caregiving and staffing to attend to patients in need – *Community resources*: Meals on Wheels; adult day care; food commodities
5	Nutritional rehabilitation	– Regular food (no special diets) – Oral liquid supplements with replacement of protein, vitamins, minerals (e.g., UltraMeal by Metagenics) – Appetite stimulant and tube feeding when appropriate

* To evaluate medications contributing to anorexia and treating it, see: "Clinical Pharmacology Online Rx list "Guide to Preferred Drug in LTC"."

Nutrigenomics

In the last 15 years since the human genome was sequenced, clinical researchers have begun to understand how differences in gene expression dictated by epigenetic influences correlate with susceptibility toward certain disease states. As geneticists worked to classify variations within the over 20,000 genes sequenced, food emerged as one of the primary modulators of gene expression. Demonstratively, the 2002 "Grandparents Study" revealed that food choices create multigenerational inheritable changes in the epigenetics of an individual, impacting the risk of developing chronic diseases such as cardiovascular disease and diabetes.[47] Nutrigenomics, which studies the relationship between nutrients and an individual's genetic single nucleotide polymorphisms (SNPs), helps to explain this phenomenon and provide actionable lifestyle changes that can bring the body into optimal health.[48]

While nutrigenomics is still in its infancy, it is part of a growing trend toward personalized medicine. As such, nutrigenomics aims to match an individual's ideal diet with his or her genes in order to optimize gene expression and treat or even prevent disease. For example, nutrigenomics seeks to examine why some individuals seem to thrive on a high-protein diet with ample saturated fat while others feel best following a diet low in protein and saturated fat. Given further evidence from high-quality, peer-reviewed studies on the varying impact of diet on individual health, the informed practitioner may wish to employ predictive gene sequencing and SNP tests in order to determine dietary guidance for a given patient.[49,50]

Prior to nutrigenomics, practitioners crudely monitored micronutrient status by ensuring that a given patient's total dietary and supplemental intake fell between the U.S. Food and Drug Administration's established (1) Recommended Dietary Allowance (RDA) and (2) Upper Limit.[48] For some nutrients, this range is very large, while for others no Upper Limit has been established. As nutritional counseling moves away from this subjective approach to a more personalized orientation through genetic sequencing, affordable, non-medical, direct-to-consumer SNP testing companies such as 23andMe are empowering patients in their health care. For example, research has identified several disease-related SNP variants in the methylenetetrahydrofolate reductase (MTHFR) gene.[51,52] Fortunately, active forms of folate such as methylfolate can treat the resultant methylation cycle derangements. However, synthetic folate (folic acid) has no role in human metabolism and can therefore cause severe problems in patients with the MTHFR SNP. Such patients have a limited capacity to convert synthetic folate into the active form for use in the conversion of methionine and homocysteine, the metabolic defect of which correlates with a higher incidence of coronary artery disease and several cancers.[53,54] Given that inexpensive vitamins and processed foods contain synthetic folate, practitioners caring for clients with the MTHFR mutation should recommend a whole-foods–based diet in order to avert the severe impact of synthetic folate on the methylation cycle for these individuals.

In addition, prescribing a diet that matches a patient's ancestry may provide the most appropriate macro- and micro-nutrient composition for his or her genetic SNPs (MTHFR and otherwise). Please refer to Oldways (http://oldwayspt.org/) for insight about traditional foods for several cultures, including the Mediterranean, African, Latin, and Asian cultures.

Therapeutic Diets

The impact of nutrients and foods on biochemical and physiological pathways illustrates the critical role that diet plays on supporting health and preventing disease.[21,55–57] Using food therapeutically to affect health is the primary goal of integrative nutrition; as such, identifying the appropriate diet for an individual patient requires understanding the patient's complete health history as well as the indications of various dietary interventions. The following therapeutic diets are those most commonly used in the integrative nutrition practice.

ANTI-INFLAMMATORY ELIMINATION DIET

Food sensitivities are a concrete driver of gut dysfunction, which often manifests as gastrointestinal as well as systemic symptoms of imbalance. By stimulating the immune system and the release of large protein molecules as well as endotoxins such as Lipopolysaccharides (LPS) food sensitivities such as non-celiac gluten sensitivity can induce intestinal permeability and affect body systems outside of the gastrointestinal tract, such as the nervous, immune, cardiovascular, and endocrine systems (refer to Chapter 16 for a discussion of intestinal permeability).[58] These intestinal consequences may have additional adverse effects on digestion and absorption that exacerbate nutritional deficiencies in the elderly population and predispose them to frailty.[32]

Though many food sensitivity tests are on the market to assay specific foods causing an IgG, IgM, or IgA reaction in the body, these tests lack the appropriate reliability and reproducibility necessary to have much clinical utility.[59–62] Consequently, the elimination diet represents the nutritional gold standard for capturing adverse interactions between an individual and food. In the elimination diet, the unique known or suspected food triggers for a given patient are removed from the diet for 4 weeks, after which time the patient sequentially reintroduces one food item at a time to the diet with a 3-day observation period to identify symptom-causing foods. In order to discern food sensitivities from an individualized elimination diet, patients require time to allow for a reduction in systemic inflammation and gut healing. This is initiated by adherence to an anti-inflammatory elimination diet.

A basic elimination diet will remove the following most common triggers:

- *Gluten*: associated with mental fog, headache, endocrine disruption
- *Dairy*: associated with gastrointestinal disturbance such as gas, bloating, pain, constipation
- *Eggs*: associated with autoimmune reactivity
- *Soy*: often a cross-reactive food with gluten and dairy
- *Corn*: often a cross-reactive food with gluten

Additional categories of foods may also be eliminated based on a patient's symptoms:

- *Nightshades* (potato, tomato, pepper, eggplant), which are indicated when joint and muscle pain are present
- *Citrus fruits* (orange, lemon, lime, grapefruit), which are indicated as a common sensitivity
- *Nuts and seeds*, which are indicated when a history of autoimmunity is present
- *Grains*, which are indicated when malabsorption and gastrointestinal inflammation are present

MEDITERRANEAN-DASH INTERVENTION FOR NEURODEGENERATIVE DELAY (MIND)

Despite the correlation between neurological protection and strict adherence to the Mediterranean and DASH (Dietary Approaches to Stop Hypertension) diets, recent studies reported that many patients have difficulty following the diets and hence may not receive a benefit.[63] Emerging research into a new dietary protocol called the Mediterranean-DASH Intervention for Neurodegenerative Delay (MIND) reveals that certain therapeutic foods may provide neurological protection, helping to slow the progression of cognitive decline in those with strict as well as moderate adherence to the diet.[63] The

Table 2.6. MIND Diet Summary

	Foods	Frequency/Dosage	Notes
Emphasize in the MIND Diet	Berries	>2/wk	Blueberries and strawberries have the strongest protective effect.
	Leafy greens	> 6 servings/week	
	Other vegetables	>1/day	
	Nuts	5 servings/wk	
	Beans	3 servings/wk	
	Fish	1 serving/wk	
	Olive oil	Daily	As primary oil
	Poultry	2 servings/wk	
	Whole grains	>3 servings/day	
	Red wine	Daily	
Limit in the MIND diet	Butter and stick margarine	<1 Tbsp/day	
	Fast and fried foods	Limit all categories to 3 servings per week.	
	Pastries		
	Cheese		
	Red meat		

Rush Memory and Aging Project, a prospective cohort study that followed almost 1,000 participants for 5 years, resolved 15 food choices that protect neurological function and reduce the risk of developing dementia and AD.[63] This study found that the risk of developing AD was decreased by "53% in participants who strictly followed the diet, and by approximately 35% in those who followed it moderately well."[63] The guidelines for the MIND diet are summarized in Table 2.6.

Multiple additional dietary interventions provide the clinician with diverse tools to address various pathological metabolic states that will respond positively to alterations in dietary choices. While Table 2.7 is not exhaustive, it represents the most commonly used therapeutic dietary interventions in geriatric nutrition. The primary therapeutic dietary interventions to address the primary risk factors are the anti-inflammatory elimination diet, the Low FODMAP diet, MIND and ketogenic diets for neurological health, the autoimmune paleo diet, the anti-candida diet, and the low amylose diet.

Table 2.7. Summary of Key Dietary Therapeutic Interventions

Diet Name	Target Population	Therapeutic Foods	Restricted Foods	Clinical Notes
Core Food Plan[64]	– Overweight/obesity – Metabolic syndrome	Whole-foods–based diet with 8+ servings of fruits and vegetables having a variety of colors, healthy fats, lean protein sources. Organic and non-GMO sources preferred.	Processed, refined foods	Patients work with allocations within 10 categories based on desired weight body composition: protein, legumes, dairy and alternatives, nuts/seeds, fats/oils, non-starchy vegetables, starchy vegetables, fruits, whole grains, beverages.
Low FODMAP[65]	– Irritable bowel syndrome – Small intestinal bacterial overgrowth	Foods high in fiber, resistant starch, starch, and simple sugars such as banana, blueberry, grapes, broccoli, green beans, Brussels sprouts, carrot, potato	Foods high in fermentable carbohydrates such as apples, watermelon, beans, milk, wheat, rye, onion, honey, sugar alcohols	– Refer to Monash University for the complete and most up-to-date list of High or Low FODMAP foods. – All animal protein allowed
Anti-Candida[66]	– Chronic fatigue – Yeast overgrowth – Thrush – Athlete's foot	– Meat, chicken, nuts – Non-starchy vegetables – Berries	– Refined sugar of any kind – Grains – Starches – Beans/pulses – High-sugar fruit	First 2–4 weeks, limit carbohydrates to 2 servings per day unless vegetarian. Limited fat due to maldigestion unless lipase supplementation

(continued)

Table 2.7. Continued

Diet Name	Target Population	Therapeutic Foods	Restricted Foods	Clinical Notes
Ketogenic Diet[67]	– Neuro-inflammation – Diabetes – Obesity – Polycystic ovarian syndrome – Cancer – Epilepsy	– Avocado – Full-fat dairy – Macadamia nuts – Coconut – Animal protein – Eggs	– Starchy vegetables limited – Grains – Refined sugar – Corn – Beans/lentils	High fat, moderate protein, and limited carbohydrate *Blood sugar*: 55–65 mg/dL *Blood ketones*: 3–5 mM (pathologic is 15–20 mM) Support with additional electrolytes as needed.
No-Amylose Diet[68]	– Chronic inflammatory response syndrome – Mold toxicity	– Protein – Milk/cheese – Fruit – Vegetables grown above ground – Nuts/seeds – Legumes/pulses – Corn	– Grains – All foods grown beneath the ground except onion – Banana – Refined sugar in any form	Removing amylose mitigates insulin spikes and subsequent insulin and leptin resistance.
Intermittent Fasting[69]	– Neuro-inflammation – Blood sugar dysregulation – Cardiovascular disease	– Coconut oil – Medium-chain triglyceride (MCT) oil – Butter-oil coffee – Bone broth	– All – Fluids encouraged	Many different cycles for intermittent: 5 days in ketosis, 2 days off; 14 hr daily fasting between dinner and breakfast; ketogenic diet 6 days a week with 1 fasting day; etc.

Autoimmune Paleo[70]	Autoimmune diseases	- Meat - Vegetables (except nightshades) - Fruits - Bone broth - Fermented foods - Animal fat - Coconut oil - Red palm oil - Olive oil	- Grains - Dairy - Legumes/pulses - Eggs - Nuts/seeds - Nightshades (tomato, potato, pepper, eggplant, paprika)	After a 4-week elimination period and symptoms improve, systematic reintroduction to identify trigger foods. Likely not all categories need to continue to be removed from diet.
Detox Food Plan[64]	- Fatigue - Metal toxicity	- Cruciferous vegetables - Nuts/seeds - Leafy greens - Eggs - Beets - Berries - Animal and plant-based protein - Gluten-free grains - Herbs (cilantro, parsley, chives)	- Dairy - Gluten - Processed foods - Refined sugar - Caffeine	Support detox pathways with fluids, green tea.

Case Study

A 79-year-old male patient came into the clinic presenting with chronic diarrhea, lack of appetite, and weight loss. He described a 30-pound weight loss precipitated by 10 loose bowel movements per day over an approximately 10-week period. He complained that food tasted like cardboard, and of loss of appetite, loss of smell and taste, nausea, confusion, sleeplessness, fatigue, a tingling sensation, muscle spasm, and depression. His past medical history included rheumatoid arthritis (RA), Sjögren's syndrome, GERD, and hypothyroidism. However, his chronic diarrhea started after he was prescribed Arava for RA. Within one week of starting Arava, the patient developed profound diarrhea and was admitted to the hospital. Arava was discontinued, but the patient's stool frequency did not decrease. He was discharged and sent home on Imodium but was readmitted after a few weeks due to worsening diarrhea symptoms and additional weight loss. Physical examination demonstrated no abdominal tenderness and no blood per rectum.

The patient underwent colonoscopy, esophagogastroduodenoscopy, and stool studies. This workup revealed moderate diverticulosis and a tear in the distal esophagus. The patient was prescribed Anusol-HC rectal suppositories and Protonix 40 mg per day. In addition, he was advised to avoid nonsteroidal anti-inflammatory drugs.

Blood test evaluation revealed hypothyroidism (very low T3, normal free T4, normal TSH), anemia (low hemoglobin of 7.1), and a positive zinc thallium test. Despite continuing the Imodium after every bowel movement, the patient still had three or four bowel movements per day.

DIAGNOSIS

The patient was diagnosed outpatient with acute protein calorie malnutrition likely due to chronic zinc deficiency.

TREATMENT

Within 1 week of supplementation with zinc carnosine, protein, a multivitamin, micro elements (UltraMeal), and a probiotic (VSL #3), the patient regained his taste and appetite and no longer needed Imodium for bowel control. After 1 month of treatment, the patient was prescribed an active form of thyroid (Cytomel 5 mcg daily) in addition to Synthroid 75 mcg daily for hypothyroidism. The patient began gaining weight and regained 20 pounds after 4 months.

SUMMARY

The patient experienced acute zinc deficiency and diarrhea triggered by Arava and complicated by anorexia. After zinc replacement, the diarrhea stopped and the patient's appetite and taste became normal. Functional hypothyroidism treatment with free T3 helped the patient to gain weight.

1. People on Arava may experience diarrhea, loss of appetite; nausea; dizziness; mental/mood changes; weight loss; high blood pressure; throat, sinus, or nose infections; hair loss; chest pain; increased/pounding heart rate; acne; itching; rash; spontaneous growths; fatigue; numbness/tingling in the hands/feet; and muscle spasm.[71]
2. Zinc is involved in catalytic activity of the enzyme dihydroorotate dehydrogenase.[72]
3. Metalloenzyme dihydroorotate dehydrogenase containing zinc is blocked by Arava.[73]
4. Lack of reliable laboratory testing prompts us to make the diagnosis on clinical grounds.
5. Zinc carnosine stabilizes small bowel integrity and stimulates gut repair processes.[74]
6. RA is frequently associated with chronic zinc insufficiency.[75]
7. The diarrhea did not resolve after discontinuing Arava since the patient was still zinc deficient.

REFERENCES

1. Brown JE, Isaacs JS, Krinke B, Lechtenberg E, Murtaugh M. *Nutrition through the life cycle.* 5th ed. Stamford, CT: Cengage Learning; 2013.
2. Minihane AM, Vinoy S, Russell WR, et al. Low-grade inflammation, diet composition and health: current research evidence and its translation. *Br J Nutr.* 2015;114(7):999–1012. doi:10.1017/S0007114515002093.
3. Rubio-Ruiz ME, Peredo-Escárcega AE, Cano-Martínez A, Guarner-Lans V. An evolutionary perspective of nutrition and inflammation as mechanisms of cardiovascular disease. *Int J Evol Biol.* 2015;2015:179791. doi:10.1155/2015/179791.
4. Negash S, Wilson RS, Leurgans SE, et al. Resilient brain aging: Characterization of discordance between Alzheimer's disease pathology and cognition. *Curr Alzheimer Res.* 2013;10(8):844–851. doi:CAR-EPUB-55024 [pii].
5. Corley J, Kyle JAM, Starr JM, McNeill G, Deary IJ. Dietary factors and biomarkers of systemic inflammation in older people: the Lothian Birth Cohort 1936. *Br J Nutr.* 2015;114(7):1088–1098. doi:10.1017/S000711451500210X.

6. Manzel A, Muller DN, Hafler DA, Erdman SE, Linker RA, Kleinewietfeld M. Role of "Western diet" in inflammatory autoimmune diseases. *Curr Allergy Asthma Rep.* 2014;14(1):404. doi:10.1007/s11882-013-0404-6.

7. Weil AT. Food as medicine: The anti-inflammatory diet. *J Holist Healthc.* 2016;13(1):8–12.

8. Nooyens AC, Milder IE, van Gelder BM, Bueno-de-Mesquita HB, van Boxtel MP, Verschuren WM. Diet and cognitive decline at middle age: the role of antioxidants. *Br J Nutr.* 2015;113:1410–1417. doi:10.1017/s0007114515000720.

9. EWG's Shopper's Guide to Pesticides in Produce. https://www.ewg.org/foodnews/list.php. Accessed December 1, 2016.

10. Keane KN, Cruzat VF, Carlessi R, De Bittencourt PIH, Newsholme P. Molecular events linking oxidative stress and inflammation to insulin resistance and β-cell dysfunction. *Oxid Med Cell Longev.* 2015;2015. doi:10.1155/2015/181643.

11. Hyman M. *Eat fat, get thin: Why the fat we eat is the key to sustained weight loss and vibrant health.* 1st ed. New York: Little, Brown and Company; 2016.

12. Thorburn AN, Macia L, Mackay CR. Diet, metabolites, and "Western lifestyle" inflammatory diseases. *Immunity.* 2014;40:833–842. doi:10.1016/j.immun

13. LeBlanc JG, Milani C, de Giori GS, Sesma F, van Sinderen D, Ventura M. Bacteria as vitamin suppliers to their host: A gut microbiota perspective. *Curr Opin Biotechnol.* 2013;24:160–168. doi:10.1016/j.copbio.2012.08.005.

14. Humphries KM, Szweda PA, Szweda LI. Aging: A shift from redox regulation to oxidative damage. *Free Radic Res.* 2006;40(12):1239–1243. doi:10.1080/10715760600913184.

15. Di Noia J. Defining powerhouse fruits and vegetables: A nutrient density approach. *Prev Chronic Dis.* 2014;11:130390. doi:http://dx.doi.org/10.5888/pcd11.130390

16. Mathers JC. Impact of nutrition on the ageing process. *Br J Nutr.* 2015:113(S1):S18–S22. doi:1017/S0007114514003237

17. Watson RR, ed. *Handbook of nutrition in the aged.* 4th ed. Boca Raton, FL: CRC Press; 2008.

18. Marshall TA, Stumbo PJ, Warren JJ, Xie XJ. Inadequate nutrient intakes are common and are associated with low diet variety in rural, community-dwelling elderly. *J Nutr.* 2001;131(8):2192–2196. http://www.ncbi.nlm.nih.gov/pubmed/11481416.

19. Gaby A. *Nutritional medicine.* Concord, NH: Fritz Perlberg Publishing; 2011.

20. Dietary Supplement Fact Sheets. National Institutes of Health. https://ods.od.nih.gov/factsheets/. Accessed December 1, 2016.

21. Murray MT, Pizzorno J, Pizzorno L. *The encyclopedia of healing foods.* 1st ed. New York: Atria Books; 2005.

22. Resveratrol. Linus Pauling Institute: Micronutrient Information Center. http://lpi.oregonstate.edu/mic/dietary-factors/phytochemicals/resveratrol#food-sources. Published January 3, 2017. Accessed January 4, 2017.

23. Lipski E. *Digestive wellness: Strengthen the immune system and prevent disease through healthy digestion.* 4th ed. New York: McGraw-Hill; 2011.

24. Nagao K, Yanagita T. Medium-chain fatty acids: Functional lipids for the prevention and treatment of the metabolic syndrome. *Pharmacol Res.* 2010;61:208–212. doi:10.1016/j.phrs.2009.11.007.

25. Nik Norulaini NA, Setianto WB, Zaidul ISM, Nawi AH, Azizi CYM, Omar AKM. Effects of supercritical carbon dioxide extraction parameters on virgin coconut oil yield and medium-chain triglyceride content. *Food Chem.* 2009;116:193–197. doi:10.1016/j.foodchem.2009.02.030.

26. Park KY, Jeong JK. Kimchi (Korean fermented vegetables) as a probiotic food. *J Med Food.* 2014;17(1):6–20. doi:10.1016/B978-0-12-802189-7.00026-5.

27. Nakamura E, Torii K, Uneyama H. Physiological roles of dietary free glutamate in gastrointestinal functions. *Biol Pharm Bull.* 2008;31(10):1841–1843. doi:10.1248/bpb.31.1841.

28. Dhana K, Koolhaas CM, Van Rossum EFC, et al. Metabolically healthy obesity and the risk of cardiovascular disease in the elderly population. *PLoS One.* 2016;11(4):1–12. doi:10.1371/journal.pone.0154273.

29. Han TS, Tajar A, Lean MEJ. Obesity and weight management in the elderly. *Br Med Bull.* 2011;97:169–196. doi:10.1093/bmb/ldr002.

30. Villareal DT, Apovian CM, Kushner RF, Klein S. Obesity in older adults: Technical review and position statement of the American Society for Nutrition and NAASO, The Obesity Society. *Am J Clin Nutr.* 2005;82:923–934. doi:10.1038/oby.2005.228.

31. Silva AO, Karnikowski MGO, Funghetto SS, et al. Association of body composition with sarcopenic obesity in elderly women. *Int J Gen Med.* 2013;6:25–29. doi:10.2147/IJGM.S36279.

32. Landi F, Calvani R, Tosato M, et al. Anorexia of aging: Risk factors, consequences, and potential treatments. *Nutrients.* 2016;8(2):1–10. doi:10.3390/nu8020069.

33. Sanford AM. Anorexia of aging and its role for frailty. *Curr Opin Clin Nutr Metab Care.* 2017;20(1):54–60. doi:10.1097/MCO.0000000000000336.

34. Chapman IM. The anorexia of aging. *Clin Geriatr Med.* 2007;23(4):735–756. doi:10.1016/j.cger.2007.06.001.

35. Hays NP, Roberts SB. The anorexia of aging in humans. *Physiol Behav.* 2006;88(3):257–266.

36. Morley JE. Undernutrition in older adults. *Fam Pract.* 2012;29(suppl 1):i89–i93.

37. Firth M, Prather CM. Gastrointestinal motility problem in the elderly. *Gastroenterology.* 2002;122(6):1688–1700.

38. Moss C. Gastrointestinal hormones: The regulation of appetite and anorexia of aging. *J Hum Nutr Diet.* 2012;25(1):3–15. doi: 10.1111/j.1365-277X.2011.01211.x.

39. Malafarina V, Uriz-Otano F, Gil-Guerrero L, Iniesta R. The anorexia of ageing: physiopathology, prevalence, associated comorbidity and mortality: A systematic review. *Maturitas.* 2013;74(4):293–302. doi: 10.1016/j.maturitas.2013.01.016.

40. Scarlata K. Small intestinal bacterial overgrowth: What to do when unwelcome microbes invade. *Today's Dietitian.* 2011;13(4):46.

41. Calvo I, Olivar J, Martinez E, Rico A, Diaz J, Gimena M. MNA(R) Mini Nutritional Assessment as a nutritional screening tool for hospitalized older adults; rationales and feasibility. *Nutr Hosp.* 2012;27(5):1619–1625. doi:10.3305/nh.2012.27.5.5888.

42. Rombeau JL, Bandini L, Barr R, et al. Bioelectrical impedance analysis in body composition measurement. National Institutes of Health. https://consensus.nih.gov/1994/1994bioelectricimpedancebodyta015html.htm. Accessed December 1, 2016.

43. Fischbach FT, Dunning MB. *A manual of laboratory and diagnostic tests*. 7th ed. Philadelphia, PA: Williams & Wilkins; 2004.

44. Marcus EL, Berry EM. Refusal to eat in the elderly. *Nutr Rev*. 1998;56(6):163–171. doi:10.1111/j.1753-4887.1998.tb06130.x.

45. Bharadwaj S, Ginoya S, Tandon P, et al. Malnutrition: Laboratory markers vs. nutritional assessment. *Gastroenterol Report*. 2016;4(4):272–280. doi:10.1093/gastro/gow013.

46. Verdery RB. Clinical evaluation of failure to thrive in older people. *Clin Geriatr Med*. 1997;13(4):769–778.

47. Kaati G, Bygren L, Edvinsson S. Cardiovascular and diabetes mortality determined by nutrition during parents' and grandparents' slow growth period. *Eur J Hum Genet*. 2002;10(June):682–688. doi:10.1038/sj.ejhg.5200859.

48. Stover PJ. Influence of human genetic variation on nutritional requirements. *Am J Clin Nutr*. 2006;83(2):436S–442S.

49. Hamdy O, Barakatun-Nisak MY. Nutrition in diabetes. *Endocrinol Metabol Clin*. 45(4):799–817. https://doi.org/10.1016/j.ecl.2016.06.010

50. Martin K, Jackson CF, Levy RG, Cooper PN. Ketogenic diet and other dietary treatments for epilepsy. *Cochrane Database Syst Rev*. 2016;2:CD001903. doi:10.1002/14651858.CD001903.pub3.

51. Levin BL, Varga E. MTHFR: Addressing genetic counseling dilemmas using evidence-based literature. *J Genet Couns*. 2016;25:901–911. doi:10.1007/s10897-016-9956-7.

52. Liew S-C, Gupta ED. Methylenetetrahydrofolate reductase (MTHFR) C677T polymorphism: Epidemiology, metabolism and the associated diseases. *Eur J Med Genet*. 2015;58:1–10. doi:10.1016/j.ejmg.2014.10.004.

53. Das UN. Nutritional factors in the prevention and management of coronary artery disease and heart failure. *Nutrition*. 2015;31:283–291. doi:10.1016/j.nut.2014.08.011.

54. Nakai K, Itoh C, Nakai K, Habano W, Gurwitz D. Correlation between C677T MTHFR gene polymorphism, plasma homocysteine levels and the incidence of CAD. *Am J Cardiovasc Drugs*. 2001;1(5):353–361. doi:10.2165/00129784-200101050-00005.

55. Escott-Stump S. *Nutrition and diagnosis-related care*. 7th ed. Philadelphia, PA: Lippincott Williams & Wilkins; 2012.

56. Jenkins DJA, Kendall CWC, Popovich DG, et al. Effect of a very-high-fiber vegetable, fruit, and nut diet on serum lipids and colonic function. *Metabolism*. 2001;50(4):494–503. doi:10.1053/meta.2001.21037.

57. Veech RL. The therapeutic implications of ketone bodies: The effects of ketone bodies in pathological conditions: Ketosis, ketogenic diet, redox states, insulin resistance, and mitochondrial metabolism. *Prostaglandins Leukot Essent Fat Acids*. 2004;70:309–319. doi:10.1016/j.plefa.2003.09.007.

58. Fasano A, Sapone A, Zevallos V, Schuppan D. Nonceliac gluten sensitivity. *Gastroenterology*. 2015;148(6):1195–1204. doi:http://dx.doi.org/10.1053/j.gastro.2014.12.049.

59. Guhsl EE, Hofstetter G, Lengger N, et al. IgE, IgG4 and IgA specific to Bet v 1-related food allergens do not predict oral allergy syndrome. *Allergy Eur J Allergy Clin Immunol*. 2015;70:59–66. doi:10.1111/all.12534.

60. Lomer MCE. Review article: The aetiology, diagnosis, mechanisms and clinical evidence for food intolerance. *Aliment Pharmacol Ther.* 2015;41:262–275. doi:10.1111/apt.13041.
61. Pasqui F, Poli C, Colecchia A, Marasco G, Festi D. Adverse food reaction and functional gastrointestinal disorders: Role of the dietetic approach. *J Gastrointest Liver Dis.* 2015;24(3):319–327. doi:10.15403/jgld.2014.1121.243.paq.
62. Soares-Weiser K, Takwoingi Y, Panesar SS, et al. The diagnosis of food allergy: A systematic review and meta-analysis. *Allergy Eur J Allergy Clin Immunol.* 2014;69:76–86. doi:10.1111/all.12333.
63. Morris MC, Tangney CC, Wang Y, Sacks FM, Bennett DA, Aggarwal NT. MIND diet associated with reduced incidence of Alzheimer's disease. *Alzheimers Dement.* 2015;11:1007–1014. doi:10.1016/j.jalz.2014.11.009.
64. Institute for Functional Medicine. https://www.functionalmedicine.org/. Accessed December 1, 2016.
65. Low FODMAP diet for irritable bowel syndrome. Monash University: Medicine, Nursing, and Health Sciences. http://www.med.monash.edu/cecs/gastro/fodmap/. Accessed December 1, 2016.
66. White E, Sherlock C. The effect of nutritional therapy for yeast infection (Candidiasis) in cases of chronic fatigue syndrome. *J Orthomol Med.* 2005;20(3):193–209. http://www.orthomolecular.org/library/jom/2005/pdf/2005-v20n03-p193.pdf.
67. Paoli A, Rubini A, Volek J, Grimaldi K. Beyond weight loss: A review of the therapeutic uses of very-low-carbohydrate (ketogenic) diets. *Eur J Clin Nutr.* 2013;67(8):789–796. doi:10.1038/ejcn.2013.116.
68. Surviving Mold. http://www.survivingmold.com/. Accessed December 1, 2016.
69. Mattson MP, Wan R. Beneficial effects of intermittent fasting and caloric restriction on the cardiovascular and cerebrovascular systems. *J Nutr Biochem.* 2005;16:129–137. doi:10.1016/j.jnutbio.2004.12.007.
70. Ballantyne S. *The Paleo approach: Reverse autoimmune disease and heal your body.* 1st ed. Las Vegas: Victory Belt Publishing Inc.; 2014.
71. Arava oral: Uses, Side Effects, Interactions, Pictures, Warnings & Dosing. WebMD. http://www.webmd.com/drugs/2/drug-16559/arava-oral/details#side-effects. Accessed January 11, 2017.
72. Forman HJ, Kennedy J. Mammalian dihydroorotate dehydrogenase: Physical and catalytic properties of the primary enzyme. *Arch Biochem Biophys.* 1978;191(1):23–31.
73. Leban J, Vitt D. Human dihydroorotate dehydrogenase inhibitors, a novel approach for the treatment of autoimmune and inflammatory diseases. *Arzneimittelforschung.* 2011;61(1):66–72. doi:10.1055/s-0031-1296169.
74. Mahmood A, FitzGerald AJ, Marchbank T, et al. Zinc carnosine, a health food supplement that stabilises small bowel integrity and stimulates gut repair processes. *Gut.* 2007;56(2):168–175. doi:10.1136/gut.2006.099929.
75. Xin L, Yang X, Cai G, et al. Serum levels of copper and zinc in patients with rheumatoid arthritis: A meta-analysis. *Biol Trace Elem Res.* 2015;168(1):1–10. doi:10.1007/s12011-015-0325-4.

3

Exercise, Frailty, and Functional Reserve: Concepts and Optimization

JOSEPH P. CLEAVER, ALICE SCHMIDT KEHAYA, AND MIKHAIL KOGAN

Introduction

When you watch television, read magazines, or scan through a multitude of online websites and social media news feeds, you will see the promotion of exercise for better health. The premise that exercise is good for you is generally accepted as common knowledge in American culture. However, many people—especially as they get older, work longer hours, and become more sedentary—fall out of a daily exercise routine.[1]

As clinicians, we know that the sedentary body becomes more prone to injury, general health declines, and the overall quality of life decreases. Evolutionarily speaking, humans are "born to move." Out of all primates, only humans seem to be well designed for prolonged endurance movement such as running or walking. Indeed, it appears that the main evolutionary advantage that allowed human ancestors to survive and thrive early on was not strength, speed, or even a larger brain. Instead, it was the combination of superior cognitive ability, combined with endurance running.[2]

The case study of Mr. R in Chapter 1 demonstrates how endurance exercise can not only lead to improvement in a patient's medical condition(s) but serve as a pivotal point for sustainable, healthy behavior that leads to well-being and life prolongation. The data supporting the health benefits of regular exercise are overwhelming and are listed in Table 3.3 at the end of the chapter. The commonly advocated goal of achieving 10,000 steps per day has been subject to dozens of randomized trials, including ones looking specifically at a geriatric population.[3]

Despite these data, most seniors don't move or exercise enough to stay healthy.[4] Lack of exercise in the elderly reduces life expectancy more so in non-overweight individuals than among overweight/obese.[5] Most people, including those over 65 years of age, tend to overestimate their activity level, making it even more urgent for health care providers to advocate for an increase in physical activity.[6] When one looks into the "blue zones"[7] described in detail in Chapter 1, it is clear that all centenarians, wherever they are, move a lot. In some cases, they are walking the equivalent of a marathon distance every day, or in other cases double or even triple marathon distances. Often this level of activity is not even considered "exercise" or something extraordinary, but just part of living life, frequently as a means of transportation or working. The idea that one would walk over 20 miles per day would strike many Americans as not only impossible but dangerous, but historically, it appears to be the optimal amount of physical activity for the human body.

Physical activity may not be the answer to immortality, yet the preponderance of evidence shows that in most individuals, regular physical activity can increase healthy lifespan up to 7 years by slowing the decline in functional capacity associated with aging and disuse.[8] Exercise participation can reverse the loss of function and increase longevity regardless of when a person becomes more physically active.[9,10]

Aerobic Exercise

The definition of exercise is a physical activity that increases your breathing and heart rate in response to increased metabolic activity. Exercise and physical activity fall into four basic categories: aerobic, strength, flexibility, and stretching. Aerobic exercise or cardiovascular exercise supports a healthy heart, lungs, brain, and immune and circulatory system, and exercise improves your overall fitness. As a result, exercise delays or prevents many diseases that are common in older adults.

VO2MAX

VO2max measures oxygen consumption and exercise capacity and has long been considered the "gold standard" for determining cardiorespiratory fitness levels. VO2max is measured in the units of mL/kg/min. Cardiorespiratory fitness and VO2max peak in adolescence and decrease approximately 1% per year in adults; the decline accelerates starting at age 65, resulting in a loss of exercise capacity by up to 50% between ages 20 and 80. Consistent aerobic training slows the age-related decline in VO2max and aerobic power by up to 50%. In fact, a study that followed consistently physically active men for 10 years showed that at age 55 they had no decline in fitness levels or aerobic capacity.

Examples of VO2max determinants include:

- Cardiac output
- Pulmonary diffusion capacity
- Red blood cell (RBC) count/oxygen-carrying capacity
- Other peripheral limitations like muscle diffusion capacity, mitochondrial number and function, and capillary density

If one of these factors is subpar, then the whole system loses a proportion of its ability to function efficiently[11] (Fig. 3.1).

Aerobic exercise lessens the vascular stiffening associated with aging since stiffening is increased by only about half as much in endurance-trained elderly persons compared to sedentary ones. Exercise can also improve the aerobic

MEN	Age (years)			
ratios	36–45	46–55	56–65	65+
excellent	>51	>45	>41	>37
good	43–51	39–45	36–41	33–37
above average	39–42	36–38	32–35	29–32
average	35–38	32–35	30–31	26–28
below average	31–34	29–31	26–29	22–25
poor	26–30	25–28	22–25	20–21
very poor	<26	<25	<22	<20
WOMEN	Age (years)			
rating	36–45	46–55	56–65	65+
excellent	>45	>40	>37	>32
good	38–45	34–40	32–37	28–32
above average	34–37	31–33	28–31	25–27
average	31–33	28–30	25–27	22–24
below average	27–30	25–27	22–24	19–21
poor	22–26	20–24	18–21	17–18
very poor	<22	<20	<18	<17

FIGURE 3.1. Maximal oxygen uptake norms for men and women (mL/kg/min).[30]

capacity of older persons by increasing cardiac output and maintaining vascular compliance and oxygen utilization.

Losses of active muscle mass or sarcopenia and viable mitochondria are contributing factors to the decline in exercise capacity. It has been postulated that mitochondrial health, number, and dysfunction are important factors in aging. Mitochondrial health plays a key role in maintaining a healthy exercise capacity.

CELLULAR RESPONSE TO EXERCISE

Aerobic training stimulates the growth of Type I slow-twitch fibers and induces the following marked adaptive changes in skeletal muscles improving VO2max:

- Capillarization
- Changes in mitochondrial density
- An increase in the activity of oxidative enzymes

The aerobic performance of muscles improved due to these changes, which are tightly connected to the functioning of coactivators belonging to the PGC-1 family (peroxisome proliferator-activated receptor [PPAR] and gamma coactivator 1). Strength training induces these adaptive changes by stimulating hypertrophy of Type II fast-twitch fibers.

Muscle Health Function, Dynapenia, and Sarcopenia

Humans possess three types of muscle—cardiac, smooth, and skeletal—with each exhibiting distinct functional and anatomical differences. Skeletal and cardiac muscles are similar in structure, for they are characterized by striations and both contract in a similar manner. While the cardiac muscle is under involuntary control, the 600 or so skeletal muscles respond to voluntary control, allowing the individual to direct force, speed, power, and movement.

Skeletal muscle consists of three fibrous tissues: the endomysium, perimysium, and epimysium wrap the muscle structures at various depths. The sarcolemma, a thin, elastic membrane, covers the surface of each muscle fiber and the sarcoplasmic reticulum and mitochondria.

Energy derived from mitochondria drives the sarcoplasmic reticulum to regulate calcium flow, creating a Ca^{++} gradient that regulates muscle contraction of the ultrastructures of actin and myosin filaments that make up a sarcomere unit. The sarcomere consists of basic repeating units between two Z lines and represents the functional unit of a muscle fiber. The actin and myosin filaments within the sarcomere contribute primarily to muscle contraction.

Neuromuscular function and the voluntary activation of skeletal muscles are carried out centrally by the cerebral cortex and peripherally by the anterior motor unit. The anterior motor neuron consists of a cell body, axon, and dendrites. The central nervous system and peripheral nervous system work in concert and coordinate the voluntary transmission of an electrochemical impulse from the spinal cord to the muscle. The cell body of the motor neuron is located in the spinal cord's gray matter and ends at the motor unit interface on the skeletal muscle. Healthy adults age 70 and older have approximately 40% fewer motor units and a 10% decline in nerve conduction velocity, reflecting the cumulative effects of aging.

Aging is associated with a significant decline in neuromuscular function and performance, accounting for a 40% to 50% reduction in muscle mass from muscle fiber atrophy and loss of motor units, even among healthy, physically active adults. Sarcopenia, defined as age-related loss of muscle mass, strength, and functional decline, is the dominant feature of age-related changes in the neuromuscular system. Large population studies have reported that sarcopenia affects over 20% of 60- to 70-year-olds; the figure approaches 50% in those over 75 years of age. While the loss of muscle mass explains a significant component of dynapenia, other factors are emerging as important contributors. In particular, changes at the level of the motor neuron and motor unit, mitochondrial function, and low-grade inflammation driven by intramuscular adipose tissue are often associated with the metabolic syndrome.

Data from the Health, Aging, and Body Composition study examined knee extensor muscle strength and a cross-section area of quadriceps muscle with computed tomography (CT) scans. The study revealed that the decrease in muscle strength seen in older adults is significantly more rapid than the concomitant loss of muscle mass, and the change in quadriceps muscle area accounts for only approximately 6% to 8% of the change of knee extensor muscle strength. Moreover, maintaining or gaining muscle mass does not prevent aging-related decreases in muscle strength. These findings indicate that the loss of muscle strength in older adults is only weakly associated with the loss of lean body mass.[12]

In addition to strength, muscle power has been identified as an important contributor to function in older adults. Power is the ability to generate as much force as possible, as quickly as possible. When the muscles in the body are used to perform high-intensity movements in short bursts, power is used. Muscle power has emerged as a strong independent indicator of self-reported independence in the elderly.[13]

Type II fast-twitch fibers are responsible for maintaining strength and power and are particularly vulnerable to atrophy and age-related loss of neuromuscular function. The loss of Type II fibers contributes to the loss of functionality and independence seen in frailty syndrome and is characterized by slow gait speed, an impaired get-up-and-go test, and weak grip strength. Type II fibers and neuromuscular function respond well to strength training. Older skeletal muscle is capable of regeneration of neuromuscular synapses and reverses the Type II muscle fiber atrophy.[14]

With the above in mind, clinicians who work with the elderly need to be able to identify patients who are frail and developing sarcopenia and refer them to programs that can slow down or reverse it. Table 3.1 lists some program suggestions.

The definition of sarcopenia is based on two parameters. The first is a low muscle mass, over two standard deviations below the mean measured in young adults (aged 18–39) of the same sex and ethnic background. The second is low gait speed (e.g., a walking speed of less than 0.8 m/s in the 4-m walking test).[15] Lastly, grip strength is an efficient and inexpensive tool to diagnose sarcopenia and is an accurate screening test as a risk predictor for the development of sarcopenia and all-cause mortality.

In addition to sarcopenia, an important concept to understand when working with the geriatric population is functional reserve (FR). Although it may not appear to be clinically relevant, it may in fact be one of the most important clinical "forests" that is so often missed behind "trees" of illnesses or symptoms. FR should be distinguished from functional reserve capacity (FRC), which is the total amount of work that can be done during continuous exercise before fatigue sets in. Unlike FR, FRC is related more to sports and performance. Poor FR is often described as frailty. The exact concept of frailty is not fully established, but as Ronan Factora from the Cleveland Clinic describes it, "Frailty has been characterized as an interaction between loss of muscle mass

Table 3.1. Programs to Reverse Sarcopenia in the Elderly

Low- to moderate-intensity exercise has been shown to decrease hypertension in adults. Non-pharmacological antihypertensive therapy is preferred in an elderly population.

Four weeks of high-intensity endurance training improved coronary vessel endothelial function in adults with coronary artery disease.

Aerobic interval training decreases left ventricular hypertrophy and improves aerobic capacity and quality of life in individuals with heart failure.

(sarcopenia), the presence of multiple chronic illnesses, and loss of functional independence."[16]

Obesity

The physical inactivity that contributes to the severity and loss of neuromuscular function also promotes weight gain and an increase in intramuscular adipose tissue, leading to the worldwide obesity epidemic.[17] A lack of leisure time activity and the intake of calorie-dense, nutritionally poor, highly processed food contribute significantly to the growing obesity crisis and the risk of shorter longevity. The life expectancy of an obese individual with a Body Mass Index (BMI) over 30 averages 7 years less than a person with a healthy BMI of less than 25. An active lifestyle and physical activity greatly affect body composition by decreasing the ratio of free fat mass to lean muscle in more active individuals.[18]

The incidence of obesity has a strong association with metabolic syndrome. Metabolic syndrome consists of obesity, insulin resistance, dyslipidemia, and hypertension leading to an increased risk of cardiovascular disease (CVD) and renal events. Approximately 34% of adults in the United States meet the criteria for metabolic syndrome. Males greater than 60 years of age are more than four times as likely, and females 60 years of age and over are more than six times as likely, than those ages 20 to 39 to meet the criteria.

A retrospective study evaluated the relationship between metabolic syndrome and functional disability in the elderly. There were 1,778 participants aged 60 to 84 years in the National Health and Nutrition Examination Survey (1999–2002). In this study, impairments in activities of daily living (ADL) were assessed and the associations between the features of metabolic syndrome and disability were evaluated. The study found a strong correlation between metabolic syndrome and functional dependence linking metabolic syndrome components with increased disability ($p = .002$).[19]

Obesity statistics in the United States are based on BMI, and a BMI greater than 30 is considered obese. However, if BMI criteria are used to identify high-risk obese populations, then we may just be seeing the tip of the risk iceberg: obesity statistics will miss a percentage of the population with similar or even greater significant health risks that are accompanying the graying of America.

Sarcopenic Obesity

White adipose tissue, once thought to be an inert energy storage tissue, is a metabolically active organ that is intricately involved in controlling a vast array of physiological processes, including lipid and glucose metabolism. Inflammation-producing adipokines (IL-6) disrupt metabolic pathways and inflame and damage endothelial cells, increasing the risk of cardiovascular disease, metabolic syndrome, and diabetes. The location of fat qualifies its functional properties and links to the body's level of health or increased risk of disease. For example, subcutaneous fat located in the hypodermis is associated with beneficial lipid profiles, while visceral fat and intramuscular fat produce more inflammatory cytokines and are linked to heart disease risk and insulin resistance. Moreover, in the elderly with a normal BMI, the intramuscular fat increases due to the migration of visceral fat to the skeletal muscle. This results in a significant increase in the ratio of body fat to lean muscle mass, while body weight remains stable. This increase in visceral fat and intramuscular fat contributes to sarcopenic obesity, dynapenia, and metabolic syndrome.

Recent evidence supports a greater loss of muscle strength than would be expected based on loss of muscle mass, indicating a deterioration of muscle quality and function. An investigation on age-related changes in leg composition by CT scan, strength, and muscle quality in healthy men and women showed that there is an age-related increase in fatty infiltration of the mid-thigh skeletal muscle in men and women. The study found that the decreases in strength were two to five times greater than the loss of muscle size, with aging implicating losses in muscle quality. Together, these findings indicate that progressive muscle weakness and an increase in muscular fat infiltration with age occur regardless of changes in muscle mass or subcutaneous fat.[20]

Exercise Prescription

Biological aging is associated with declines in the neuromuscular and cardiovascular systems, resulting in an impaired capacity to exercise and even perform daily functions. Strength training and endurance training promote specific neuromuscular and cardiovascular adaptations.

Designing healthy exercise programs for an older population requires a specific set of goals addressing the functional challenges that are encountered in a less-fit group. Muscle fiber regeneration and muscle hypertrophy increase the motor unit recruitment capacity and motor unit firing rate. Focus on increasing power and balance improves function and reduces all-cause risk. A combination of strength training and endurance training in an older population is the most effective way to enhance both neuromuscular and cardiorespiratory functions and consequently to preserve the functional capacity, quality of life, and possibly longevity.

The physiological adaptations to exercise in the elderly are similar to those observed in an untrained young population. The exercise prescription should be designed in such a way that the patient will be motivated to exercise. For example, a highly social patient may feel more comfortable in an exercise class setting; others may be more likely to thrive in a solo- or dual-participant exercise program. Consider these factors when issuing an exercise prescription for patients.

The first step is to establish functional goals, which include any or all of the following:

- Weight loss
- Metabolic health (blood sugar, insulin)
- Cardiovascular health
- Functional ADLs
- Strength
- Power

Next, determine the proportion of aerobic exercise versus strength training, which may include:

- Treadmill stress test—An exercise stress test usually involves the patient walking on a treadmill or riding a stationary bike while the heart rhythm, blood pressure, and breathing are monitored.
- VO2max—VO2max, or maximal oxygen uptake, is one factor that can determine an athlete's capacity to perform sustained exercise and is linked to aerobic endurance. VO2max refers to the maximum amount of oxygen that an individual can utilize during intense or maximal exercise.
- 1RM (one repetition max) is the maximum amount of weight that one can lift for a given exercise. Using the 1RM, you can determine the patient's maximum strength of muscles based upon the exercises being performed.
- Grip strength—Grip strength is the force applied by the hand to pull on or suspend from objects and is a specific part of hand strength. Optimal-sized objects permit the hand to wrap around a cylindrical shape with a diameter from 1 to 3 inches. The grip strength test is advocated for all practices to use if you cannot use all five of these tests for practical reasons. Grip strength takes a minute to do and can be part of any physical exam.

- Leg extension strength—The leg extension strength test is an isometric strength test as a measure of lower body strength. This test is part of the protocol for the Groningen Fitness Test for the Elderly. Its purpose is to measure lower body strength. The equipment required includes a table and a specially constructed box with two arm supports, connected to a screen.

There are three major categories in an older patient population:

1. Frail and focused on decreasing falls to improve function, independence, chair rise, walk test, grip strength untrained—Supervised exercise is recommended for this group.
2. Healthy non-frail non-exercisers—general aerobic and stress test— Target risks while designing the exercise program for this group.
3. Health non-frail exercisers—optimal exercise to maintain function strength/power, metabolic health, healthy weight, cardiovascular health—Encourage this group to continue exercising and strive to meet personal goals.[21,22]

Exercise in the preservation of cardiorespiratory fitness and FR in response to exercise varies and is influenced by:

- Muscle mass and strength
- Percentage of body fat
- Heredity
- Quantity and choice of exercise

Most people tend to focus on one activity or type of exercise and think they're doing enough. Each type of exercise adds different synergistic benefits, and programs with varied physical activity can achieve superior results. For example, a balance between strength training that improves strength, power, and neuromuscular facilitation and cardiovascular exercise that decreases low-grade inflammation and endothelial function will yield superior functional benefits by improving metabolic and cardiovascular health and physical function. Also, muscle strength is inversely proportional to risk factors for cardiovascular disease—most notably lowered blood pressure, improved insulin sensitivity, decreased inflammatory markers (i.e., hsCRP), improved lipid profile, lower body fat, and decreased abdominal girth.[23] Lastly, the volume and intensity of exercise together induce a positive dose-related physiological and risk reduction response.[24]

Geriatric Exercise Prescription Made Practical

The following section discusses general principles of exercise prescription for geriatric patients. The specific exercise prescription for each geriatric condition is outside the scope of this chapter and is covered in some detail throughout this book. Tai chi, yoga, and specific body movement prescriptions like Alexander Technique are covered separately in Chapter 6, Manual and Movement Therapies.

Before an exercise prescription is made, providers should evaluate each patient's individual fitness level, preferences, daily schedule, and therapeutic goals. Before the appointment, patients can fill out forms related to their exercise readiness, including a questionnaire available from the Canadian Society of Exercise Physiology at http://www.csep.ca/view.asp?ccid=517.[25]

An effective exercise recommendation should include FITT-PRO (frequency, intensity, type, time, and progression of exercise) within disease-specific guidelines (Table 3.2).[26,27]

While this model provides broad recommendations and can be used for virtually every patient, there are number of limitations. First, balance is not specifically emphasized here. Balance training is critical to decrease the risk of falls. Second, adherence to any exercise program can be limited due to multiple factors, such as chronic illnesses resulting in severe symptoms that may include fatigue, lack of motivation, fear of trauma, and others.

For balance, we favor tai chi and yoga. These gentle exercises are rapidly gaining popularity, tend to be low cost, and do not require comprehensive, highly specialized programs and facilities. Teachers are available in most communities, and the space needed for these activities is usually just a big enough room with appropriate flooring. Resolving barriers to exercise often requires patience and time. Using a health coach who is well versed in motivational skills and experienced in working with the elderly can be essential, but is not covered by Medicare. Engaging physical therapists can also be key, but their use is limited to patients with existing medical conditions, and they are routinely covered only for a few visits. Referral to physical therapy must have a specific medical reason; referral for general geriatric conditions such as weakness, deconditioning, and poor balance is appropriate and can be used.

Adherence with an exercise prescription can be enhanced with social elements and exercises associated with a high degree of enjoyment and satisfaction. This requires a good understanding of the patient's interests. While social dances can be a wonderful exercise for one person, they will be stressful and disengaging for another. Dance therapy has great potential for the geriatric population. Unfortunately, the evidence supporting dance therapy is not

Table 3.2. Guidelines and Recommendations for Prescribing Exercise

Type of Exercise	Description & Recommendation	Example
Aerobic exercise	Repetitive activity of large muscle groups that sustains an elevated heart rate of 65–75% maximum for age. Goal of 20–60 minutes of aerobic exercise on 3 or more days per week.	Brisk walking, jogging, yard work, aerobics class, swimming, or biking for 30 minutes on 5 days each week. Increase duration, intensity, or frequency as patient progresses.
Resistance training	Moving limbs against resistance such as body weight, bands. or weights. Goal of two or three resistance exercise sessions each week.	Body weight calisthenics (body-weight squats, push-ups, sit-ups), free weight training (bench press, bicep curls, calf raises), or weight machine circuit training. Three sets total: 15 → 10 → 5 repetitions. Increase weight or add repetitions as patient progresses.
Flexibility training	Movement of a joint through its complete range of motion. Goal of two or three flexibility sessions per week.	Provide patients with stretching handouts or other resources (websites, videos). Flexibility techniques can be static or dynamic. Hold static stretches gently for 20–30 seconds each.
Balance training	Exercise that prevents falls by maintaining stability during physical activity. Goal of two or three balance exercise routines per week.	Tai chi, yoga, single-leg exercises. Balance training can be incorporated into weekly resistance and flexibility training.
Lifestyle modifications	Making changes to a patient's existing daily routine to increase physical activity. Goal of gradually implementing lifestyle changes.	Park at the back of a parking lot, use stairs for one or two flights instead of the elevator, walk or bike to run errands that are close to home, meet up with friends for "exercise dates."

robust, with the notable exception of Parkinson's disease. The evidence shows some physical benefits as well as increased social engagement, positive effects of music, improved coordination, and memory stimulation.[28]

Lack of direct comparison of different types of dances makes it pretty much open to the local availability of teachers and the patient's preference. In recent years Zumba, an exercise adaptation of Latin dances, has become one of the most popular class exercises in the world. Zumba Gold was specifically designed for geriatric populations and is now available in many community centers and gyms. The health benefits of Zumba Gold are in the early phases of research.[29]

Regardless of the type of initial exercise prescription, the clinician's job is to continue ongoing reassessment and support of the patient's exercise routine. Table 3.3 summarizes the benefits of exercise for age-related diseases and syndromes.

Table 3.3. Benefits of Exercise for Age-Related Diseases and Syndromes

Cardiovascular Benefits	
Improves hypertension[31,32]	Low- to moderate-intensity exercise has been shown to decrease hypertension in adults. Nonpharmacologic antihypertensive therapy is preferred in an elderly population.
Decreased risk of coronary artery disease[33]	Four weeks of high-intensity endurance training improved coronary vessel endothelial function in adults with coronary artery disease.
Improves symptoms of congestive heart failure[34]	Aerobic interval training decreases left ventricular hypertrophy, improves aerobic capacity and quality of life in individuals with heart failure.
Improves lipid profile[35]	Endurance exercise in elderly participants produced decreases in total and LDL cholesterol levels.
Improves fitness[36]	Strength, power, aerobic capacity, and flexibility were improved in participants in their 70s who followed exercise regimens.
Musculoskeletal Benefits	
Decreases fall risk[37]	Eccentric exercise programs significantly improved strength, balance, and stair-descent abilities in frail elderly study participants.
Maintains bone mineral density[38]	Postmenopausal women who completed 1 year of high-intensity strength training exercises maintained total body bone mineral content and achieved small increases in bone density of the femoral neck and lumbar spine.

Table 3.3. Continued

Improves osteoarthritis pain and stiffness[39,40]	Older adults who completed a program of aerobic, resistance, and tai chi exercise had improvements in symptoms of osteoarthritis of the knee.
Protects against low back pain[41]	Being engaged in strenuous activity was shown to be significantly protective against low back pain in the elderly population.

Neurological and Psychological Benefits

Improves symptoms of depression[42,43]	After a 1-year endurance exercise program, older adults self-reported positive changes in morale. Similarly, older adults who participated in moderate-intensity strength training showed increases in mood and self-confidence.
Improves overall cognitive function[44]	People aged 60–75 years who completed aerobic training showed significant improvement in executive performance on cognitive tasks.
Improves sleep quality[45]	Implementing moderate-intensity exercise improved self-rated sleep quality in older adults.
Improves Parkinson disease symptoms[46]	After a 12-week rehabilitation exercise program, patients with Parkinson disease had improved scores for motor symptoms and overall quality of life.

Endocrinological Benefits

Decreases risk of obesity[47]	According to a meta-analysis of exercise program studies, exercise leads to a decrease in weight and prevents obesity across all age groups.
Increases insulin sensitivity[48]	Aerobic exercise in elderly people who are obese improves glucose metabolism, decreases visceral fat, and reverses insulin resistance.
Decreases incidence of type II diabetes and lowers hemoglobin A1C[49,50]	Increased physical activity has been shown to prevent diabetes and lower hemoglobin A1C in patients with diabetes.
Improves symptoms of hot flashes in postmenopausal women	16 weeks of moderate-intensity exercise improved self-reported symptoms of hot flashes. Objective measures such as sweat rate and vasodilation were also improved.[51]

Other Benefits

Decreases mortality (all-cause)[52]	A comparison of adults with variable physical activity levels showed a significant reduction in all-cause mortality in adults with high fitness activity levels.

ACKNOWLEDGMENT

The authors thank Jennifer Filzen for help with the editing of the chapter.

WEBSITE RESOURCES

ACSM Fit Society Page (click Publications and Other Media): http://www.acsm.org

CDC Physical Activity for Everyone: http://www.cdc.gov/nccdphp/dnpa/physical/index.htm

ICAA: Common Questions and Answers About Exercise: http://www.icaa.cc/FacilityLocator/Doctors/physiciantools.htm

Shape Up America!: http://www.shapeup.org

Canadian Society of Exercise Physiology: http://www.csep.ca/

REFERENCES

1. Sims J, Smith F, Duffy A, Hilton S. The vagaries of self-reports of physical activity: a problem revisited and addressed in a study of exercise promotion in the over 65s in general practice. Fam Pract. 1999;16(2):152–157.
2. Rowe GC, Safdar A, Arany Z. Running forward: new frontiers in endurance exercise biology. Circulation. 2014;129(7):798–810.
3. Garvey WT, Mechanick JI, Brett EM, et al. American Association of Clinical Endocrinologists and American College of Endocrinology Comprehensive Clinical Practice Guidelines for Medical Care of Patients with Obesity. Executive summary. Complete guidelines available at https://www.aace.com/publications/guidelines. Endocr Pract. 2016;22(7):842–884.
4. Troiano RP, Berrigan D, Dodd KW, Mâsse LC, Tilert T, Mcdowell M. Physical activity in the United States measured by accelerometer. Med Sci Sports Exerc. 2008;40(1):181–188.
5. Coombs N, Stamatakis E, Lee IM. Physical inactivity among older adults: implications for life expectancy among non-overweight and overweight or obese individuals. Obes Res Clin Pract. 2015;9(2):175–179.
6. Sims J, Smith F, Duffy A, Hilton S. The vagaries of self-reports of physical activity: a problem revisited and addressed in a study of exercise promotion in the over 65s in general practice. Fam Pract. 1999;16(2):152–157.
7. Buettner D. The Blue Zones, 9 Lessons for Living Longer from the People Who've Lived the Longest. Washington, DC: National Geographic Books; 2012.
8. Franco OH, De laet C, Peeters A, Jonker J, Mackenbach J, Nusselder W. Effects of physical activity on life expectancy with cardiovascular disease. Arch Intern Med. 2005;165(20):2355–2360.

9. Blair SN, Kohl HW, Barlow CE, Paffenbarger RS, Gibbons LW, Macera CA. Changes in physical fitness and all-cause mortality. A prospective study of healthy and unhealthy men. JAMA. 1995;273(14):1093–1098.
10. Paffenbarger RS, Hyde RT, Wing AL, Hsieh CC. Physical activity, all-cause mortality, and longevity of college alumni. N Engl J Med. 1986;314(10):605–613.
11. Wagner PD. New ideas on limitations to VO2max. Exerc Sport Sci Rev. 2000;28(1):10–14.
12. Snijder MB, Visser M, Dekker JM, et al. Low subcutaneous thigh fat is a risk factor for unfavourable glucose and lipid levels, independently of high abdominal fat. The Health ABC Study. Diabetologia. 2005;48(2):301–308.
13. Foldvari M, Clark M, Laviolette LC, et al. Association of muscle power with functional status in community-dwelling elderly women. J Gerontol A Biol Sci Med Sci. 2000;55(4):M192–M199.
14. Cadore EL, Pinto RS, Bottaro M, Izquierdo M. Strength and endurance training prescription in healthy and frail elderly. Aging Dis. 2014;5(3):183–195.
15. Muscaritoli M, Anker SD, Argilés J, et al. Consensus definition of sarcopenia, cachexia and pre-cachexia: joint document elaborated by Special Interest Groups (SIG) "cachexia-anorexia in chronic wasting diseases" and "nutrition in geriatrics". Clin Nutr. 2010;29(2):154–159.
16. Available at: http://www.clevelandclinicmeded.com/medicalpubs/diseasemanagement/preventive-medicine/aging-preventive-health/. Accessed February 1, 2017.
17. Yang L, Colditz GA. Prevalence of overweight and obesity in the United States, 2007–2012. JAMA Intern Med. 2015;175(8):1412–1413.
18. Pollock ML, Mengelkoch LJ, Graves JE, et al. Twenty-year follow-up of aerobic power and body composition of older track athletes. J Appl Physiol. 1997;82(5):1508–1516.
19. Liaw FY, Kao TW, Wu LW, et al. Components of metabolic syndrome and the risk of disability among the elderly population. Sci Rep. 2016;6:22750.
20. Delmonico MJ, Harris TB, Visser M, et al. Longitudinal study of muscle strength, quality, and adipose tissue infiltration. Am J Clin Nutr. 2009;90(6):1579–1585.
21. Cadore EL, Pinto RS, Lhullier FL, et al. Physiological effects of concurrent training in elderly men. Int J Sports Med. 2010;31(10):689–697.
22. Cadore EL, Izquierdo M. How to simultaneously optimize muscle strength, power, functional capacity, and cardiovascular gains in the elderly: an update. Age (Dordr). 2013;35(6):2329–2344.
23. Ruiz JR, Sui X, Lobelo F, et al. Association between muscular strength and mortality in men: prospective cohort study. BMJ. 2008;337:a439.
24. Wen CP, Wai JP, Tsai MK, et al. Minimum amount of physical activity for reduced mortality and extended life expectancy: a prospective cohort study. Lancet. 2011;378(9798):1244–1253.
25. Swain DP, ACSM, Brawner CA. ACSM's Resource Manual for Guidelines for Exercise Testing and Prescription. Philadelphia: Lippincott Williams & Wilkins; 2012.
26. American College of Sports Medicine Position Stand. Exercise and physical activity for older adults. Med Sci Sports Exerc. 1998;30(6):992–1008.
27. Mcdermott AY, Mernitz H. Exercise and older patients: prescribing guidelines. Am Fam Physician. 2006;74(3):437–444.

28. Mcneely ME, Duncan RP, Earhart GM. A comparison of dance interventions in people with Parkinson disease and older adults. Maturitas. 2015;81(1):10–16.

29. Dalleck LC, Roos KA, Byrd BR, Weatherwax RM. Zumba Gold(*): are the physiological responses sufficient to improve fitness in middle-age to older adults? J Sports Sci Med. 2015;14(3):689–690.

30. Available at: http://www.topendsports.com/testing/norms/vo2max.htm. Accessed February 1, 2017.

31. Hagberg JM, Park JJ, Brown MD. The role of exercise training in the treatment of hypertension: an update. Sports Med. 2000;30(3):193–206.

32. Nguyen QT, Anderson SR, Sanders L, Nguyen LD. Managing hypertension in the elderly: a common chronic disease with increasing age. Am Health Drug Benefits. 2012;5(3):146–153.

33. Hambrecht R, Wolf A, Gielen S, et al. Effect of exercise on coronary endothelial function in patients with coronary artery disease. N Engl J Med. 2000;342(7):454–460.

34. Wisløff U, Støylen A, Loennechen JP, et al. Superior cardiovascular effect of aerobic interval training versus moderate continuous training in heart failure patients: a randomized study. Circulation. 2007;115(24):3086–3094.

35. Frankel JE, Bean JF, Frontera WR. Exercise in the elderly: research and clinical practice. Clin Geriatr Med. 2006;22(2):239–256.

36. Greig CA, Young A, Skelton DA, Pippet E, Butler FM, Mahmud SM. Exercise studies with elderly volunteers. Age Ageing. 1994;23(3):185–189.

37. Lastayo PC, Ewy GA, Pierotti DD, Johns RK, Lindstedt S. The positive effects of negative work: increased muscle strength and decreased fall risk in a frail elderly population. J Gerontol A Biol Sci Med Sci. 2003;58(5):M419–M424.

38. Nelson ME, Fiatarone MA, Morganti CM, Trice I, Greenberg RA, Evans WJ. Effects of high-intensity strength training on multiple risk factors for osteoporotic fractures. A randomized controlled trial. JAMA. 1994;272(24):1909–1914.

39. Ettinger WH, Burns R, Messier SP, et al. A randomized trial comparing aerobic exercise and resistance exercise with a health education program in older adults with knee osteoarthritis. The Fitness Arthritis and Seniors Trial (FAST). JAMA. 1997;277(1):25–31.

40. Song R, Lee EO, Lam P, Bae SC. Effects of tai chi exercise on pain, balance, muscle strength, and perceived difficulties in physical functioning in older women with osteoarthritis: a randomized clinical trial. J Rheumatol. 2003;30(9):2039–2044.

41. Hartvigsen J, Christensen K. Active lifestyle protects against incident low back pain in seniors: a population-based 2-year prospective study of 1387 Danish twins aged 70–100 years. Spine. 2007;32(1):76–81.

42. Hill RD, Storandt M, Malley M. The impact of long-term exercise training on psychological function in older adults. J Gerontol. 1993;48(1):P12–P17.

43. Tsutsumi T, Don BM, Zaichkowsky LD, Delizonna LL. Physical fitness and psychological benefits of strength training in community dwelling older adults. Appl Human Sci. 1997;16(6):257–266.

44. Kramer AF, Hahn S, Cohen NJ, et al. Ageing, fitness and neurocognitive function. Nature. 1999;400(6743):418–419.

45. King AC, Oman RF, Brassington GS, Bliwise DL, Haskell WL. Moderate-intensity exercise and self-rated quality of sleep in older adults. A randomized controlled trial. JAMA. 1997;277(1):32–37.

46. Cholewa J, Boczarska-jedynak M, Opala G. Influence of physiotherapy on severity of motor symptoms and quality of life in patients with Parkinson disease. Neurol Neurochir Pol. 2013;47(3):256–262.

47. Shaw KA, Gennat HC, O'Rourke P, Del Mar C. Exercise for overweight or obesity. Cochrane Database of Systematic Reviews 2006, Issue 4. Art. No.: CD003817. DOI: 10.1002/14651858.CD003817.pub3.

48. O'Leary VB, Marchetti CM, Krishnan RK, Stetzer BP, Gonzalez F, Kirwan JP. Exercise-induced reversal of insulin resistance in obese elderly is associated with reduced visceral fat. J Appl Physiol. 2006;100(5):1584–1589.

49. Helmrich SP, Ragland DR, Leung RW, Paffenbarger RS. Physical activity and reduced occurrence of non-insulin-dependent diabetes mellitus. N Engl J Med. 1991;325(3):147–152.

50. Sigal RJ, Kenny GP, Wasserman DH, Castaneda-Sceppa C, White RD. Physical activity/exercise and type 2 diabetes: A consensus statement from the American Diabetes Association. Available at: http://care.diabetesjournals.org/content/29/6/1433.short. Accessed January 10, 2017.

51. Bailey TG, Cable NT, Aziz N, et al. Exercise training reduces the acute physiological severity of post-menopausal hot flushes. J Physiol (Lond). 2016;594(3):657–667.

52. Blair SN, Kohl HW, Paffenbarger RS, Clark DG, Cooper KH, Gibbons LW. Physical fitness and all-cause mortality. A prospective study of healthy men and women. JAMA. 1989;262(17):2395–2401.

4

Preventive Geriatrics

RONAK MEHTA, MARIATU KOROMA-NELSON,
ELIZABETH R. MACKENZIE, AND BIRGIT RAKEL

Introduction

Societies worldwide are challenged by the ongoing growth in health care expenditures and the changing patterns in the demand for health care.[1] These contemporary health care systems face difficulties in solving these challenges, as they have originally been designed to solve single, acute, and mainly short-term diseases.[2] Worsening this situation, ongoing specialization and technological improvements have led to fragmentation of care delivery and resulted in a substantial increase in health care expenditures that negatively affects the provision of integrated long-term care and support for the chronically ill and for elderly people with complex care needs.[3-5]

Epidemiological research shows that in the United States, approximately 80% of all persons aged 65 and older have at least one chronic condition, and 50% have at least two, and this can lead to severe disability in this patient population.[6,7] Chronic illness and its appropriate management is an increasingly important issue as many aspects of mortality among older adults may be preventable through a change in lifestyle behaviors. Studies show that tobacco use, poor diet, and physical inactivity directly reflect the leading causes of death (i.e., heart disease, malignant neoplasm, cerebrovascular disease, and chronic lower respiratory disease) in aging adults.[8] However, researchers have determined that public health interventions can decrease disability among older persons with the goal of helping them to live independently, which would reduce health care costs.[9]

Caloric Restriction and Intermittent Fasting

Few studies have been done on the correlation between diet and supplements and longevity. According to the National Institute for Aging, calorie restriction and intermittent fasting have been shown to increase lifespan in vitro. The Comprehensive Assessment of Long-term Effects of Reducing Intake of Energy (CALERIE) study has shown a decreased incidence of chronic diseases like cancer in overweight individuals on a calorie-restricted diet. Please read Chapter 2 for more details on nutrition.

Exercise

Along with nutrition, it is important to establish and encourage an exercise or movement regimen with patients for healthy aging. Although there is no standard "one size fits all" exercise regimen that is recommended, the minimal duration recommended is 10 minutes a day; for additional health benefits, 300 minutes of moderate training per week or 150 minutes of vigorous-intensity exercise per week is suggested.[10] Additional recommendations include incorporating 3 or more days per week of balance exercises to help prevent falls.[10] Practitioners should take a holistic approach to exercise and movement by suggesting a combination of strength and resistance training, aerobic activity, balancing exercises, and group exercises.[11] Exercises that have been noted to provide beneficial outcomes in the aging population include yoga, tai chi, and qi gong. Studies have shown that strength training is beneficial for postural control in elderly people and is a safe way to improve strength and functional capabilities in sedentary elderly people.[11] Strength training can also help reduce pain and improve overall function as well as prevent falls and loss of deconditioning.[12] Movement exercises such as yoga, tai chi, and qi gong can also facilitate the patient's mind–body connection and improve flexibility and balance. Research has also shown that exercise can improve psychological well-being, including anxiety and depression, and reduces the risk of cognitive decline and dementia.[11]

Although it is important to emphasize exercise in the aging population, it is essential to be mindful of acute and chronic limitations patients may have. Geriatric patients with limitations on mobility can still enjoy exercise and movement therapies individualized to their current situation.[13] Please refer to Chapter 3 for more details.

Mind Body

In 1979 Ellen Langer published an article that would become the basis for her book *Counterclockwise*. In it, she presented findings from a study suggesting that the mind appears to have a significant impact on measurable dimensions of aging.[14] Langer and her colleagues led a group of older adult volunteers on a journey back in time by bringing them to a retreat area in which the surroundings depicted the era of their youth. The participants were encouraged to speak and act as if it were 20 years earlier. "Psychological and physical measures were taken before and after the intervention to see if such a mental context change could produce observable improvements in physical health and cognitive capability."[15] Remarkably, a significant number of measures indicated positive changes associated with adopting a young mindset, such as joint flexibility and near-point vision. These findings flew in the face of conventional understandings of aging and human development and raised important questions about the mind–body connection and physical aging.

Cognitive Function, Neuroplasticity, and Brain Structure

Beginning with Davidson et al.,[16] brain-imaging studies performed on persons who meditate have yielded intriguing new findings about brain plasticity suggesting that brain structure, neurocircuitry, and cerebral blood flow all respond over time to mental activity and that this plasticity endures across the lifespan.[17-20]

One study of 20 healthy adults who meditated (compared with matched controls) found that meditation practice was associated with increased cortical thickness, with differences in prefrontal cortical thickness being most pronounced among older meditators, suggesting that meditation protects against age-related cortical thinning.[21] Hölzel et al.[22] reported that an 8-week mindfulness-based stress reduction intervention was associated with a change in the gray matter concentration in regions of the brain that have a role in learning, memory, emotional regulation, self-referential processing, and perspective taking. Moss et al.[23] found that an 8-week meditation program in a cohort of adults (aged 52–77) with memory loss resulted in positive changes in mood and anxiety; these changes were associated with changes in cerebral blood flow.

Cellular Aging, Telomere Length, and Gene Expression

Epel et al.[24] hypothesized that meditation practice may reduce stress arousal and therefore promote telomere maintenance and cell health. Several studies have reported an association between meditation and telomerase activity.[25-27] In a randomized trial of healthy women, Epel at al.[28] compared the effects of a meditation retreat with the effects of a relaxing vacation among non-meditators, novice meditators, and regular meditators and found that although all the women showed improvements in well-being, the regular meditators showed a trend over time toward increased telomerase activity compared with the other groups.

A number of studies suggest that meditation may affect gene expression in salubrious ways, especially those regulating oxidative stress, inflammation, and cellular aging.[29] Dusek at al.[30] found evidence that the Relaxation Response (RR), which they define as including meditation, yoga, qi gong, tai chi, progressive relaxation, and biofeedback, elicits changes in gene expression in both short-term and long-term practitioners. Sharma et al.[31] assessed gene expression, oxidative stress, DNA damage, and cell aging and apoptosis in 42 practitioners of Sudarshan Kriya (SK; pranayama breathing practices from the yoga tradition) and 42 healthy controls. They found that persons who practiced SK exhibited "better antioxidant status both at the enzyme activity and RNA level." SK practitioners also showed better stress regulation and immune status. The authors concluded that this practice may "exert effects on immunity, aging, cell death, and stress regulation. See Chapter 9 for details of utilizing mind–body and meditative methods in geriatric practice.

Toxic Exposures

While recommendations to avoid tobacco use and excessive alcohol consumption are part of the standard of care for elders, there are no specific recommendations regarding counseling patients to avoid environmental exposures. The U.S. Environmental Protection Agency (EPA) works to ensure that negative impacts on human health from man-made and naturally occurring toxins are avoided or minimized. Clinicians who do not specialize in this issue should establish close working relationships with environmental physicians and should refer patients to high-quality resources that can help them minimize toxic exposures. The Environmental Working Group (http://www.ewg.org/), a not-for-profit organization, provides a number of practical tools, some reviewed in this book. The "Dirty Dozen" eating guide, which lists foods that should be consumed only if they have been grown organically due to their heavily polluted state, is one such tool and is highly valuable in clinical practice since many patients ask about this subject. Also, the federal Office of Disease Prevention and Health Promotion offers detailed information on essential environmental issues such as air and water quality, toxic waste, indoor and outdoor pollution, and global environmental health issues (https://www.healthypeople.gov/2020/topics-objectives/topic/environmental-health).

Drug Metabolism

Cytochrome P450 is composed of enzymes found mainly in the liver and involved in the production of substances in the human body as well as multiple types of metabolic involvement, such as biochemical reactions. Substances can work on the cytochrome P450 system as inducers or inhibitors. An example of this is St. John's wort. St. John's wort is a potent inducer of cytochrome P450 enzyme, and specifically CYP3A4, and therefore lowers the effect of oral contraceptives, anticoagulant medications like warfarin, and immunosuppressants like cyclosporine.[32] Goldenseal can also decrease the effect of many drugs. Garlic has both inductor and inhibitor properties and as an inducer can decrease the effect of HIV medications. Gingko may decrease the effect of some blood pressure medication like diltiazem because of its inhibitory effect on cytochrome P450.[32] It is essential to be mindful of changes in drug metabolism with aging since older people tend to take more medications and metabolize them more slowly, increasing the risk of drug interactions and side effects.

POLYPHARMACY

Thirty-six percent of older persons take at least five prescription medications and 64% take dietary supplements.[33] Twenty-eight percent of older adults' hospital admissions are due to adverse drug events.[33] Physiological changes that impact drug metabolism includes changes in the gut, skin, liver, and kidney. In the stomach, there is decreased gastric emptying, decreased gastric motility, and decreased surface absorption; all of these changes impact drug absorption slightly. On the skin, the increased body fat and decreased lean body mass prolong the distribution of drugs. The decreased liver size and the decreased flow of blood also influence the metabolism of drugs through the liver. In the kidney, there is decreased blood flow and a decreased filtration rate, which slows kidney clearance of drugs and leads to potential toxicity. The serum albumin level also decreases, which increases the concentration of drug in the blood.[34] Given all this, it is essential to minimize the number of medications that the elderly are exposed to.

BEERS CRITERIA

Some medications are well known to be high risk for use in the elderly. The most commonly used tools to identify such medications are the Beers criteria, the Screening Tool of Older Persons' Potentially Inappropriate Prescriptions (STOPP), and the Screening Tool to Alert Doctors to the Right Treatment (START).

The 2015 American Geriatric Society (AGS) Beers criteria list medication indications, medications to avoid, and medications to use with caution among older adults, divided by specific diseases.[35] High-risk medications with strong recommendations to avoid among elders are heart medications (amiodarone, nifedipine), antidepressants (amitriptyline, paroxetine), sulfonylureas (glyburide), barbiturates, proton pump inhibitors, growth hormone, and oral estrogen.[36,37] Medications with moderate risk with strong recommendations are anticholinergic medications (diphenhydramine [Benadryl], benztropine, scopolamine), insulin sliding scale, muscle relaxants, nonsteroidal anti-inflammatory drugs (NSAIDS, like ibuprofen, ketorolac), stomach medications like metoclopramide and mineral oils), appetite stimulants (megestrol), nonbenzodiazepine sleep aids (zolpidem, zaleplon, eszopiclone), benzodiazepines, first- and second-generation antipsychotics, digoxin, heart medications (terazosin, doxazosin), and blood thinners (ticlopidine, dipyridine). We recommend that all clinicians who work with elders should be very familiar with the Beers criteria. The free online resource can be found here: https://www. guideline.gov/summaries/summary/49933.

DRUG–HERB INTERACTIONS

Among elders, nutritional and herbal supplements are most commonly used for arthritis, immune stimulation, and cardiovascular support.[38] Nearly 50% of community-dwelling geriatric patients had at least one drug–herb interaction. Lobelia herbs interact with lithium. Red rice yeast can cause toxicity if used together with statin cholesterol medications. Black cohosh can interact with tamoxifen and doxorubicin. St. John's wort can interact with medications like antidepressants, oral contraceptives, transplant medications, and heart medications (Table 4.1).

Some herbs should be used with caution and should be avoided in some conditions. Garlic and bilberry are not recommended in patients with gastrointestinal problems. Red yeast rice should be avoided in those with liver diseases. Kava may lead to liver damage. Cabbage should be used in limited amounts among individuals with high blood pressure and thyroid disease.[39]

For busy clinicians, the Natural Database is a good online resource that can quickly identify possible drug–herb interactions (http://naturaldatabase. therapeuticresearch.com/).

Table 4.1. Common Drug–Herb Interactions

Name of Herb	Drug it interacts with	Type of interaction
Bilberry	Aspirin, insulin, Plavix, ticlopidine	Increased risk of side effects and bleeding
Cinnamon	Diabetes medications	May increase the risk of low blood sugar
Dandelion	Metronidazole	Nausea
Ginger	Antidepressants, anticoagulants (blood thinners), antipsychotics (benzodiazepines), quinidine	Increased risk of side effects and toxicity
Green tea	Anticoagulants, theophylline, drugs that block hormones (anti-androgens)	Increased risk of side effects
Ginkgo	Anticoagulants, aspirin, antidepressants, vitamin E, garlic	Increased seizure threshold and serotonin syndrome. Increased risk for bleeding
Ginseng	Blood pressure medications, anticoagulant, digoxin, hormone replacement (estrogenic drugs)	Causes increased blood pressure, sleepiness; blocks estrogen
Licorice	High blood pressure medications	Increased risk of hypertensive crisis
Kava	Sleeping medications, alcohol, antipsychotics	Increased risk of lethargy and confusion
St. John's wort	Antidepressants	Increased risk for adverse effect
Psyllium	Digoxin, diuretics, antidepressants, lithium, anticoagulants	Potentiate side effects
Yohimbe	Blood pressure medications	May increase risk of low blood pressure

Based on information from Meng and Lui 2014.[45]

Geriatric Screening Tests

The most common chronic diseases among older adults are arthritis, cancer, heart disease, hypertension, and diabetes. According to the U.S. Preventive Services Task Force (USPSTF), fall risk is decreased by geriatric assessment, exercise, physical therapy, and vitamin D supplementation. Recommendations for screening for older adults are controversial and vary by functional status and comorbidities (Table 4.2). The USPSTF recommends mammography every 1 to 2 years between ages 50 and 74, but the American College of Obstetrics and Gynecology (ACOG) recommends starting at age 40.

Table 4.2. Geriatric Screening Recommendations

Tests	USPSTF	CDC	Other	AGS	Age	Interval
DEXA scan	Yes	Yes		Yes	≥65–85	2 years
Colorectal cancer	Yes	Yes		Yes	≥50–85	
Mammography	Yes, ages 50–74	Yes	ACOG, starting at age 40	Up to age 80	≥40/ 50–74	1–2 years
Lung cancer	Smoking history— low-dose computed tomography (LDCT)	Yes	Medicare part B covers age 55–77		55–80years	Annual
Pap smear	No	No		No, except if never screened before	21–65	Every 1–3 years
Prostate exam	No		Insufficient evidence (I) for age ≥75	Annual digital rectal exam		
Abdominal ultrasound		Recommended	American College of Cardiology, men ≥ 60 with family history		Male smokers age 65–75	
Dementia	Cannot recommend based on benefits or risk		American Academy of Family Physicians, cannot recommend based on benefits or risk			If reports of cognitive problems may screen using Minicog, SLUMS, MMSE, or MOCA

(continued)

Table 4.2. Continued

Tests	USPSTF	CDC	Other	AGS	Age	Interval
Visual test	I	I		Yes		Annually
Complete physical	Every 2 years	Every 2 years		Yes		
Hypertension	Yes	Yes		Yes		Annually
Diabetes	Yes	Yes		Yes		Annually
Fall	No	No		Yes		Annually. May use TUG
Hearing test	No	No		Yes		
Depression	Yes	Yes		Yes		Annually
Smoking cessation	Yes	Yes		Yes		
Alcohol use	Yes	Yes		Yes		

Abbreviations: SLUMS, St. Louis University Mental Status Examination; MMSE, Mini Mental Status Exam; MOCA, Montreal Cognitive Assessment; TUG, Times Up and Go test; AGS, American Geriatric Society; USPSTF; U.S. Preventive Services Task Force; CDC, Centers for Disease Control and Prevention; ACOG, American College of Gynecology.

Table 4.3. Vaccine Recommendations

Vaccines	Intervals	Types	Effectiveness
Influenza	Annually	Inactivated trivalent or quadrivalent	Controversial. Decreased hospital admissions.
Pneumococcal	≥ 65 years—2 vaccines	PCV13 and PPSV23	Decreased morbidity and mortality
Herpes zoster	Once if given after age 60	Live	Decreased morbidity
Tetanus and diphtheria	Every 10 years	TD or Tdap	No specific geriatric evidence

Immunizations

According to the Centers for Disease Control and Prevention, the recommended vaccines in this population are for influenza, herpes zoster, tetanus, diphtheria, and pneumonia (Table 4.3).[40]

The inactivated form of influenza vaccine is recommended annually. The herpes zoster vaccine is given once if administered after age 60. The tetanus and diphtheria vaccine is given as a booster every 10 years. A Cochrane review concluded that polysaccharide vaccines are effective in reducing the incidence of pneumococcal disease among adults older than 55, but the PPSV23 does not appear to reduce the incidence of pneumonia or death in adults. Evidence shows that inactivated influenza virus vaccines overall decrease mortality and hospital admission among elders, but the effectiveness was mainly among institutionalized seniors.[41]

In an evaluation of vaccine safety, a 2011 systemic review from the Institute of Medicine reported high evidence for an association of seasonal influenza vaccine and arthralgia, myalgia, malaise, fever, and pain at the injection site. There was no evidence supporting an association between influenza and pneumococcal vaccines and cardiovascular events in the elderly.[41] The evidence was insufficient to make conclusions regarding the association of vaccines with multiple sclerosis, transverse myelitis, and acute disseminated encephalomyelitis.[42]

Models of Geriatric Care

Geriatric Resources for Assessment and Care of Elders (GRACE) is an interdisciplinary team that prepares an individualized care plan incorporating protocols that have been developed for the treatment of 12 targeted geriatric conditions.[38] The GRACE model is mainly driven by nurse practitioners and social workers using community and social resources to help individuals age in place. The literature shows that the GRACE intervention decreases the number of hospital admissions and emergency room visits (Table 4.4).

Table 4.4. Models of Geriatric Care

Name of Care	Type of Care	Team	Insurance	
GRACE	Home-based primary care	Geriatrician, primary care physician, nurse practitioner, social worker, nurse, mental health support	Medicare, Medicaid Veteran Affairs (VA)	Individualized, uses community resources, focuses on geriatric syndrome
PACE	Home and adult day center	Physician, nurse practitioner, social worker, nurse, physical therapy, occupational therapy, dietician, pharmacy, transport	Medicare and Medicaid	Requires family or caregiver collaboration
Patient-centered medical home	Outpatient	Primary provider, specialist, nurse	Medicare, Medicaid, private insurance	Coordination of care
ACE	Inpatient	Nurse practitioner, social worker, nurse	Variable, but typically all insurances	Maintain activities of daily living
NICHE	Inpatient and outpatient	Nurses	Variable	Focused on nursing training and interventions
HELP	Inpatient	Geriatric nurse, elder specialists, volunteer, geriatrician	Variable	Prevent delirium

Geriatric emergency care	Emergency room	Physician, nursing staff	All insurances	Incorporates geriatric assessment, discharge planning, and community resources
Hospital at Home model	Outpatient	Physicians, nursing staff	Variable	Avoid hospital admission and receive hospital care at home. Cost-effective.
Palliative care	Inpatient and outpatient	Palliative Care team,	All insurances	Refer to chapter 31 for detailed overview
Nursing home	Short-term subacute rehabilitation and Long-term Care.	Physician, nurse, nursing assistance, social worker, dietician, physical therapy, occupational therapy, Speech Therapy	Medicaid, private pay	Non-skilled medical and nonmedical care of debilitated older adults. Refer to chapter 28 for detailed overview

Table 4.5. Useful Online Resources

Environmental Working Group (EWG): http://www.ewg.org/
Healthy People: https://www.healthypeople.gov/2020/topics-objectives/topic/environmental-health
Natural Database: http://naturaldatabase.therapeuticresearch.com/
BEER criteria for geriatric high-risk medications: https://www.guideline.gov/summaries/summary/49933

The Program of All-Inclusive Care for the Elderly (PACE) is a day program that prevents institutionalization and helps individuals who meet the criteria for a nursing home to receive care at home. PACE is a collaborative program requiring family or caregiver support. It allows caregivers to maintain employment during the day while the patient is in a PACE center.

A patient-centered medical home provides comprehensive primary care for people of all ages and with all medical conditions, with an emphasis on coordinated care.

The Nurses Improving Care to Health-system Elders (NICHE) is a patient-centered model to improve hospital care processes for older adults, with a focus on nursing programs and protocols shown to improve care among older adults.[43]

Acute Care for Elders (ACE) concentrates on helping hospitalized older adults maintain or achieve functional independence in basic activities of daily life. ACE units were associated with decreased hospital readmissions, greater independence in activities of daily living, less frequent discharge to a nursing home, and decreased health care expenses.[44]

The Hospital Elder Life Program (HELP) is designed to prevent delirium and functional decline among hospitalized older patients.

The Care Transitions Intervention Model provides chronically ill patients with "transition coaches" who help them move effectively from hospital to home. The Palliative Care Consultation Model focuses on averting unwanted medical interventions for adults with life-limiting illnesses.[38]

Table 4.5 provides a list of useful online resources for preventive geriatrics.

ACKNOWLEDGMENTS

The authors thank the following for research assistance: Diana Cardenas, Caroline Huber, and Glenn Shrum.

REFERENCES

1. Spoorenberg SLW, Uittenbroek RJ, Middel B, Kremer BPH, Reijneveld SA, Wynia K. Embrace, a model for integrated elderly care: Study protocol of a randomized controlled trial on the effectiveness regarding patient outcomes, service use, costs, and quality of care. *BMC Geriatr.* 2013;13(1):62. doi:10.1186/1471-2318-13-62.

2. World Health Organization. *Innovative Care for Chronic Conditions: Building Blocks for Action.* Geneva, Switzerland; 2002.

3. Institute of Medicine. *Best Care at Lower Cost: The Path to Continuously Learning Health Care in America* (Smith M, Saunders R, Stuckhardt L, McGinnis JM, eds.). Washington, DC: National Academies Press; 2012.

4. Organisation for Economic Co-operation and Development (OECD). *Health Reform: Meeting the Challenge of Ageing and Multiple Morbidities.* 2011. doi:10.1787/9789264122314-en.

5. Nolte E, Knai C, Hofmarcher M, et al. Overcoming fragmentation in health care: Chronic care in Austria, Germany and The Netherlands. *Health Econ Policy Law.* 2012;7(1):125–146. doi:10.1017/S1744133111000338.

6. Marengoni A, Angleman S, Melis R, et al. Aging with multimorbidity: A systematic review of the literature. *Ageing Res Rev.* 2011;10:430–439. doi:10.1016/j.arr.2011.03.003.

7. Vogeli C, Shields AE, Lee TA, et al. Multiple chronic conditions: Prevalence, health consequences, and implications for quality, care management, and costs. *J Gen Intern Med.* 2007;22(Suppl 3):391–395. doi:10.1007/s11606-007-0322-1.

8. Spalding MC, Sebesta SC. Geriatric screening and preventive care. *Am Fam Physician.* 2008;78(2):206–215.

9. Centers for Disease Control and Prevention (CDC). Public health and aging: Trends in aging—United States and worldwide. Available at cdc.gov.

10. *Global Recommendations on Physical Activity for Health.* Geneva: World Health Organization; 2010.

11. Cvecka J, Tirpakova V, Sedliak M, Kern H, Mayr W, Hamar D. Physical activity in elderly. *Eur J Translational Myology.* 2015;25(4):249–252. doi:10.4081/ejtm.2015.5280.

12. Paterson D, Warburton D. Physical activity and functional limitations in older adults: a systematic review related to Canada's Physical Activity Guidelines. *Int J Behav Nutr Phys Activ.* 2010; 7(38).

13. Bickley LS, Szilagyi PG, Boshkov L. *Bates' Guide to Physical Examination and History-taking with Access Code.* 11th ed. Philadelphia: Wolters Kluwer Health/ Lippincott Williams & Wilkins; 2012.

14. McCabe Ruff, Kelley et al. The role of mindfulness in healthcare reform: A policy paper. *Explore: The Journal of Science and Healing.* 2009;5(6):313–323.

15. Langer E, Chanowitz B, Palmerino M, Jacobs S, Rhodes M, Thayer P. Nonsequential development and aging. In C. Alexander & E. Langer (Eds.), *Higher Stages of Human Development* (pp. 114–136). New York: Oxford University Press, 1990.

16. Davidson RJ, Kabat-Zinn J, Schumacher J, et al. Alterations in brain and immune function produced by mindfulness meditation. *Psychosom Med.* 2003;65(4):564–570.

17. Chiesa A, Calati R, Serretti A. Does mindfulness training improve cognitive abilities. A systematic review of neuropsychological findings. *Clin Psychol Rev.* 2011;31(3):449–464.

18. Fox KCR, Nijeboer S, Dixon ML, et al. Is meditation associated with altered brain structure? *Neurosci Biobehav Rev.* 2014;43:48–73.

19. Lutz A, Brefczynski-Lewis J, Johnstone T, Davidson RJ. Regulation of the neural circuitry of emotion by compassion meditation: Effects of meditative expertise. *PloS One.* 2008;3(3):e1897.

20. Newberg AB, Wintering N, Waldman MR, et al. Cerebral blood flow differences between long-term meditators and non-meditators. *Conscious Cogn.* 2010;19(4):899–905.

21. Lazar SW, Kerr CE, Wasserman RH, et al. Meditation Experience is associated with increased cortical rhickness. *Neuroreport.* 2005;16(17):1893.

22. Hölzel BK, Carmody J, Evans KC, et al. Stress reduction correlates with structural changes in the amygdala. *Social Cognitive and Affective Neuroscience.* 2010;5:11–17.

23. Moss A, Wintering N, Roggenkamp H, et al. Effects of an 8-week meditation program on mood and anxiety in patients with memory loss. *J Alternative Complementary Med.* 2012;18(1):48–53.

24. Epel E, Daubenmier J, Moskowitz JT, Folkman S, Blackburn E. Can meditation slow rate of cellular aging? Cognitive stress, mindfulness, and telomeres. *Ann NY Acad Sci.* 2009;1172:34–53.

25. Carlson LE, Beattie TL, Giese-Davis J, et al. Mindfulness-based cancer recovery and supportive-expressive therapy maintain telomere length relative to controls in distressed breast cancer survivors. *Cancer.* 2015;121(3):476–484.

26. Jacobs TL, Epel ES, Lin J, et al. Intensive meditation training, immune cell telomerase activity, and psychological mediators. *Psychoneuroendocrinology.* 2011;36(5):664–681. doi:10.1016/j.psyneuen.2010.09.010. Epub 2010 Oct 29.

27. Lengacher CA, Reich RR, Kip KE, et al. Influence of mindfulness-based stress reduction (MBSR) on telomerase activity in women with breast cancer (BC). *Biol Res Nursing.* 2014;16(4):438–447.

28. Epel ES, Puterman E, Lin J, et al. Meditation and vacation effects have an impact on disease-associated molecular phenotypes. *Translational Psychiatry.* 2016;6:e880; doi:10.1038/tp.2016.164.

29. Innes KE, Selfe TK, Brown C, Rose KM, Thompson-Heisterman A. The effects of meditation on perceived stress and related indices of psychological status and sympathetic activation in persons with Alzheimer's disease and their caregivers: A pilot study. *Evid Based Complement Altern Med.* 2012;2012:927509.

30. Dusek JA, Otu HH, Wohlhueter AL, et al. Genomic counter-stress changes induced by the Relaxation Response. PLoS One. 2008;3(7):e2576. doi:10.1371/journal.pone.0002576

31. Sharma H, Datta P, Singh A, et al. Gene expression profiling in practitioners of Sudarshan Kriya. *J Psychosom Res.* 2008;64:2013–2018.

32. Saxena A, Tripathi KP, Roy S, Khan F, Sharma A. Pharmacovigilance: Effects of herbal components on human drugs interactions involving cytochrome P450. *Bioinformation.* 2008;3(5):198–204. http://doi.org/10.6026/97320630 003198.

33. Qato DM, Wilder J, Schumm L, Gillet V, Alexander G. Changes in prescription and over-the-counter medication and dietary supplement use among older adults in the United States, 2005 vs 2011. *JAMA Intern Med.* 2016;176(4):473–482. doi:10.1001/jamainternmed.2015.858.

34. Klotz U. Pharmacokinetics and drug metabolism in the elderly. *Drug Metabolism Reviews.* 2009;41(2):67–76. http://doi.org/10.1080/03602530902722679.

35. Heidelbaugh JJ. Proton pump inhibitors and risk of vitamin and mineral deficiency: evidence and clinical implications. *Therapeutic Advances in Drug Safety.* 2013;4(3):125–133. http://doi.org/10.1177/2042098613482484

36. American Geriatrics Society. Updated Beers Criteria. *J Am Geriatr Soc.* 2015;63:2227–2246. http://doi.org/10.1111/jgs.13702

37. O'Mahony D, O'Sullivan D, Byrne S, O'Connor MN, Ryan C, Gallagher P. STOPP/START criteria for potentially inappropriate prescribing in older people: version 2. *Age Ageing.* 2015 Mar;44(2):213–218. doi: 10.1093/ageing/afu145.

38. American Geriatric Society. www.americangeriatrics.org

39. Rouhi-Boroujeni H, Rouhi-Boroujeni H, Gharipour M, Mohammadizadeh F, Ahmadi S, Rafieian-Kopaei M. Systematic review on safety and drug interaction of herbal therapy in hyperlipidemia: a guide for internist. *Acta Biomed.* 2015 Sep 14;86(2):130–136. PMID: 26422426

40. Centers for Disease Control and Prevention. www.cdc.gov

41. Lang PO, Mendes A, Socquet J, Assir N, Govind S, Aspinall R. Effectiveness of influenza vaccine in aging and older adults: Comprehensive analysis of the evidence. *Clinical Interventions in Aging.* 2012;7:55–64. http://doi.org/10.2147/CIA.S25215.

42. Nicholas JA, Hall WJ. Screening and preventive services for older adults. *Mt Sinai J Med.* 2011;78(4):498–508. http://doi.org/10.1002/msj.20275.Screening.

43. The NICHE models of care: www.nicheprogram.org/models-of-care/

44. Counsell SR, Holder CM, Liebenauer LL, et al. Effects of a multicomponent intervention on functional outcomes and process of care in hospitalized older patients: a randomized controlled trial of Acute Care for Elders (ACE) in a community hospital. *J Am Geriatr Soc.* 2000;48(12):1572.

45. Meng Q, Liu K. Pharmacokinetic interactions between herbal medicines and prescribed drugs: focus on drug metabolic enzymes and transporters. *Curr Drug Metab.* 2014;15(8):791–807.

5

Acupuncture and Traditional Chinese Medicine (TCM)

ANGELA GABRIEL AND TIFFANY C. HOYT

In ancient times the Yellow Emperor, Huang Di [said], "I've heard that in the days of old everyone lived one hundred years without showing the usual signs of aging. In our time, however, people age prematurely living only fifty years. Is this due to a change in the environment, or is it because people have lost the correct way of life?"

Qi Bo replied, "In the past people understood the principle of balance, of yin and yang. They ate a balanced diet at regular times, arose and retired at regular hours. They maintained well-being of body and mind; thus it is not surprising that they lived over one hundred years. These days people have changed their way of life. They fail to regulate their lifestyle and diet and sleep improperly. So it is not surprising that they look old at fifty and die soon after."

The Yellow Emperor's Classic of Medicine, ca. 220 C.E.[1]

Case Study

An 84-year-old woman had undergone chemotherapy for breast cancer 20 years earlier, which left her with dry eyes and photophobia, with little relief from conventional treatments. She also complained of lower back soreness and occasional night sweats. Her memory was poor, and she often felt confused and depressed. Her sleep was disrupted by frequent urination, and her urine was dark yellow.

Her family arranged a visit to a traditional Chinese medicine (TCM) practitioner. Upon examination her radial pulses were found to be rapid and hard. Her tongue was small, dark red, and dry without coat, with a long vertical crack in the center. She had bright red flags in her cheeks. Her tongue, pulse, and the malar flush are all indications of yin deficiency with internal fire as well as blood stasis, kidney jing deficiency, and unsettled shen. Treatment included biweekly acupuncture sessions for 10 weeks with a short daily qi gong practice. She also took an individualized Chinese herbal formula for 5 weeks.

After several weeks the patient reported her eyes were more moist, and she no longer had to use eye drops during the night. Her nighttime bathroom visits also had reduced from three to four times nightly to zero to one, which improved the refreshing quality of her sleep. Her low back soreness was moderately improved as she continued with qi gong. She felt calmer and less depressed and began to participate in various group activities at her facility. She still had poor memory and felt confused occasionally, but at other times she was more present and alert. She opted to have acupuncture once a month for maintenance, and requested a qi gong practice group to be organized at her facility.

Introduction

Chinese medicine is a comprehensive medical system with its own understanding of physiology and pathology, and methods of diagnosis and therapy. For over 2,000 years it has been developed and retooled. Political and economic changes within the Chinese empire occurred concomitantly with changes in medicine. Unlike Western biomedicine Chinese medicine never rejected its foundational theories but strove to incorporate all of its accumulated philosophy into its present shape.[2] Most recently it has started accommodating Western medicine's contributions.

In the 20th century, the Chinese government, embarrassed by what it felt was "backward" medicine, prohibited Chinese medicine, but due to enormous internal pressure, the government reversed its policy shortly thereafter. The newly renamed Traditional Chinese Medicine (TCM) was codified, standardized, and taught in dedicated universities. In 1972, with U.S. President Richard Nixon's trip to China, Western journalists returned with stories of miraculous acupuncture treatments, and Chinese medicine burst into American consciousness.

While the Western media have frequently romanticized TCM as an exogenous, exotic practice (see Woody Allen's 1988 film *Alice*), at its heart it is a down-to-earth medicine (Table 5.1[3]). TCM's goal is to ensure optimal daily functioning. Trained practitioners chart progress through a consistent, evaluative review of systems such as sleep quality, digestion, excretion, appetite, and pain. Improvement over time is based on the patient's subjective feelings of

Table 5.1. Key Concepts in Chinese Medicine

Concept	Description
Natural Cycles	The earliest Chinese medicine physicians based their observations of human health and illness on what they saw in nature: 24-hour cycle of the day 28-day cycle of the moon 4-season cycle of the year 60-year cycle of growth and decline
Yin and Yang	First appearing in the *Yi Qing*—compiled in the eighth century BCE—this concept describes a cycle with two polar points, often depicted by the tai jitu. These principles are opposite, mutually dependent and inter-transforming. The law of the transformation of yin and yang is an elegant description of the process of homeostasis.
Balance in Mind–Body	When the mind and the body are in a balanced state, and synchronized with nature, people will enjoy health and happiness. "Balance" is not an esoteric concept at all, but rather it describes the pragmatic smooth functioning of daily bodily systems and shows up as regular, refreshing sleep, hearty appetite at appropriate intervals, regular satisfying bowel movements, and relative freedom from pain.
The Three Treasures: *Jing, qi, shen*	• *Jing* or "vital essence" is inherited material from parents and ancestors; as it decreases, chronic degenerative diseases occur. • *Qi* (pronounced *chee*) or bodily "energy" is acquired and spent daily from food, water, clean air, REM sleep, and a positive mental attitude. Like blood, and lymph, it flows in wide channels (or meridians) from the core to the peripheries, and like water it suffuses all the tissues of the body. • *Shen* or "mind" describes the potential and intention a person brings to daily activities. The mind affects all aspects of life, from the etheric (the personality) to the physical (sleep quality).
Causes of Disease	There are three main causes of illness: internal, external and other: • *Internal causes* correspond to dysregulated or unresolved emotions. • *External causes* were based on climatological conditions entering the body. Because early physicians had no concept of germ theory, they extrapolated that pathological factors entered the body through the orifices. Today these pathological factors are still used to describe illness, but they exist in tandem with the modern concept of viruses and bacteria. • *Other causes*: poor diet, trauma, parasites and poisons, overworking, and incorrect medical treatment

functioning rather than through quantitative test results, although today many TCM practitioners are trained to use blood and hormone panels to verify the results of the treatments. In China today, the health care model strives to integrate TCM with Western biomedical treatments for best medical outcomes and highest standards of quality of life.

TCM Therapies

ACUPUNCTURE AND MOXIBUSTION

Of the many TCM therapies, acupuncture is by far the best known in the West.[4] Acupuncture uses very fine filiform needles, usually made of stainless steel, at precise must be used a single time on a single point and then disposed of. Moxibustion—a less well known but highly effective technique—uses moxa (*Artemesia argyri*), an herbal wool from the common mugwort plant that has been processed. Used on acupuncture points for therapeutic boosting, it is essential for frail consumers. Moxa therapy is especially important for all aging persons as it builds yang qi and can slow the decline of essence.[5]

DIETARY THERAPY

Dietary therapy is the most important of all the acupuncture-related therapies. In fact, diet is one of the best ways to make a significant difference in a person's health as well as to prevent illness. Every diet should be specifically tailored to a person's constitution. Dietary changes can be therapeutic for medical conditions, either acute or chronic: for example, a person with an acute, productive cough would benefit from the reduction of dairy, sugar, raw foods, and iced drinks, and the addition of mild pungent spices to food, until the condition clears.[6,7] Another patient presenting with low energy and poor appetite would benefit from nutrient-dense bone broth, consumed daily over time.[8] Unfortunately many patients in North America, particularly those who are house-bound, lack access to high-quality meats and produce, traditional products, and freshly prepared meals.

TCM principles state that eating fresh, properly cooked light meals, without a lot of fat, salt, or sugar, cooked rather than raw, is better for a weaker digestion. The standard American diet is heavy, with cloying, difficult-to-digest fried foods, mucus-producing dairy, and glucose- and salt-enriched processed foods. It lacks the wide variety of tastes that TCM principles state should be eaten at each meal: salty, sweet, sour, pungent or spicy, bitter, bland, astringent. In fact, the therapeutic taste of bitter is often entirely absent from the American diet.

TUINA/THERAPEUTIC MASSAGE

Tuina is a specific type of manual manipulation that relies on TCM foundational principles to treat disease. While it may look superficially like massage, it also addresses skeletal dysregulation in a manner similar to chiropractic. Through careful therapeutic stimulation muscles are energized so that blood and qi flow to areas of stagnation, which is of particular benefit to a sedentary population. Tuina has been studied as a treatment for a range of both external conditions (pain, reduced range of motion) and internal conditions, including disorders of the respiratory, digestive, and circulatory systems.[9]

CHINESE HERBAL MEDICINE

Herbal medicine has been practiced in China for thousands of years and is still the most common TCM practice in Asia today. The oldest materia medica extant lists botanicals, minerals, and animal parts to be used for various symptoms. Early formularies established the principles of polypharmacy: formulas in which "chief herbs" were combined in working pairs to potentiate their positive effects, with "assistant herbs" to mitigate their negative effects and "envoy" herbs to direct the benefits of the therapy to the correct location. Many of the oldest formulas still being used today have been tested on millions of people.[10] Today animal substances are regulated in the West. Formulas produced in North America must adhere to Good Manufacturing Practices (GMP) for quality assurance that the medicinals are properly identified and batch tested for heavy metals.[11]

A TCM herbalist will take a detailed personal history before prescribing a formula tailored specifically for a patient. In the process he or she will take into consideration not only the patient's chief complaint, but also the constellation of his or her accompanying symptoms, dietary considerations, and information from an objective assessment. For the elderly, in general, many of these formulas focus on augmenting qi, blood, and jing and improving blood circulation,[12] which can greatly help increase quality of life.

QI GONG AND TAI CHI

Qi gong (pronounced *chee gung*) is a mind–body exercise that combines gentle movement, breathing techniques, and visualization or meditation. Types of qi gong range from a completely static practice (meditation with little movement) to more dynamic forms (of which tai chi is an example), providing a variety of therapeutic exercises including those that can be performed by bedridden or wheelchair-bound persons.

The success of this therapy relies on the TCM assumption that focused, fluid movements practiced regularly increase the circulation of blood and qi to specific areas of the body. When practiced daily, movement increases range of motion, loosens frozen joints, and improves blood circulation to the peripherals and balance. Performed over a period of time qi gong may remediate the effects of aging and stave off further deterioration. Group or individual daily exercise can easily become part of a health maintenance plan.

Medical qi gong is practiced by medical therapists who are trained in TCM theory to work with individuals on a case-by-case basis. In China, medical qi gong has been studied for a broad range of symptoms including hyper- and hypotension, rheumatoid arthritis, dermatological conditions, diabetes, peripartum diseases, cancer, necrosis of the head of the femur, Parkinson's disease, Ménière's syndrome, cataracts, glaucoma, myopia, amblyopia, leukemia, and iatrogenic tinnitus.[13] Trained instructors of qi gong and practitioners of medical qi gong can be found at The Qigong Institute, http://www.qigonginstitute.org/ and various other qi gong organizations.

Approach to Treatment

A TCM diagnosis relies on history taking, oral interview, palpation of the radial pulses, and visual examination of the tongue. If there is pain, there may be orthopedic assessment. The constellation of signs and symptoms and additional findings will paint an overall picture called a "pattern of disharmony." Identification of the pattern is essential for treatment. All patterns include a cause and generate a treatment plan.

TCM does not treat disease but goes to the root cause of the complaint. For example, three migraine sufferers may have three different underlying causes, or "disharmonies." The underlying cause is seen as the "root" of the problem, and the symptom manifesting itself (the migraine) as the "branch." When both the root and the branch are treated together, there is a better chance the symptom will not recur.

TCM sees the symptoms of aging as a depletion of vital essence. Gentle tonifying and invigorating techniques play a part in every treatment when working with this population. With each population there are treatment considerations to be taken into account, and the geriatric population is no exception. For example, thinning skin and decreased muscle mass increase the likelihood of bruising with acupuncture. This population frequently takes multiple medications, so the risk of undesirable interactions from polypharmacy complicates the prescription of Chinese herbal medicine, although many traditional Chinese herbal formulas call for the use of anodyne medicinals, such as reishi mushroom (*Ganoderma*), American ginseng (*Panax quinquefolius*), and gou ji berries (*Fructus lyceum barbium*), in geriatric formulas.[14]

Evidence-Based Medicine and Acupuncture

Of all the TCM therapies in the West, acupuncture remains the most sought-after treatment, although Chinese mind–body practices such as tai chi and qi gong have also elicited scientific interest in recent years. As a result, most scientific resources have been allocated to its study. Acupuncture research focuses on two main areas: understanding its biomedical mechanisms and investigating its effectiveness for specific medical conditions in clinical trials.

Many studies in animal and human models have demonstrated that acupuncture can produce a variety of profound biological responses. These responses can occur locally—in the tissues surrounding the site of needle insertion—or at a distance, mediated by sensory neurons within the central nervous system.[15] Central biomedical mechanisms of acupuncture are supported by following studies:

- Studies have demonstrated that levels of endorphins, epinephrine, encephalin, serotonin, nitric oxide, prostaglandins, TNF-alpha, and other mediators were modulated during and following acupuncture treatment.[16]
- Brain imaging studies such as functional magnetic resonance imaging (MRI) reveal changes in brain activity caused by acupuncture interventions.[17,18]

- Acupuncture intervention had been shown to upregulate gene expression.[19]
- The area of integrating acupuncture with systems biology approach and functional medicine can become a major research topic.[20,21]
- Acupuncture needles affect skin and connective tissue such as muscle fibers, tendons, and fascia mechanically and through activation of local neurons and vasculature.[22]
- Holistic effects of acupuncture treatment have become a focus of recent studies.[23]

These responses facilitate tissue healing, decrease pain sensory threshold,[24] regulate the central nervous system, reduce stress, and optimize the body's healing resources. The search for biological mechanisms explaining acupuncture continues. The National Center for Complementary and Integrative Health considers certain areas of acupuncture research as a higher priority. These include studies elucidating and quantifying possible biological mechanisms of acupuncture and electro-acupuncture.

Studying the clinical effects of acupuncture had been challenging because clinical trials often differ in terms of technique, types of control methods, the number of acupuncture points, the number of sessions, and the duration of those sessions. Randomized clinical trials (RCTs), especially double-blind randomized trials, are difficult to conduct due to the active involvement of the therapist and imperfection of control techniques. Moreover, results may be influenced by a patient's beliefs and expectations about his or her treatment.[25,26]

Even taking these methodological challenges into consideration, small but statistically significant differences between classically administered acupuncture and "sham" acupuncture have been repeatedly demonstrated in many high-quality RCTs. Larger statistical differences were found when acupuncture was compared to standard care.[27]

There have been very few studies, especially RCTs, focused on the geriatric population specifically. However, many health conditions commonly afflicting elders have been studied in the wider population, and there is adequate evidence that acupuncture is effective, safe, and cost-effective. These conditions include low back pain, knee and hip pain, headache, insomnia, constipation, depression, memory loss, and Parkinson's disease, to name a few.[28–34]

One last but not the least important topic of acupuncture studies is safety. According to the National Center for Complementary and Alternative

Medicine (NCCAM), "numerous surveys show that of all the complementary and holistic medical practices, of which there are many, acupuncture enjoys the most credibility in the medical community." It is essential that acupuncture and any other Chinese medical therapy is delivered by a qualified practitioner.[35,36]

Cognitive Health, Pain Conditions, Quality of Life

One of the most distressing health issues for older adults and their families is the decline of mental abilities and emotional instability. Decline of cognitive function affects memory, thinking, self-expression, judgment, and behavior. Dementia, Alzheimer's disease, and vascular cognitive impairment are currently leading senior health care problems. Seniors also often suffer from mood disorders: depression, anxiety, irritability, agitation, and sleep issues. TCM offers sophisticated explanations and treatments for emotions and their excesses. Acupuncture, herbal therapy, qi gong, and meditation can restore central balance to daily life. A number of studies demonstrate the effectiveness of TCM in slowing symptoms of cognitive decline.[37-40] More evidence supports the role of TCM therapies in improving mood, alleviating depression, and improving sleep.[41-44]

There are additional intangibles that make therapeutic touch ideal for seniors, particularly those who no longer live with family or spouses. Active listening, touch, relaxation, and positive feedback are essential components to therapeutic interaction, and in the care of seniors this can be game-changing.[45-48]

Pain is a frequent complaint within the aging population. "Where there is free flow, there is no pain; where there is pain, there is no free flow."[49] TCM explains pain as a blockage of free-flowing qi and blood to the affected area. The affected area ceases to freely flow itself and then manifests as a "frozen" joint or in reduced range of motion.

Fortunately, there are more positive studies on the treatment of pain with acupuncture than any other single condition. Pain in the lower back, hip, and knee, as well as arthritis, is a leading source of stress for the elderly. Acupuncture presents a viable alternative or addition to the pharmaceutical approach. Opiates or nonsteroidal anti-inflammatories taken daily to treat chronic pain have long been known to have deleterious effects on the digestive, renal, and immune systems.[50,51]

Bodily Functions

Other issues seniors face may be less urgent but do impact quality of life. Constipation, poor digestion, poor sleep, frequent urination, low energy, hypertension, and poor appetite are all daily, nagging annoyances for persons who have ample time to dwell on them. All of these conditions have been treated successfully with TCM.[52] Moreover, TCM therapies are easily incorporated into existing care plans.[53] When acupuncture, massage, qi gong, and tai chi are prescribed, they are always in addition to conventional therapies.

Credentialing

Acupuncture is a rigorously regulated field of medicine. Most states require formal training, standardized testing, certification, and licensure. Training involves a 4-year master's degree in acupuncture (M.S. Ac.) or acupuncture and Chinese herbal medicine (M.S. OM) from an accredited institution with 1,500 to 2,300 hours of didactic and clinical work.[54] An acupuncturist must also pass a written and practical state and/or national board examination for licensure. Curricula for these programs include foundations of Chinese medical theory, anatomy and physiology, and introduction to Western medicine. Herbal medicine training includes courses in physiology, basic chemistry, pharmacology, and pharmacokinetics.

Currently, 43 states require certification by the National Certification Commission for Acupuncture and Oriental Medicine (NCCAOM). California administers its own examination, the California Licensing Examination. To maintain NCCAOM certification and renew their state license, acupuncturists must also complete continuing education courses (CEUs) in areas of professional development and ethics.

Licensed acupuncturists (L.Ac.) do not necessarily have NCCAOM certification. Medical doctors and veterinarians can be granted certification by one of their professional organizations after completion of an acupuncture course and do not have to complete extensive training or pass the NCCAOM board examination.

Consumers interested in locating trained and licensed acupuncturists can consult the NCCAOM "Find a Practitioner directory" on the NCCAOM website, or use a private company—Acufinder.com. Medical doctors certified to use acupuncture in their practice can be located through their professional organization search engine. Not all insurance providers cover acupuncture treatments and not all acupuncturists accept insurance. This should be verified directly with the insurance provider.

REFERENCES

1. Ni M. *The Yellow Emperor's Classic of Medicine: A New Translation of the Neijing Suwen with Commentary.* Boston: Shambhala Press; 1995.
2. Unschuld P. *Medicine in China: A History of Ideas* (Comparative Studies of Health Systems and Medical Care). Berkeley, CA: University of California; 2010.
3. Maciocia G. *The Foundations of Chinese Medicine, A Comprehensive Text.* Edinburgh, UK: Elsevier Health Sciences; 2015.
4. https://www.aaaomonline.org/news/248468/National-Health-Statistics-Report-Estimated-over-3-million-people-receive-acupuncture-a-year.-.htm
5. Wilcox L. *Moxibustion: A Modern Clinical Handbook.* Boulder, CO: Blue Poppy Press; 2009.
6. Leggett D, Trenshaw K. *Helping Ourselves, A Guide to Traditional Chinese Food Energetics.* Totnes, UK: Meridian Press; 1995.
7. Flaws B. *The Tao of Healthy Eating, Dietary Wisdom According to Traditional Chinese Medicine.* Boulder, CO: Blue Poppy Enterprises, Inc.; 1998.
8. http://www.westonaprice.org/health-topics/broth-is-beautiful/
9. http://www.tui-na.com/tuina.html "Orthodox Tui-Na Treatment." The World Tui-Na Association. Retrieved July 24, 2012.
10. Chen JK, Chen TT, Crampton L. *Chinese Medical Herbology and Pharmacology.* City of Industry, CA: AOM Press; 2004.
11. Annals of Traditional Chinese Medicine: Volume 2 Current Review of Chinese Medicine, Quality Control of Herbs and Herbal Material, Edited by: Ping-Chung Leung, Harry Fong, and Charlie Changli Xue, Singapore, World Scientific Publishing Company, 2006.
12. Yan D. *Aging and Blood Stasis: A New Approach to Geriatrics*, 1st Edition. Boulder, CO: Blue Poppy Press; 1999.
13. Zhang H. *The Cases of Chinese Special Medicine* (Vol. 1). Beijing, China: People's China Publishing House; 1997.
14. Sperber G. *Integrated Pharmacology, Combining Modern Pharmacology with Chinese Medicine.* Boulder, CO: Blue Poppy Enterprises, Inc.; 2007.
15. Acupuncture. NIH Consensus Statement Online 1997 Nov 3-5; 15(5):1–34.
16. Wang Y, Yin LM, Xu YD, Lui YY, Ran J, Yang YQ. The research of acupuncture effective biomolecules: retrospect and prospect. *Evid Based Complement Alternat Med.* 2013;20:608026.
17. Huang W, Pach D, Napadow V, et al. Characterizing acupuncture stimuli using brain imaging with FMRI—a systematic review and meta-analysis of the literature. *PLoS One.* 2012;7(4):e32960.
18. Chae Y, Chang DS, Lee SH, et al. Inserting needles into the body: A meta-analysis of brain activity associated with acupuncture needle stimulation. *J Pain.* 2013;14(3):215–222.

19. Shiue HS, Lee YS, Tsai CN, Hsueh YM, Sheu JR, Chang HH. Gene expression profile of patients with phadiatop-positive and -negative allergic rhinitis treated with acupuncture. *J Altern Complement Med.* 2010;16(1):59–68.

20. Zhang A, Sun H, Yan G, Cheng W, Wang X. Systems biology approach opens door to essence of acupuncture. *Complement Ther Med.* 2013;21(3):253–259.

21. Ding X, Yu J, Yu T, Fu Y, Han J. Acupuncture regulates the aging-related changes in gene profile expression of the hippocampus in senescence-accelerated mouse (SAMP10). *Neurosci Lett.* 2006;399(1-2):11–16.

22. Langevin HM, Yandow JA. Relationship of acupuncture points and meridians to connective tissue planes. *Anat Rec.* 2002;269(6):257–265.

23. Yang JW, Li QQ, Li F, Fu QN, Zeng XH, Liu CZ. The holistic effects of acupuncture treatment. *Evid Based Complement Alternat Med.* 2014;2014:739708.

24. Baeumler PI, Fleckenstein J, Takayama S, Simang M, Seki T, Irnich D. Effects of acupuncture on sensory perception: A systematic review and meta-analysis. *PLoS One.* 2014;9(12):e113731.

25. Lundeberg T, Lund I, Sing A, Näslund J. Is placebo acupuncture what it is intended to be? *Evid Based Complement Alternat Med.* 2011;2011:932407.

26. Vase L, Baram S, Takakura N, et al. Specifying the nonspecific components of acupuncture analgesia. *Pain.* 2013;154(9):1659–1667.

27. Macpherson H, Vertosick E, Lewith G, et al. Influence of control group on effect size in trials of acupuncture for chronic pain: A secondary analysis of an individual patient data meta-analysis. *PLoS One.* 2014;9(4):e93739.

28. Vickers AJ, Cronin AM, Maschino AC, et al. Acupuncture for chronic pain: Individual patient data meta-analysis. *Arch Intern Med.* 2012;172(19):1444–1453.

29. Shergis JL, Ni X, Jackson ML, et al. A systematic review of acupuncture for sleep quality in people with insomnia. *Complement Ther Med.* 2016;26:11–20.

30. Chan YY, Lo WY, Yang SN, Chen YH, Lin JG. The benefit of combined acupuncture and antidepressant medication for depression: A systematic review and meta-analysis. *J Affect Disord.* 2015;176:106–117.

31. Yin fan A, Zhou K, Gu S, Ming li Y. Acupuncture is effective for chronic knee pain: A reanalysis of the Australian Acupuncture Trial. *Altern Ther Health Med.* 2016;22(3):32–36.

32. Chen FP, Chang CM, Shiu JH, et al. A clinical study of integrating acupuncture and Western medicine in treating patients with Parkinson's disease. *Am J Chin Med.* 2015;43(3):407–423.

33. Zhou J, Peng W, Xu M, Li W, Liu Z. The effectiveness and safety of acupuncture for patients with Alzheimer disease: a systematic review and meta-analysis of randomized controlled trials. *Medicine (Baltimore).* 2015;94(22):e933.

34. Linde K, Allais G, Brinkhaus B, Manheimer E, Vickers A, White AR. Acupuncture for tension-type headache. *Cochrane Database Syst Rev.* 2009;(1):CD007587.

35. Vincent C. The safety of acupuncture. *BMJ.* 2001;323(7311):467–468.

36. Xu S, Wang L, Cooper E, et al. Adverse events of acupuncture: A systematic review of case reports. *Evid Based Complement Alternat Med.* 2013;2013:581203.

37. Chen LP, Wang FW, Zuo F, Jia JJ, Jiao WG. Clinical research on comprehensive treatment of senile vascular dementia. *J Tradit Chin Med.* 2011;31(3):178–181.
38. Xu-feng W, Min D. An updated meta-analysis of the efficacy and safety of acupuncture treatment for vascular cognitive impairment without dementia. *Curr Neurovasc Res.* 2016;13(3):230–238.
39. Zhou J, Peng W, Xu M, Li W, Liu Z. The effectiveness and safety of acupuncture for patients with Alzheimer disease: a systematic review and meta-analysis of randomized controlled trials. *Medicine (Baltimore).* 2015;94(22):e933.
40. Tadros G, Ormerod S, Dobson-Smyth P, et al. The management of behavioural and psychological symptoms of dementia in residential homes: does Tai Chi have any role for people with dementia? *Dementia (London).* 2013;12(2):268–279.
41. Zuppa C, Prado CH, Wieck A, Zaparte A, Barbosa A, Bauer ME. Acupuncture for sleep quality, BDNF levels and immunosenescence: a randomized controlled study. *Neurosci Lett.* 2015;587:35–40.
42. Shergis JL, Ni X, Jackson ML, et al. A systematic review of acupuncture for sleep quality in people with insomnia. *Complement Ther Med.* 2016;26:11–20.
43. Wu J, Yeung AS, Schnyer R, Wang Y, Mischoulon D. Acupuncture for depression: a review of clinical applications. *Can J Psychiatry.* 2012;57(7):397–405.
44. Zhang ZJ, Chen HY, Yip KC, Ng R, Wong VT. The effectiveness and safety of acupuncture therapy in depressive disorders: systematic review and meta-analysis. *J Affect Disord.* 2010;124(1-2):9–21.
45. Simoncini M, Gatti A, Quirico PE, et al. Acupressure in insomnia and other sleep disorders in elderly institutionalized patients suffering from Alzheimer's disease. *Aging Clin Exp Res.* 2015;27(1):37–42.
46. Couilliot MF, Darees V, Delahaye G, et al. Acceptability of an acupuncture intervention for geriatric chronic pain: An open pilot study. *J Integr Med.* 2013;11(1):26–31.
47. Dong X, Bergren SM, Chang ES. Traditional Chinese Medicine use and health in community-dwelling Chinese-American older adults in Chicago. *J Am Geriatr Soc.* 2015;63(12):2588–2595.
48. Dello Buono M, Urciuoli O, Marietta P, Padoani W, De Leo D. Alternative medicine in a sample of 655 community-dwelling elderly. *J Psychosom Res.* 2001;50(3):147–154.
49. Flaws B. *Statements of Fact in Traditional Chinese Medicine*, 1st Edition. Boulder, CO: Blue Poppy Press; 1994.
50. Pergolizzi J, Böger RH, Budd K, et al. Opioids and the management of chronic severe pain in the elderly: consensus statement of an International Expert Panel with focus on the six clinically most often used World Health Organization Step III opioids (buprenorphine, fentanyl, hydromorphone, methadone, morphine, oxycodone). *Pain Pract.* 2008;8(4):287–313.
51. Lazzaroni M, Bianchi porro G. Gastrointestinal side-effects of traditional non-steroidal anti-inflammatory drugs and new formulations. *Aliment Pharmacol Ther.* 2004;20(Suppl 2):48–58.

52. Lao L, Ning Z. Integrating traditional Chinese medicine into mainstream health-care system in Hong Kong, China-A model of integrative medicine in the HKU-SZ Hospital. *J Integr Med*. 2015;13(6):353–355.

53. Singer J, Adams J. Integrating complementary and alternative medicine into main-stream healthcare services: the perspectives of health service managers. *BMC Complement Altern Med*. 2014;14:167.

54. http://www.acaom.org/

6

Manual and Movement Therapies

ILANA SEIDEL

The Alexander Technique and the Feldenkrais Method

Anne McDonald

CASE STUDY

Dick, a 78-year-old, 6-foot-4 semiretired scientist and businessman came to me for help with low back pain, body awareness, and balance due to a recent fall. Dick was also aware of his worsening "stooping" posture. "I walk into a room and feel self-conscious of my height," he said. "After my presentations, I'm tense, sore, and exhausted. I would like to enter a room full of strangers and feel confident and relaxed."

Employing Alexander and Feldenkrais techniques of movement and attention, I had him enter my office three times: first, exaggerating his stoop, as well as any other body movements or thoughts accompanying that posture; second, entering in a different way of his choosing while noticing any physical and psychological effects; and third, with a pause before opening the door to give himself the first direction used in the Alexander Technique: *Release the neck to allow the head to move forward and up.* When asked what he then noticed, he replied that he moved more slowly, he exhaled as he opened the door, and, surprised, he said, "I looked around and noticed paintings and plants I hadn't seen before. I felt lighter. I was actually proud about being tall!"

For 6 months Dick continued with biweekly lessons of gentle hands-on and verbal guidance on a massage table and simple activities such as transferring from sitting to standing, walking, and reaching. Since learning these techniques, he reported that he had not fallen, his presentations were less stressful, and his low back pain was significantly reduced.[1]

INTRODUCTION

Falls are the leading cause of fatal and non-fatal injuries for older Americans, threatening safety, quality of life, and independence. The Alexander Technique (AT) and Feldenkrais Method (FM) teach seniors how to move safely and avoid potential falls as well as address other health issues of aging, including musculoskeletal pain, stress-related muscular tension, and neurological movement disorders.[2,3] The evidence for the effectiveness of AT and FM is growing, especially in the areas of balance, functional mobility, and quality of life in adults with Parkinson's disease, multiple sclerosis, dementia, and post-stroke, along with evidence for effective pain management in chronic back, neck, and shoulder pain.

The AT and FM are educational practices that use movement and attention to improve sensorimotor processing. By improving the ability to process information from internal and external environments, these practices enhance perception, increasing our accuracy of knowing where we are in space and how we are moving and thinking. With more reliable processing "students," as clients are called, learn to identify and inhibit habitual tension patterns that can induce pain and limit effective movement. Using unique and gentle hands-on and verbal techniques, AT and FM practitioners help their students improve sensory awareness; identify and inhibit postural and movement tension patterns; and develop better moving capabilities.

Frederick Mathias Alexander (1869–1955) and Moshe Feldenkrais (1904–1984), originators of the AT and FM, respectively, developed their work by healing their own injuries after careful self-observation of physical and cognitive patterns. Alexander, an Australian Shakespearian actor and equestrian, cured his severe laryngitis during his stage performances. Feldenkrais, an Israeli physicist and martial artist, changed his way of walking to cure debilitating knee pain. Through their experiential processes both men improved their sensory processing and developed a more accurate and reliable sensorimotor feedback system. They were able to be engaged in an activity and, at the same time, they could be aware of where their bodies were in space and how they were moving, feeling, and thinking.

APPLICATIONS

Getting up from a chair, walking down the aisle in a movie theater, and reaching for something are daily activities that pose challenges for many older adults. These daily challenges are often associated with poor balance and fear of falling, which creates increased muscular tension, stress, and pain. After prolonged use, the extra muscular tension used to guard against a potential fall and the fearful way of thinking become habitual movement and thought patterns, contributing to deficits in proprioceptive acuity and attention-to-task. As a result, declines in sensorimotor performance occur, causing the senior to limit or even eliminate favorite activities from his or her life. This in turn creates weakness, isolation, and most importantly, a loss in confidence. The AT and FM address these issues using the key components of pausing, learning a new skill, and choice.

Pausing

The crucial moment for both methods is the moment right before the action begins. The AT and FM teach students to pause, or inhibit, the impulse to do what they are intending to do and recognize a subtle preparation or pre-set that occurs, such as a preparatory muscular tightening; a compression of the spine; fixing a joint; or holding the breath. The ability to stop and prevent this habitual pre-set enables the student to "not do" the old way of reacting and learn a new skill: the skill of moving with awareness, conscious control, and confidence.[4]

Learning a New Skill

Learning how to perform daily activities with less muscular effort, in a more balanced, coordinated manner, is a challenging new skill to acquire. Research shows that challenging activity strengthens neuronal connections and that sustained engagement in novel, cognitively demanding activity enhances motivation, confidence, and memory function in older adults.[5] Learning new ways to perform daily activities initially requires students to become aware of how they are moving versus how they *perceive* they are moving. For example, we may feel like we are standing upright, but in reality, we are bent forward. Employing the methods of AT and FM, students improve their kinesthetic and proprioceptive awareness and thereby acquire practical tools needed to identify inappropriate habitual patterns and change the manner in which they use their mental and physical capabilities.

Choice

Relearning basic movements gives seniors a choice to respond differently in a given situation. For example, before stepping off a curb, older adults can react in their old habitual manner of use or they can pause and choose a safer, more balanced and efficient way of acting. Empowering seniors with options, or conscious choices, provides the possibility of change; more importantly, having choice generates a sense of freedom and control, on which health and well-being are dependent. Learning and applying the AT and FM allows seniors to create more choices, giving them the tools to take charge of their own health.

TRAINING

Certified AT teachers complete a 1,600-hour teacher training program over a minimum of 3 years with a student/teacher ratio no greater than five to one. Training courses must meet the requirements set by the American Society for the Alexander Technique (AmSAT). Certified FM practitioners graduate from an accredited Feldenkrais Professional Training Program established by the Feldenkrais Guild of North America (FGNA), a professional organization of Feldenkrais practitioners in the United States. Training includes 800 hours over 4 years. Both AmSAT and FGNA require continuing education and establish and maintain Standards of Practice and a Code of Professional Conduct. To locate certified practitioners and access research and resources, visit www.AmSATonline.org and www.feldenkrais.com. The AT and FM are offered in several settings, including wellness and chronic pain clinics; athletic facilities; martial arts, yoga, and dance studios; university performing arts departments; and private practices. Select health insurance companies will reimburse for the AT and FM if provided by a licensed occupational or physical therapist.

RESOURCES

Recommended books include *Awareness Through Movement: Easy-To-Do Health Exercises to Improve Your Posture, Vision, Imagination, and Personal Awareness* by Feldenkrias (HarperOne; 2009) and *The Use of the Self: Its Conscious Direction in Relation to Diagnosis, Functioning and the Control of Reaction* by Alexander (Methuen & Co., 1932).

Chiropractic Care

Eric J. Roseen

CASE STUDY

John, a 70-year-old professor, presented with severe non-radiating low back pain and associated neck stiffness after a fall 5 weeks previously. His primary care physician prescribed anti-inflammatory medication and recommended physical therapy. However, John reported only marginal pain relief with this regimen and continued having difficulty getting out of bed, getting dressed, and performing most other activities of daily living. Per diagnosis of lumbosacral strain, John received chiropractic care twice weekly for 3 weeks and then once weekly for an additional 2 weeks. Treatment included gentle joint mobilization and soft tissue treatment of the spine and hips; his chiropractor also taught him exercises to do at home to improve his core strength and balance. While progress was initially slow, by the eighth visit his pain resolved, and he returned to all normal activities.

INTRODUCTION

Doctors of Chiropractic (DCs) are experts in the management of musculoskeletal health, with an emphasis on spinal conditions. Chiropractic care begins with a thorough evaluation and diagnosis of a patient's health concerns. While chiropractic care is often associated with spinal manipulative therapy, DCs provide a wide variety of in-office manual and exercise-based therapies. The majority of Americans experiencing a new episode of back or neck pain consult either a chiropractor (40%) or a primary care physician (34%) first.[1] However, DCs also care for other musculoskeletal complaints, such as hip or shoulder pain; help patients begin new exercise programs; and promote general well-being. Chiropractors also promote healthy behaviors though educating patients on various topics such as stretching, general exercise, ergonomics, and a healthy diet.

Best practice guidelines have been described for chiropractic care in older adults.[2] Chiropractors are well equipped to care for older adults through managing acute and chronic pain syndromes, improving physical function, and limiting disability. They also play an important role in screening for fall risk and preventing falls through improving back and lower extremity function. DCs offer multiple nonpharmacological approaches (e.g., joint manipulation, soft tissue techniques, exercise therapy), which may be important in preventing and reducing polypharmacy. An overview of geriatric practice-specific issues can be found in Bougie's section in Haldeman's *Principles of Chiropractic Practice of Chiropractic* (McGraw-Hill, 2005).

MANIPULATION, MOBILIZATION, AND OTHER MANUAL THERAPIES

A joint clinical guideline from the American College of Physicians and the American Pain Society recommends spinal manipulation for adults with acute or chronic low back pain. Manipulation or mobilization is also helpful for treating neck pain, migraines, cervicogenic headaches, cervicogenic dizziness, and some extremity joint conditions, such as osteoarthritis.[3] Manipulative therapy may involve *high-velocity low-amplitude* forces to spinal segments and supporting soft tissues. *Mobilization,* a low-velocity option of stretching spinal or extremity joints (e.g., hip and wrist), may be provided instead per patient preference or for patients with significant osteoporosis. Additional low-force techniques may be appropriate, such as *flexion-distraction mobilization* or *instrument-assisted manual treatment* (e.g., Activator Method). Soft tissue treatments such as *myofascial release* and *trigger point therapy* are commonly applied. Applying one or more manual and/or exercise therapies may collectively improve joint biomechanics and stimulate multiple peripheral and central nervous system mechanisms that address pain.

Primary care providers referring patients to chiropractic care should first screen for red flag symptoms that may indicate serious, albeit rare, conditions. For example, back pain patients should be screened for fracture, infection, cancer, or cauda equina syndrome. For those who do not exhibit these symptoms, chiropractic care may be effective. Serious adverse events to chiropractic care are very rare (1.46/10,000,000 manipulations[4]). Minor transient side effects, such as a temporary increase in pain or stiffness, are common.

TAILORING SELF-CARE STRATEGIES TO OLDER ADULTS

Older adults may have concerns about performing general exercise safely or avoid exercise due to fear of reinjury. DCs can help modify activities to a patient's comfort level and provide reassurance on how to safely start new physical activities. DCs identify functional deficits (e.g., restricted movement and weakness) and educate patients on what they can do at home to recover faster and prevent reinjury. They often recommend that patients engage in community-based exercise programs that offer additional social support, such as tai chi, yoga, or one-on-one exercise training with a personal trainer.

RESEARCH AND RESOURCES

Multiple randomized controlled trials have assessed the effectiveness of chiropractic care for older adults with back and neck pain.[2,5] The chiropractic research community has identified continued research in older adults as a high-priority area. The American Chiropractic Association provides information on patient resources, publications and research at http://www.acatoday. org. A reading list of key research publications recommended by the World Federation of Chiropractic can be found at https://www.wfc.org. For health professionals involved in the care of the older patient, Gleberzon's textbook, *Chiropractic Care of the Older Patient* (Butterworth-Heinemann, 2001), is a good resource.

TRAINING AND LICENSURE

The DC degree is a 4-year clinical doctorate. The Council of Chiropractic Education (CCE) is responsible for accrediting all DC programs in the United States. The CCE sets standards for the curriculum, faculty and staff, facilities, patient care, and research. The CCE requires DC students complete 4,667 contact hours, including 1,405 hours of clinical internship. DC students are required to take at least one geriatrics course; considerations for older adults are integrated into courses where students learn to apply treatment techniques.[6] Comprehensive information about CCE accreditation standards, policies, and bylaws can be found at http://www.cce-usa.org.

Chiropractors must pass four national board examinations administered by the National Board of Chiropractic Examiners, after which they may apply for licensure in all 50 states. As portal of entry providers, patients typically do not need a referral to see a DC and almost all major insurance companies have plans that cover chiropractic care, including Medicare and Medicaid.

Therapeutic Massage

Mary Starich

CASE STUDY

Betty sought massage therapy at the age of 78, at first hoping to reduce edema in her left leg. Her venous insufficiency and the condition of the soft tissue in her leg contraindicated effleurage and moderate-depth massage therapy, but she was a candidate for a broad-handed, lighter touch. Her edema could not be resolved with massage therapy, but Betty received nurturing, companionship, and relaxation from her weekly 30- to 45-minute touch sessions. Following sessions, she would often say, "I feel so relaxed and I think I'm standing up straighter when I use my walker now."

INTRODUCTION

Consumer survey statistics compiled by the American Massage Therapy Association identify 52% of the American adults who received a massage between July 2014 and July 2015 sought therapeutic bodywork for medical or health-related reasons, including pain management, muscle stiffness, rehabilitation, or general health.[1] A broad use survey of alternative therapies used by American outpatients at geriatric clinics in St. Louis, Missouri, revealed that 35.7% of elderly clinic patients who used alternative therapies chose massage therapy to help them manage problems associated with their back, hips, joints, or arthritic changes.[2] Among those using massage, 85.8% of respondents perceived that their bodywork treatments helped their specific problem.[2] A variety of randomized studies have been conducted that point to specific efficacy of moderate-pressure massage to reduce pain, improve range of motion for arthritic patients, and positively affect mood.[3] Though not restricted to the elderly, many of these studies address the effect of massage on conditions that are faced during normal aging. It is generally accepted that massage therapy promotes relaxation, reduces muscular tension, improves circulation, increases flexibility, and reduces anxiety.

CLINICAL APPLICATIONS

The joint pain and limited mobility that accompany osteoarthritis often lead to the reduction or elimination of regular physical activity among aging seniors.

For active seniors and individuals with good connective tissue health, the body of existing evidence suggests that the application of moderate-pressure massage therapy will provide more benefit than light-pressure massage for low back pain, neck pain, osteoarthritis of the joints, and rheumatoid arthritis. Field et al. have published multiple, small-sample, randomized controlled studies demonstrating the effectiveness of 15 to 30 minutes of moderate-pressure massage in treating pain and reduced range of motion associated with arthritis of the knee, hand, neck, and upper limbs.[3]

Social isolation, anxiety, and depression may also show improvement with moderate-pressure massage. Individuals experiencing depression often exhibit high cortisol, low serotonin, and low dopamine levels. Moderate-pressure massage, as compared to light-pressure work, stimulates increased vagal activity and a parasympathetic nervous system response characterized by lower heart rate and reduced anxiety.[3] Receiving regular 15- to 30-minute massage sessions lowers salivary and urinary cortisol levels in adults with varying health conditions.[3]

Agitation experienced by those suffering from Alzheimer's disease and dementia improves with massage of the head, shoulders, and hands.[4] Massage is viewed as a safer alternative to antipsychotics or physical restraint, and a massage program is relatively easy to implement in a long-term care setting if contact staff are willing to learn appropriate techniques. Rose's text, *Comfort Touch: Massage for the Elderly and Ill* (Wolters Kluwer, 2010), provides a comprehensive discussion of massage for the elderly and is written for massage therapists, nurses, and other allied health professionals.

CONTRAINDICATIONS

For active individuals with good skin elasticity, healthy muscle, and robust connective tissue, contraindications are few, though geriatric patients should be assessed on a case-by-case basis. For example, moderate-depth and Swedish massage may require limited duration (20–30 minutes) for individuals with congestive heart failure or venous insufficiency even when symptoms are well managed. Light touch and gentle holding are more appropriate for patients with late-stage congestive heart failure. A few common acute situations that contraindicate massage are skin ulcers or open sores, unidentified rashes, fever, dizziness, severe agitation, healing fractures, vigorous leg massage for bedridden individuals, and a recent history of deep vein thrombosis. For the medically fragile who demonstrate a visibly thinner epidermal layer, deep-tissue and moderate-depth work should generally be avoided. The reader is referred to more comprehensive texts discussing massage therapy and various pathologies, including Werner's *Massage Therapist's Guide to Pathology* (Wolters Kluwer, 2015).

TRAINING AND REFERRAL RESOURCES

As of 2016, 44 states and the District of Columbia either require licensure of massage therapists or provide voluntary state certification.[1] Investigation of county or local credentialing mechanisms may be required in states that do not regulate massage therapy to identify properly trained professionals. In the absence of any local government credentialing body, the National Certification Board for Therapeutic Massage & Bodywork provides a board certification process for massage therapists and offers an online therapist locator (http://www.ncbtmb.org/tools/find-a-certified-massage-therapist).

Massage therapists generally have an average of 671 hours of initial training and take an average of 20 hours of continuing education per year.[1] Graduation from a massage school that is in good standing with the Commission on Massage Therapy Accreditation (http://comta.org) also ensures a basic level of competence as agreed on by industry professionals. Specialized continuing education classes in geriatric massage are provided nationwide by Day-Break Geriatric Massage Institute (http://www.daybreak-massage.com/). Patients and family caregivers can be directed to the American Massage Therapy Association (http://amtamassage.org) massage locator tool, which typically provides detailed practice information for individual therapists, the modalities each practices, and contact information. The Associated Bodywork and Massage Professionals (ABMP; https://www.abmp.com/public) also provides a basic locator tool. Connecting with local assisted living and graduated living facilities may also provide a rich referral source of experienced geriatric massage therapists.

Osteopathic Manipulative Medicine

Maryclaire O'Neill

CASE STUDY

Mrs. L. Bridges, an active 73-year-old female, presented for osteopathic evaluation for persistent headaches that began after a fall with head injury. Imaging cleared her of fracture and intracranial hematoma, but she continued to experience daily headaches, which were exacerbated by looking down. Upon examination, her osteopathic physician noted somatic dysfunction in the head, neck, and sacral regions and subsequently applied myofascial, articulatory, and cranial techniques to release these structural restrictions. After three sessions of osteopathic manipulation Mrs. Bridges' headaches resolved.

INTRODUCTION

Osteopathic medicine, founded in 1874 by Andrew Taylor Still, MD, DO, a Civil War physician looking for an alternative to the often ineffective or harmful orthodox medical practices of his day, encompasses a distinct system of health care that takes a whole-person approach based on four tenets: (1) The body is a unit: the person is a unit of body, mind, and spirit; (2) The body is capable of self-healing, self-regulation, and health maintenance; (3) Structure and function are reciprocally interrelated; and (4) Rational treatment is based upon an understanding of the basic principles of body unity, self-regulation, and the relationship between structure and function. The "rational treatment" of Doctors of Osteopathy (DOs) may include manual techniques to apply the philosophy of these tenets.

Osteopathic Manipulative Medicine (OMM), also known as Osteopathic Manipulative Treatment (OMT), comprises numerous and varied manual techniques applied to muscles, fascia, and bones to restore the homeostatic action of arteries, veins, lymphatics, nerves, and cerebrospinal fluid, based on Still's teaching that disease is the effect of an abnormal anatomical state with subsequent physiological breakdown and decreased host adaptability. Modern studies in reflex neurophysiology readily demonstrate the effects of *somatovisceral and viscerosomatic reflexes* on host function. For example, myofascial trigger points located in the pectoralis muscle may cause a cardiac dysrhythmia via a somatovisceral reflex, while the pain referral pattern of gallbladder colic from T7-T8 visceral afferent innervation to T7-T8 somatic innervation, felt in the right subscapular region, demonstrates a viscerosomatic reflex.[1] Further, emerging research in the field of *biotensegrity* shows fascia to be an extensive connective tissue network that not only covers all organs, muscles, bones, nerves, and blood vessels but also interfaces with individual cells at the extracellular matrix (ECM). Mechanical stimulation at the ECM activates *mechanotransduction*, a process whereby applied force leads to changes in intracellular biochemistry and gene expression. Biotensegrity explains how "mechanical forces applied during OMT could lead to effects at the cellular level, providing a platform for future research on the mechanisms of action of osteopathic manipulative treatment."[2]

RESEARCH

Addressing the reciprocal relationship of structure and function, OMT can be applied to improve any health condition. While the nature of OMT is not conducive to the gold standard of randomized double-blind placebo-controlled (RDBPC) trials, several non-RDBPC studies demonstrate the relevance of OMT for the elderly patient. A 2014 study showed OMT to be "a cost-effective adjunctive treatment of pneumonia shown to reduce patients' length of hospital stay, duration of intravenous antibiotics, and incidence of respiratory failure or death when compared to subjects who received conventional care alone."[3] Another study, investigating the "benefits elderly nursing home residents may receive from preventative OMT designed to optimize structure and function and enhance their bodies' homeostatic mechanisms, found that twice monthly OMT reduced the number of hospitalizations and decreased medication usage."[4] In one of many studies showing the effectiveness of OMT for pain, patients receiving spinal OMT for low back pain were found to use less physical therapy and require significantly less pain medication than those in the standard-care cohort.[5] Research on the therapeutic effects of cranial osteopathy for various conditions that can affect geriatric patients is accessible at http://cranialacademy.org/research/bibliography/.

CRANIAL OSTEOPATHY

Osteopathy in the cranial field, discovered by William G. Sutherland, DO, a student of Still's, assesses and treats the *primary respiratory mechanism* (PRM), which is based on anatomic-physiological interactions involving the central nervous system, fluctuations of cerebrospinal fluid, the articular mobility of cranial bones, intraspinal membrane connections, and sacral mobility. The *biodynamic* approach to cranial osteopathy, developed by James Jealous, DO, approaches the PRM by addressing embryonic-development-motion-forces that continue throughout the life cycle as forces of development, growth, and healing. It bears mentioning that cranial-sacral therapy, while sharing a historical background with cranial osteopathy, is a therapeutic touch modality practiced by non-medical practitioners and, as such, has different certification, licensing, and billing requirements.

TRAINING AND RESOURCES

A DO is a doctoral degree for physicians and surgeons. DOs have equivalent rights, privileges, and responsibilities as medical doctors (MDs) and are licensed to practice the full scope of medicine in all states. Like their MD counterparts, DOs attend 4 years of medical school followed by a residency in their chosen specialty, which may be any of the allopathic specialties, or Neuromusculoskeletal Medicine (NMM) and OMM. Over the course of training all DOs receive 300 to 500 hours of instruction in osteopathic philosophy and practice, including manual techniques. This allows any licensed DO to focus his or her practice on OMM without a specific residency or board certification required. An estimated 20% of all DOs use OMM occasionally in their practice, while 2% use OMM primarily. Most insurance companies, including Medicare and Medicaid, reimburse for osteopathic manipulation under ICD-10 billing codes.

A few postgraduate programs offer training in OMM not just to DOs but also to MD, dental, and physical therapy candidates, including Michigan State University College of Osteopathic Medicine, the University of New England College of Osteopathic Medicine, the Osteopathic Cranial Academy, and the Sutherland Cranial Teaching Foundation. As part of a 2014 agreement for single graduate medical education accreditation, future MDs may receive osteopathic training within residency if participating in a program with osteopathic recognition. This new system, with a June 30, 2020, transition completion date, will replace the current dual-accreditation processes now offered through the American Osteopathic Association (AOA) and the Accreditation Council for Graduate Medical Education.

To locate DOs registered with the AOA, visit http://doctorsthatdo.org. Recommended books for further reading include Kuchera's *Osteopathic Considerations in Systemic Dysfunction* (Greydon Press, 1994) and *Foundations of Osteopathic Medicine* (Wolters Kluwer, 2011).

Rolfing® Structural Integration

Mary Starich

CASE STUDY

Richard first sought Rolfing® Structural Integration (Rolfing® SI) at the age of 62, hoping to reduce pain in his body from numerous sports injuries and to address tingling and numbness in his left leg that led him to use a cane more frequently during activities of daily living. He reported a serious ski injury 15 years earlier that required orthopedic reconstruction of his left acetabulum and eventual total hip arthroplasty. He received a Rolfing® SI 10-series over 20 weeks, during which his left-sided sciatica dissipated. Upon completion of his sessions, Richard no longer carried a cane, as he experienced better balance and stability in walking and standing. He explained, "The pain that was once unbearable from the rebuilding of my left hip is now tolerable because of Rolfing®. It changed my body and I am moving and sleeping comfortably again."

INTRODUCTION

Developed by Ida Pauline Rolf (1896–1979), Rolfing® SI is a system of bodywork and sensorimotor re-education focused on optimizing the body's overall biomechanical efficiency in lieu of addressing localized pain. As the body experiences improved alignment and freer movement, however, many chronic musculoskeletal conditions are attenuated or alleviated. Rolf's text, *Rolfing: Reestablishing the Natural Alignment and Structural Integration of the Human Body for Vitality and Well-Being* (Healing Arts Press, 1989) asserts that individuals develop habitual structural patterns over their lifetime to adapt to the stress of functioning in gravity.[1] The efficiency or inefficiency of adaptive movement and postural patterns significantly contributes to one's overall health and quality of life. Rolf presented specific visual ideals, which included alignment of the major body units (head, thorax, pelvis, knees, and feet) along a vertical "gravity line," and served as indicators of a well-integrated human structure.[1–3] The manipulation techniques developed by Rolf address restrictions in the myofascia and other connective tissues to assist the individual through gradual, often profound, changes toward optimal alignment and function.

For individuals new to Rolfing® SI, a series of 10 treatments is typically suggested, each session focusing on improving biomechanical efficiency in a particular part of the body. In addition to session goals, each session addresses soft tissues around the spine and neck to promote adaptability for vertebrae to realign in response to changes in other regions.[2] The Rolfer™ typically applies sustained moderate or deep direct pressure to selected soft tissues in order to release fascial restrictions. Rolfing® SI is unique in viewing and balancing segmental relationships in the body as they relate to functioning in gravity. Additional discussion of fascial release and structural balance is provided in a recent text by Earls and Meyers, *Fascial Release for Structural Balance* (North Atlantic Books, 2010).

Although there are no clinical studies in the literature focusing on the effects of SI specifically on health conditions of the elderly, a handful of clinical studies have appeared in the literature since 1981, the majority of them completed since 2000.[2] The most recent and most relevant to geriatrics are a Harvard randomized pilot trial (N = 46) examining SI as an adjunct therapy to outpatient rehabilitation for chronic, nonspecific low back pain and a randomized pilot study following the effects of Rolfing® SI and acupuncture at the University of São Paulo School of Medicine.[4,5] When paired with outpatient rehabilitation, Rolfing® SI resulted in statistically significant improvement in disability in the short term compared to outpatient rehabilitation alone.[5] In treating fibromyalgia, Rolfing® SI and Rolfing® SI paired with acupuncture demonstrated significant reductions in pretreatment levels of pain intensity, anxiety, and depression and improved quality of life immediately following treatment and at a 3-month follow-up.[5]

As a supportive modality to geriatric medicine, Rolfing® SI may have a more lasting impact than massage therapy on a variety of musculoskeletal pain conditions, such as back pain, neck pain, osteoarthritis of the spine and appendicular joints, frozen shoulder, fibromyalgia, later stages of postsurgical recovery (knee, hip, spine, and abdominal surgeries), and trauma due to falls. Rolfing® SI is not recommended for severe pathologies or acute injury—for example, disk herniation, spinal stenosis, significant labral or meniscal tears, and abdominal hernias. In the case of advancing stenosis or spine pathology that will eventually require surgery, Rolfing® SI might offer a nonpharmacological pain management tool, but the optimization of biomechanical efficiency is difficult to achieve when acute conditions exist. In these situations, medical massage therapy is likely to be equally effective.

Contraindications are similar to those for massage therapy. Individuals with a fragile epidermal layer or nearing end of life will not likely enjoy or benefit from Rolfing® SI and may be better served by cranial osteopathy or Cranial Sacral® techniques.

Finally, it is also important to recognize that SI does not purport to completely solve serious maladaptation or restore completely normal function after surgery or accident. Instead, the methodology seeks to bring the human structure to the highest level of integrated function possible, given the existing circumstances (e.g., Richard's case study).

Patients and their families can find contact information for local Rolfers™ using the practitioner locator tool on the Rolf Institute® website (www.rolf.org). Certified Rolfers™ with no prior bodywork training complete a minimum of 600 hours of basic instruction and supervised clinical training. Advanced Certified Rolfers™ take an additional 192 hours of supervised clinical training, which emphasizes work with individuals who have already received a 10-series. Many practitioners will have additional certification in Rolf Movement® Integration. Initially structural integration was only provided by therapists trained at the Rolf Institute®. Since the 1990s, however, other comparable training programs have emerged, including the Guild for Structural Integration (http://www.rolfguild.org) and Kinesis Myofascial Integration (http://www.anatomytrains.com/kmi). The International Association of Structural Integrators® (http://www.theiasi.net) also maintains a searchable directory of affiliated structural integrators.

Tai Chi

Aaron A. Davis

CASE STUDY

Mr. Begaye is a 67-year-old Navajo man who lives alone. He has worked for years as a rancher, sustaining countless orthopedic injuries in work and from other events in his life, and now suffers from osteoarthritis and chronic pain. For years he has been dependent on pain medications to carry out his work and activities of daily living. A relative suggested tai chi after reading an article in a popular magazine, and Mr. Begaye began performing 10 minutes of tai chi movements roughly once a day. After several months he reports to his family doctor that he now has increased mobility and requires far less pain medication than he did a year ago. He also finds it has been a useful practice for reducing anxiety and the thoughts of helplessness he has related to the recent loss of loved ones and the poor health of his aged mother.

INTRODUCTION

T'ai Chi Ch'uan (taijiquan), more commonly known in the West as tai chi, was developed as a martial art at least 700 years ago. The true origins of tai chi are unclear, but in the most popular version of its creation it is believed that the creator, Zhang Sanfeng, a Taoist monk and practitioner of Shaolin Kung fu, observed a crane fighting a snake. He became mesmerized by the subtle movements each animal used to evade and to attack. This experience led him to translate his knowledge of Shaolin Kung fu and Taoism into a martial art with a soft, internal focus, and from this tai chi is thought to have developed. Zhang Sanfeng is said to have characterized tai chi as follows: "In every movement every part of the body must be light, a gel, and connected in a sequence, the postures continuous, the movement rooted in the feet, released through the legs, focused in the waist and expressed in the fingers."

Whatever the true origins of tai chi, over the past several hundred years many styles have evolved, including the traditional Chen, Yang, Wu, and Sun styles, as well as contemporary styles that combine elements of the new and the traditional. While tai chi is still practiced as a martial art, in the early 20th century a focus was placed on promoting the health benefits of the practice, and this emphasis ultimately found global appeal and widespread acceptance in the West.

Typical tai chi classes and programs involve a series of slow, gentle, continuous movements performed with an emphasis on deep mindfulness and focused breathing. The participants often are not required to wear special uniforms, as in other martial arts, and instead wear loose comfortable clothing. It is considered safe for people in varying states of health, but as with all other exercise, participants are advised to speak with their physicians before beginning. While it is recommended that beginners attend classes to learn, there are DVD and online videos for those who may be housebound or intimidated by groups or a classroom setting. Because of the physical nature of tai chi, videos are recommended over books for those wishing to learn the concepts and movements, and classes are ultimately the preferred option.

RESEARCH

The health benefits of tai chi have been studied extensively, with a large body of research, including large-scale meta-analyses and randomized trials, with evidence supportive of the health claims promoted by tai chi practitioners. Research has been particularly focused on those health benefits afforded to the elderly and conditions affecting the elderly, as the slow, gentle movements of many tai chi classes are highly accessible to those with physical immobility, even those limited to a wheelchair. In the group setting, tai chi can provide a social environment, especially for those living alone. The robust body of literature allows providers to confidently prescribe tai chi as an effective intervention.

Fall Reduction and Physical Function

According to the Centers for Disease Control and Prevention, the cost of falls in the United States is estimated to be $34 billion in direct medical costs. A

2009 Cochrane Review found that tai chi, including home-based programs, was useful to prevent falls in the elderly.[1] A randomized controlled trial published in the *New England Journal of Medicine* found that tai chi was useful in preventing falls in patients with Parkinson's disease.[2] Relatedly, patients with osteoarthritis had a 30% improvement in balance, pain relief, and overall function after a prescribed tai chi program,[3] while another randomized controlled trial demonstrated that patients with knee arthritis who participated in 60 minutes of tai chi had significant reduction in pain and improvement of physical function.[4]

Cognition, Sleep, and Psychological Health

Studies demonstrate that tai chi could be useful to preserve or enhance cognitive function in older patients, especially executive functioning.[5] Tai chi has been shown to decrease cellular inflammation and gene encoding of pro-inflammatory markers responsible for senile insomnia. Researchers at UCLA took a large group of seniors with depression, refractory to treatment with medication, and prescribed 2 hours of tai chi weekly. Findings showed that in 10 weeks their depression symptoms were markedly improved compared with those who did not participate in tai chi.[6] Meta-analysis demonstrates that tai chi is effective in improving symptoms of mental health issues, including depression and anxiety.[7,8]

Rehabilitation

Tai chi has also demonstrated efficacy as a rehabilitation strategy for patients with catastrophic illness such as myocardial infarction, with measurable physiological gains after 12 weeks of a prescribed program.[9]

TRAINING AND RESOURCES

Unlike in China, tai chi is not strictly regulated in the United States. Just as there are many styles, systems, and even brands of tai chi actively taught, there are as many schools of training for those who wish to become instructors. The Taoist Tai Chi Society of the USA promotes the benefits of tai chi and offers resources for finding classes. It is a member of the International Taoist Tai Chi Society and offers pathways to those interested in becoming tai chi instructors. More information on these resources can be found at www.taoist.org.

Tai Chi For Health is a comprehensive program founded by family physician and tai chi expert Dr. Paul Lam and is endorsed by both the Arthritis Foundation and the Centers for Disease Control and Prevention, as well as many international agencies. This program offers classes, workshops, and videos for home practice. A formal training program is offered for those interested in teaching the certified programs offered by Tai Chi For Health. Additionally, Dr. Lam has written the book *Teaching Tai Chi Effectively: Simple and Proven Methods to Make Tai Chi Accessible to Everyone* (2006). More information can found at taichiforhealthinstitute.org.

For a concise reference regarding the overall health benefits of tai chi, readers may consult Wayne's *The Harvard Medical School Guide to Tai Chi* (Harvard Health Publications, 2012).

Yoga and Yoga Therapy

Yael Flusberg

CASE STUDY

Lidia Velazquez, an active single 66-year-old female with a love for the arts, is close to her three sisters, but all live abroad. Lidia was nervous that retirement from a 30-year international career would leave her without social support and open to depression, which she had struggled with when she had breast cancer 7 years earlier. She decided to try out two yoga classes: one for cancer survivors offered weekly at the hospital, and a laughter yoga group that met monthly at her local library. A year later she reports having learned much about herself: "I feel more whole now that I am listening to my body. Who would have thought that the effects of one hour a week would be so tangible?"

INTRODUCTION

With its emphasis on mindfulness, health promotion, and well-being, yoga can be a potent low-cost tool for physical and psychological wellness in the older patient. It is particularly useful in chronic conditions; during times of stress, transition, or trauma; and as a complement to conventional therapies. Yoga can help older patients access their own resources for reducing stress, improving self-efficacy and independence, and building resiliency. According to the "2016 Yoga in America Study" conducted by Yoga Journal and Yoga Alliance, the number of yoga practitioners in the United States grew by 20% a year over the last 4 years, almost doubling to 36 million. Most people, including seniors, come to yoga because they want to feel better and take greater charge of their health. Twenty-one percent of all practitioners are now over the age of 60. Yoga practitioners see themselves as stronger (75% vs. 57% of non-practitioners), enjoying better balance (80% vs. 64%), and having greater mental clarity (86% vs. 77%). Multiple studies have shown the beneficial impact of yoga for the older adult, including positive effects on osteopenia, osteopenia, osteoarthritis, and related issues; mobility, strength, and stability; chronic pain; cognitive wellness; attitudes about aging; loss and grief; maintaining independence in daily living; engaging in self-care; and cultivating social connections.

YOGA PRINCIPLES

Yoga is a system of philosophies, principles, and practices derived from the Vedic tradition of the Himalayas more than 2,500 years ago. It is founded on the principle that intelligent practice and self-inquiry can influence physical, psychological, and social well-being. Practitioners cultivate a sense of wholeness and harmony using a range of practices designed to increase awareness and generate a clear and calm mind. These practices include postures and movement, breath awareness and breathing exercises, meditation, and relaxation.

Physical postures consist of stretches, poses, and dynamic movement that are coordinated with the breath and increase flexibility, strength, balance, and focus. *Breath awareness and management exercises* help practitioners control the rate, depth, and direction of the breath, which affects respiratory function, the autonomic nervous system, and mood. *Meditative and relaxation* components of yoga emphasize mental alertness and calmness. These range from meditations where one follows the breath, scans bodily sensations, or listens to sounds; to guided visualizations and imagery (such as yoga nidra, which enjoys widespread popularity in the U.S. military, where it is known as iRest); to the use of chants (mantra) and hand gestures (mudras). Researchers theorize that yoga alters cognition by promoting adaptive thinking and decreasing repetitive, negative thoughts.[1,2]

YOGA VERSUS YOGA THERAPY

One consideration for the doctor "prescribing" yoga is whether to refer patients to a yoga classes facilitated by a yoga teacher, or to a yoga therapist who will offer one-on-one consultation and/or group classes in which partici-pants share a condition or seek a similar therapeutic outcome.

Yoga teachers are accredited at the 200-hour or 500-hour level by the Yoga Alliance and meet strict standards, including ethics and continuing educa-tion. A good teacher will be able to choose appropriate practices that meet the needs, interests, and abilities of students, and modify for injury and other health conditions. In addition to mainstream yoga classes, yoga teachers may offer special classes or workshops relevant to the geriatric population (e.g., chair yoga for seniors, yoga for cardiovascular health).

A yoga therapist explicitly offers yoga with a therapeutic intent, adapting yoga to specific health problems and populations. Yoga therapists are creden-tialed as yoga teachers first, and then complete at least an additional 800 hours in the philosophy, theory, process, and application of yoga therapy, including working as part of a health care team. The International Association of Yoga Therapists (www.iayt.org) is finalizing the national credentialing process in the United States, which should be in place for all yoga therapists by the end of 2016.

One of the most highly regarded therapeutic yoga programs focusing on seniors is offered to registered yoga teachers by Duke Integrative Medicine (https://www.dukeintegrativemedicine.org/programs-training/professionals/therapeutic-yoga-for-seniors/). The two co-leaders of that training, Kimberly Carson and Carol Krucoff, started http://yoga4seniors.com, which includes a way to search for teacher graduates of the "Therapeutic Yoga for Seniors" pro-grams, as well as access yoga research and other pertinent resources.

METHODS OF DELIVERY

There are many ways for seniors to do yoga, depending on their temperament, learning style, interests, and needs. Classes or private sessions are often the most helpful for the beginner or those facing a new condition or life situation, as well as for those who need or prefer ongoing instruction or social interac-tion and support. Others prefer to practice on their own, with a DVD, or to take online classes. Dr. Loren Fishman's *12 Pose Daily Regimen for Osteoporosis* (http://sciatica.org/yoga/12poses.html) is a simple place to start, as is *Structural Yoga Therapy: Adapting to the Individual* by Mukunda Stiles (first print 2000, RedWheel/Weiser), a comprehensive reference with user-friendly resources on how to start a yoga practice appropriate for differing body types and needs. For ongoing information, techniques, and summaries of latest studies, seniors may consider subscribing to *Yoga for Healthy Aging* at http://yogaforhealthy-aging.blogspot.com.

YOGA RESEARCH

The evidence for yoga's therapeutic value continues to grow and includes studies in areas of interest to older adults and their health care providers.

Osteoporosis-Related Fractures

The United States currently spends $19 billion on the more than 2 million annual fragility fractures and the 500,000 hospitalizations these entail. Hip fractures are often considered a "sentinel event," indicating a general and irreversible decline in many aspects of health. In a 10-year study using a 12-minute daily protocol of 12 yoga postures that focused on strength and balance of 741 adults who underwent DEXA scans before and after, bone quality improved in the spine, hips, and femur of the 227 moderately and fully compliant patients. Since the medications for bone loss are associated with spontaneous fracture, atrial fibrillation, slowed healing, gastric distress, osteonecrosis, scleritis, and episcleritis, and since yoga improved posture, balance, coordination, gait, range of motion, and strength, and reduced levels of anxiety and risk of falling, it appears to be a dramatically low-cost and less dangerous alternative and a safe and effective means of preventing osteoporosis-related fracture.[3]

Postural Control and Mobility

Several studies have shown improvement with therapeutic yoga, although stronger studies are needed. In an 8-week therapeutic yoga pilot program focusing on postural control, mobility, rising from the floor, and gait speed in 13 community-living older adults with a mean age of 81, improvements in postural control (as measured by the Berg Balance Scale) and gait (as measured by fast gait speed) indicated that research subjects benefited from the yoga intervention. In a similar small pilot study, 13 residents of a retirement facility took twice-weekly yoga classes for 12 weeks. Improvements in postural control and mobility and Timed Up and Go gait (as measured by fast gait speed) indicated that research participants benefited from the therapeutic yoga intervention.[4,5]

Sleep and Depression

In a 6-month study conducted in eight senior activity centers in Taiwan with 139 participants ages 60 and up, a 70-minute "silver yoga" class was given three times a week. Most of the mental health indicators of the participants in the experimental group had significantly improved after the silver yoga interventions, and many of the indicators improved after 3 months of intervention and were maintained throughout the 6-month study.[6]

Psychological Health and Cognition

In a 6-week study of 98 older adults ages 65 to 92 living in two North Florida facilities, chair yoga participants improved more than both exercise and control participants in terms of anger, anxiety, depression, well-being, and self-efficacy for daily living. Another study sought to determine the effect of yoga on cognitive function, fatigue, mood, and quality of life in healthy seniors ages 65 to 85. One hundred thirty-five either did yoga, did walking, or were waitlisted. The yoga intervention did not show improvement in cognitive function but did show improvement in physical measures, as well as a number of quality-of-life measures related to sense of well-being and energy and fatigue compared to controls.[2,7]

REFERENCES

Alexander Technique and Feldenkrais Method

1. Little P, Lewith G, Webley F, et al. Randomised controlled trial of Alexander technique lessons, exercise, and massage (ATEAM) for chronic and recurrent back pain. *BMJ*. 2008 Aug 19;337:a884. doi:10.1136/bmj.a884.
2. Stallibrass C, et al. Randomized controlled trial of the Alexander Technique for idiopathic Parkinson's disease. *Clin Rehab*. 2002;16:707–718.
3. Teixeira-Machado L, Araújo FM, Cunha FA, et al. Feldenkrais method-based exercise improves quality of life in individuals with Parkinson's disease: A controlled, randomized clinical trial. *Altern Ther Health Med* 2015 Jan-Feb;21(1):8–14.
4. Jones FP. Method for changing stereotyped response patterns by the inhibition of certain postural sets. *Psychol Rev*. 1965;72(3):196–214.
5. Park DC, Lodi-Smith J, Drew LM, et al. The impact of sustained engagement on cognitive function in older adults: The Synapse Project. *Psychol Sci*. 2014;25(1):103–112.

Chiropractic

1. Kosloff TM, Elton D, Shulman SA, Clarke JL, Skoufalos A, Solis A. Conservative spine care: opportunities to improve the quality and value of care. *Popul Health Manag*. 2013;16(6):390–396.

2. Hawk C, Schneider M, Dougherty P, Gleberzon BJ, Killinger LZ. Best practices recommendations for chiropractic care for older adults: Results of a consensus process. *J Manipulative Physiol Ther.* 2010;33(6):464–473.

3. Bronfort G, Haas M, Evans R, Leininger B, Triano J. Effectiveness of manual therapies: the UK evidence report. *Chiropr Osteopat.* 2010;18:3.

4. Gouveia LO, Castanho P, Ferreira JJ. Safety of chiropractic interventions: A systematic review. *Spine.* 2009;34(11):405–413.

5. Gleberzon BJ. A narrative review of the published chiropractic literature regarding older patients from 2001–2010. *J Can Chiropr Assoc.* 2011;55(2):76–95.

6. Killinger LZ. Chiropractic and geriatrics: A review of the training, role, and scope of chiropractic in caring for aging patients. *Clin Geriatr Med.* 2004;20(2):223–235.

Massage

1. AMTA website http://www.amtamassage.org/infocenter/economic_industry-fact-sheet.html, Updated February 2016. Accessed March 8, 2016.

2. Flaherty J, Takahashi R, Teoh J, et al. Use of alternative therapies in older outpatients in the United States and Japan: Prevalence, reporting patterns, and perceived effectiveness. *J Gerontol Med Sci.* 2001;56A(10):M650–M655.

3. Field T. Massage therapy research review. *Complement Ther Clin Pract.* 2014;20:224–229.

4. Moyle W, Murfield J, O'Dwyer S, Van Wyk S, The effect of massage on agitated behaviours in older people with dementia: a literature review. *J Clin Nurs.* 2013;22(5–6):601–610.

Osteopathic Medicine

1. Chila AG. *Foundations of Osteopathic Medicine.* Philadelphia, PA: Wolters Kluwer Health/Lippincott Williams & Wilkins; 2011.

2. Swanson RL. Biotensegrity: A unifying theory of biological architecture with applications to osteopathic practice, education, and research—A review and analysis. *J Am Osteopath Assoc.* 2013;113:34–52.

3. Yao S, Hassani J, Gagne M, George G, Gilliar W. Osteopathic manipulative treatment as a useful adjunctive tool for pneumonia. *J Vis Exp.* 2014;87:e50687. doi:10.3791/50687.

4. Snider KT, Snider Johnson JC, Hagan C, Schoenwald C. Preventative osteopathic manipulative treatment and the elderly nursing home resident: A pilot study. *J Am Osteopath Assoc.* 2012;112(8):489–501.

5. Andersson GBJ, Lucente T, Davis A, Kappler R, Lipton J, Leurgans S. A comparison of osteopathic spinal manipulation with standard care for patients with low back pain. *N Engl J Med.* 1999;341:1426–1431 doi:10.1056/NEJM199911043411903

Rolfing

1. Rolf I. *Rolfing: Reestablishing the Natural Alignment and Structural Integration of the Human Body for Vitality and Well-Being*, rev. ed. Rochester, VT: Healing Arts Press; 1989.
2. Jacobson E. Structural integration, an alternative method of manual therapy and sensorimotor education. *J Altern Complement Med.* 2011;17(10):891–899.
3. Jacobson E, Structural integration: Origins and development. *J Altern Complement Med.* 2011;17(9):775–780.
4. Jacobson E, Meleger A, Bonato P, et al. Structural integration as an adjunct to out-patient rehabilitation for chronic nonspecific low back pain: A randomized pilot clinical trial. *Evid Based Complement Alternat Med.* 2015;2015:813418.
5. Stall P, Kosomi J, Faeli C, et al. Effects of structural integration Rolfing method and acupuncture on fibromyalgia. *Rev Dor Sao Paulo.* 2015;16(2):96–101.

Tai Chi

1. Li F, et al. Tai chi and postural stability in patients with Parkinson's disease. *N Engl J Med.* 2012;366(6):511–519.
2. Gillespie LD, Robertson MC, Gillespie WJ, et al. Interventions for preventing falls in older people living in the community. *Cochrane Database of Systematic Reviews Reviews.* 2012; doi:10.1002/14651858.cd007146.pub3
3. Song R, Lee EK, Lam P, Bae S. Effects of tai chi exercise on pain, balance, muscle strength, and perceived difficulties in physical functioning in older women with osteoarthritis: A randomized clinical trial. *J Rheumatol.* 2003 Sep;30(9):2039–2044.
4. Wang C, Schmid CH, Hibberd PL, et al. Tai chi is effective in treating knee osteoarthritis: A randomized controlled trial. *Arthritis Rheumatism.* 2009;61(11):1545–1553.
5. Wayne PM, Walsh JN, Taylor-Piliae RE, et al. The impact of tai chi on cognitive performance in older adults: A systematic review and meta-analysis. *J Am Geriatr Soc.* 2014;62(1):25–39.
6. Irwin MR, Olmstead R, Breen EC. Cognitive behavioral therapy and tai chi reverse cellular and genomic markers of inflammation in late-life insomnia: A randomized controlled trial. *J Biol Psychol.* 2015 Nov 15;78(10):721–729.
7. Lavretsky H, Alstein LL, Olmstead RE, et al. Complementary use of tai chi chih augments escitalopram treatment of geriatric depression. *Am J Geriatr Psychiatry.* 2011;19(10):839–850.
8. Wang F, Lee EK, Wu T, Yeung AS. The effects of tai chi on depression, anxiety, and psychological well-being: A systematic review and meta-analysis. *Int J Behav Med.* 2014;21(4):605–617.
9. Nery RM, Zanini M, de Lima JB, et al. Tai chi chuan improves functional capacity after myocardial infarction: A randomized clinical trial. *Am Heart J.* 2015;169(6):854–860.

Yoga

1. Sharma M, Haider T, Knowlden AP. Yoga as an alternative and complementary treatment for cancer: A systematic review. *J Altern Complement Med.* 2013;19:870–875.

2. Uebelacker LA, Epstein-Lubow G, Gaudiano BA, Tremont G, Battle CL, Miller IW. Hatha yoga for depression: Critical review of the evidence for efficacy, plausible mechanisms of action, and directions for future research. *J Psychiatry Practices.* 2010 January;16(1):22–33.

3. Fishman L, et al. Twelve-minute yoga regime reverses osteoporotic bone loss. *Topics in Geriatric Rehabilitation.* 2016;32(2):81–87.

4. Kelley KK, et al. The effects of a therapeutic yoga program on postural control, mobility, and gait speed in community-dwelling older adults. *J Altern Complement Med.* 2014 Dec;20(12):949–954.

5. Oken BS, et al. Randomized, controlled, six-month trial of yoga in healthy seniors: Effects on cognition and quality of life. *Alternative Therapies Health Medicine.* 2006;12(1):40–47.

6. Chin K-M, et al. Sleep quality, depression state, and health status of older adults after silver yoga exercises: Cluster randomized trial. *Int J Nurs Studies.* 2009;46(2):154–163.

7. Bonura KB, Tenenbaum G. Effects of yoga on psychological health in older adults. *J Physical Activity Health.* 2014;11(7):1334–1341.

7

Energy Modalities and Aromatherapy

LUANN JACOBS, MARY KENDELL, AND YAEL FLUSBERG

As we continue to make medical advances that prolong life, the quality of that life lived becomes equally important. Furthermore, health care for the elderly often involves the direct, hands-on, often day-to-day assistance of family members, and they too need organized systems for relief and support in order to promote well-being in their elderly dependents. In light of these considerations, the first part of this chapter provides an overview of the role of biofield healing modalities for the treatment of the elderly. The second part covers aromatherapy.

Energy Modalities

Alice Berg, Luann Jacobs, MA-CCC/SLP, RMT,
and Yael Flusberg, E-RYT 500, RMT, MS

SUBTLE ENERGY AND BIOFIELD THERAPY

Throughout history and across the globe, different cultures have espoused the existence of subtle energies (e.g., Chinese *chi/qi*, Japanese *ki*, Indian *prana*, Western *Holy Spirit*, Hawaiian *Mana*, Hebrew *Ruarch*, New Zealand Maori *Wairua*) that permeate and animate all life.[1-3] Perceiving and manipulating disruptions in these subtle energies forms the basis of many traditional and contemporary energy healing practices.[3,4] Nevertheless, the existence of these subtle energies, or the "biofield" as it is sometimes called, continues to be a matter of debate. Though different forms of biofield healing exist involving known mechanisms of energy transfer (e.g., magnetic therapy and near-infrared light therapy), traditional and other modified biofield healing methods (e.g., Reiki, external qi gong therapy [EQT], therapeutic touch [TT], healing touch [HT], polarity therapy, acupuncture) seem to involve a putative (not directly measurable) form of energy transfer that defies the conventional laws of physics.[5]

Practitioners of biofield healing modalities use intention and their hands positioned on or above a recipient in order to harmonize and balance the recipient's subtle energy field, thereby—through an as yet undefined mechanism—facilitating the removal of blockages that contribute to pain and illness.[4] By restoring harmony and balance to the recipient's energy field, biofield therapy presumably stimulates the recipient's innate healing forces and promotes body–mind health and relaxation.[4,6] While some recipients experience observable biofield healing results immediately, other recipients experience restoration of balance progressively and over time.

Both the biofield healing practitioner and the recipient may sense subtle energy as warmth, cold, vibration, tingling, or pulsations.[7] Interestingly, the transmitted energy mediating this effect is not impeded by barriers that block conventional electromagnetic fields (e.g., Faraday Cage barrier, or lead for x-ray energy). Moreover, the transmitted energy is not subject to the inverse square law whereby the energy force dissipates as a function of the inverse square of the distance.[5] In other words, whereas one feels less heat the farther one steps away from a fire, subtle energy does not seem to lose intensity as it moves away from the initial source. This, in turn, enables practitioners to access and manipulate the biofield of recipients at a distance that may be far from close physical proximity. The magnetic resonance imaging (MRI) study in which practitioners performed intermittent distance energy healing from an electromagnetically shielded room on receivers located in an optically isolated room found significant and immediate activation of certain areas of the brain in the recipients compared to controls.[8]

Though many question the existence of the biofield, researchers have measured and visualized what may represent the human biofield through the Superconducting Quantum Interference Device (SQUID magnetometer), Kirlian photography, and gas discharge visualization, the latter of which claims utility as a diagnostic device of human disease.[9,10] Biophoton (ultra-weak light) emissions have also emerged as a measurable and intrinsic property of all life with unique signatures in the healthy, chronic disease, and meditative states.[5,11–13] Whether the interaction between practitioner and recipient biofields in proximity or at a distance involves quantum entanglement (which is beyond the scope of this chapter) or some other means remains to be determined.[5,8]

Biofeedback is an important component in understanding biofield therapies. Just as fever and a high white blood count serve as biometric feedback indicative of infection, the energy transferred through biofield therapy serves as biofeedback to the software of body–mind–spirit, helping to signal shifts in feeling states (depression), emotions (anxiety), tension abatement, and perceptions of pain,[14] and enabling the practitioner and recipient to restore homeostasis and balance to the biofield. These changes can be measured through heart-rate variability (HRV) demonstrating shifts in the autonomic nervous system (ANS).[14]

BIOFIELD HEALING AND THE ELDERLY

Whether a "believer" or "skeptic," the informed health care provider must have at least a basic appreciation of biofield modalities and what they could offer since many patients, particularly those with chronic diseases for which conventional medicine offers no "cure," seek alternative therapies, with or without the knowledge of the conventional provider.[4] In 2012 U.S. adults spent $421.6 million on biofield therapies despite poor insurance reimbursement (only 8% of reporting persons).[13,15,16] Owing to patient demand and satisfaction, hospitals, clinics, and other institutionalized settings, particularly those focusing on palliative care, are increasingly integrating bioenergy healing into their list of services.[1] Isolated studies suggests that in the geriatric population biofield therapies may mitigate pain and anxiety, improve mood and well-being, offer relaxation, speed wound healing, improve immune function, lower blood pressure, and improve functional status.[1,6,7,11,15,17–22] In conventional medical practice, current interventions for many age-associated chronic health concerns (e.g., chronic pain, arthritis, cardiovascular disease, Parkinson's disease, dementia, anxiety, depression) focus on symptom management using medications, the side effects of which may put the elderly at risk for cascade iatrogenesis.

Unlike pharmaceutical or even botanical medicine, biofield therapy is noninvasive, reported safe for most populations, and does not put the recipient at risk for complex drug interactions.[23] In addition, biofield therapy may offer psychosocial benefits to the elderly population, enhancing personal empowerment, cognitive function, and emotional wellness in order to promote resilience and well-being amidst the challenges of aging, illness, and loss of loved ones.

POPULAR BIOENERGY HEALING THERAPIES

Among the current roster of energy healing therapies, reiki, TT, HT, EQT, and aromatherapy have become increasingly accepted in integrative medical practice. Reiki, internal qi gong, and aromatherapy are practices that patients can also learn themselves, helping to empower them in their healing process while increasing their potential exposure to the modality.

For both reiki and TT, the practitioner applies gentle touch (mediated through direct physical contact or a few inches above the recipient's body through "field interactions" between the practitioner and recipient) to different parts of the recipient's body in order to alleviate disruptions in the recipient's biofield. In addition to restoring balance to the biofield, practitioner-delivered reiki and TT also benefit recipients through the therapeutic value of touch itself, the science and understanding of which have only recently begun to garner attention.[24] Research indicates that the elderly, particularly those in institutionalized settings, are especially receptive to caring presence and expressive touch, which has been shown to improve heart rhythm, lower blood pressure, reduce anxiety, reduce pain, and enhance well-being.[25]

EQT incorporates meditation, relaxation, physical movement, and breathing exercises. Unlike reiki and TT, the EQT practitioner usually does not place hands directly on the recipient.

BIOFIELD HEALING RESEARCH

Though biofield healing has been practiced for thousands of years, empirical research investigating the clinical utility and effectiveness of these modalities has not occurred until recently,[15] and biofield therapy clinical research in humans has involved mostly small pilot studies.[2,4,11,15,26]

Although preclinical studies on cells in culture, plants, and animals have their own issues of reproducibility, translation to human function, and equivalent treatment dosage, they are easier to control and have shown benefits of biofield therapy for wound healing, accelerated growth, and even cancer reduction.[14] In contrast, a Cochrane Review that investigated the effect of therapeutic touch on wound healing in humans from randomized and quasi-randomized controlled trials concluded that further research is warranted given a high risk of bias in the included studies, of which only half reported significance in accelerating healing.[27] On the other hand, a systematic review by Jain and Mills[4] that included all available controlled trials on proximal biofield therapy (without specifying randomization or distinguishing contact touch from off-body delivery) found moderate evidence that contact therapeutic touch reduces negative behaviors related to dementia, moderate to strong evidence that biofield therapies mitigate pain in different patient populations, and conflicting evidence that biofield therapies reduce anxiety and fatigue in cancer populations, among other outcomes. Another systematic review by Thrane and Cohen evaluating the effect of reiki on pain and anxiety found large effect sizes for some patient populations.[11] However, a recent Cochrane Review that likewise investigated the utility of reiki for pain and anxiety found equivocal results that were compounded by the unclear risk of bias among the three randomized controlled trials included.[2]

The following case reports provide a rich repository of anecdotal and qualitative evidence that show the potential of biofield healing to help the elderly achieve holistic wellness in body, mind, and spirit.[28,29]

CASE STUDIES

Reiki in an Urban Senior Living Facility

Janice was 85 years old and had been living for 6 months in a senior living facility when she asked her medical doctor and her reiki therapist to help her start a reiki program there. Janice's previous work history was in nursing and massage, but she felt the stillness of the reiki touch would be perfect both for the residents who were vibrant and active like herself and for those residents who were restricted physically and mentally, and possibly the staff would be open to learning reiki for their own self-care and to help the residents.

The reiki therapist and doctor devised both an initial Level One training program and an Institutional Review Board–approved assessment study for 10 residents and staff who volunteered to be participants. While reiki has been reported previously to induce a sense of calmness, to decrease anxiety, and to improve well-being in different medical settings, very few studies looked at its effect on elderly patients with multiple chronic conditions and their caregivers. The objective of this study was to assess the effect of reiki therapy on quality of life and HRV of elderly residents and staff members. The participants (eight residents and two staff members) attended a one-day reiki training and a reiki share group for 2 hours a week for 12 weeks, and were also asked to do daily self-care reiki.

Assessments showed improved HRV and a tendency toward a slower heart rate while receiving reiki. Eighty percent of the participants reported they would like to continue with the reiki share group. The single-focus group identified recurring themes of caring for the self, helping others in a new way, reiki as a spiritual practice, nonverbal way to connect with others, and improved staff job satisfaction.[30,31]

Caregiver Burnout

Deborah, age 54, became the supervising caregiver for both her parents when their decline in health necessitated moving them to an assisted living facility. Her mother developed Alzheimer's and her father terminal cancer. The struggle of working full time in a high-pressure law firm and visiting her parents after work and on weekends to supervise appropriate staff compliance and to provide company to her parents, as they were far from their home and other family and friends, had worn her down. She came to an integrative medicine clinic for relief from insomnia, fatigue, overall pain, and burnout. Deborah was diagnosed with fibromyalgia and irritable bowel syndrome (IBS). Her doctor recommended acupuncture for balancing her energy, a dietary program with a nutritionist to address her IBS, and three sessions with the reiki/biofeedback therapist to assess her response to touch and its effect on her mood and sleep.

Acupuncture sessions proved helpful for increasing her energy. The dietary program was less successful because of the amount of time needed for shopping and preparing food, but she did try to implement a few changes and found it helpful. However, acupuncture and reiki sessions became her go-to treatments. She continued acupuncture two or three times per week and reiki sessions every 2 weeks for several months. Deborah described feeling rested, peaceful, and more hopeful about her situation with her mother. She learned reiki for self-care and became an avid daily reiki user to help her sleep. As her mother became less able to communicate verbally, Deborah learned how to do reiki touch with her mother. Deborah found she looked forward to her visits as she could be with her mother without having the pressure of communicating and could see her mother visibly relax and her agitation diminish in response to the touch.

Deborah continued to use and study reiki and, after the death of both parents, she elected to offer reiki to others by participating in a hospital reiki volunteer program for 2 years once weekly. Deborah moved through all the stages of healing: from searching for a better way and learning the difference between curing and healing, to maintaining balance through daily self-care practices, and then to serving others as she regained her health.

BIOFIELD PRACTITIONER CREDENTIALING AND LICENSING

There is no single standardized approach to training or credentialing for each of the bioenergy modalities. There are school-specific training guidelines for each modality and at each level of advanced training within the modality. For example, reiki training has four levels, the most advanced being Master Teacher. At Master Teacher level the practitioner can both do treatments and teach self-care and treatment of others. Generally speaking, clients seeking an effective bioenergy practitioner should ask a few key questions:

- What is your experience history?
- Who have you trained with?
- How long have you spent in training?

- Can you tell me about your modality?
- What credentials or licenses have you achieved (e.g., a nurse who knows therapeutic touch)?

Here are some informational website recommendations for each of the biofield modalities discussed in this chapter: http://therapeutic-touch.org/, http://reikiinmedicine.org/, http://nqa.org/, http://www.healingtouchprogram.com/, https://www.heartmath.org

Aromatherapy

Mary Kendell, MS, WHNP-BCV

The use of aromatic plants as medicine has been documented throughout history and across the globe. Aromatherapy by definition is the use of essential oils for healing. Once a part of herbal medicine, modern-day aromatherapy is derived from the steam distillation of the essential oils found in the stems, leaves, flowers, seeds, roots, or bark of plants. In the case of citrus fruits, cold pressing of the fruit's rind is used to obtain the essential oil.

Essential oils are a complex mixture of many natural constituents derived from the whole plant.[1] According to Mills, the sum of the parts of plants is greater than the total.[2] If the most active constituent is synthesized from a plant, it may have a much different effect or even a negative effect compared to that of the whole plant. The complex interaction of plant constituents allows a single oil to have multiple therapeutic uses. Oregano oil, for example, has demonstrated antimicrobial as well as fungicidal activity in vitro and in vivo.[3] Oregano has also been found effective in the treatment of parasitic infections.[4] Additionally, plant constituents, when present in the whole oil, seem to act as "quenchers" of unwanted side effects, allowing the oil to be used effectively without causing harm.[5]

THERAPEUTIC USES

Some of the known therapeutic properties of essential oils include the following (Table 7.1):[1 p.76]

- Antiseptic, antibacterial, antiviral, antifungal
- Wound healing and granulation promoting

Table 7.1. Essential Oils and Their Most Common Uses

	Frankincense	Lavender	Lemon	Melaluca	Wild Orange	Oregano	Peppermint	Rosemary	Hawaiian Sandalwood
Analgesic		x							
Anti-anxiety		x			x				X
Antibacterial				x	x	x		x	
Antidepressant		x	x	x	x		x	x	X
Antifungal			x	x	x	x		x	
Antihistamine	x	x	x						
Anti-inflammatory	x	x		x	x	x	X		X
Antioxidant	x		x						X
Antiparasitic						x			
Antiseptic	x		x	x		x			
Antiviral			x	x		x			X
Cognitive	x	x	x				X	x	X
Digestive issues			x		x	x	X		X
Diuretic			x		x			x	
Energizing			x		x		X		

Fatigue						X		
Headaches	x					X	x	
Immune-enhancing	x		x		x			
Insomnia		x		x				
Muscle aches		x	x		X	X		X
Skin problems (eczema, psoriasis, insect bites, cuts, ulcers, scars, rashes)	x		x			X		X
Respiratory issues	x	x			x		x	X
Urinary tract infections						x		X

From references 6 and 14.

- Analgesic, anti-inflammatory, antitoxic, hyperemic
- Relaxing, sedative, antidepressant
- Immunostimulant, hormonal
- Insecticidal, repellant
- Mucolytic, expectorant
- Deodorant

The improvement of cognitive function is another area in which essential oils can be of therapeutic value.[6]

HOW ARE ESSENTIAL OILS USED?

Although the word "aroma" implies the inhalation of a substance, the components of essential oils can also be absorbed topically both internally and externally and through ingestion. For the geriatric population, multiple delivery options give essential oils a distinct advantage over many therapies, as the therapeutic effects of essential oils can be obtained through whatever form best meets the needs of the individual. Each delivery method has its own physiological process and will offer certain advantages and disadvantages.

Inhalation

A key determinant in behavior, smell is now recognized as one of the most important senses in humans. Whether we are aware of it or not, when we breathe we inhale aroma. Inhalation is the fastest and easiest way of getting essential oils into the body. Inhalation of essential oils results in absorption into the bloodstream via the alveoli of the lungs. The sense of smell is a chemical reaction that has an immediate effect on the brain. "*Odors can affect our brain by influencing the production of endorphins and noradrenaline*".[7] [p.21] This holds true even if a person has a decreased sense of smell. A study by Henkin and Levy[7] found that "*odors induced*" central nervous system (*CNS*) "*activation in patients with congenital hyposmia, which distinguishes olfaction from vision and audition since neither light nor acoustic stimuli induce CNS activation*". The findings of this study support the efficacy of the use of aromatherapy in the geriatric population, where a decreased sense of smell is common.[8]

Numerous studies using inhalation aromatherapy have shown positive outcomes in cognition, mood states, stress and anxiety reduction, and improved sleep.[9–14] Aromatherapy via inhalation can occur actively through the intentional use of an aroma stick, cotton balls, tissue, a piece of cloth placed at the nostrils, or the simple cupping of hands over the nose and mouth after essential oils have been applied. Other methods include the use of steam or nebulizers or the wearing of an aroma ribbon or necklace. More passive inhalation occurs when someone is in a room where oils are being diffused. Dosing via inhalation is difficult to determine, but toxicity resulting from inhaled vapor is unlikely under normal conditions.[5 P.49]

Topical Application

Topical application of essential oils is most often done in conjunction with some form of massage. However, essential oils can also be used to facilitate tissue granulation and promote wound healing. The ability of essential oils to penetrate the skin and the amount of systemic absorption that occurs depend on several factors. The use of carrier oils can decrease absorption while the use of occlusive dressings can enhance absorption. Thin or damaged skin and vasodilation, as occurs with massage, will enhance absorption. While essential oils are safe to inhale undiluted, some need to be diluted to avoid skin irritation. Caution is advised when using citrus oils topically as photosensitivity can occur. Essential oils should never be placed in the eyes or ears. If other medications are being used topically, essential oils should be applied to a different part of the body.

Dermal dosing of essential oils depends on several factors, including the quantity of the oil applied, the dilution of the oil in vehicle, the total area of skin covered, the health and integrity of the skin, the age of the recipient, the amount of occlusion after massage, and the type of essential oil used. The percentage of dilution used for massage can vary from 1% to 5%, with an average being 2% to 3%.[5 P.47]

Oral Use

Many essential oils are not safe for oral use. Tree oils such as birch, cedar wood, and cypress, for example, are just a few of the oils that should never be ingested.[14] Hot oils such as oregano, clove, and cinnamon, while safe for ingestion, are known to be irritating to mucous membranes so they should be diluted with honey or water or placed in a gelatin capsule prior to ingestion.[6 P.29]

Essential oils are very concentrated and usually prescribed as number of drops given. However, as drop size can vary, dosing is stated in milliliters. The recommended dose for oral use of essential oils is 0.05 to 1.3 ml per 24 hours.[5 P.50]

NOT ALL OILS ARE ALIKE

Essential oils are widely available and can vary considerably in price and quality. Pure essential oils tend to be more expensive than those obtained in the grocery store, but the cost per dose is still much less than that of prescription medications.

Not all essential oils can be used therapeutically. Non-therapeutic oils are most commonly diluted with alcohol or a carrier oil, or adulterated with insecticides during growing or in production by adding a cheaper oil. Oils are graded by their intended use and range from synthetic (used for perfumes, lotions, etc.), to food grade (used for flavorings in food) to therapeutic grade (used in clinical practice). *"If essential oils are being used clinically, they should be from a reputable supplier who can state the following: country of origin, botanical name, part of the plant, wild crafted or organic, method of extraction, batch number, expiration date, and chemotype (when relevant)".*[6 p. 31]

Essential oils should be supplied in colored bottles containing integral droppers and should be clearly marked 100% pure. Basic safety precautions should also be included in the labeling. Supplemental facts and dosing recommendations should be present in the labeling if the oil can be used internally.

REGULATION OF PRODUCT AND PROFESSION

In the United States, aromatherapy is unregulated and unlicensed both in practice and product. When referring a client to an aromatherapist, it is wise to assess his or her credentials. Certification courses vary in length and content. The National Association of Holistic Aromatherapy has set standards for aromatherapy education and accredits schools that meet those standards. Although not mandatory, the Aromatherapy Registration Council offers a national examination to applicants who have completed training at an accredited school.

While inhaled and topical uses of essential oils are quite common and considered safe, ingestion of essential oils should be done only under the direct supervision of a trained expert.

SUMMARY

Essential oil use can be an effective option or adjunct in the treatment of many geriatric health care needs. Advantages of using essential oils include flexibility in delivery methods, low cost compared with many prescription medications, and a high safety profile when used properly.

RESOURCES

The following websites and books contain useful information about aromatherapy:

- National Association of Holistic Aromatherapy—naha.org
- American Holistic Nurses Association—ahna.org
- Aromatherapy Registration Council—aromatherapycouncil.org
- Essential Oil University—essential oils.org
- International Journal of Clinical Aromatherapy—www.IJCA.net
- http://roberttisserand.com/blog/
- Buckle J. *Clinical Aromatherapy: Essential Oils in Healthcare*. 3rd edition. Churchill Livingstone; 2015.
- Tisserand R, Young R. *Essential Oil Safety*. 2nd edition. Churchill Livingstone; 2013.

REFERENCES

Energy Modalities

1. Dufresne F, Simmons B, Vlachostergios PJ, et al. Feasibility of energy medicine in a community teaching hospital: An exploratory case series. *J Altern Complement Med*. 2015;21(6):339–349. http://doi.org/10.1089/acm.2014.0157
2. Joyce J, Herbison GP. Reiki for depression and anxiety. *Cochrane Library*. 2015(4): 1–34. http://doi.org/10.1002/14651858.CD006833.pub2
3. Rindfleisch JA. Human energetic therapies. In Rakel D, ed., *Integrative Medicine*, 3rd ed. Philadelphia, PA: Saunders; 2012:980–987.
4. Jain S, Mills PJ. Biofield therapies: Helpful or full of hype? A best evidence synthesis. *Int J Behav Med*. 2010;17(1):1–16. http://doi.org/10.1007/s12529-009-9062-4
5. Ives JA, Jonas WB.). Energy Medicine. In Micozzi MS, ed., *Fundamentals of Complementary and Alternative Medicine*, 5th ed. St. Louis: Elsevier;2015:197–212.
6. Wardell DW, Engebretson J. Biological correlates of reiki touch healing. *J Adv Nurs*. 2001;33(4):439–445. http://doi.org/0.1046/j.1365-2648.2001.01691.x
7. Bukowski EL. Short report: The use of self: Reiki for stress reduction and relaxation. *J Integrative Med*. 2015;13(5):336–341. http://doi.org/10.1016/S2095-4964(15)60190-X
8. Achterberg J, Cooke K, Richards T, Standish LJ, Kozak L, Lake J. Evidence for correlations between distant intentionality and brain function in recipients: A functional magnetic resonance imaging analysis. *J Altern Complement Med*. 2005;11(6):965–971. http://doi.org/10.1089/acm.2005.11.965
9. Anderson JG, Taylor AG. Biofield therapies in cardiovascular disease management. *Holistic Nursing Practice*. 2011;25(4):199–204. http://doi.org/10.1097/HNP.ob013e3182227185

10. McCormack GL. Using non-contact therapeutic touch to manage post-surgical pain in the elderly. *Occupational Therapy International.* 2009;16(1):44–56. http://doi.org/10.1002/oti.264

11. Thrane S, Cohen SM. Effect of reiki therapy on pain and anxiety in adults: An in-depth literature review of randomized trials with effect size calculations. *Pain Manag Nurs.* 2014;15(4):897–908.

12. Hammerschlag R, Levin M, McCraty R, et al. Biofield physiology: A framework for an emerging discipline. *Global Advances in Health and Medicine.* 2015;4(suppl): 35–41. http://doi.org/10.7453/gahmj.2015.015.suppl

13. Van Wijk R, Van Wijk EPA. The search for a biosensor as a witness of a human laying on of hands ritual. *Alternative Therapies in Health and Medicine.* 2003;9(2):48–55. Retrieved from http://search.proquest.com/openview/2cbfb71ab81a2df2d768a-2139d7a5efa/1?pq-origsite=gscholar

14. Childre D, Martin H. *The Heartmath Solution, The HeartMath Institute's Revolutionary Program for Engaging the Power of the Heart's Intelligence.* HarperOne Publishing, August 2000.

15. Jain S, Hammerschlag R, Mills P, et al. Clinical studies of biofield therapies: Summary, methodological challenges, and recommendations. *Global Advances in Health and Medicine.* 2015;4(suppl):58–66. http://doi.org/10.7453/gahmj.2015.034. suppl

16. Nahin RL, Barnes PM, Stussman BJ, Bloom B. Costs of complementary and alternative medicine (CAM) and frequency of visits to CAM practitioners: United States, 2007. *National Health Statistics Reports.* 2009;(18):1–14.

17. Bowden D, Goddard L, Gruzelier J. A randomised controlled single-blind trial of the efficacy of Reiki at benefitting mood and well-being. *Evidence-Based Complementary and Alternative Medicine.* 2011;2011:1–8. http://doi.org/10.1155/2011/381862

18. Fazzino DL, Griffin MTQ, McNulty RS, Fitzpatrick JJ. Energy healing and pain: A review of the literature. *Holistic Nursing Practice.* 2010;24(2):79–88. http://doi.org/10.1097/HNP.0b013e3181d39718

19. Gronowicz G, Bengston W, Yount G. Challenges for preclinical investigations of human biofield modalities. *Global Advances in Health and Medicine.* 2015;4(suppl):52–57. http://doi.org/10.7453/gahmj.2015.013.suppl

20. Mackay N, Hansen S, McFarlane O. Autonomic nervous system changes during reiki treatment: A preliminary study. *J Altern Complement Med.* 2004;10(6): 1077–1081. http://doi.org/10.1089/acm.2004.10.1077

21. Mirel L, Carper K. MEPS statistical brief # 429: Trends in health care expenditures for the elderly, age 65 and over: 2001, 2006, and 2011. 2014, AHRQ – Agency for Healthcare Research and Quality: https://meps.ahrq.gov/data_files/publications/st429/stat429.pdf

22. Cabrera E, Sutcliffe C, Verbeek H, et al. Non-pharmacological interventions as a best practice strategy in people with dementia living in nursing homes. *Eur Geriatr Med.* 2015;6(2):34–150. http://doi.org/10.1016/j.eurger.2014.06.003

23. Henneghan AM, Schnyer RN. Biofield therapies for symptom management in palliative and end-of-life care. *Am J Hospice Palliat Care.* 2013;32(1):90–100. http://doi.org/10.1177/1049909113509400

24. Linden DJ. *Touch: The Science of Hand, Heart, and Mind.* Viking., Penguin Books, January 2016.

25. Bush E. The use of human touch to improve the well-being of older adults. *J Holistic Nurs.* 2001;19(3):256–270. http://doi.org/10.1177/089801010101900306

26. Hammerschlag R, Marx BL, Aickin M. Nontouch biofield therapy: A systematic review of human randomized controlled trials reporting use of only nonphysical contact treatment. *J Altern Complement Med.* 2014;20(12):881–892. http://doi.org/10.1089/acm.2014.0017

27. O'Mathúna DP, Ashford RL. Therapeutic touch for healing acute wounds. *Cochrane Database of Systematic Reviews.* 2014;7(7). http://doi.org/10.1002/14651858.CD002766.pub3

28. Gregory S, Verdouw J. Therapeutic touch: Its application for residents in aged care. *Australian Nurs J.* 2005 Feb;12(7):23–25. Retrieved from http://www.healthyoutlook.com.au/images/0502_clin_update.pdf

29. Woods DL, Dimond M. The effect of therapeutic touch on agitated behavior and cortisol in persons with Alzheimer's disease. *Biological Research for Nursing.* 2002;4(2):104–114. http://doi.org/10.1177/1099800402238331

30. Elliott S. Dacher MD. *Whole Healing: A Step by Step Program To Reclaim Your Power To Heal.* Plume Publishing, August 1997.

31. Willis E, Martinez M, Jacobs L, Kogan M. Reiki share group within a retirement community: A novel approach to enhance wellbeing, resident-staff communication, and staff's job satisfaction. Poster Presentation AHHA/ICIM Conference, 2010.

Aromatherapy

1. Steflitsch W, Steflitsch M. Clinical aromatherapy. *J Mens Health.* 2008;5(1):74–85.

2. Mills S. *Out of the Earth.* London: Viking Arkana; 1991.

3. Manohar V, Ingram C, Gray J, et al. Antifungal activities of origanim oil against candida albicans. *Mol Cell Biochem.* 2001;228(1):111–117.

4. Anthony JP, Fyfe L, Smith H. Plant active components—a resource for antiparasitic agents? *Trends in Parasitiology.* 2005;21(10):462–468.

5. Tisserand R, Young R. *Essential Oil Safety,* 2nd ed. Edinburgh: Churchill Livingstone; 2014. http://roberttisserand.com/blog/

6. Buckle J. *Clinical Aromatherapy: Essential Oils in Healthcare.* St. Louis: Churchill Livingstone; 2015.

7. Henkin RI, Levy LM. Functional MRI of congenital hyposmia: Brain activation to odors and imagination of odors and tastes. *J Comp Assist Tomogr.* 2002;26(1):39–61.

8. Lafreniere D, Mann N, Anosmia: Loss of smell in the elderly. *Otolaryngol Clin North Am.* 2009;42:123–131.

9. Jimbo D, Kimura Y, Taniguchi M, Inoue M, Urakami K. Effect of aromatherapy on patients with Alzheimer's disease. *Psychogeriatrics.* 2009;9:173–179.

10. Sayorwan W, Ruangrungsi N, Piriyapunyporn T, Hongratanaworkit T, Kotchabhakdi N, Vorasith S. Effects of inhaled rosemary oil on subjective feelings and activities of the nervous system. *Scientia Pharmaceutica.* 2013;81:531–542.

11. Johannessen B. Nurses' experience of aromatherapy use with dementia patients experiencing disturbed sleep patterns. *Complementary Therapies in Clinical Practice.* 2013;19:209–213.

12. Koulivand PH, Ghadiri MK Gorji A. Lavender and the nervous system. *Evidence-Based Complementary and Alternative Medicine.* 2013;2013:1–10.

13. Chien LW, Cheng SL, Liu CF. Effect of lavender aromatherapy on autonomic nervous system in midlife women with insomnia. *Evidence-Based Complementary and Alternative Medicine.* 2012;2012:1–8.

14. *Modern Essentials Usage Guide: A Quick Guide to the Therapeutic Use of Essential Oils.* Orem, UT: AromaTools; 2014.

8

Naturopathic Medicine

DEIRDRE ORCEYRE AND MEREDITH BULL

Introduction

Naturopathic medicine is an approach to health care that emphasizes prevention and supports the body's inherent self-healing processes to achieve optimal wellness. It utilizes a therapeutic order that primes physicians to address the foundational aspects of health and to implement treatments that target all aspects of the patient, not just symptoms or diagnoses. The naturopathic approach often results in effective and sustainable health care outcomes, in part because the philosophy is one that empowers patients to take an active role in their health. Its function in geriatrics is invaluable. The geriatric patient is often complex with a unique set of concerns; these patients benefit greatly from the time and detail involved in the patient-centered, naturopathic approach, as well as the autonomy such an approach provides in one's health.

History

The roots of naturopathic medicine extend from physicians in the early 19th century known as *Nature Doctors*.[1] These doctors practiced *Nature Cure* medicine that combined diet, botanical medicine, exercise, and massage with *water cure* practices—the use of hot and cold water applications (i.e., hydrotherapy), movement, and fresh air to invoke a healing response in the body. Nature Cure treatment methods were introduced to the United States in the late 19th century by Benedict Lust, who was cured in Germany by a nature doctor after his American physicians assured him of an imminent death. He returned to America in 1896 to establish the early naturopathic profession, which included Nature Cure, homeopathy, and spinal manipulations, and was the founder of the first naturopathic educational institution in 1901: the American School of Naturopathy in New York. Dr. Henry Lindlahr furthered the naturopathic profession, taking a rational, scientific approach to naturopathic practices through careful observations. He saw the preventable path to chronic illness and focused his efforts educating others about the importance of lifestyle modification in the prevention of disease; the establishment of *naturopathic medicine* is attributed to his practices.

Naturopathic medicine waxed and waned throughout the early 20th century. The National University of Natural Medicine in Portland, Oregon, founded in 1956, is the oldest remaining naturopathic medical school.[2] It wasn't until 1978 that another naturopathic medical school was founded, the still-thriving John Bastyr College of Naturopathic Medicine, now known as Bastyr University in Seattle, Washington. The naturopathic profession has grown exponentially since this time.

Philosophy

There are six principles of naturopathic medicine (Table 8.1). The core tenet is that of *vis medicatrix naturae*, or the healing power of nature, and is perhaps what distinguishes the profession most from conventional medicine. *Vis medicatrix naturae* refers to the innate healing mechanisms within living organisms, a process naturopathic medicine strives to support rather than suppress. It is from this tenet that the Therapeutic Order from which naturopathic physicians practice was developed (Fig. 8.1). This hierarchy of therapies encourages physicians to first consider the determinants of health in order to identify any obstacles to healing. These obstacles may be present in diet, lifestyle, psychoemotional state, environment, socioeconomic factors, or a combination thereof. After addressing these foundational aspects, therapies higher in the Therapeutic Order and perceived "invasiveness" are considered.

Naturopathic medicine views the body system as constantly working to maintain health; a disturbance to the optimal health state results in bodily responses attempting to restore balance.[3] Symptoms are not viewed as the entirety of the illness itself but rather manifestations of this restorative reaction. Suppression of the symptoms is avoided with the view that this may lead to chronicity of the condition or even create fertile ground for other disease processes. Rather, attention is paid to the initiating insult—the "root cause" or

Table 8.1. Principles of Naturopathic Medicine

The Healing Power of Nature: *Vis Medicatrix Naturae*	Naturopathic medicine recognizes an inherent self-healing process in people that is ordered and intelligent. Naturopathic physicians act to identify and remove obstacles to healing and recovery, and to facilitate and augment this inherent self-healing process.
Identify and Treat the Causes: *Tolle Causam*	The naturopathic physician seeks to identify and remove the underlying causes of illness rather than to merely eliminate or suppress symptoms.
First Do No Harm: *Primum Non Nocere*	Naturopathic physicians follow three guidelines to avoid harming the patient: • Utilize methods and medicinal substances which minimize the risk of harmful side effects, using the least force necessary to diagnose and treat; • Avoid, when possible, the harmful suppression of symptoms; and • Acknowledge, respect, and work with individuals' self-healing process.
Doctor as Teacher: *Docere*	Naturopathic physicians educate their patients and encourage self-responsibility for health. They also recognize and employ the therapeutic potential of the doctor–patient relationship.
Treat the Whole Person	Naturopathic physicians treat each patient by taking into account individual physical, mental, emotional, spiritual, genetic, environmental, social, and other factors.
Prevention	Naturopathic physicians emphasize the prevention of disease by assessing risk factors, heredity and susceptibility to disease, and by making appropriate interventions in partnership with their patients to prevent illness.

House of Delegates Position Paper: Definition of Naturopathic Medicine. American Association of Naturopathic Physicians, 2011. www.naturopathic.org. Accessed January 2017.

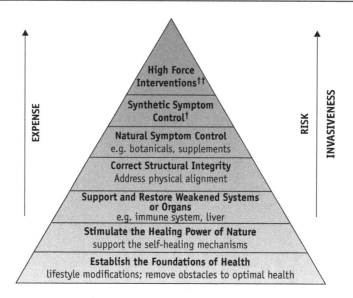

FIGURE 8.1. The Naturopathic Therapeutic Order.
Adapted from AANMC – need permissions
† Use of pharmacologic and synthetic substances
†† Surgery, suppressive drugs (e.g., immune suppression), chemotherapy, radiation

underlying imbalance. Thus, naturopathic physicians target treatment to the body and not the disease, as guided by the Therapeutic Order (see Fig. 8.1). An example of this philosophy may be illustrated in Box 8.1 in the treatment of atopic dermatitis.

Box 8.1. Naturopathic Management of Atopic Dermatitis

Medical dermatology typically uses topical or even oral steroids to control the inflammatory symptoms such as itching, redness, and pain involved in atopic dermatitis. Naturopathic medicine sees this suppression of the symptoms as a superficial and temporary solution that ignores any deeper pathologies such as food sensitivities, nutrient deficiencies, microbiome imbalances, environmental allergens, emotional or lifestyle stressors, and so forth. Addressing underlying aspects as they pertain to the individual aligns with the Therapeutic Order and may include food elimination and challenge diets, nutritional and botanical supplementation to support emotional, digestive, or skin health, biofeedback and relaxation techniques, and others. The need for immediate symptom relief may be addressed with topical botanicals and other non-pharmacological agents before considering the higher-force intervention of steroid therapy.

Naturopathic philosophy recognizes that aging is a natural process in health and something that should not be dismissed or rejected. In the treatment of the geriatric patient, the focused approach on health primes the physician to *work with* the unique challenges of aging in order to optimize wellness as much as possible. This begets proactive treatment aimed at supporting patients through the aging process.

Credentials

NATUROPATHIC EDUCATION

At present, there are seven accredited naturopathic programs in North America (Box 8.2). These institutions confer the Doctor of Naturopathic Medicine degree (ND or NMD), granting graduates eligibility for licensure as primary care physicians upon passing board examinations.

Box 8.2. Accredited Naturopathic Programs in Canada and the United States*

Bastyr University
  Kenmore, WA
Bastyr University—California Campus
  San Diego, CA
National University of Natural Medicine
  Portland, OR
National University of Health Sciences
  Lombard, IL
Southwest College of Naturopathic Medicine
  Tempe, AZ
University of Bridgeport—College of Naturopathic Medicine
  Bridgeport, CT
Canadian College of Naturopathic Medicine
  Toronto, ON
Boucher Institute of Naturopathic Medicine
  New Westminster, BC

Association of Accredited Naturopathic Medical Colleges. www.aanmc.org.

* Naturopathic programs outside of these institutions are not accredited and do not confer a licensable doctorate degree. As of January 2017, the University del Turado in Puerto Rico is undergoing accreditation review by the CNME and is slated to become the eighth accredited naturopathic program.

Doctors graduating from an accredited naturopathic program may be titled either naturopathic doctor or naturopathic physician, depending on licensure. ND medical training in the United States is a four-year medical program requiring an undergraduate degree and specific basic science prerequisites, similar to other medical schools. Most programs in the United States begin with 2 years of foundational naturopathic philosophy in conjunction with basic and clinical sciences such as biochemistry, anatomy with cadaver lab, physiology, immunology, pathology, and so forth. The final 2 years focus on internal medicine subjects, including coursework in geriatrics. The naturopathic education includes over 1,200 hours of clinical rotations in private and community-based patient care centers.[4,5]

With their general and preventive health care education, naturopathic students learn to diagnose and treat the most common complaints seen in primary care according to conventional standards, in addition to learning therapeutic approaches to initiate when standards of care have failed or when patients wish to pursue alternatives. This additional education includes extensive coursework in dietary modifications, nutritional biochemistry, supplement use, botanical medicine, counseling, homeopathy, and physical medicine. In the state of Arizona and in the Canadian province of Ontario, regulations mandate that students learn acupuncture, and thus graduates from schools in those areas learn this skill as well. It is common for naturopathic students to pursue training in various additional modalities such as Chinese medicine, massage, craniosacral therapy, ayurvedic practices, and countless others.

Unlike conventional counterparts, residencies for naturopathic medicine are not federally funded. Due to the reliance on private funding, there are only enough residencies for roughly 15% to 20% of the graduating naturopathic students each year.[6] At this time, there is no board certification in geriatrics or other population specialties, but many naturopathic physicians work with geriatric patients as part of a family practice setting.

LICENSURE

Nineteen states and the District of Columbia, Puerto Rico, the U.S. Virgin Islands, and five Canadian provinces currently license NDs (Table 8.2). Scope of practice, such as the ability to prescribe pharmaceuticals or to perform physical adjustments, varies by state or province. Licensure in all

Table 8.2. U.S. and Canadian Provinces that License Naturopathic Physicians

UNITED STATES

Alaska	Kansas	North Dakota
Arizona	Maine	Oregon
California	Maryland	Pennsylvania
Colorado	Massachusetts	Utah
Connecticut	Minnesota	Vermont
District of Columbia	Montana	Washington
Hawaii	New Hampshire	US Territories: Puerto Rico, U.S. British Virgin Islands

CANADA

Alberta	Manitoba	Saskatchewan
British Columbia	Ontario	

Association of Accredited Naturopathic Medical Colleges. www.aanmc.org.

50 states and expansion of licensure in Canada are active goals of the American and Canadian naturopathic associations. Securing licensure allows naturopathic practitioners to practice to the full extent of their training and helps to clearly identify medically trained naturopathic physicians from NDs without medical education.

MEDICARE

NDs are currently not included under Medicare's definition of physician.[7] This has negative consequences for patients, especially those who have chosen a naturopathic physician as their primary care provider and can no longer receive covered care. Patients may see their naturopathic physician separately and pay out of pocket for services, but the naturopathic physician would be unable to order necessary laboratory work or imaging, or to even make referrals to specialists, nursing homes, hospice services, or in-home care. This inconvenience and the out-of-pocket costs from not having Medicare coverage alienate the burgeoning aging population, which is already short of primary care providers and would benefit tremendously from the health-based approach of naturopathic medicine.

The Naturopathic Approach

ASSESSMENT

The geriatric assessment for naturopathic physicians does not differ greatly from that of conventional standards. The same physical examinations, preventive screening measures, and laboratory tests are performed by licensed naturopaths, although some naturopathic physicians may choose to employ additional alternative diagnostic techniques, especially when the routine physical examination is not adequate to evaluate a presenting condition. The difference in the treatment of the geriatric patient is most notably in the time spent during the office visit, affording the naturopathic physician the ability to offer more comprehensive care, especially in the identification of obstacles in everyday living that may be preventing the patient from achieving his or her health goals. This additional time provides greater insight into not only the physical state but mental, emotional, and spiritual health as well, components likely contributing to physical manifestations.

NATUROPATHIC MODALITIES

Nature Cure

The Nature Cure methods of hydrotherapy, fresh air, movement, and diet are foundational components of naturopathic medicine. While modern naturopathic physicians are trained to today's conventional standards of care, the roots of the medicine are not forgotten, and these aspects of Nature Cure are addressed in every visit as basic determinants of health. Proper hygiene; time spent outdoors, preferably in nature with good air quality and moderate sun exposure; daily exercise, which may be as simple as walking; and eating a variety of foods—these are all aspects the naturopathic physician re-establishes into patients' daily activities, especially as patients age.

Nutrition

Naturopathic medical education includes comprehensive coursework in nutrition and nutritional biochemistry. This equips the naturopathic physician with a greater understanding of the importance of nutrition in health and bodily processes and puts nutrition at the forefront of naturopathic

> **Box 8.3. Physiological Changes to the Gut in the Elderly that Impact Nutrition Status**
>
> Gastric atrophy
> Decreased stomach acid production
> Slowed gut motility
> Decrease in microbiome diversity
>
> Vitamin B12, iron, and calcium may be most affected by these changes.[8-11]

clinical thinking and assessment. Pharmaceutical use, normal physiological changes to the gastrointestinal system that come with aging (Box 8.3), mental state, and socioeconomic status can all disrupt nutritional status. The naturopathic physician will assess for all this and more in the intake, as part of the physical examination, and through laboratory testing. This attention to nutrition often results in dietary recommendations as part of the treatment plan. In addition to making sure macro- and micronutrient needs are met and digestive and absorptive functioning is optimized, NDs may include trials of food elimination and reintroduction, especially those known to promote inflammatory processes (e.g., red meat,[12,13] added sugar[14,15]) or those suspected of causing systemic issues (i.e., food allergies and sensitivities).

Homeopathy

Homeopathy is a highly complex system of medicine that goes beyond the scope of this chapter. It is an energetic modality that utilizes infinitesimal amounts of organic material dosed based on an individual's constitution and symptoms. The naturopathic education includes coursework in homeopathy, and NDs may use it as part of the treatment plan. For the geriatric patient, homeopathy is a wonderfully gentle treatment to incorporate adjunctively to support overall health, or to use acutely to help promote the healing process.

Physical Medicine

A large part of the naturopathic education involves instruction in physical medicine, skills useful for addressing the "Correct Structural Integrity" component of the therapeutic order discussed in Figure 8.1. The scope of these physical modalities is broad and includes therapeutic exercise, spinal manipulations, massage techniques, hydrotherapy, therapeutic ultrasound, electric stimulation, and more. Possessing skills in physical medicine allows the naturopathic physician to address many complaints directly in the office and decreases the need for referrals to specialists. For the geriatric patient with mounting physical complaints, this can be very beneficial.

Supplements and Nutraceuticals

Dietary supplements are the complementary health approach most commonly used by adults age 50 and up.[16] While supplements and nutraceuticals are at times heavily utilized within naturopathic practice, it is important to recognize that their implementation falls further up the Therapeutic Order; they are to be used in conjunction with the foundational aspects of health, or reserved for use after these have been addressed. As the nutraceutical industry expands, naturopathic physicians are the foremost authority in addressing concerns over the quality of these products.

Botanical Medicine

The use of botanicals is paramount in naturopathic medicine. Therapeutic benefit comes from quality herbal preparations and accurate dosing, aspects often missed by the untrained. Contrary to what some may believe, much research exists in the herbal medicine field, although funding for large-scale clinical studies tends to be limited. Safety and efficacy are generally guided by animal or small-scale human studies as well as thousands of years of time-tested use. Mechanism-of-action studies often support the use of traditional botanicals, confirming benefits touted for centuries. Most practitioners of botanical medicine recognize that there is a synergistic effect among the various constituents of a plant, often more gentle and sometimes more effective than the use of an isolated ingredient. Botanical medicine is dosed via teas, powdered herb, tinctures, oils, and topical applications, and the naturopathic practitioner is proficient in the utility of these preparations as well as in any potential drug–herb interactions.

Please review Table 8.3 for information on commonly used botanicals.[17-20]

Table 8.3. Commonly Used Botanicals

Herb	Main Constituents and Therapeutic Actions	Use	Dose
Marshmallow *Althea officinalis* Part used: root	Mucilage; emollient to GI mucosa	Inflammation of GI (GERD, IBD, gastric ulcers, etc.)	*Cold infusion:* 2–4 grams per cup cold water, infused overnight; 1 cup TID
Astragalus *Astragalus membranaceus* Part used: root	Flavonoids, polysaccharides; immune function, antiviral activity	Adjunctive therapy for autoimmune diseases, acute and chronic viral infections, general immune support	*Standardized extract:* 1–2 gram qd *Tincture:* 5 ml of 1:5 extract BID
Oatstraw *Avena sativa* Part used: milky oat seed	Polysaccharides, alkaloids; anxiolytic	Anxiety, nervous disorders (psychological and physical), nicotine withdrawal	*Infusion:* 1 gram per cup water TID *Tincture:* 5 ml TID of 1:5 extract
Boswellia *Boswellia serrata* Part used: bark, root	Volatile oil, resins; anti-inflammatory	Arthritis, IBD	*Standardized extract:* 200–400 mg TID, with meals
Hawthorn *Crataegus mongyna* Part used: berries, leaf, flower	Flavonoids, oligomeric procyanidins; Antioxidant, positive inotropic	Adjunctive therapy for heart disease, cardiac insufficiency, valvular disease, ischemia, moderate HTN	*Infusion:* 1.5–3.5 grams qd *Standardized extract:* 1 g TID–QID

(continued)

Table 8.3. Continued

Herb	Main Constituents and Therapeutic Actions	Use	Dose
Deglycyrrhizinated* Licorice (DGL) Glycyrrhiza glabra Part used: rhizome	Flavonoids, polysaccharides; inflammation modulator, emollient to GI mucosa	GERD, gastric ulcers, GI inflammation	Standardized extract: 1.2–4.6 grams qd
Lemon Balm Melissa officinalis Part used: flowering tops, leaves	Volatile oils, flavonoids; carminative, mild sedative, antiviral	Flatulence, IBS, anxiety, insomnia, herpesvirus infections	Infusion: 1.5–4.5 grams per cup water BID Tincture: 2–5 mL TID of 1:5 extract
Passionflower Passiflora incarnata Part used: flowering tops, leaves	Alkaloids, flavonoids; antispasmodic, sedative	Insomnia, anxiety, IBS	Infusion: 1–2 grams per cup BID–TID Tincture: 1–3 mL TID of 1:5 extract
Saw Palmetto Serenoa repens Part used: berry	Fatty acids, sterols; inhibition of 5α-reductase	BPH for prostates <50 g in size	Standardized extract: 320 mg qd

*Glycyrrhizin and glycyrrhetinic acid are main constituents of licorice that offer a number of additional benefits. However, these components may also contribute to increased cortisol levels, increased blood pressure, and potassium loss; DGL forms are commonly used to eliminate these potential side effects.

Environmental Medicine

Naturopathic medicine recognizes that the environment plays a tremendous role in health. Home and occupational environments may unknowingly expose individuals to noxious agents, often without any indication that these exposures are behind their health complaints. Because practitioners are alert to these environmental hazards, they will often consider testing for heavy metal exposures and various xenobiotics in the patient encounter. When treating geriatric patients, it is imperative to rule out environmental toxicities as a contributor to cognitive and neurological complaints as well as any decline in kidney and liver function.

Box 8.4 lists further resources on naturopathic medicine.

REFERENCES

1. Kirchfeld F, Boyle W. *Nature Doctors, Pioneers in Naturopathic Medicine*. Portland, OR: Medicina Biologica; 1994.
2. *A Brief History of NUNM*. National University of Natural Medicine. www.nunm. edu. Accessed January 2017.
3. Zeff JL, Snider P, Myers SP. A hierarchy of healing: The Therapeutic Order. In: Pizzorno JE, Murray MT. *Textbook of Natural Medicine*, 4th ed. Edinburgh: Elsevier Health Sciences; 2012:22–26.

4. *The Curriculum.* Association of Accredited Naturopathic Medical Colleges. www.aanmc.org. Accessed January 2017.
5. *Doctor of Naturopathic Medicine: Clinical Training.* Bastyr University. www.Bastyr.edu. Accessed January 2017.
6. *CNME-Approved Naturopathic Residency Application 2017-18.* Association of Accredited Naturopathic Medical Colleges. aanmc.org. Accessed January 2017.
7. *Glossary and Acronyms.* Centers for Medicare & Medicaid Services. www.cms.gov
8. Claesson MJ, Jeffery IB, Conde S, et al. Gut microbiota composition correlates with diet and health in the elderly. *Nature.* 2012;488(7410):178–184. doi:10.1038/nature11319
9. Krasinski SD, Russell RM, Samloff IM, et al. Fundic atrophic gastritis in an elderly population. *J Am Geriatr Soc.* 1986;34:800–806.
10. Rémond D, Shahar DR, Gille D, et al. Understanding the gastrointestinal tract of the elderly to develop dietary solutions that prevent malnutrition. *Oncotarget.* 2015;6(16):13858–13898.
11. Russell RM. Factors in aging that affect the bioavailability of nutrients. *J Nutr.* 2001;131(4 Suppl):1329S–1400S.
12. Ley SH, Sun Q, Willett WC, et al. Associations between red meat intake and biomarkers of inflammation and glucose metabolism in women. *Am J Clin Nutr.* 2014;99(2):352–360. doi:10.3945/ajcn.113.075663.
13. Song M, Garrett WS, Chan AT. Nutrients, foods, and colorectal cancer prevention. *Gastroenterology.* 2015;148(6):1244–1260.e16. doi:10.1053/j.gastro.2014.12.035.
14. Beilharz JE, Maniam J, Morris MJ. Diet-induced cognitive deficits: The role of fat and sugar, potential mechanisms and nutritional interventions. *Nutrients.* 2015;7(8):6719–6738. doi:10.3390/nu7085307.
15. DiNicolantonio JJ, Lucan SC. The wrong white crystals: Not salt but sugar as aetiological in hypertension and cardiometabolic disease. *Open Heart.* 2014;1(1):e000167. doi:10.1136/openhrt-2014-000167.
16. Clarke TC, Black LI, Stussman BJ, et al. *Trends in the use of complementary health approaches among adults: United States, 2002–2012.* National Health Statistics Reports, no 79. 2015. Retrieved from www.cdc.gov
17. Select monographs from Bastyr University Department of Botanical Medicine.
18. Bone K, Mills S., *Principles and Practice of Phytotherapy,* 2nd ed. Edinburgh: Churchill Livingstone/Elsevier; 2013.
19. Hoffman, D. *Medical Herbalism: The Science and Practice of Herbal Medicine.* Rochester, VA: Healing Arts Press; 2013.
20. Yarnell E. *Natural Approach to Gastroenterology,* 2nd ed. East Wenatachee, WA: Healing Mountain Publishing; 2011.

9

Spirituality and Mind–Body Medicine in Geriatrics

CHRISTINA M. PUCHALSKI
AND PATRICIA A. BLOOM

Today's health care systems still focus primarily on the physical dimensions of health, yet increasingly clinicians, patients, and society in general are recognizing that health and illness are multidimensional and include the mind and spirit, not only the body. In recent years two related fields have emerged: "mind–body medicine" and "spirituality and health." Both fields focus on the importance of the mind and spirit in the attainment of health and in coping with illness. Spirituality and health focuses on the inner life of people and how they find meaning, purpose, and connectedness to the significant or sacred. Spirituality is a fundamental element of human experience. It encompasses the individual's search for meaning and purpose in life and the experience of the transcendent. Spirituality also encompasses the connections one makes with others, himself or herself, and nature, and to the sacred realms, inside as well as outside of traditional religion. Viewed in this way, spirituality can be a key factor in how people cope with illness, experience healing, and achieve a sense of coherence. A global consensus derived definition of spirituality is

> Spirituality is a dynamic and intrinsic aspect of humanity through which persons seek ultimate meaning, purpose, and transcendence, and experience relationship to self, family, others, community, society, nature, and the significant or sacred. Spirituality is expressed through beliefs, values, traditions, and practices.[1]

Spiritual practices might include personal or religious rituals, meditation, journaling, art, and other types of mind–body interventions. In this chapter, we will give an overview of spiritual care in geriatrics care and describe mindfulness-based interventions.

There is a significant body of literature that highlights the role of spirituality in aging. As we age, spirituality plays a more dominant role in our lives than when we were younger. As our awareness of our own mortality becomes more obvious as we age, the questions about meaning, purpose, and connection become more critical for us. The diagnosis of chronic or life-threatening illness can lead to spiritual struggles for patients. The turmoil may be short for some patients and protracted for others as they attempt to integrate the reality of their diagnosis with their spiritual beliefs. The journey may result in growth and transformation for some people and in distress and despair for others, and in both for many people. In a recent study of 203 older patients, 65.0% reported some spiritual distress and 22.2% reported at least one severe unmet spiritual need.[2] Spiritual distress is associated with depression, poor health outcomes, poorer recovery of independence of activities of daily living, and increased mortality in elderly patients.

But spirituality can also be a resource of strength for many people. Studies have demonstrated that spirituality can result in increased spiritual well-being and less depression and anxiety, thus leading to improved health outcomes.[3] An intervention study in which the test group received a unit on spiritual well-being that included spiritual and mind–body resources demonstrated these same outcomes, especially quality of life.[4]

Over the last 25 years guidelines have been developed in multidisciplinary spiritual care, with spiritual care being defined as

> That care which recognizes and responds to the needs of the human spirit when faced with trauma, ill health or sadness, and can include the need for meaning, for self-worth, to express oneself, for faith support, perhaps for rites or prayer or sacrament, or simply for the sensitive listener. Spiritual care begins with encouraging human contact in compassionate relationship, and moves in whatever direction need requires.[5]

Preeminent consensus panels, including the National Quality Forum (2006) and the National Consensus Project for Quality Palliative Care (2009), include spiritual care as one of eight clinical practice guidelines in palliative care settings.[6,7]

Spirituality in Coping, Health Functioning, and Hope

Spirituality is an important coping strategy for the elderly population, who experience age-related losses, disabilities, physical illness, and mortality confronted in old age. Spirituality brings a sense of connectedness to self, to others, and to the significant or sacred. This attachment and commitment of spiritual values and belief system might offer a greater social resource for the elderly that promotes positive relationships with other people and higher social and psychological well-being. In a cross-sectional study of medically ill hospitalized older adults, religiousness and spirituality significantly predicted greater social support, better cognitive function, fewer depressive symptoms, and greater cooperativeness.[8]

Daaleman et al. found that spirituality, but not religiosity, was an important predictor of self-appraised good health.[9] Several studies demonstrated that spiritual well-being and spiritual practices were associated with better overall health and a lower incidence of depression.[10,11] Spirituality is an important source of hope and comfort that improves resiliency in older people. Spiritual distress and higher religious struggle was associated with higher mortality, supporting the need to address spiritual distress in patients.[12]

Spiritual Stage of Aging

As people age they face may existential and spiritual issues as the reflect on their final phase of life. *Gerotranscendence* is a relatively new term used to describe the developmental spiritual stage associated with older age. Tornstam et al. developed the gerotranscendence theory as a positive development toward a transcendent outlook on life, "a shift in metaperspective, from a materialistic and rational vision to a more cosmic and transcendent one, normally followed by an increase in life satisfaction."[13]

In this stage, people begin to detach from those parts of their life such as titles, money, the acquisition of things, and even illness or debility in favor of a more focused attention on those things that matter most: legacy building and mentorship, relationships, as well as a new understanding of fundamental existential issues. Three dimensions of gerotranscendence have been described through empirical testing: cosmic transcendence (universe), solitude transcendence (self), and coherence transcendence (social and personal relationships).

Spiritual Distress of the Aging and Dying

Some spiritual issues are prominent in the older or the dying person. These are considered sources of spiritual distress and are cited in the NCCN guidelines for the diagnosis "spiritual or existential distress."[14] This spiritual distress is often manifested as intense suffering for the patient. It is critical that clinicians are able to diagnose spiritual distress and attempt to alleviate it. Unlike treating physical pain with medications, there are no quick or standardized solutions to the care of people's spiritual or existential suffering. But having a clinician present to listen to the patient talk about his or her suffering and express compassion and care is an important step in helping patients cope with their suffering. The role of the clinician is to help the patient give voice to that suffering. In externalizing the distress and talking about it, the patient often comes to a resolution on his or her own. In aging or in chronic illness, people can face these issues many times. There is no linear stage in which one experiences hope and never again feels hopeless. Spiritual journeys are dynamic and fluid. Issues are revisited many times, but over time there is some resolution. The spiritual issues faced by chronically ill and dying patients are summarized in Table 9.1.

Table 9.1. Spiritual Concerns of Aging

Spiritual Issues of Aging	Key Feature from History
Lack of meaning and purpose	Lack of meaning Concerns about afterlife Questions about the existence and meaning of suffering
Despair/hopelessness	Despair as absolute hopelessness No hope or value of life
Not being remembered	Separated from community No sense of relatedness
Guilt/shame	Feeling that one has done something wrong or evil Feeling that one is bad or evil
Anger at God/others	Displaced anger toward religious representatives or others Inability to forgive
Abandonment by God/others	Lack of love, loneliness
Feeling out of control	Deep sense of lack of control over physical and mental function
Spiritual or existential suffering	Loss of faith or meaning
Reconciliation	Need for forgiveness or reconciliation from self or others
Grief/loss	The feeling and process associated the loss of person, health, relationship

Spirituality in Geriatrics Care

Several models have been developed for interprofessional spiritual care.[6] The essence of these models is that spirituality is a required domain of whole-person care: physical, emotional, social, and spiritual. Thus, all clinicians should address all these domains with the recognition that trained and certified clinical chaplains are the experts in the spiritual clinical domain. While referral to a chaplain is key to good spiritual care, it is particularly important to involve all health care providers (e.g., physicians, nurses, social workers) in generalist spiritual care—that is, the practice of compassionate care and the integration of spirituality in their routine medical care practice. In clinical care chaplains are the spiritual care specialists and other clinicians are the spiritual care generalists. Because spiritual care is about the manner in which care will be given, it involves empathy, compassion, respect, sensitivity, and comfort. Spiritual care also involves building trusting, intimate, and meaningful relationships. Out of these relationships with their clinicians, patients may be able to find meaning, hope, and resilience in the middle of suffering.

The basics of spiritual care in the clinical settings include (1) listening actively to what patients and their families are saying (both verbally and nonverbally), (2) identifying the patient's religious or spiritual concerns through a spiritual screening, a history that clinicians do, or a full assessment by a chaplain, and (3) responding to those concerns, either directly or by referral.[6] The first step in communicating about spiritual issues is to listen to spiritual themes such as meaning, hope, relationships, religious beliefs, and values. By actively listening, the health care provider will be able to know the patient's full story and to recognize his or her spiritual concerns. The clinician can listen for how important the patient's spirituality is in his or her life and whether the it affects his or her health.

Once spiritual distress or issues are identified, they need to be addressed as part of the assessment and treatment plan. Clinicians can also document the patient's spiritual and psychosocial resources of strength and note those in the assessment and plan. This plan should be based on the biopsychosocial and spiritual model of care, or what many have called "whole-person care" (Table 9.2).[15]

The first part of the treatment plan for any patient is what all clinicians can do. This includes compassionate presence and deep listening to the patient's concerns and witnessing to the suffering of the patient. To witness means creating the environment of trust where the patient can feel comfortable to share his or her deepest concerns and be listened to with respect and compassion. Use of silence can be a powerful intervention; in the silence the patient

Table 9.2. Whole-Person Assessment and Treatment Plan

	Ms. Katie Brown is a 86-year-old woman status post hip replacement. She also has hypertension and insomnia. She is nervous about physical therapy but mostly about her independence after surgery. She is a self-described Catholic who also has found Buddhist practices important to her, but she has not meditated in many years and would like to start again. She also has some conflicts about her lack of adherence to the full traditions of the Catholic church and is exploring returning to a spiritual community.
Physical	Rehabilitation, encourage adherence to physical therapy Continue with current medications for pain and blood pressure
Emotional	Stable, good resources, is coping well
Social	Referral to social work for discharge planning and counseling about her concerns regarding maintaining her independence
Spiritual	Continued presence of the team, referral to chaplain for further exploration of her spiritual conflicts, recommend a mindfulness-based teacher to work with her on meditation as a resource for well-being and sleep and stress management

can reflect on his or her pain and give voice to the deep suffering within. Reflective inquiry can be used to help patients explore their inner concerns. Clinicians can reinforce spiritual and psychosocial resources of strength. They can also connect patients to community resources. Clinicians should always consider a referral to a chaplain or other spiritual care professional.

There are several other tested interventions that are based on meaning-making and life review, as there is a growing shared understanding that these two techniques are important spiritual processes that can manifest in a variety of ways.

Examples of spiritual health intervention are summarized in Table 9.3.

Table 9.3. Spiritual Health Interventions

Intervention	*Examples of Evidence*
Spiritual reminiscence	References 16, 17, 18
Meditation, prayer	References 19, 20, 21
Gratitude	Reference 22
Forgiveness/reconciliation	References 23, 24
Meaning oriented therapy	Reference 25
Dignity therapy	Reference 26
Organized religious activities	References 27, 28

Mindfulness

Mind–body medicine, and particularly mindfulness practices, has had a growing presence in clinical practice and research, but its application specifically to the older adult population has lagged behind. *Mindfulness Research Monthly* (www.goAMRA.org), a survey of published mindfulness science, demonstrates an exponential growth in the number of its citations. There were 641 in 2015, but a recent scholarly review by Geiger et al. of the benefits of mindfulness for older adults included only 15 studies published between 1980 and 2014 that had sufficient methodological quality for inclusion.[29] Overall research evidence, as well as that pertaining specifically to older adults, suggests benefit for a wide spectrum of geriatric issues and underscores the need for more scientifically rigorous research in this area. These issues include prevention and amelioration of age-associated diseases, alleviation of pain, prevention of cognitive decline, improvement in the well-being of caregivers, and improvement of psychological and emotional well-being. For whatever reason older adults seek training in mindfulness practices, in my (P.B.) experience they often come to experience the ways in which the practices lead them into the realm of spirituality, as defined earlier in the chapter.

What Is Mindfulness?

Mindfulness is the act of paying attention to the present moment in an open and non-reactive way. Most religions have some form of mindfulness (or meditation) practice; many of the mindfulness practices being taught today have roots in Eastern spiritual traditions but have been stripped of their religious connotations. One of the most widely taught methods of mindfulness practice is Mindfulness-Based Stress Reduction (MBSR), a curriculum developed by Jon Kabat-Zinn, PhD, at the University of Massachusetts in 1979. MBSR involves a weekly 2.5-hour class for 8 weeks, an all-day retreat, and home practice, during which participants learn to do sitting and walking meditation, the body scan, and simple yoga or "mindful movement" sequences. Participants use the attention skills and insights gained to respond more skillfully to life's stresses. MBSR is now taught in over 750 health-related centers around the world. Mindfulness-Based Cognitive Therapy (MBCT) is an application of MBSR to traditional cognitive-behavioral therapy developed by British/Canadian psychologists John Teasdale, Zindel Segal, and Mark Williams.

Numerous adaptations of MBSR, called Mindfulness-Based Interventions (MBIs), have evolved for particular groups. Mindfulness-Based Elder Care

(MBEC), developed by Lucia McBee, LCSW, has adapted mindfulness and other integrative techniques into the care of frail elders.[30] Other integrative modalities such as yoga, tai chi, and qi gong may be included under the umbrella of mindfulness practices and are discussed elsewhere in this text.

Evidence for Mind–Body Interventions in Geriatric Care

MBSR and MBCT, and adaptations of them, are the most widely used MBIs in research concerning mindfulness for older adults. Adaptations include shorter classes, elimination or modification of movement practices, and a reduced amount of required homework practice.

MINDFULNESS FOR PHYSICAL AND PSYCHOLOGICAL CONDITIONS AND EMOTIONAL WELL-BEING

A significant body of mindfulness research suggests the potential for MBIs to reduce the burden of age-associated chronic diseases. Evidence based on meta-analyses of randomized controlled trials exists for the ability of mindfulness to lower blood pressure and to improve the psychological symptoms and quality of life in cancer patients. Randomized controlled trials also support the ability of MBIs to reduce pain in a number of chronic pain syndromes, improve diabetic control, and improve symptoms of irritable bowel syndrome,[31] and reduce morbid events in high-risk patients with coronary artery disease.[32] A meta-analysis of studies of MBIs for psychological conditions supports the benefits of mindfulness for anxiety, depression, and pain.[33] These studies of adult participants suggest benefit in terms of the overall burden of disease and distress in older adults, but data from studies specifically targeting older adults are less robust.

MINDFULNESS FOR CHRONIC PAIN IN OLDER ADULTS

Morone et al.'s positive study of mindfulness for older adults with chronic low back pain[34] supports the findings of Goyal et al.'s meta-analysis of studies for adults of all ages,[33] but more studies are needed. Practical use of mind–body modalities for chronic pain are reviewed in detail in Chapter 12.

MINDFULNESS FOR CAREGIVERS

Caregiver burden is associated with an increased risk for depression, adverse health outcomes, dementia, and death. McBee and Bloom offer a review of the evidence supporting the benefits of MBIs both for informal caregivers (family and friends) and for paid professional caregivers, for whom the stresses of caring for complex geriatric patients may lead to burnout.[35]

REFERENCES

1. Puchalski CM, Vitillo R, Hull SK, Reller N. Improving the spiritual dimension of whole person care: Reaching national and international consensus. *J Palliat Med.* 2014 Jun 1;17(6):642–656.
2. Monod S, Martin E, Spencer B, Rochat E, Bula C. Validation of the Spiritual Distress Assessment Tool in older hospitalized patients. *BMC Geriatr.* 2012 Mar 29;12(1):13.
3. Salsman JM, Fitchett G, Merluzzi TV, Sherman AC, Park CL. Religion, spirituality, and health outcomes in cancer: A case for a meta-analytic investigation. *Cancer.* 2015 Nov 1;121(21):3754–3759.
4. Ferrell B, Sun V, Hurria A, Cristea M, Raz DJ, Kim JY, et al. Interdisciplinary palliative care for patients with lung cancer. *J Pain Symptom Manage.* 2015;50(6):758–767.
5. *Spiritual Care Matters: An Introductory Resource for all NHS Scotland Staff.* Edinburgh: NHS Education for Scotland, 2009.
6. Puchalski C, Ferrell B, Virani R, Otis-Green S, Baird P, Bull J, et al. Improving the quality of spiritual care as a dimension of palliative care: the report of the consensus conference. *J Palliat Med.* 2009;12(10):885–904.
7. National Consensus Project for Quality Palliative Care. *Clinical Practice Guidelines for Quality Palliative Care, 2009.* Pittsburgh, PA: National Consensus Project for Quality Palliative Care, 2012;2.
8. Jafari N, Roth K, Puchalski C. Spiritual Care. In: Halter JB, Ouslander JG, Studenski S, High KP, Asthana S, Supiano MA, & Ritchie C (eds.), *Hazzard's Geriatric Medicine and Gerontology, 7e.* New York: McGraw-Hill, 2016:885–896.
9. Daaleman TP, Perera S, Studenski SA. Religion, spirituality, and health status in geriatric outpatients. *Ann Fam Med.* 2004 Jan-Feb;2(1):49–53.
10. You KS, Lee H, Fitzpatrick JJ, et al. Spirituality, depression, living alone, and perceived health among Korean older adults in the community. *Arch Psychiatr Nurs.* 2009;23(4):309–322.
11. Singh D, Kedare J. A study of depression in medically ill elderly patients with respect to coping strategies and spirituality as a way of coping. *J Geriatr Mental Health.* 2014;1(2):83.

12. Manning LK. Enduring as lived experience: Exploring the essence of spiritual resilience for women in late life. *J Relig Health.* 2014 Apr;53(2):352–362.

13. Tornstam L. Gerotranscendence: The contemplative dimension of aging. *J Aging Studies.* 1997;11(2):143–154.

14. Holland JC, Bultz BD. (2007). The NCCN guideline for distress management: A case for making distress the sixth vital sign. *Journal of the National Comprehensive Cancer Network*, 2007;5(1):3–7.

15. Puchalski C, Ferrell B. *Making Health Care Whole: Integrating Spirituality into Patient Care.* West Conshohocken, PA: Templeton; 2011.

16. MacKinlay E, Trevitt C. *Facilitating Spiritual Reminiscence for People with Dementia.* London, United Kingdom: Jessica Kingsley Publishers; 2015.

17. Wu LF, Koo M. Randomized controlled trial of a six-week spiritual reminiscence intervention on hope, life satisfaction, and spiritual well-being in elderly with mild and moderate dementia. *Int J Geriatr Psychiatry.* 2016 Feb 1;31(2):120–127.

18. MacKinlay E, Trevitt C. Living in aged care: Using spiritual reminiscence to enhance meaning in life for those with dementia. *Int J Mental Health Nurs.* 2010;19(6):394–401.

19. Helm HM, Hays JC, Flint EP, Koenig HG, Blazer DG. Does private religious activity prolong survival? A six-year follow-up study of 3,851 older adults. *J Gerontol A Biol Sci Med Sci.* 2000 Jul;55(7):M400–M405.

20. Benson H. *The Relaxation Response.* New York: William Morrow & Co.; 1975.

21. Koenig HG, McCullough ME, Larson DB. *Handbook of Religion and Health.* New York: Oxford University Press; 2001.

22. Wood AM, et al. Gratitude and well-being: A review and theoretical integration. *Clinical Psychology Review.* 2010;30:890–905.

23. Worthington EL, Jr. *Dimensions of Forgiveness: Psychological Research and Theological Perspectives.* Philadelphia: Templeton Foundation Press; 1998.

24. McCullough ME, Pargament KI, Thoresen CE, eds. *Forgiveness: Theory, Research, and Practice.* New York: Guilford; 2000.

25. Breitbart W, Heller KS. Reframing hope: Meaning-centered care for patients near the end of life. *J Palliative Med.* 2003;6:979–988.

26. Chochinov HM, Hack T, Hassard T, Kristjanson LJ, McClement S, Harlos M. Dignity therapy: A novel psychotherapeutic intervention for patients near the end of life. *J Clin Oncol.* 2005 Aug 20;23(24):5520–5525.

27. Hewson P, Rowold J, Sichler C, Walter W. Are healing ceremonies useful for enhancing quality of life? *J Altern Complement Med.* 2014;20(9):713–717.

28. Hewson PD, Rowold J. Do spiritual ceremonies affect participants' quality of life? A pilot study. *Complementary Therapies in Clinical Practice.* 2012;18(3):177–181.

29. Geiger PJ, Boggero IA, Brake CA, et al. Mindfulness-based interventions for older adults: A review of the effects on physical and emotional well-being. *Mindfulness.* 2016;7(2):296–307.

30. McBee L. *Mindfulness-Based Elder Care: A CAM Model for Frail Elders and Their Caregivers.* New York: Springer Publishing Co; 2008.

31. Carlson LE. Mindfulness-based interventions for physical conditions: A narrative review evaluating levels of evidence. *ISRN Psychiatry*. Volume 2012, Article ID 651583;2012:1–21.

32. Schneider RH, Grim CE, Rainforth MV, et al. Stress reduction in the secondary prevention of cardiovascular disease: Randomized, controlled trial of transcendental meditation and health education in Blacks. *Circ Cardiovasc Qual Outcomes*. 2012 Nov;5(6):750–758.

33. Goyal M, Singh S, Sibinga EM, et al. Meditation programs for psychological stress and well-being: A systematic review and meta-analysis. *JAMA Internal Med*. 2014;174(3):357–368.

34. Morone NE, Greco CM, Moore CG, et al. A mind-body program for older adults with chronic low back pain: A randomized clinical trial. *JAMA Internal Med*. 2016;176(3):329–337.

35. McBee L, Bloom P. Is aging a disease? Mental health issues and approaches for elders and caregivers. In Shonin E, et al (eds.), *Mindfulness and Buddhist-Derived Approaches in Mental Health and Addiction: Advances in Mental Health and Addiction*. Switzerland: Springer International Publishing; 2016:348–353.

10

Men's Health

GEORGE MUÑOZ AND MIKHAIL KOGAN

Case Studies

Mike T. is a 62-year-old executive who is experiencing some decreased energy, and despite working out 3 or 4 days a week and taking vitamins and protein shakes, he can't lose weight or improve his plateaued strength. He has also been experiencing decreased libido in the last 9 to 12 months. As part of his yearly annual physical, he says he would like direction and evaluation of his symptoms, and his wife has urged him to "get checked out." He presents to you and upon further questioning admits that he also has erectile dysfunction, which is new since last year. How would you approach Mike's clinical issues, and what options would you consider reasonable for him? What nutraceuticals would you recommend? What about testosterone hormone replacement and its benefits and risks? Would you advise prostate monitoring? Is there any other specific testing to consider with his erectile dysfunction?

Gary G. is a 65-year-old insurance broker who is complaining of increasing difficulty with urination and increased urinary frequency and wants to know what to do. He looked online and is concerned about prostate cancer versus benign prostatic hypertrophy. He is now quite overweight, and last year he was exhibiting some symptoms of pre-metabolic syndrome on examination and based on laboratory results. This year, his waist is 42 inches, and he has mild hyperglycemia with a fasting blood sugar level of 104 mg/dl, an HsBA1C of 6.8%, elevated fasting triglyceride levels, and a fasting insulin of 30 units. His current prostate-specific antigen (PSA) level is 3.5, which is 0.5 higher than 2 years ago and currently at 25% free PSA. He wants to know what to do and is ready to follow your advice completely. What testing, recommendations, supplements, and medications are reasonable to consider for Gary? What is the relationship with pro-inflammatory metabolic syndrome, prostate health, and testosterone hormone levels? Is replacing testosterone enough for Gary to reach goals of optimal healthy aging?

Why Men's Health?

Many men underutilize health care for a number of reasons, including habit, societal or personal bias, fear, denial, and even a macho attitude of "unless I'm bleeding" or "unless it's falling off, I will just carry on." Some of these beliefs are deeply engrained and if not adjusted can result in an unnecessary and even dangerous delay in seeking care for potentially dangerous conditions. Because the general health system is mostly concerned with prevention of common chronic maladies such as cardiovascular disease, less time is usually spent on men's sexual health and prevention than for their counterpart in women's gynecologic care. Hence, men are more sideline observers to the entire health care process, using services only for "problems." If no problems are perceived, then they see no reason to seek a preventive or wellness type of visit and discuss more intimate questions about sexuality, prostate health, and other personal health matters with a health practitioner with whom they have established a bond over time.

Paradoxically, there is now a plethora of advertisements in media of all types and social discussions about male sexual performance, with an emphasis on testosterone deficiency or erectile dysfunction that supposedly can be cured like a headache just by taking the correct little pill. Unfortunately, many times, the general discussion that should accompany these themes is missing. Possible side effects, comorbidities, prostate health, prostate cancer evaluation, goals of testosterone therapies, and overall sexual health, including not only physical but psychological aspects, are glossed over as though only testosterone or a missing ingredient contained within the magic pill could possibly be the singular issue or deficiency in these conditions.

The aim of this chapter is to review nutrition, hormones, natural substances, and integrative aspects to men's health specific to the geriatric population. This segment of the population is growing, and they are more active and want to remain so for as long as possible. Older men therefore are entitled to and demand healthy options and lifestyle education and interventions to meet their future goals, mirroring their female counterparts.[1]

Nutrition Specifics for Men

Men in general have different caloric requirements than woman, but the geriatric male also has different requirements than the younger middle-aged male and the young pre-andropause male, who may be quite a bit more active. Senior women require about 1,500 calories per day versus senior men, who require about 2,200 calories daily for low-activity individuals. This requirement increases according to activity levels and would be about 2,800 calories per day for a very active male. In general, for each level of activity, low, moderate, or high, men require about 400 calories more than women.[2] While there are various healthy eating patterns, including the Mediterranean Diet, Paleo, and even more plant-based diets, individual discretion and preference will obviously play a role in the food patterns any individual selects. In general, reducing red meat consumption and consuming more plant-based foods, fish, and chicken with healthy oils is one general recommendation. The healthy fats from avocado, fatty wild fish (salmon, mackerel, cod, kippers), and other sources should be consumed in moderation. Other sources of monounsaturated fats such as nuts (walnuts, almonds, pistachios) are also recommended along with up to 6 teaspoons of healthy fatty oils (extra-virgin olive oil, coconut oil, avocado oil). How much protein to consume varies with exercise, body frame, and anabolic versus catabolic state. A healthy male who is exercising regularly can consume more calories and higher amounts of protein and unprocessed carbohydrates. However, for a sedentary individual who has a waist size greater than 40 inches and high triglycerides and is prediabetic or diabetic, then total carbohydrate restriction is advised, along with increased vegetable and fiber consumption and limitation of potentially pro-inflammatory red meat and saturated fats.

Flexibility and Balance

For men, a lifelong focus on flexibility is less likely than for women; for this reason, aging men seeking a healthy life are encouraged to consistently add a flexibility regime into their daily life as part of their regular exercise. Tissue flexibility along with spinal flexibility can be trained through repetitive consistent exercises and stretches, which improve biomechanics, gait, posture, and movement. In the event of a sudden jolt, fall, or impact, added flexibility reduces the risk of injury. Martial art disciplines such as tai chi, yoga, and Pilates are all good examples.[3-5]

In addition to flexibility, balance is an often overlooked but critical part of aging male physiology. Good balance is one of the key aspects of fall prevention. All of the above-listed methods that help flexibility also improve balance.[5-7] Please refer to Chapters 3 and 23 for additional information on exercise and falls.

Mind–Body Role for the Healthy Aging Male

The role of the mind–body connection is critical for everyone, but clearly for the aging male, who by sociological determinants and life-table analysis would have a shorter lifespan than his female counterpart.[8] Through the various mind–body constructs, including breathwork, meditation, and movement disciplines such as tai chi, qi gong, yoga, and the like, men may explore mindfulness, movement, and synchronous breathing.

Another key concept for the aging healthy male is the need to maintain a purpose. Everyone needs a purpose, so why is this concept perhaps more relevant in the aging male? Men who maintain a purpose that is congruent with their vision of existence, a soul's purpose, if you will, have an increased chance to remain vital. This is especially true if a spouse or life partner were to pass. Mentoring, meaningful volunteering, and continued learning are ways to keep one's brain, intellect, curiosity, value, and initiative for global societal and personal contributions active even after retirement.

Sexuality

Men's sexuality and sexual health are considered hallmarks of overall health. The same is true of the aging male. Anatomically, cardiovascular health and functionally, endothelial and neurological function, and mental health are pillars of healthy men's sexuality.[9,10] Erectile dysfunction (ED) appears to be a societal focus and is of great importance to all males, including the aging man. Loss of adequate blood supply due to atherosclerosis or neurogenic causes (diabetes, spinal caudal nerve impingement, or iatrogenic causes such as prostate cancer surgery complications) can be physical causes of impotence.[11] Aside from these situations, psychogenic causes include stress, a poor relationship, or other psychosocial factors that may require psychological or psychiatric intervention.[11] The aging male looks to maintain healthy sexual function primarily by maintaining an overall healthy lifestyle, as has been outlined in many sections and chapters of this book.

Erectile Dysfunction

PATHOPHYSIOLOGY

ED is a highly important aspect of men's health, including the aging male. Its impact on quality of life, self-esteem, and relationships cannot be overstated. For this reason, ED is considered a quality-of-life condition for which even the National Institute of Health has weighed in with an official descriptor that includes "an inability to achieve or maintain an erection sufficient for satisfactory sexual performance."[12] An aging male's sexual function entails a complex series of biological activities intertwined with and potentially affected by psychological factors and interactions that either do or don't result in an erection. The interplay of these biological functions and their effect on neurotransmitters, smooth muscle, and endothelial function or dysfunction result in blood flow changes to the cavernous sinusoids. Molecular changes in the endothelium and cell to cell, involving potent chemicals such as nitrous oxide, result in these and other physiological changes of smooth muscle altering venous return flow and ultimately an erection.

The potential causes of ED are many and reflect an assessment of overall health; cardiovascular risk assessment factors, including obesity, smoking, inactivity, and elevated lipids; diabetes; and the entire array of psychosocial situations, past and present, that can alter this complex physiological process. A careful history and safe environment for the male patient is critical to establish what factors, physiological and psychological, are playing a role in the ED landscape. Polypharmacy and drug-induced causes also need to be assessed, including common medications such as antihistamines, selective serotonin reuptake inhibitors, and even some cardiac medications such as beta blockers. Standardized metrics for assessing sexual health regarding ED exist and include the IIEF-3.[13]

THERAPY

First-line pharmacotherapies for ED include all the drugs in the phosphodiesterase-5 (PDE5) inhibitor class, sildenafil and its subsequent alternatives, vardenafil, and tadalafil. Sildenafil's marked efficacy has been well established.[14] Since that study was released, enhanced and other non-FDA uses of this class of drugs have exploded due to their potent effects on endothelial cell function; they have been used to promote wound healing and in some cases of severe primary hypertension. For geriatric males, however, the rule that always applies in integrative medicine remains true. Despite the efficacy of the PDE5 class of drugs, both the patient and physician should focus their attention on all the key anti-inflammatory lifestyle elements reviewed in other chapters in this book. All pro-inflammatory conditions, metabolic syndrome, obesity, and diabetes should be treated aggressively. Finally, the role of andropause and testosterone deficiency, when indicated by symptom assessment and confirmed by serum assessment of free testosterone, may or should be corrected as well.

Aphrodisiac botanicals are a topic of interest globally and have been over the ages. From the Andes, maca (*Lepidium meyenii*) is a root botanical that has aphrodisiac and fertility properties and has been used for hundreds and perhaps thousands of years.[15,16] A well-known botanical from Asia, *Panax ginseng*, has been studied for use in ED with positive results, despite the dosing variations in many studies.[17] Its overall safety and relatively low cost make it a worthwhile consideration. Finally, leveraging the nitrous oxide pathway, L-arginine looks to improve endothelial function as a strategy for ED. While trial data are mixed, the other benefits of L-arginine include its use as a vasodilator with blood pressure–lowering effects and improvement in heart failure, peripheral vascular disease, and heart disease. While the Mayo Clinic gives it a grade of C, its high safety profile and possible additional beneficial effects make it worth a try.[18] The typical supplemental dose is about 3 to 8 gm/day and is safe. The typical Western diet contains about 5 gm of L-arginine.[19] Of note, L-arginine should not be combined with PDE5 inhibitors. In one small study, adding 40 mg of pycnogenol further increased the efficacy of L-arginine.[20]

As with other conditions, ED lends itself to treatment with psychotherapy, acupuncture, and stress-reducing programs utilizing mind–body interventions. The benefit of acupuncture in psychogenic ED was impressive at about 68% in one study, so it should be considered a viable treatment approach.[21]

Prostate Health

Prostate health is a key aspect of the aging male's health concerns. From a practical and genitourinary standpoint, benign prostatic hypertrophy (BPH) is common part of normal aging and impacts daily life for the aging male. Advances in pharmacotherapy and urological procedures can significantly improve the symptoms of BPH if needed.[22] Medications include the alpha-1 blocking drugs such as tamsulosin and alfuzosin as well as the 5a reductase inhibitors, finasteride and dutasteride. All can be used to reduce severe symptoms of BPH that have not responded to natural supplements such as *Pygeum africanum*, lycopene, saw palmetto, flower pollen, stinging nettle, red clover, turmeric (curcumin), and numerous others marketed widely. The best-studied herbal for BPH, saw palmetto, is typically used at 160 mg twice daily but has not been shown to be effective, even at much higher doses.[23] However, the above botanicals appear to be safe, and given the typically mild symptoms at early stages, a trial of botanicals can make sense. Also, botanicals with spasmolytic activity can be helpful; these include *Ammi visnaga* fruit (1 ml tid, with a mild sedative effect), *Valeriana* spp root (2–3 ml tid, also associated with mild sedation), and *Gelsenium sempervirens* root (10 gtt tid, also associated with sedation).[1]

It is also worth noting that some exercises may aggravate prostate function, such as excessive bike riding for many hours on a rigid seat. Accommodations, padding, and moderation and reduction of this activity are recommended if prostate symptoms increase in conjunction with bicycling. Similar issues may be seen with long-distance runners; use of an appropriate athletic supporter is recommended in these settings to minimize symptoms.

Bone Health

The prevention, recognition, and treatment of osteoporosis in men involves a multitiered approach and a change in mindset toward being proactive rather than solely reactive. Geriatric integrative men's health requires a focus on this specific aspect of men's health as the emphasis historically has been on women as the sole or primary individuals with osteoporosis. In 2008 statement the American College of Physicians recommended "that clinicians periodically perform individualized assessment of risk factors for osteoporosis in older men."[24] Indeed, testosterone-deficient men of any age should be considered for screening for osteoporosis.[25,26] Additionally, if family history, prior fractures, endocrine metabolic conditions (thyroid dysfunction, hyperparathyroidism, vitamin D deficiency, hyper-adrenal states, certain drug exposures [warfarin, seizure medications, chronic use of antacids and proton pump inhibitors]), spinal deformity and kyphosis, or a history of steroid exposure exist or there are other fixed risk factors such as immobility, rheumatoid arthritis, or nutritional deficiency as a result of colitis or Crohn's disease, then screening should be performed.

Why is bone health so important to the aging male? First, it has been well established that from a morbidity and mortality perspective, osteoporosis and resultant complications are of high importance and generally underpublicized in men.[27] This important fact relating to aging men is either not widely known or severely understated, and hence the need for more impactful clinical emphasis, education, and prevention. Premature andropause is associated with a decrease in bone mass and an increased risk of osteopenia and osteoporosis as is the case for the normal aging andropausal male. The same risk factors that are applicable to women apply to the aging male as well and are reviewed in detail in Chapter 15.

Vitamin D3 or 25-hydroxy vitamin D3 merits its own detailed discussion as an important overall health factor for the aging male. There are a few key points worth mentioning. First, there is no consensus as to what the optimal daily dose is or what the serum level of vitamin D3 should be across the board. The Institute of Medicine's 2010 recommendation doubled the recommended daily dosage for adults up to age 70 to 600 international units daily; the IOM recommended that individuals 71 years old and older should consume 800 international units daily.[28] Similarly, the "tolerable upper limit" was raised from 2,000 international units to 4,000 international units daily for individuals 9 years old and up, which speaks to the general safety of its use in population health. There are many experts on vitamin D who believe that these recommendations are significantly too low, and there is a growing consensus that levels of 40 to 60 ng/ml are more consistent with optimal bone and overall health; others recommend still higher levels between 60 and 80 ng/ml for optimal health because of evidence cited for cancer reduction in both men and women. It is noteworthy that the IOM recommendations are focused on bone health and not the other known associated benefits of vitamin D, including cancer reduction, cardiovascular and immune benefits, and reduced fall risk. Additionally, it should be noted that the vitamin D receptor has over 2,000 binding sites along the entire human genome and therefore plays a genomic transcriptional role in gene expression that is ubiquitous.[29] However, it is impractical for most individuals to avail themselves of natural sunlight in nonpeak hours for 30 minutes daily without the use of sunblock.[30] For this reason, vitamin D3 supplementation is considered a must for the aging male unless natural daily sunlight exposure is consistently practiced.

Vitamin D is a pro-hormone and binds to the vitamin D receptor that is genetically predetermined. The free hormone level will be the active hormone, as is the case with other complex steroid types or sex hormones. Many people will require between 2,000 and 10,000 international units daily; the dosage needs to be customized based on the indication, body size, and absorption. Ongoing monitoring of serum levels of vitamin D3 is required. Having said this, though, it is very difficult to overdose on vitamin D3. The current 30 to 100 ng/ml dosage offers a wide therapeutic range to classify as "normal," yet the optimal clinical benefits many times are seen at higher-than-recommended levels when monitoring bone marker suppression as a therapeutic endpoint. Overdose symptoms in an adult would need to be in the range of 200 to 300 ng/ml, and upper zone levels of 80 to 100 ng/ml are generally quite safe. If concern exists, urinary measurement of calcium may be carried out to preclude potential stone formation in at-risk individuals. For additional management details refer to Chapter 13 on osteoporosis.

Testosterone Deficiency

Testosterone deficiency (TD) is a clinical condition and not solely a laboratory-determined diagnosis. Signs and symptoms can be physical, psychological, and sexual. Prevalence rates around 38% to 39% have been reported for men 45 years and older, with a general rule of thumb that levels of free testosterone (the bioactive form) fall at about 1.4% per year in men age 39 to 70.[31]

Complementary and alternative medicine interventions for TD mirror what was stated above for ED. The primary focus is on maintaining an optimal lifestyle that includes balanced exercise with about 50/50 resistive training and cardio at the optimal recommendations weekly, good and restful deep sleep, mind–body interventions for stress reduction, and conventional focus and therapy for all pro-inflammatory conditions (metabolic syndrome, hypertension, diabetes, etc.). Irrespective of this healthy lifestyle, some men will experience symptoms of TD that include fatigue, decreased libido, ED, decreased muscle strength, or ineffective training results despite vigorous attempts, along with mood and sleep disturbances.[32] Additional symptoms or conditions associated with TD include decreased lean body mass, decreased bone mass, and increased body fat, a triad the aging male wants to avoid for optimal health and aging.[33]

Physical symptoms include diminished muscle mass, strength, and bone mineral density, and an increase in the 3 "F's," fragility, fat, and fatigue. None of these are desirable for the optimally aging male. **Sexual symptoms** include diminished libido, morning awakening erections (a surrogate of health, adequate testosterone level, and cardiovascular health), ED, and sexual performance. **Psychological symptoms** include decreased mood and impaired cognition, memory, and overall sense of well-being. These conditions are avoidable with proper testosterone replacement in the aging male.[34]

After TD has been diagnosed the use of testosterone replacement therapy should be considered. The manner of replacement depends on patient and physician preferences or experience. Options include transdermal delivery or injectable forms of testosterone or pellets, as oral replacement in general is too toxic. Furthermore, the other metabolic surrogate associations of TD, including metabolic syndrome, insulin resistance, and hypertension, are noteworthy and another reason to address this hormonal deficiency state in the aging male.[35,36]

Treatment of TD should be focused on restoring levels back to normal physiological or optimal youthful levels of free testosterone, not simply for that person's age and not by total testosterone measurement. By doing so, the treating physician optimizes the health of the aging male and restores normal youthful physiological functions and helps to slow the aging process along with a whole-person, mind, body, and spirit approach. Physicians should avoid prescribing dosages that exceed the normal optimal physiological amounts of youth. Doing so increases the risk of side effects such as aggressiveness, excessive acne, increased blood viscosity, hemoglobin, hematocrit above 50%, and red blood cell counts and can create a pro-inflammatory state with diminishing returns. Dosing targets proposed in the literature range from 300 to 1,050 ng/ml of total testosterone.[37] The exact level of testosterone therapy needs to be individualized for patients as there is no clear consensus, but again, optimal youthful levels with minimal clinical side effects should be the goal.

There are several testosterone preparations available, including injectable, testosterone cypionate or depo-testosterone (200 mg/cc) and enanthate (Delatestryl) and mixed esters and very-long-acting compounds, both in brand-name and in compounded forms. Testosterone undecanoate injections (Nebido, Aveed)) are used when infrequent administration is desired, usually 4–5 injections/year. Transdermal delivery gels (Androgel, Testim), patches (Androderm, Testoderm TTS), or compounded creams and gels alsoexist for clinical use as well as buccal, sublingual, and scrotal patches. Oral therapies are not approved or widely used in the United States.

Injectable testosterone cypionate of 200 mg/cc in doses of 0.3 to 0.5 cc twice weekly are usual and customary for most individuals. Twice-weekly dosing tends to reduce the high peak and low trough that can occur with weekly, every other week, or monthly dosing, avoiding the excessive rebound and withdrawal effects experienced by men given high and infrequent dosing. Once a stable dose has been achieved by monitoring symptoms, effect, and free levels of testosterone, PSA, and any other hormone being replaced in men (e.g., DHEA, HCG, or thyroid), monitoring can be done every 3 months.[38] Prior to that, monthly determinations or even more frequent measurements of testosterone may be needed to fine-tune doses.

What about some of the controversies we and aging males may hear about testosterone replacement therapy related to safety? A common misconception is that testosterone causes prostate cancer.[39] To date, there is no association between testosterone levels and prostate cancer development.[40] Aging men should therefore be reassured accordingly. From a practical standpoint, the mainstay of monitoring should be focused on the prostate health and hematological bone marrow response with subsequent increase in red blood cells and potential serum viscosity. Hematocrits higher than 50% merit close follow-up and levels of 52% to 55% merit dose reduction, dose holds, or possibly discontinuation pending blood donation as a therapeutic intervention. Adequate hydration recommendations by the patient and physician dose adjustments are possibilities to consider. Prostate guidelines include monitoring every 3 to 6 months, and if the PSA is rising at a slope of more than 1.0 per year and the free PSA percentage is less than 20 to 25, then a prostate biopsy and advanced imaging and urologic examination should be considered, along with a temporary hold of testosterone replacement.[38]

Cardiovascular events have recently been points of controversy in some poorly controlled studies where the causality of the testosterone intervention has not been proven. As cited by Morgantaler recently, "*A recent retrospective study reporting increased risk of cardiovascular events and death with testosterone therapy has received extensive media attention. However, the authors' conclusions are highly questionable given the extensive data manipulation and serious methodological errors. Indeed, a rich body of literature strongly suggests that testosterone therapy offers cardiovascular benefits.*"[41] The many cardiovascular benefits of testosterone therapy, including reduced inflammation and insulin resistance and secondary benefits on endothelial function, are all desirable for the aging man. These salutary effects tip the scales significantly in favor of testosterone replacement as a central offering for the aging male, especially when coupled with an optimal lifestyle.

A brief word about Dehydroepiandrosterone (DHEA) and thyroid replacement in aging men. First, with respect to DHEA, this androgen hormone has various benefits, as does testosterone, in improving metabolism, reducing insulin resistance, and increasing lean mass, and additionally has beneficial immune-modulating effects.[42] Optimal youthful levels for the aging male are between 100 and 300 mcg/dl of DHEA-sulfate, and doses between 25 and 75 mg once or twice daily of bioavailable micronized DHEA are recommended. Additional benefits include improvement in bone mass, although this is not an FDA-approved use.

Thyroid hormone is also underrated in the aging male as part of the overall hormone evaluation. Undiagnosed and underdiagnosed thyroid disorders are relatively common and tend to occur in concert with metabolic syndrome, obesity, and insulin resistance and in patients with classic hypothyroid symptoms, including fatigue, constipation, and cold intolerance, and with skin, hair, and nail changes. Measuring TSH to determine if a patient is hypothyroid is inadequate. The clinical symptoms and direct measurement of the active thyroid hormones, free T3 and free T4, are essential as well as reverse T3 for conversion to assess bioconversion pathways. Replacement with levothyroxine (Synthroid) alone provides only T4 and may prove inadequate for some patients; they may need T3 replacement as well, using either a brand-name product (Cytomel) or compounded thyroid formulas containing both T3 and

T4. The body requires T3 for function and the brain utilizes T4. Optimal T3 levels should be near 4.0 and free T4 should be close to 1.5. Borderline TSH levels of 4.0 to 5.0 may be associated with significant hypothyroid symptoms, and precise T3 and T4 determinations many times indicate low or suboptimal levels of these thyroid hormones that when corrected to youthful ranges improve the patient significantly. Correcting underactive thyroid conditions produces a benefit in terms of energy, mental state, mood, metabolism, lipid profiles, and overall function, a reduction in body fat, and weight loss. Aging men with depressive symptoms should be assessed for subclinical or overt hypothyroidism along with testosterone and DHEA deficiencies as part of their overall wellness and whole-body approaches. For a detailed discussion on thyroid hormone replacement please refer to Chapter 14.

Summary

The healthy aging man has various options to choose for the prevention of structural bone health, fall prevention, and optimal metabolic state. These options result in reduced inflammation and body fat and increased muscle mass, strength, and vitality. A healthy libido, healthy sexual function, and enhanced mood and cognition are all attainable with proper exercise, optimal nutrition, and proper deep restful sleep. The understanding of testosterone replacement as a bioidentical therapeutic and preventive medicine intervention fits into the overall paradigm to achieve healthy aging for men.

REFERENCES

1. Spar, M, Munoz G. *Integrative Men's Health*. Oxford: Oxford University Press; 2014.
2. NIH Seniors Health. https://nihseniorhealth.gov/eatingwellasyougetolder/knowhowmuchtoeat/01.
3. Farinatti PT, Rubini EC, Silva EB, Vanfraechem JH. Flexibility of the elderly after one-year practice of yoga and calisthenics. *Int J Yoga Therap*. 2014;24:71–77. http://www.ncbi.nlm.nih.gov/pubmed/25858653.
4. Azevedo S De, Simas J, Machado Z, Jonck V. The effect of Pilates method on elderly flexibility. *Fisioter em Mov*. 2014;27(2):181–188. doi:10.1590/0103-5150.027.002.AO03.
5. Huang Y, Liu X. Improvement of balance control ability and flexibility in the elderly Tai Chi Chuan (TCC) practitioners: A systematic review and meta-analysis. *Arch Gerontol Geriatr*. 2015;60(2):233–238. doi:10.1016/j.archger.2014.10.016.
6. Schmid AA, van Puymbroeck M, Koceja DM. Effect of a 12-week yoga intervention on fear of falling and balance in older adults: A pilot study. *Arch Phys Med Rehabil*. 2010;91(4):576–583. doi:10.1016/j.apmr.2009.12.018.

7. de Oliveira Francisco C, de Almeida Fagundes A, Gorges B. Effects of Pilates method in elderly people: Systematic review of randomized controlled trials. *J Bodyw Mov Ther.* 2015;19(3):500–508. doi:10.1016/j.jbmt.2015.03.003.

8. Seifarth JE, McGowan CL, Milne KJ. Sex and life expectancy. *Gend Med.* 2012;9(6):390–401. doi:10.1016/j.genm.2012.10.001.

9. Kaiser FE. Sexuality in the elderly. *Urol Clin North Am.* 1996;23(1):99–109. doi:10.1016/S0094-0143(05)70296-2.

10. Jagus CE, Benbow SM. Sexuality in older men with mental health problems. *Sex Relatsh Ther.* 2002;17(December 2012):271–279. doi:10.1080/14681990220149077.

11. Shamloul R, Ghanem H. Erectile dysfunction. *Lancet.* 2013;381(9861):153–165. doi:10.1016/S0140-6736(12)60520-0.

12. NIH Consensus Conference. NIH Consensus Development Panel on Impotence. *Impot JAMA.* 1993;270(4):83–90. doi:10.1001/jama.1993.03510010089036.Text.

13. Rosen RC, Cappelleri JC, Smith MD, Lipsky J, Peña BM. Development and evaluation of an abridged, 5-item version of the International Index of Erectile Function (IIEF-5) as a diagnostic tool for erectile dysfunction. *Int J Impot Res.* 1999;11(6): 319–326. doi:10.1038/sj.ijir.3900472.

14. Salonia A, Rigatti P, Montorsi F. Sildenafil in erectile dysfunction: a critical review. *Curr Med Res Opin.* 2003;19(4):241–262. doi:10.1185/030079903125001839.

15. Zenico T, Cicero AFG, Valmorri L, Mercuriali M, Bercovich E. Subjective effects of *Lepidium meyenii* (Maca) extract on well-being and sexual performances in patients with mild erectile dysfunction: A randomised, double-blind clinical trial. *Andrologia.* 2009;41(2):95–99. doi:10.1111/j.1439-0272.2008.00892.x.

16. Patel DK, Kumar R, Prasad SK, Hemalatha S. Pharmacologically screened aphrodisiac plant: A review of current scientific literature. *Asian Pac J Trop Biomed.* 2011;1(Suppl. 1). doi:10.1016/S2221-1691(11)60140-8.

17. Nocerino E, Amato M, Izzo AA. The aphrodisiac and adaptogenic properties of ginseng. *Fitoterapia.* 2000;71(Supp. 1). doi:10.1016/S0367-326X(00)00170-2.

18. MayoClinicArginineReview.http://www.mayoclinic.org/drugs-supplements/arginine/evidence/HRB-20058733

19. Böger RH. The pharmacodynamics of L-arginine. *Altern Ther Health Med.* 2014;20(3):48–54. doi:10.3945/ajcn.110.005132.1.

20. Stanislavov R, Nikolova V. Treatment of erectile dysfunction with pycnogenol and L-arginine. *J Sex Marital Ther.* 2003;29(3):207–213. doi:10.1080/00926230390155104.

21. Engelhardt P, Daha L, Zils T, Simak R, Kö Nig K, Pflü Ger H. Acupuncture in the treatment of psychogenic erectile dysfunction: first results of a prospective randomized placebo-controlled study. *Int J Impot Res.* 2003;15:343–346. doi:10.1038/sj.ijir.3901021.

22. van Rij S, Gilling P. Recent advances in treatment for benign prostatic hyperplasia. *F1000Research.* 2015;4(0):1–7. doi:10.12688/f1000research.7063.1.

23. Crawford-Faucher A. Saw palmetto extract ineffective for BPH symptoms. *Am Fam Physician.* 2012;85(12):1202. doi:10.1370/afm.1385.

24. Qaseem A, Snow V, Shekelle P, Hopkins R, Forciea MA, Owens DK. Screening for osteoporosis in men: A clinical practice guideline from the American College of Physicians. *Ann Intern Med.* 2008;148(9):680–684.

25. Fink HA, Ewing SK, Ensrud KE, et al. Association of testosterone and estradiol deficiency with osteoporosis and rapid bone loss in older men. *J Clin Endocrinol Metab.* 2006;91(10):3908–3915. doi:10.1210/jc.2006-0173.

26. Martin AC. Osteoporosis in men: a review of endogenous sex hormones and testosterone replacement therapy. *J Pharm Pract.* 2011;24(3):307–315. doi:10.1177/0897190010397716.

27. Haentjens P, Magaziner J, Colón-Emeric CS, et al. Meta-analysis: Excess mortality after hip fracture among older women and men. *Ann Intern Med.* 2010;152(6): 380–390. doi:10.7326/0003-4819-152-6-201003160-00008.

28. 2010 IOM report—Vitamin D intake recommendation. http://www.nationalacademies.org/hmd/Reports/2010/Dietary-Reference-Intakes-for-Calcium-and-Vitamin-D.aspx

29. Ramagopalan SV, Heger A, Berlanga AJ, et al. A ChIP-seq defined genome-wide map of vitamin D receptor binding: Associations with disease and evolution. *Genome Res.* 2010;20(10):1352–1360. doi:10.1101/gr.107920.110.

30. Terushkin V, Bender A, Psaty EL, Engelsen O, Wang SQ, Halpern AC. Estimated equivalency of vitamin D production from natural sun exposure versus oral vitamin D supplementation across seasons at two US latitudes. *J Am Acad Dermatol.* 2010;62(6). doi:10.1016/j.jaad.2009.07.028.

31. Gray A, Feldman HA, Mckinlay JB, Longcope C. Age, disease, and changing sex hormone levels in middle-aged men: Results of the Massachusetts Male Aging Study. *J Clin Endocrinol Metab.* 1991;73(5):1016–1025. doi:10.1210/jcem-73-5-1016.

32. Schulman CC, Fusco F, Martin Morales A, Tostain J, Vendeira P, Zitzmann M. Testosterone deficiency: A common, unrecognised syndrome? *Eur Urol Suppl.* 2009;8(9):772–777. doi:10.1016/j.eursup.2009.05.003.

33. Dandona P, Rosenberg MT. A practical guide to male hypogonadism in the primary care setting. *Int J Clin Pract.* 2010;64(6):682–696. doi:10.1111/j.1742-1241.2010.02355.x.

34. Petak SM, Nankin HR, Spark RF, Swerdloff RS, Rodriguez-Rigau LJ. American Association of Clinical Endocrinologists Medical Guidelines for clinical practice for the evaluation and treatment of hypogonadism in adult male patients—2002 update. *Endocr Pract.* 2002;8(6):440–456.

35. Zitzmann M. Testosterone deficiency, insulin resistance and the metabolic syndrome. *Nat Rev Endocrinol.* 2009;5(12):673–681. doi:10.1038/nrendo.2009.212.

36. Kupelian V, Page ST, Araujo AB, Travison TG, Bremner WJ, McKinlay JB. Low sex hormone-binding globulin, total testosterone, and symptomatic androgen deficiency are associated with development of the metabolic syndrome in nonobese men. *J Clin Endocrinol Metab.* 2006;91(3):843–850. doi:10.1210/jc.2005-1326.

37. Miner MM, Sadovsky R. Evolving issues in male hypogonadism: Evaluation, management, and related comorbidities. *Cleve Clin J Med.* 2007;74 Suppl 3. doi:10.3949/ccjm.74.Suppl_3.S38.

38. Rhoden EL, Morgentaler A. Risks of testosterone-replacement therapy and recommendations for monitoring. *N Engl J Med.* 2004;350(5):482–492. doi:10.1056/NEJMra022251.

39. Morgentaler A. Testosterone and prostate cancer: What are the risks for middle-aged men? *Urol Clin North Am.* 2011;38(2):119–124. doi:10.1016/j.ucl.2011.02.002.

40. Calof OM, Singh AB, Lee ML, et al. Adverse events associated with testosterone replacement in middle-aged and older men: A meta-analysis of randomized, placebo-controlled trials. *J Gerontol A Biol Sci Med Sci.* 2005;60(11):1451–1457.

41. Morgentaler A, Miner MM, Caliber M, Guay AT, Khera M, Traish AM. Testosterone therapy and cardiovascular risk: advances and controversies. *Mayo Clin Proc.* 2015;90(2):224–251. doi:10.1016/j.mayocp.2014.10.011.

42. Cameron DR, Braunstein GD. The use of dehydroepiandrosterone therapy in clinical practice. *Treat Endocrinol.* 2005;4(2):95–114. doi:10.2165/00024677-200504020-00004.

11

Women's Health

MARY KENDELL
AND MARGIE WENTZEL

Clinical Case

Barbara is a 55-year-old married mother of two daughters in their late teens. She is a full-time salaried nurse. In addition to her 40 hours per week, her job requires her to be on call 8 hours per week and to attend frequent professional trainings during her off hours. As the oldest and closest daughter to her parents, Barbara has taken on additional responsibilities for their care, including driving them to medical appointments and medication management.

Lately Barbara has been experiencing poor sleep, increasing anxiety, inability to "keep it together," and intermittent hot flashes. She has also noticed discomfort during sexual activity and a significant drop in her libido that is affecting her relationship with her spouse. As a nurse, she is well aware that she will soon go through menopause. However, as a breast cancer survivor of 5 years, she is uncertain as to how she can manage her already annoying symptoms. Barbara comes to you for advice.

Introduction

With a current U.S. life expectancy of 78.8 years, today's woman will spend more than one third of her life postmenopause.[1,2] When discussing the female geriatric patient, it is tempting to focus on menopause solely as a biophysical event. Although the hormonal changes that occur are the same for all women, the experience of menopause will be as unique as the woman herself.

It will be modulated as much by the physiological changes that occur in her body as it will be by her cultural upbringing, thoughts and attitudes about this time in her life, and her current life stressors.[3] Menopause, therefore, should be viewed and evaluated as a bio-psycho-social event. Understanding what underlies a menopausal complaint offers the care provider opportunities for an integrative approach to symptom management, including education and counseling. Helping women understand what is occurring in their bodies can reduce anxiety and facilitate the development of healthy perceptions and positive attitudes toward this phase of life.

By definition, menopause begins 12 months after the cessation of menstruation. The average age of menopause is 52 years. Menopausal symptoms can appear up to 6 years before the final menstrual period and can last for a variable number of years after menopause. This time period is known as the *menopausal transition.*[4] During this time, women can experience a wide range of symptoms such as hot flashes, insomnia, mood changes, irregular periods, and weight gain. As hormone levels fluctuate, symptoms will wax and wane in severity. Table 11.1 lists the effects of estrogen loss on the menopausal female.

Table 11.1. Effects of Estrogen Loss on the Menopausal Female

Body Part/System	Effects of Estrogen Loss
Body Weight	Weight gain of 5 lbs (related to aging and lifestyle changes more than menopause)
Skin	Increased skin thickness and elasticity Loss of collagen Increased laxity, wrinkling, and dyspigmentation Delayed wound healing
Hair	Hair loss (female pattern hair loss [FPHL]); also called androgenic alopecia Telogen effluvium
Eyes	Dry eyes Cataracts (prevalence higher than men of same age)
Ears	Hearing loss; loss of reproductive hormones may contribute
Mouth/Teeth	Gingival thinning/recession causes increase in periodontal inflammation and susceptibility to oral lesions. Decreased bone mineral density is associated with tooth loss and periodontal disease.
Fertility	Decreases with advancing age Age-related symptoms (fibroids, tubal factor, endometriosis) Diminished ovarian reserve

Table 11.1. Continued

Body Part/System	Effects of Estrogen Loss
Uterine Bleeding	90% of women experience 4 to 8 years of cycle changes before menopause (heavier flow of longer duration). Early perimenopause: disturbances in timing and regulation of ovulation Late perimenopause: decreased ovulation
Vasomotor Symptoms	Hot flashes in up to 75% of women for 6 months to 2 years; some women may have symptoms for 10 years or longer
Genitourinary Syndrome of Menopause/ Symptomatic Vulvovaginal Atrophy	Genital dryness, burning, and irritation Lack of vaginal lubrication Impaired sexual function
Urinary Incontinence	Urinary urgency, dysuria, recurrent urinary tract infections
Sexual Function	Dyspareunia due to vaginal atrophy
Sleep Disturbances	Reduced sleep quality due to hot flashes Insomnia, sleep apnea, and restless legs syndrome Common symptom of depression
Headache	Tension type Migraines without aura Migraines with aura associated with increased risk of stroke
Cognition	Poor concentration, memory, and trouble multitasking (during menopausal transition and early postmenopause) May be related due to sleep disturbances and midlife stressors
Psychological Symptoms	Depressed mood Anxiety Decreased sense of well-being History of premenstrual syndrome or postpartum depression is a strong risk factor. Midlife stressors often coincide with the menopausal transition.

While hormonal depletion is universal, not all women will experience the same level of physical or psychological impact from their loss of hormones. Women's perceptions of and attitudes toward this milestone will vary based on their individual health and the quality of their personal relationships.[2,5] These factors, if negative, correlate with an increased amount of symptom reporting by women.[2]

Common symptoms of hormonal loss include vasomotor symptoms (hot flashes and night sweats), mood swings, loss of libido, and genitourinary symptoms (vaginal dryness, dyspareunia, urinary complaints). While estrogen therapy has the most documented efficacy in the management of menopausal symptoms, many women, for a variety of reasons, can't or would prefer not to use hormone replacement therapy (HRT). Regardless of her choice of therapy, symptom management should start with simple strategies and progress to more difficult lifestyle changes. Pharmacotherapeutics should be considered once other strategies have been deemed ineffective.

Vasomotor Symptoms

Vasomotor symptoms are the result of fluctuating estrogen levels in the body. Hot flashes often begin in the menopausal transition period and can last for months or years after menopause. Approximately 75% of women will complain of hot flashes and/or night sweats, making it the most common complaint of menopause.[6] The frequency and severity of hot flashes will vary from one woman to another. Signs and symptoms of hot flashes include:

1. Sudden onset of an intense feeling of heat
2. Heart palpitations
3. Sweating, sometimes followed by cold chills
4. Other symptoms, including acute anxiety, nausea, and dizziness

When these symptoms occur at night, they often result in sleep disturbances, which, in turn, can lead to changes in mood, including irritability and depression.[6]

In evaluating hot flash complaints, it is important to remember that various medical conditions and medications can cause similar symptoms. A thorough physical evaluation and medication review should be undertaken before assuming that hormonal fluctuations are the only underlying etiology for vasomotor symptoms.

Initial management of vasomotor symptoms should include encouraging women to keep track of when and under what circumstances their symptoms occur. This information can guide education about triggers and provide counseling opportunities regarding lifestyle changes.

Commonly identified triggers for hot flashes include cigarette smoking, caffeine, spicy foods, alcohol, anxiety, and stress. Avoiding these triggers and making simple lifestyle changes can help significantly in the management of hot flashes.

The ills of cigarette smoking are well documented. Educating women regarding the correlation between smoking and hot flashes may provide the motivation necessary for smoking cessation.

The initial reported findings of the Women's Health Initiative (WHI) resulted in a sharp decrease in the use of HRT for menopausal symptom management. As a consequence, there has been an increased interest in the use of foods and herbal products containing phytoestrogens. Based on their isoflavone content, soy foods have been particularly popular. To date, no study has assessed the efficacy of these foods utilizing objective measures. Of the small number of studies that have been done using subjective measures, results have been conflicting, so the efficacy of soy foods for the management of menopausal symptoms remains unclear.[7] Diet changes recommended for vasomotor symptom management include staying well hydrated and consuming foods high in tryptophan. Tryptophan is an amino acid necessary for the production of serotonin. In combination with good carbohydrates such as whole grains, consuming foods high in tryptophan will increase the amount of amino acids available for serotonin production. Serotonin plays a key role in mood and has been shown to improve vasomotor symptoms.[8] Foods high in tryptophan include eggs, cheese, chicken, turkey, and soy products.

A result of the use of light box therapy in the treatment of seasonal affective disorder and other mood disorders is an increase in serotonin levels. Recommendations for the timing and amount of Lux exposure vary depending on the disorder being treated.[9] Research indicates that regular exercise, including yoga and tai chi, may be beneficial in improving menopausal symptoms, including mood and vasomotor symptoms.[10,11]

Women should be encouraged to stay well hydrated with cool beverages and wear non-constrictive, breathable, and quick-drying materials. Dressing in layers is another useful strategy. Arriving early to work meetings or social gatherings will allow women to position themselves in the coolest place in the room.

Bedtime strategies include a cool shower before bed, colds packs under a pillow, a fan, turning down the thermostat, and using light cotton clothing and bedding. Having a glass of cold water available on the nightstand may also be useful. Sleep can be further improved with regular exercise and by following the recommendations for good sleep hygiene, including having a consistent hour for sleep and awakening (even on the weekend) and sleeping in a quiet, dark room devoid of all LED readouts.[12] Use of lavender oil, by diffusion or placed topically, may also improve sleep quality.[13] A systematic review and meta-analysis of 31 randomized controlled trials found that acupuncture is associated with a significant reduction in sleep disturbances in women experiencing menopause-related sleep problems.[14]

Central to all other strategies is the management of anxiety and stress. According to a 6-year study published in *Menopause*, hot flashes are tightly linked with anxiety. The study found that women with the highest levels of anxiety were five times more likely to report hot flashes.[15]Strategies to manage stress and anxiety are abundant in the literature. Examples include regular exercise, meditation, yoga, breathwork, and learning to say "no" without feeling guilty.

If avoiding triggers and making lifestyle changes are inadequate to manage vasomotor symptoms and estrogen is not an option, it may be useful to look at non-hormonal prescription medications. Prescription medications used in the management of vasomotor symptoms include antihypertensives, anticonvulsants, and antidepressants.[16] The most commonly used class of non-hormonal prescription medications is the antidepressants, specifically the selective serotonin reuptake inhibitors (SSRIs). A 2014 meta-analysis of 11 randomized controlled trials found that SSRIs were associated with a statistically significant decrease in hot flash frequency.[17] As these medications are classified as antidepressants, they may have the added benefit of improving the mood changes that often occur during menopause. Unfortunately, the use of SSRIs can introduce unwanted side effects such as reduced sexual desire, difficulty reaching orgasm, insomnia, diarrhea, nervousness or agitation, and drowsiness.[18] Prior to being prescribed an SSRI, women must be counseled about potential side effects so they can weigh the benefits against the risks. Counseling regarding side effects will also help women discern between a medication side effect and a new menopausal symptom.

The most popular over-the-counter supplements for vasomotor symptom management include black cohosh, red clover, evening primrose oil, and dong quai. Current studies in the literature do not support the efficacy of their use.[19,20] Concerns have been raised regarding potential side effects related to the use of these supplements.[21]

Skin Changes After Menopause

The integumentary system can be affected by the menopausal transition, as is every other body system. Lack of estrogen and progesterone, and a subsequent increase in testosterone levels, can cause thinning of the skin, increased vascularity, acne, a decrease in skin laxity, and an increase in pigmented lesions. Wound healing may also be impaired.[22] Hair can be affected, including a loss of scalp hair and an increase in unwanted facial hair. Wrinkling of the skin and scalp hair loss can be of great concern to the geriatric patient, as they are noticeable to others and affect body image.[23] It is important for the clinician to be aware of how these changes affect the postmenopausal woman and to be supportive of positive lifestyle changes.

Electrolysis is the only FDA-approved form of permanent hair removal.[24] However, there are many other treatments available in retail or spa settings, as well as in the health care provider's office. These treatments may include epilators (needle, electrolysis, tweezers), waxing, sugaring, threading, and shaving.[25] Laser treatments are used for the removal of unwanted hair and pigmented lesions and intense pulsed light (IPL) therapy for hair removal and treatment of hyperpigmented skin.[26] Oral HRT may decrease the growth of unwanted facial hair.

Scalp hair loss can be treated with locally applied minoxidil, and some sources recommend vitamin and mineral supplementation with zinc, vitamin E, and biotin.[27,28] A healthy diet, moderate exercise, and stress reduction are also strategies for reducing menopause-related hair loss.

Discontinuation of smoking and a decrease in sun exposure can minimize the skin changes of dryness, lax skin, wrinkles, and hyperpigmentation, and offer the patient some control over these postmenopausal effects. Women may also wish to take advantage of Botox and other filler injectables. Adequate oral hydration, a healthy diet, wearing sun-protective clothing, and moisturizing skin are also important ways to minimize skin changes. Moisturizers may contain estrogen or progesterone, and overuse can result in hormone imbalance.[29]

Breast Health

Breast pain or tenderness, which may be referred to as mastalgia or mastodynia, is caused by fluctuations in estrogen and progesterone in perimenopausal women. Many women complain of breast pain similar to when they were premenstrual during their reproductive years. Touching the breast can be exquisitely painful, and this can impact sexual response and activity in the menopausal woman. In addition, skin changes in menopause can create lax connective tissue, which causes the breasts to sag and be uncomfortable. Treatments for breast pain include discontinuation of smoking, decrease in caffeine intake (including coffee, tea, sodas, and chocolate), heat or cold application, and vitamin supplementation (vitamins B and E).[30] Oral evening primrose oil at doses of 500 to 1,000 mg/day has also been used to decrease the pain. However, evidence for these supplements is weak. Purchasing a bra that is properly fitted can relieve pain as well as enhance body image by providing support to the breast tissue. The health care provider can be helpful in providing referral to a specialist in fitting bras, for both menopausal women and breast cancer survivors.

Screening for breast cancer is of utmost importance to the menopausal population. Please see Chapter 4 for more details. Breast cancer becomes more prevalent after menopause because of the loss of beneficial estrogen. The WHI found an increase in the incidence of breast cancer in women who used estrogen and progestin.[32] Current recommendations are for the limited use of HRT in the lowest possible dosage for the shortest period of time. Breast cancer survivors of all ages may suffer symptoms similar to menopause because of the use of aromatase inhibitor therapy for hormone-dependent tumors. Non-hormonal therapies are being used with greater success for these symptoms.[33,34]

Genitourinary Problems

Genitourinary symptoms affect up to 50% of perimenopausal and menopausal women.[35,36] They can be chronic and progressive and are unlikely to improve over time. Genitourinary syndrome of menopause (GSM) is the current terminology used to comprehensively refer to menopausal symptoms of the lower genital tract in response to declining estrogen levels that are not better accounted for by another diagnosis. It is a term that encompasses symptoms such as vulvovaginal dryness, burning, and irritation, decreased lubrication with sexual activity, dyspareunia, decreased arousal or orgasm, postcoital bleeding, dysuria, and urinary frequency or urgency.[37]

Symptoms of GSM can have a profound impact on quality of life and relationships. The importance of screening for GSM at every comprehensive visit cannot be stressed enough. Screening should include questions regarding symptoms of vaginal dryness or irritation, pain or bleeding with sexual activity, changes in response or function, as well as bladder function, including urinary frequency, urgency, and incontinence. Treatment strategies for GSM are numerous and sometimes overlapping and range from simple lifestyle changes to complex therapies and medication or counseling.

Management of a vulvovaginal complaint requires a good understanding of genital anatomy and physiology. Estrogen loss at menopause results in physiological, vascular, neurological, and histological changes of the lower genital tract.[28] Estrogen loss decreases small blood vessel circulation, leading to a reduction in vaginal secretions and in turn to decreased lubrication and an increase in vaginal pH.[38] As a result, the tissues of the vulva and the lining of the vagina become thinner, drier, and less elastic or flexible. These changes can manifest as complaints of vaginal infections that may be real or perceived; vaginal dryness, which may or may not be associated with lubrication, pain, or bleeding with sexual activity; or changes in arousal and orgasmic capacity.

After a vaginal infection has been ruled out, management of vulvovaginal complaints can include counseling regarding simple lifestyle changes, over-the-counter (OTC) products, or prescription medications. Women can be counseled that anything interfering with small blood vessel circulation, including cigarette smoking, antihistamines, high blood pressure, or lack of exercise, can reduce genital lubrication.[39,40] Regular sexual activity has been shown to improve vulvovaginal health. Regular sexual activity with a partner or with use of a vibrator will improve blood circulation and genital lubrication.[40,41] Adequate oral intake of water is essential to all skin turgor.

Avoidance of daily use of sanitary products, talc, and all soaps will help decrease irritation and the drying out of delicate vulvar tissues. Women should be counseled to use only plain warm water for genital hygiene and educated in the use of genital lubricants and moisturizers.

Lubricants are useful for sexual activity because they reduce friction.[1] Lubricants should contain one or more of the following ingredients:

- Aloe vera
- Carrageenan (made from sea algae)
- Hydroxyethylcellulose or cellulose polymer
- Dimethicone or dimethiconol
- Vitamin E

The following ingredients should be avoided:

- Oil of any kind, including olive oil, mineral oil, and jojoba oil
- Glycerin
- Menthol, or peppermint
- Cinnamon
- Capsaicin
- Beeswax
- Chlorhexidine gluconate
- Products labeled as warming or cooling
- Vaseline/petroleum jelly
- Wild yam

For severe dryness, the best choice for a sexual lubricant is one that is 100% silicone. These only have dimethicone and dimethiconol in them. This type of lubricant stays slippery because it does not soak into the skin. Silicone lubricants seal in available moisture but do not hydrate.

Tissue turgor can be improved by using moisturizers on the vulva and in the vagina on a daily basis. Moisturizers can help increase comfort during day-to-day activities by hydrating the tissue and sealing that moisture in place. They can be massaged on the vulva any time dryness and irritation is experienced and can be used in place of a lubricant during sexual activity; with use of an applicator, 1 to 3 ml can be placed in the vagina at bedtime.

While there is a variety on the market, some moisturizers have ingredients that may cause problems. Moisturizers should contain one or more of the following ingredients:

- Hyaluronic acid
- Aloe vera
- Vitamin E

These ingredients should be avoided:

- Oils, including olive, mineral, jojoba, and palm kernel oil
- Glycerin
- Beeswax and other waxes

Essential oilsAnother common vulvovaginal complaint is dyspareunia. Pelvic floor dysfunction (PFD) may be the result of sexual pain from vaginal dryness or it may be the underlying cause of sexual pain. The prevalence of PFD is 36% to 49% after 60 years of age.[42] When sexual pain complaints persist despite well-estrogenized tissue, PFD should be suspected. Associated symptoms may include complaints of constipation and/or urinary frequency or urgency and a feeling of tightness or narrowing at the introitus or within the vaginal canal.[43] Evaluation of PFD is done by gently palpating along both sides of the vaginal canal and noting differences in pelvic floor tension and where a woman identifies pain. Management includes referral to a physical therapist trained in the treatment of PFD. See Table 11.2 for information on finding physical therapists in your area. Compounded vaginal diazepam suppositories, 10 mg at bedtime for 1 month, have been shown to markedly improve pelvic floor hypertonicity.[44] As low vitamin D levels are correlated with PFD, women should have their vitamin D levels checked.[42] Supplementation to the optimal range of 50 to 70 ng/ml is encouraged if levels are low.

Worldwide, lower urinary tract symptoms (LUTS) are the most common complaints in women of all ages, and their prevalence increases with age. Risk factors contributing to LUTS include race, childbirth, weight, chronic cough, gynecologic surgery such as hysterectomy, depression, and profession.[45] For

Table 11.2. Resources

Agency for Healthcare Research and Quality website provides up-to-date, evidence-based clinical practice guidelines.
https://www.guideline.gov

A Woman's Touch Sexuality Resource Center website offers products and educational materials to support sexual health and help people resolve concerns about sexual function Operated by two women, a physician and a social worker.
https://sexualityresources.com

Women's Health American Physical Therapy Association website provides downloadable educational handouts on a number of issues including pelvic floor dysfunction. The website also provides a locator to identify certified women's health physical therapists by state and ZIP code.
www.womenshealthapta.org/pt-locator/

North American Menopause Society website provides an abundance of information and resources for the practitioner and the patient.
https://www.menopause.org

---

the menopausal woman, declining estrogen levels and PFD may also contribute to LUTS.[46] Symptoms of LUTS include urgency, frequency, recurrent urinary tract infections, nocturia, dysuria, and incontinence. While there is evidence that systemic estrogen therapies worsen urinary symptoms, local estrogen appears to have a beneficial impact on reducing urge incontinence and recurrent urinary tract infections.[38,46]

Although Kegel exercises are often recommended, PFD may be an issue of hypo- or hypertonus. Referral to a pelvic floor physical therapist is preferred. Pelvic floor rehabilitation may involve manual therapy and/or neuromuscular retraining through biofeedback.[43] General therapies that can be recommended include weight loss, avoidance of bladder irritants such as alcohol and caffeine, and adequate daytime hydration, with decreased fluid intake starting in the early evening. The urology literature offers more in-depth discussion of medications and devices available to manage specific urologic complaints.

For all GSM symptoms, local application of estrogen should be considered. Unlike oral estrogen, local estrogen therapy avoids the "hepatic first-pass effect" and has minimal systemic absorption.[38] According to the 2016 Cochrane Database for Systematic Reviews, "there was no conclusive evidence of a difference in the main adverse events (endometrial thickness, breast disorders and total adverse events) between oestrogenic preparations versus each other or placebo."[47] Additionally, the review found there was no difference in efficacy between vaginal preparations when compared with each other.

Sexual Response

Sexual desire and response represent a complex interplay of biopsychosocial factors. For the menopausal woman, declining levels of estrogen can result in physical changes including decreased vasocongestion, inadequate lubrication, less expansion of the vagina, and fewer muscle contractions during orgasms.[39] For some women these physical changes can affect every phase of the sexual response cycle. Frustration may be experienced when arousal becomes difficult. Pain may be experienced during sexual activity, and satisfaction may be affected when orgasm becomes less intense or is not achieved. Often, a loss of desire is the end result. Other social factors that may affect a woman's sexual desire include the quality of her intimate relationship, her personal attitudes and beliefs about sex and sexual activity, and the presence of other life stressors, including her general health.

Evaluation of sexual complaints in menopause should include a thorough history, medication review, and physical examination. Once this has been completed, clinicians are in a unique position to offer education and counseling for sexual complaints that go beyond the offering of estrogen therapy. In the perimenopausal phase, normalizing and providing anticipatory guidance related to menopausal changes may relieve anxiety and open the door to understanding and acceptance as well as future conversations with the practitioner. An explanation of the sexual response cycle as circular rather than linear could provide a woman with motivation for sexual activity beyond feelings of desire. Suggestions for the use of vibrators to enhance stimulation and lubricants or moisturizers to decrease friction and pain may provide permission for a woman to incorporate novelty into her intimate relationship. Education in mindfulness may help a woman let go of outside stressors and allow her to be fully present and more satisfied with her sexual activity. If necessary, discussion that redefines intimacy as something other than vaginal/penile intercourse should be undertaken.

Hormone Replacement Therapy

When estrogen is an option for the management of vasomotor symptoms, the use of HRT should be tailored to a woman's medical history, her individual needs, and her lifestyle. It is beyond the scope of this chapter to thoroughly discuss the many aspects of HRT. In brief, the initial results of the 2002 WHI called into question the safety as well as the efficacy of HRT for the management of any chronic disease state.[48] Since that time, there has been much debate regarding the timing for initiation of HRT as well as length of use. There is also controversy and misunderstanding regarding the terms "synthetic" versus "natural" or bioidentical hormones.

Guidelines set forth by the North American Menopause Society (NAMS) advise that HRT be used in the lowest dose for the shortest duration necessary to manage menopausal symptoms. Currently, the primary indication for HRT use is the management of vasomotor symptoms.[28] Regardless of source, all hormones used to manage menopausal symptoms are synthetically derived. Technically, whether the source is a pregnant mare's urine or a soy or yam plant, synthetically derived hormones are also all natural. The distinction among the types of hormones has more to do with how chemically similar they are to a woman's endogenous hormones than it has to do with their source. Conjugated estrogens and progestins are chemically and structurally different than hormones produced in the body. The different chemical structure of these compounds has caused concern that they do not necessarily behave the same way in the body as endogenous hormones.[49]

Bioidentical hormones (17 beta-estradiol, estrone, estriol, and progesterone) refer to synthesized plant-based compounds that have the same chemical and molecular structure and therefore function identically to hormones that are produced in the body. Several FDA-approved products on the market meet this definition. Brand names and type of preparations are listed in Table 11.3.[49]

Despite the availability of bioidentical FDA-approved medications, custom-compounded HRT therapies are popular. According to proponents of custom-compounded bioidentical hormones, blood levels can be more accurately monitored, allowing for more precise and individualized management of menopausal symptoms. Opponents argue that because no testing has been done to prove active ingredients or predictable absorption rates of custom compounds, their efficacy is questionable. Currently, FDA approval for these medications is lacking.[50,51]

Regardless of the type of HRT chosen for symptom management, counseling related to the risks, benefits, and side effects is essential. While baseline hormonal testing is recommended prior to the initiation of HRT, no specific recommendations for the frequency of follow-up testing could be found. Ideally, a woman would return at 3 and 6 months after initiation of HRT and then annually if her symptoms have stabilized. The need for hormonal testing could then be based on clinical presentation. Close follow-up by the clinician is key to successful HRT. For additional information on hormonal testing please refer to Chapter 25.

Table 11.3. FDA-Approved Bioidentical Hormones

Type	Brand Names	Preparations
Estrogens		
17 beta-estradiol/plants	Estrace	Oral tablet
	Alora, Climara, Esclim Estraderm, Vivelle, Fempatch, Estelle solo, Menostar, others	Patches
	Estrogel, Divigel Elestrin	Transdermal gel
	Estrasorb	Topical cream
	Estrace	Vaginal cream
	Estring	Vaginal ring
	Evamist	Spray
Estradiol acetate	Femring	Vaginal ring
Estradiol hemihydrate	Vagifem	Vaginal tablet
Micronized Progesterone		
	Prometrium	Tablet
	Prochieve 4%	Vaginal gel

This information on moisturizers and lubricants is reprinted with permission from a patient handout entitled "Vulvovaginal Atrophy Patient Information Sheet." Dated September 2014, the handout was developed by Ellen Barnard, MSSW, Anne Ford, MD, and Paul Smith, MD. *A Woman's Touch Sexuality Resource Center: www.sexualityresources.com*

Summary

As the human lifespan increases, the increasing length of time that a woman spends in postmenopause makes this stage of life more than an afterthought. Health care providers need to be well versed in the bio-psycho-social aspects of menopause. An abundance of literature discusses the symptoms and treatment of menopause with Western medicine as well as with integrative medicine. The agreement about the best strategies is limited. Randomized clinical trials do not prove many integrative approaches to be any more effective than placebo.[34] However, women should be offered information about all safe interventions so that they can make decisions about which treatment works best for them. An integrative approach to menopause management offers individualized treatments in keeping with a woman's health needs, values, and beliefs.

REFERENCES

1. Xu JQ, Murphy SL, Kochanek KD, Bastian BA. Deaths: Final data for 2013. National Vital Statistics Reports; vol. 64, no. 2. Hyattsville, MD: National Center for Health Statistics; 2016.
2. Yanikkerem E, Koltan S, Tamay A, Dikayak S. Relationship between women's attitude towards menopause and quality of life. *Climacteric* [serial online]. December 2012;15(6):552–562. Available from: Academic Search Complete, Ipswich, MA. Accessed June 7, 2016.
3. Jones EK, Jurgenson JR, Katzenellenbogen JM, Thompson SC. Menopause and the influence of culture: Another gap for Indigenous Australian women? *BMC Women's Health.* 2012;12(43): doi:10.1186/1472-6874-12-43
4. Coney P. Menopause. http://emedicine.medscape.com/article/264088-overview#a1. 2015.
5. Osarenren N, Ubangha MB, Nwadinigwe IP. Attitudes of women to menopause: Implications for counseling. *Edo Journal of Counseling.* 2009;2(2):155–164.
6. Bachman GA. Menopausal vasomotor symptoms: a review of causes, effects and evidenced-based treatment options. *J Reprod Med.* 2005;50(3):155–165.
7. Levis S, Griebeler ML. The role of soy foods in the treatment of menopausal symptoms. *J Nutr.* 2010 Dec;140(12): 2318s–2321s.
8. Young SN. How to increase serotonin in the human brain without drugs. *J Psychiatry Neurosci.* 2007 Nov;32(6):394–399.
9. Parry BL, Maurer EL. Light treatment of mood disorders. *Dialogues in Clinical Neuroscience.* 2003;5(4):353–365.
10. Daley AJ, Stokes-Lampard HJ, MacAurthur C. Exercise to reduce vasomotor and other menopausal symptoms: A review. *Maturitas.* 2009;63(3):176–180.
11. Innes KE, Selfe TK, Vishnu A. Mind-body therapies for menopausal symptoms: A systematic review. *Maturitas.* 2010;66(2):135–149. doi:10.1016/j.maturitas.2010.01.016.
12. http://healthysleep.med.harvard.edu/healthy/getting/overcoming/tips
13. Karadag E, Samancioglu S, Ozden D, Bakir E. Effects of aromatherapy on sleep quality and anxiety of patients. *Nursing In Critical Care* [serial online]. July 27, 2015; available from: MEDLINE Complete, Ipswich, MA. Accessed September 24, 2016.
14. Chiu H, Hsieh Y, Tsai P. Acupuncture to reduce sleep disturbances in perimenopausal and postmenopausal women: A systematic review and meta-analysis. *Obstet Gynecol.* [serial online]. March 2016;127(3):507–515. Available from: MEDLINE Complete, Ipswich, MA. Accessed January 15, 2017.

15. Freeman E, Sammel M, Lin H, et.al. The role of anxiety in menopausal hot flashes. *Menopause*. 2005;12(3):258–266.

16. Stoppler MC. Alternative treatments for hot flashes of menopause. Medicinenet website. http://www.medicinenet.com/alternative_treatments_for_hot_flashes/page3.htm. Updated August 19, 2016; accessed December 9, 2016.

17. Shams T, Firwana B, Habib F, et al. SSRIs for hot flashes: A systematic review and meta-analysis of randomized trials. *J Gen Intern Med*. 2014;29(1):204–213.

18. Higgins A, Nash M, Lynch AM. Antidepressant-associated sexual dysfunction: impact, effects, and treatment. *Drug Healthc Patient Saf*. 2010;2:141–150. Published online 2010 Sep 9.

19. Pachman DR, Jones JM, Loprinzi CL. Management of menopause-associated vasomotor symptoms: Current treatment options, challenges and future directions. *Int J Womens Health*. 2010;2:123–135.

20. Geller SE, Shulman LP, van Breemen RB, et al. Safety and efficacy of black cohosh and red clover for the management of vasomotor symptoms: A randomized controlled trial. *Menopause NY*. 2009;16(6):1156–1166. doi:10.1097/gme.0b013e3181ace49b.

21. Adnan MM, Khan M, Hashmi S, Hamza M, AbdulMujeeb S, Amer S. Black cohosh and liver toxicity: Is there a relationship? *Case Reports in Gastrointestinal Medicine*, 2014, Article ID 860614. doi:10.1155/2014/860614

22. Australian Menopause Society. Menopause and Body Changes. Information Sheet. November 2014, www.menopause.org/au. Accessed Sept. 27, 2016.

23. Hall G, Phillips TJ. Estrogen and skin: The effects of estrogen, menopause and HRT on the skin. *J Am Acad Dermotol*. 2005 Oct;53(4):555–568.

24. Jesitus J. Electrolysis successful where laser hair removal fails. *Dermatology Times*. 2011, Sept. 1. Accessed Dec. 3, 2016.

25. Herman J, Rost-Roszkowska M, Skoticka-Graca U. Skin care during the menopause period: Noninvasive procedures of beauty studies. *Advances in Dermatology and Allergology/Postepy Dermatologii I Alergologii*. 2013;30(6):388–395.

26. Goldberg DJ. Current trends in intense pulsed light. *J Clin Aesthetic Dermatol*. 2012;5(6):45–53. Accessed online Sept. 27, 2016.

27. www.health.harvard.edu. Treating female pattern hair loss. *Harvard Women's Health Watch*. 2015, Dec. 9. Accessed Dec. 3, 2016.

28. Shrifren JL, Glass MLS. The North American Menopause Society recommendations for clinical care of midlife women. *Menopause*. 2014; 21(10):1038–1062. doi:10.1097/gme.0000000000000319

29. www.breastcancer.org/researchnews. Dec. 17, 2008. Some moisturizers contain estrogen even though ingredients don't list it. Accessed Dec. 3, 2016.

30. Pruthi S, Wahner-Roedler DL, Torkelson CJ, et al. Vitamin E and evening primrose oil for management of cyclic mastalgia: A randomized pilot study. *Alter Med Review*. Apr 2010;15(1):59–67.

32. Chlebowski RT, Anderson GS, Gass M, et al. Estrogen and progestin and breast cancer incidence and mortality in postmenopausal women. *JAMA*. 2010 Oct 20;304(15):1684–1692.

33. Biglia N, Bounous VE, Sgro LG, D'Alonzo M, Peccchio S, Nappi RE. Genitourinary syndrome of menopause in breast cancer survivors: Are we facing new and safe hopes? *Clin Breast Cancer.* 2015 Dec;15(6):413–420.

34. North American Menopause Society. Position Statement: Nonhormonal management of menopause-associated vasomotor symptoms. *Menopause.* 2015;22(1):1155–1174.

35. Parish SJ, Nappi RE, Krychman ML, et al. Impact of vulvovaginal health on postmenopausal women: a review of surveys on symptoms of vulvovaginal atrophy. *Int J Womens Health.* 2013;5:437–447.

36. Erekson EA, Li FY, Martin DK, Fried TR. Vulvovaginal symptoms prevalence in postmenopausal women and relationship to other menopausal symptoms and pelvic floor disorders. *Menopause.* 2016;23(4):368–375.

37. Portman DJ, Gass MLS. Genitourinary syndrome of menopause: New terminology for vulvovaginal atrophy from the International Society for the Study of Women's Sexual Health and The North American Menopause Society. *Menopause.* 2014;21(10): DOI: 10.1097/gme.0000000000000329

38. Krause M, Wheeler TL, Snyder TE, Richter HE. Local effects of vaginally administered estrogen therapy: A review. *J Pelvic Med Surg.* 2009;15(3):105–114.

39. Kuzmarov IW, Bain J. Sexuality in the aging couple, Part 1: The aging woman. *Geriatrics and Aging.* 2008;11(10):589–594.

40. www.sexualityresources.com

41. Levin R. Sexual activity, health and well-being: The beneficial roles of coitus and masturbation. *Sexual & Relationship Therapy* [serial online]. February 2007;22(1):135–148.

42. Navaneethan PR, Kekre A, Jacob KS, Varghese L. Vitamin D deficiency in postmenopausal women with pelvic floor disorders. *J Mid-Life Health.* 2015;6(2):66–69. doi:10.4103/0976-7800.158948.

43. Faubion SS, Shuster LT, Bharucha AE. Recognition and management of nonrelaxing pelvic floor dysfunction. *Mayo Clin Proc.* 2012;87(2):187–193. doi:10.1016/j.mayocp.2011.09.004.

44. Carrico DJ, Peters KM. Vaginal diazepam use with urogenital pain/pelvic floor dysfunction. *Urol Nurs.* 2011;31(5):279–284.

45. Bilgic D, Beji NK. Lower urinary tract symptoms in women and quality of life. *Int J Urol Nurs.* 2011;4:97–105. doi:10.1111/j.1749-771X.2010.01100.x

46. Roberts H, Hickey M. Managing the menopause: An update. *Maturitas.* Apr 2016;86:53–58.

47. Lethaby A, Ayeleke RO, Roberts H. Local oestrogen for vaginal atrophy in postmenopausal women. *Cochrane Database of Systematic Reviews* 2016, Issue 8. Art. No.: CD001500. DOI: 10.1002/14651858.CD001500.pub3.

48. Manson JE, Chlebowski RT, Stefanick ML, et al. The Women's Health Initiative hormone therapy trials: Update and overview of health outcomes during the intervention and post-stopping phases. *JAMA.* 2013;310(13):1353–1368. doi:10.1001/jama.2013.278040

49. Files JA, Ko MG, Pruthi S. Bioidentical hormone therapy. *Mayo Clin Proc.* 2011;86(7):673–680. doi:10.4065/mcp.2010.0714.

50. Bioidentical Hormone Therapy. The North American Menopause Society. https://www.menopause.org/publications/clinical-practice-materials/bioidentical-hormone-therapy Accessed Nov. 30, 2016.

51. What Are Bioidentical Hormones. Harvard Health Publications. http://www.health.harvard.edu/womens-health/what-are-bioidentical-hormones. Updated Dec. 4, 2015. Accessed Dec. 1, 2016.

12

Pain

MARC BRODSKY AND ANN E. HANSEN

Persistent pain can be defined as an unpleasant sensory and emotional experience that continues for a prolonged period of time and that may or may not be associated with a recognizable disease process. Older people are more likely to suffer from arthritis, bone and joint diseases, and other chronic pain conditions.[1] Depression, anxiety, decreased socialization, sleep disturbance, impaired ambulation, and increased health care utilization and costs are associated with pain in older people. Older people with pain may also have associated gait disturbance, slow rehabilitation, and adverse effects from multiple drug prescriptions. Any persistent pain that has an impact on physical function, psychological function, or other aspects of quality of life should be recognized as a significant problem.[1]

Osteoarthritis of the Knee

S.S. is an 84-year-old male with knee pain. In assessing his knee pain, a standardized approach may guide history taking (Table 12.1).[1] A constructive collaboration between the patient and physician on the initial visit begins an ongoing therapeutic alliance.[2]

HISTORY

SS's right-sided knee pain gradually worsened over the previous few years. Onset was atraumatic and was attributed to the cumulative effects of an active life that included military duty on a ship and hobbies that included snowmobile riding. The intensity of his pain ranged from 4/10 to 6/10.

Table 12.1. American Geriatric Society (AGS) Recommendations for History Taking and Physical Exam of an Older Adult with Persistent Pain

History taking of adult with persistent pain

- Intensity, character, frequency, location, duration, ameliorating and exacerbating factors

- Description of pain in relation to impairments in physical and social function in ADLs, IADLs, sleep, appetite, energy, exercise, mood, cognitive function, interpersonal and intimacy issues, social and leisure activities, and overall quality of life

- Analgesic history, including effectiveness and side effects of any current and previously used medications, over-the-counter medications, complementary methods

- A quantitative assessment of pain should be recorded by the use of a standardized scale that is sensitive to cognitive, language, and sensory impairments.

- A multidimensional pain instrument that evaluates pain in relation to other domains should be considered.

- Patients should be asked about symptoms and signs that may indicate pain, including nonverbal pain-related behaviors to include recent changes in activities and functional status.

- Patient attitudes and beliefs regarding pain and its management, as well as knowledge of pain management strategies, should be discussed.

- Satisfaction with current pain treatment should be determined and concerns should be identified.

- Documentation of current medications, including herbal medications, and history of any adverse effects of medications

- Documentation of past medical history, past surgical history, review of systems, and family history
  - Cognitive function should be evaluated for new or worsening confusion

- Social history
  - Evaluation of psychological function, including mood, self-efficacy, pain coping skills, helplessness, and pain-related fears
  - Evaluation of social support, caregivers, family relationships, work history, cultural environment, spirituality, and health care availability
  - Assessment for sleep disturbance that may be associated with persistent pain
  - Assessment of alcohol use

Physical exam of an older patient with persistent pain

- Physical examination should include careful examination of the site of the reported pain, common sites for pain referral, and common sites of pain in older individuals.

Table 12.1. Continued

- Focus on the musculoskeletal system may identify myofascial pain, fibromyalgia, inflammation, deformity, and posture.

- Evaluation of neurological system should search for weakness, hyperalgesia, hyperpathia, allodynia, numbness, parasthesia, or other neurological impairment.

- Initial assessment should include observation of physical function such as measures of ADLs, performance measures such as range of motion, get-up-and-go test, or others.

- Pertinent laboratory and other diagnostic tests should only be done if they affect decisions about treatment.

Character was described as a deep ache. Frequency was every day. Location was anterior knee without radiation. Duration was for minutes to hours after exacerbating factors that include walking. His symptoms improved with relative rest and application of ice to his knee.

The pain limited his walking to a quarter-mile. He did not note impairments in activities of daily living (ADLs) or instrumental activities of daily living (IADLs), sleep, appetite, energy, mood, cognitive function, intimacy issues, or social function. He reported that relief from his knee pain would allow him to participate in hobbies such as walking with his wife and dog at a beach park. The patient stated that he believed that his pain is related to years of wear and tear. He believed that it is safe to be physically active and that his knee pain could improve. Instead of medications and more physical therapy treatments, S.S. preferred home remedies, topical agents, and informal cognitive strategies such as social gatherings, spending time with family and friends, and humor.[3]

Since S.S. first noted his knee pain, he had been evaluated by his primary care physician and an orthopedic surgeon. His workup included a knee x-ray that demonstrated degenerative joint disease. He was referred to physical therapy, which offered some temporary relief of his symptoms. He did not get lasting relief with medications, which included acetaminophen, nonsteroidal anti-inflammatory medications, and tramadol. S.S. perceived that complementary treatments, particularly acupuncture, were low risk and could help him to get some relief from his pain and improve his quality of life. He perceived conventional therapies such as "addictive" pain medications and surgery as high risk with associated adverse effects that could cost him his independence.

S.S. used acetaminophen as needed for pain. He also took medications for his comorbidities, which included hypertension, high cholesterol, sleep apnea, and ulcerative colitis. His surgical history was significant for hiatal hernia repair and cholecystectomy. His review of systems was unremarkable other than his knee pain issues. His family history was noncontributory.

S.S. described his mood as "happy-go-lucky." He denied depressed mood or helplessness. He coped with his knee pain by using humor to lower pain levels and to keep an optimistic frame of mind. S.S. lived with his wife and has children and friends in the area. He was a retired U.S. Navy baker and subsequently worked as an entrepreneur. He did not smoke. He drank a shot of Scotch each day. His sleep has improved since using a continuous positive airway pressure (CPAP) mask for his sleep apnea. He described himself as spiritual though he is not active in a religious congregation. S.S. was treated by his primary care physician to manage his chronic conditions, and his health maintenance preventive measures were up to date, including treatment for vision and hearing loss.

PHYSICAL EXAMINATION

A standardized approach may guide the physical examination for older adults with pain (see Table 12.1).[1] On physical examination, the patient quickly arose from his chair in the waiting room and ambulated to his examining room without assistance of a cane or walker. Gait was steady. With the patient in a supine position, the right knee was examined compared to the left knee. The right knee demonstrated an effusion and otherwise no deformity. On palpation, trigger points in the muscles surrounding the knee were tender to palpation. Range of motion was decreased on right knee flexion compared to the left knee. The physical examination was otherwise normal, including no weakness, hyperpathia, allodynia, numbness, paresthesia, or other neurological impairment. No other diagnostic tests were ordered given that the results of the tests would not affect decisions about treatment.

ASSESSMENT AND EVIDENCE-BASED TREATMENT OPTIONS

Classifying persistent pain in pathophysiological terms may help the clinician select therapy and determine prognosis. This patient's medical history and physical examination findings suggested a diagnosis of osteoarthritis and associated myofascial pain of the surrounding muscles.

Nociceptive pain may be somatic or visceral and is caused by stimulation of pain receptors. Nociceptive pain may result from impending or ongoing tissue damage or inflammation. Examples include inflammatory arthritis, degenerative arthritis, myofascial pain syndrome, and ischemic pain.[1]

Biochemical Pharmacological Therapies

For nociceptive pain, as experienced by the majority of older patients with osteoarthritis, a stepwise pharmacological approach may be considered. Because of its favorable safety profile, acetaminophen is the first-line therapy for older adults with mild to moderate pain. Despite its safety profile, however, unintentional overdose is a leading cause of hepatotoxicity.[2,4]

Geriatric pain guidelines recommend that oral nonsteroidal anti-inflammatory drugs (NSAIDS) be used with caution on a short-term basis given their cardiovascular and gastrointestinal side effects. A trial of an opioid is recommended for older patient with persistent pain that has not responded to other treatments or when significant pain-related functional impairments are present despite treatment. Risks associated with opioids for chronic non-cancer pain in older adults, however, may include falls and fall-related injuries, hospitalizations, and all-cause mortality.[2,4]

The physiological changes that accompany aging result in altered pharmacokinetics. In older persons there is a relative increase in body fat and a relative decrease in lean body mass, which causes increased distribution of fat-soluble drugs. This also increases the half-life of such medications. The volume of distribution of water-soluble compounds is decreased in older patients, which means a smaller dose is required to reach a given target plasma concentration. There is also a predictable reduction in glomerular filtration rate and tubular secretion with aging, which causes decreased clearance of medications in the geriatric population. All of these changes are important to consider when choosing dosages of medications for older patients.[5]

When starting a medication, guidelines recommend beginning with the lowest anticipated effective dose, monitoring on the basis of expected absorption and known pharmacokinetics of the agent, and titrating the dose on the basis of likely steady-state blood levels and clinically demonstrated effects. A careful surveillance plan can determine whether treatment goals are being met. Medications should only be continued so long as treatment goals are being met.[4]

In addition to medication, the following treatment options may optimize management of pain in this patient with osteoarthritis of the knee: (1) non-pharmacological biochemical, (2) biomechanical, and (3) bioenergetics (Table 12.2).[6]

Table 12.2. Cochrane Database Systematic Reviews of Non-pharmacological Biochemical Treatments, Biomechanical Treatments, and Bioenergetics Therapies for Osteoarthritis of the Knee

Nonpharmacologic biochemical therapies	
Mineral baths	Scientific evidence is weak because of the poor methodological quality and the absence of an adequate statistical analysis and data presentation. "Positive findings" should be viewed with caution.
Topical herbal therapies	Arnica gel probably improves symptoms as effectively as a gel containing an NSAID, but with no better (and possibly worse) adverse event profile. Comfrey extract gel probably improves pain, and Capsicum extract gel probably will not improve pain or function at the doses examined in this review. Further high-quality, fully powered studies are required to confirm the trends of effectiveness identified in studies so far.
Glucosamine	Pooled results from studies using a non-Rotta preparation or adequate allocation concealment failed to show benefit in pain and WOMAC function, while those studies evaluating the Rotta preparation showed that glucosamine was superior to placebo in the treatment of pain and functional impairment resulting from symptomatic osteoarthritis.
S-Adenosylmethionine (SAMe)	The effects of SAMe on both pain and function may be potentially clinically relevant and, although effects are expected to be small, deserve further clinical evaluation in adequately sized randomized, parallel-group trials in patients with knee or hip osteoarthritis. Meanwhile, routine use of SAMe should not be advised.
Chondroitin	Chondroitin had a lower risk of serious adverse events compared with control. More high-quality studies are needed to explore the role of chondroitin in the treatment of osteoarthritis. The combination of some efficacy and low risk associated with chondroitin may explain its popularity among patients as an over-the-counter supplement.
"Oral herbal therapies": Boswellia, avocado–soyabean unsaponifiables (ASU)	Extracts of *Boswellia serrata* show trends of benefits that warrant further investigation in light of the fact that the risk of adverse events appears low. There is no evidence that ASU significantly improves joint structure, and there is limited evidence that it prevents joint space narrowing. Structural changes were not tested for with any other herbal intervention. Further investigations are required to determine optimal daily doses producing clinical benefits without adverse events.

Table 12.1. Continued

Biomechanical therapies	
Heat and ice	Ice massage compared to control had a statistically beneficial effect on range of motion, function, and knee strength. Cold packs decreased swelling. Hot packs had no beneficial effect on edema compared with placebo or cold application. Ice packs did not affect pain significantly, compared to control, in patients with osteoarthritis. More well-designed studies with a standardized protocol and adequate number of participants are needed to evaluate the effects of thermotherapy.
Acupuncture	Sham-controlled trials show statistically significant benefits; however, these benefits are small, do not meet our predefined thresholds for clinical relevance, and are probably due at least partially to placebo effects from incomplete blinding. Waiting list–controlled trials of acupuncture for peripheral joint osteoarthritis suggest statistically significant and clinically relevant benefits, much of which may be due to expectation or placebo effects.
Bioenergetic therapies	
Transcutaneous electricity	The current systematic review is inconclusive, hampered by the inclusion of only small trials of questionable quality. Appropriately designed trials of adequate power are warranted.
Magnetic fields	Current evidence suggests that electromagnetic field treatment may provide moderate benefit for osteoarthritis sufferers in terms of pain relief. Further studies are required to confirm whether this treatment confers clinically important benefits in terms of physical function and quality of life.

Mind–Body Therapies

Cognitive coping strategies are designed to modify factors such as helplessness, low self-efficacy, and catastrophizing, which increase pain and disability. Cognitive strategies may include distraction methods to divert attention from pain, such as imagery, focal point, and counting methods; mindfulness methods to enhance acceptance of pain, such as meditation; and methods for altering self-defeating thought patterns that contribute to pain and psychological distress, such as altering underlying beliefs and attitudes.[1]

Depression may be associated with pain in the older person. Recommending interventions to emphasize a positive attitude, for example by encouraging a patient to socialize and to reconnect with longstanding artistic or religious interests, may help neutralize the patient's feeling of hopelessness.[2]

Cognitive strategies may be combined with behavioral strategies to reduce pain and improve function. Behavioral strategies may help patients to control pain by pacing their activities, increasing their involvement in pleasurable activities, and using relaxation methods.[1]

Strategies to counter negative treatment expectations include (1) remaining readily available to respond to questions and concerns with each intervention, (2) providing an effective backup or rescue pain medication during each new analgesic period, and (3) listening to the patient and offering realistic expectations. These strategies help reassure the patient with persistent pain that he or she will not be abandoned.[2]

Lifestyle

Addressing function and fall risk is important for all older adults, particularly those with persistent pain. Geriatric pain management guidelines recommend that all older patients with persistent pain participate in a physical activity regimen that includes strengthening, flexibility, balance, and endurance exercises. Patients should also be questioned about primary sleep disturbance that may be associated with persistent pain.[1]

TREATMENT APPROACH

Linking potential treatment benefits with an important patient goal may be helpful. The patient identified his goals as (1) maximizing function and minimizing risk for falls and injury and (2) getting ideas for pain management.[2] Incremental goals for obtaining pain relief were pain relief that allows for restful sleep, pain relief at rest, and tolerable pain with activity.[3]

Risks and benefits of various treatment options to achieve the patient's goals were discussed. The patient preferred to begin with lifestyle interventions, such as emphasizing a positive attitude by engaging in activities with family and friends to help neutralize his feeling of hopelessness. The patient also began a physical activity regimen that included strengthening, flexibility, balance, and endurance exercises.[7] He was compliant with his CPAP mask, which had improved his sleep.

The patient continued taking acetaminophen, which provided some relief. He was concerned about the effects of an anti-inflammatory medication given his cardiac risk factors, and he was concerned about the side effects of more potent pain medications. The patient discussed his internet research about the therapeutic effect of topical capsaicin, a vanilloid receptor subtype 1 agonist, and dietary supplementation with curcumin and ginger, both with cyclooxygenase-2 inhibition. The treatment plan included topical capsaicin 0.1% up to four times a day. The patient also started taking curcumin and ginger, 1 gram a day of each, or an equivalent 1/5 teaspoon of both turmeric, which contains curcumin, and ginger with cooking. He continued taking glucosamine and chondroitin.

The patient also opted for acupuncture. In addition to weekly acupuncture sessions for the first 4 weeks, self-help efforts including acupressure were reinforced at every patient encounter. After 4 weeks of the treatment regimen, the follow-up visits were gradually spread out to each month. Regular visits helped to reassess improvement or worsening of the condition, medication side effects, and patient compliance. Positive and negative effects of therapeutic modalities and medications were noted and the treatment plan was modified as appropriate.[8] Through this strategy, the patient was able to reduce his pain level, feel more stable on his feet, and more actively participate in his hobbies.

At each visit, the therapeutic alliance was reinforced by mutually agreed-upon treatment goals, realistic expectations, commitment on the part of both the patient and physician, availability of the physician for advice, reassurance and support during flares, mutual respect, and a reciprocal bond generated by both parties who had an emotional investment in the outcomes of treatment.[2]

Low Back Pain

In most cases, chronic low back pain does not have a specific underlying cause such as cancer, spinal infections, fractures, or ankylosing spondylitis. More commonly it is multifactorial. Chronic low back pain may be classified by impact, and impact can be described by pain intensity, pain interference with normal activities, and functional status.[9]

Chronic low back pain may be the result of multiple biological and behavioral etiologies. Anatomical and functional changes in the central nervous system may develop over time with persistent pain from multifactorial pathologies of the spine, intervertebral disks, ligaments, joint capsules, and muscles.[9]

A thorough history may include precipitating factors, a diary of daily activities with attention to habits and ergonomics contributing to pain, and psychosocial stressors. The history may reveal "red flags" that suggest more serious underlying pathology such as cauda equine syndrome, neurological dysfunction, infection, or cancer. The evaluation may also identify "yellow flags," psychosocial factors associated with progression to persistent disabling conditions such as comorbid psychiatric illness and inability to work.[10]

Physical examination findings may add useful information to the history. The examination may include a functional assessment of strength and flexibility, as well as palpation to identify any tender muscles. Focused examination features for chronic low back pain to rule out more serious reversible causes include straight leg raise for patients with leg pain; hip internal rotation as a measure of hip arthritis, a potential cause of low back pain; and lower extremity strength. The evaluation may also explore potential contributing conditions such as thyroid or menstrual/menopausal-related endocrine imbalances and concomitant knee pain. Laboratory or imaging tests have limited indication as they are weakly associated with patient symptoms and function in patients with history and physical examination findings suggestive of degenerative spine changes.[9]

Lifestyle-based mind–body interventions and exercise may be prudent first-line treatments for persistent low back pain. Mind–body therapies such as yoga, mindfulness-based stress reduction (MBSR), and cognitive-behavioral therapy have demonstrated efficacy as a component of a low back pain treatment plan.[15,16] If the examination identifies myofascial trigger points or trunk muscle weakness, comprehensive muscle pain protocols, first described in the medical literature in the 1960s, may be effective in giving patients relief from persistent muscular low back pain. These protocols may include therapeutic exercises aimed at correcting deficits in muscle strength and flexibility.[11–14]

In addition to mind–body self-care practices and exercise, spinal manipulation and acupuncture have demonstrated modest benefits for treatment of acute and chronic back pain. Massage may be effective for patients with chronic low back pain as well.[17]

HISTORY

Patient R.M., an 80-year-old female, presents with low back pain. She underwent surgery for a herniated disk 2 years prior to her initial visit for chronic low back pain symptoms. A neurosurgeon referred her for an epidural injection when her pain symptoms continued after the surgery. She declined physical therapy, which did not provide lasting relief in the past. Subsequent to her epidural, she was prescribed a cyclooxygenase-2 inhibitor, which did not provide adequate relief. She noted the most benefit from her chiropractic treatments.

R.M. reported that the intensity of her back pain ranges from 4/10 to 8/10. Character is described as soreness. Frequency was every day. Location was across the low back with radiation down the back of both legs to the knees. Duration was for minutes to hours after exacerbating factors that include standing and house cleaning. Her symptoms improved with sitting, lying down, and applying ice.

The pain limited her walking to 10 minutes with assistance of a cane and interfered with her active lifestyle that includes hosting friends and family to dinner parties in her home. The patient attributed her pain to 38 years of owning a diner and being responsible for all aspects of its operations other than the grill duties, which her husband supervised.

R.M. took a cyclooxygenase-2 inhibitor or acetaminophen as needed for pain in addition to her medications for hypertension. Nutritional supplements included a multivitamin, vitamin D, olive leaf extract for her "immune system," red yeast rice for her "cholesterol," vitamin C, glucosamine, chondroitin, methyl sulfonyl methane (MSM), fish oil, coenzyme Q10, and vitamin B12. Her surgical history was significant for right hip replacement in addition to her spine surgery.

R.M. described her mood as happy, though she reports that pain could make her feel irritable. She denied depressed mood or helplessness. She coped with her pain by reminding herself that she would be able to get relief from her pain with rest. R.M. lived with her husband and grown son. She did not smoke or drink alcohol. Her sleep was restorative, though it could be interrupted a few times each night to get up to urinate. She was active in her religious congregation.

PHYSICAL EXAMINATION

The patient got out of her chair in the waiting room with assistance of the arm of the chair and her cane. She ambulated to the examining room with the assistance of a cane. On palpation, trigger points and acupuncture points overlying the gluteus maximus muscle were tender to palpation. All muscle groups of the lower extremity demonstrated normal strength. Straight leg test was negative.

ASSESSMENT AND EVIDENCE-BASED TREATMENTS

In a discussion of lifestyle interventions, the patient reaffirmed how her positive attitude and longstanding religious interests helped her better frame frustration from her pain and preserve her sense of hope. In particular, she found comfort in prayer for health of family and friends. Prayer improved her sleep, which was one of the factors that helped her to get relief from her pain symptoms. She was instructed on a daily stretching exercise program to improve range of motion and to reverse muscle weakness. Proper footwear minimized the load on her low back and protected her from falls. Active patient involvement in these measures fostered self-reliance and control over pain.[1]

In addition to her self-care and continued chiropractic treatments, the patient also opted to begin treatment with trigger point injections to treat the myofascial pain component of her condition. The patient was also instructed on how to perform acupressure on points in the back of the calf to ease her symptoms. She decided to postpone acupuncture treatments and massage for the time being for financial considerations since the procedure was not covered by her medical insurance.

After 4 weeks of the treatment regimen, the follow-up visits were gradually spread out to each month. She also continued her chiropractic treatments. The patient followed up more frequently for flares and would spread out the appointments if she was able to function optimally with adequate comfort. Through this strategy, the patient was able to achieve her goals. She no longer noted pain in her legs, and her back pain improved to the point that she was able to perform her regular housework and to prepare her house to host guests.

Myofascial Neck Pain and Headache

Persistent pain in older adults is most often attributable to musculoskeletal causes, usually involves multiple sites, and often occurs with other comorbidities. Persistent pain in adults is similar to other geriatric syndromes in that it results via a multifactorial pathway from accumulated impairments in multiple systems.[2]

Aside from chronic neck pain, myofascial pain of the head and neck may contribute to or be associated with other conditions such as whiplash symptoms,[18] migraine and tension headaches,[19] temporomandibular joint pain,[20] fibromyalgia,[21] and cancer-related pain.[22–24]

Myofascial pain syndrome is diagnosed by history and physical examination findings that demonstrate major and minor criteria for myofascial trigger points (Table 12.3).[25,26] Trigger points, a diagnostic feature of myofascial pain syndrome, are most commonly identified in the upper trapezius muscle in chronic myofascial neck pain. Trigger points associated with chronic neck

Table 12.3. Centers for Medicare & Medicaid Services (CMS) Major
and Minor Criteria for Myofascial Trigger Point

Major Criteria (all four required)	Minor Criteria (at least one of four required)
A. Regional pain complaint B. Pain complaint or altered sensation in the expected distribution of referred pain from a trigger point C. Taut band palpable in an accessible muscle with exquisite tenderness at one point along the length of it D. Some degree of restricted range of motion, when measurable	A. Reproduction of referred pain pattern by stimulating the trigger point B. Altered sensation by pressure on the tender spot C. Local response elicited by snapping palpation at the tender spot or by needle insertion into the tender spot D. Pain alleviated by stretching or injecting the tender spot

pain are less prevalent in the levator scapulae, sternocleidomastoid, and temporalis muscles.[27]

HISTORY

B.A. is a 65-year-old male with neck pain and headache. An amateur pianist and university mathematics professor, he was in a state of good health until two years prior, when he first noticed left-sided neck pain after sleeping with his neck in an awkward position. As his neck pain continued, he developed daily generalized headaches. These headaches were severe enough to interfere with his routine daily activities and prevented him from playing the piano and composing music.

The patient's primary care physician eventually prescribed an opioid pain medication after he obtained no relief with acetaminophen, NSAIDS, and tramadol. The headaches subsided with pain medication but returned within a few hours, requiring him to take another dose. He awakened every morning with a headache and repeated the cycle of taking the opioid and other pain medications, followed by recurrent headache symptoms, followed by taking more medication, up to six times a day.

The patient was referred to a neurologist for evaluation after his symptoms persisted 3 to 6 months. A computed tomography (CT) scan showed no abnormality of the brain that would cause the headaches, but the findings suggested chronic sinusitis.

The neurologist diagnosed the patient with rebound headaches due to the frequent use of pain medications. He advised the patient to discontinue the opioid and limit his other pain medications and prescribed a course of oral steroids.

The patient was referred to an otolaryngologist, who prescribed medications for chronic sinusitis. The patient's symptoms were refractory to these measures as well as treatment by an allergist. The patient subsequently underwent sinus surgery.

After the patient's condition did not improve with sinus surgery, he had further evaluation of his continuing headaches with a magnetic resonance imaging (MRI) scan. The MRI demonstrated incidental findings of previous strokes from hypertension. The patient was subsequently started on a beta blocker to treat his hypertension and as headache prophylaxis.

The patient had temporary relief of his symptoms with the medications, but he began having headaches again within the next few months. Over the next year, his headaches worsened to the point that he was evaluated by a second neurologist. The neurologist made a diagnosis of tension headaches as well as rebound headaches, as the patient had resumed taking an anti-inflammatory agent every day.

As the patient's severe and ongoing neck pain raised the possibility of carotid artery dissection, an MRI/magnetic resonance angiography (MRA) scan of the head and neck was performed. That study demonstrated incidental findings consistent with cerebrovascular and carotid disease and degenerative cervical spine changes. At this point, the patient opted for an approach not limited to medications and surgery to get relief from his chronic neck pain and headaches.

PHYSICAL EXAMINATION

A thorough physical examination, which included laying hands on the patient, was performed. Cervical and thoracic muscles demonstrated trigger points. Neck range of motion was also decreased.

ASSESSMENT

In the past this patient had undergone an extensive evaluation for neck pain and headaches. He had been diagnosed with tension headache, rebound headaches, osteoarthritis of the cervical spine, previous strokes from high blood pressure, and chronic sinusitis. His multifactorial chronic pain condition was refractory to multiple medications and surgery.

The biomedical concept of allostasis helps explain this patient's pattern of symptoms under a unifying cause. Allostasis, or adaptation to maintain homeostasis, is mediated in part by secretion of glucocorticoids and the activity of the autonomic nervous system, neurotransmitters, and inflammatory cyto-kines. Prolonged stress or stress that overwhelms the system's resiliency can cause pathophysiology.[28]

In the history, the patient identified cervical muscle strain as the initial insult that led to a cascade of infrastructure decline. Rage caused by intense conflicts in his personal life potentially influenced his pain through biological, behavioral, and emotional mechanisms.

As a musician, he was also at risk for a unique set of psychosocial, environ-mental, and mechanical stresses.[29] In this case, overloading repetitive micro-trauma from poor ergonomics that the patient described while playing the piano and composing may have perpetuated his condition.

TREATMENT APPROACH

The initial visit included a discussion to explore how the patient might incorpo-rate positive lifestyle changes related to exercise, diet, social support, stress and anger management, sleep hygiene, and other self-care strategies to restore resil-iency. The therapeutic plan consisted of trigger point injections of the trape-zius and splenius capitis muscle (Fig. 12.1) and acupuncture. Self-care included

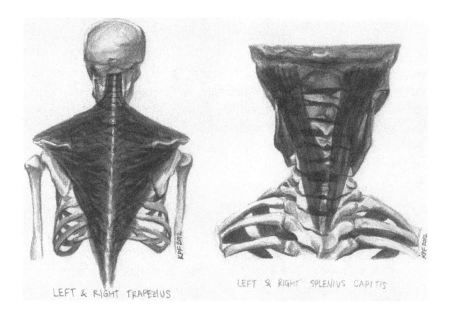

FIGURE 12.1. Trapezius (*left*) and splenius capitis (*right*) muscles (Courtesy of Katrina Franzen).

yoga for exercise and stress reduction and daily acupressure of Chinese medicine acupoints relevant for neck pain.

To minimize microtrauma from the patient's participation in music, he received treatments from an Alexander Technique therapist.[30] Alexander Technique and the Feldenkrais Method both use imagery and sensory feedback from the therapist along with muscle relaxation and neuromuscular re-education. Both forms may help this patient to "unlearn" improper use of muscle functions and rehabilitate the body by optimal muscle activity in the proper alignment and technique.[31]

The beta blocker was continued for his hypertension and headache prophylaxis. A low-dose muscle relaxant 1 hour before bedtime was considered as needed for muscle spasm, which may have also contributed to sleep disruption and headaches.

The patient initially received weekly treatments and gradually implemented his self-care program into his routine. Over time, he came to terms with his rage, managed the conflicts in his personal life, and noted improved sleep. After several weeks of treatment, the patient stated that he had near-complete resolution of his symptoms and was able to increasingly reconnect with his music. He was able to recognize early warning signs of depletion and took action through lifestyle behaviors and therapies to prevent flares, restore resiliency, and optimize function and quality of life.

Neuropathic Pain

Neuropathic pain results from injury to the peripheral or central nervous system. Common features of neuropathic pain are damage to thermonociceptive neuronal pathways, hyperalgesia and allodynia in areas of secondary hyperalgesia in nonaffected contiguous areas, and poor response to opioids. Examples include postherpetic neuralgia, diabetic neuropathy, trigeminal neuralgia, post-stroke central or thalamic pain, and post-amputation phantom limb pain.[3]

HISTORY

M.D. is a 68-year-old female with post-herpetic neuralgia. She was treated for shingles with antiviral mediations and opioids 5 weeks prior to her initial visit. She noted worsening symptoms with associated skin redness and burning pain over the last week that began after she applied heat to the area. The patient stated that she was visiting from out of town and serving on a church mission for the next 3 months. She described the character of the pain as burning, duration as constant, and intensity as severe. Symptoms worsened in an upright position and improved with lying down and holding a pillow to her chest.

PHYSICAL EXAMINATION

The skin demonstrated warmth and erythema overlying a healing rash on her right chest. She was afebrile. A trigger point was appreciated in the neck, and range of motion of the neck was decreased.

ASSESSMENT

This patient presented with post-herpetic neuralgia. In addition, she had findings suspicious for a secondary skin infection in the area of the healing rash.

Individual variation to neuropathic pain requires a customized approach to analgesics and adjuvant analgesics. Drugs for neuropathic pain are classified as topical analgesics, adjuvant analgesics, and opioids. Adjuvant analgesics are classified as tricyclic antidepressants, other antidepressants, anticonvulsants, antiarrhythmics, and other drugs.[3,4]

If a medication is included in the treatment plan, the lowest anticipated effective dose may be started. Then the therapeutic effect and any side effects may be monitored based on expected absorption and pharmacokinetics of the agent and titrated on the basis of likely steady-state blood levels and clinically demonstrated effects.[1,4]

TREATMENT APPROACH

On the initial visit, inspection of the affected thoracic area was suggestive of superficial skin infection. The patient was treated with antibiotics, which resolved the erythema and improved pain to some degree. The patient was treated with a trigger point injection of the right trapezius muscle, which improved her neck pain and range of motion, though her thoracic neuropathic pain persisted. A trial of acupuncture did not improve her pain.

The patient declined a trial of alpha-lipoic acid, benfotiamine, and acetyl-L-carnitine in preference of "something stronger," though she was concerned with opioid side effects.[32–34] Acetaminophen did not provide any relief. The patient did not tolerate a lidocaine patch, which irritated her skin.

The patient opted for a tricyclic antidepressant with goals to support exercise, enjoy activities, and get a good night's sleep.[1] A low dose taken before bedtime was prescribed for the short term to minimize the potential risks of visual, urinary, and gastrointestinal anticholinergic adverse effects as well as orthostasis and atrioventricular blockade cardiovascular adverse effects.[4]

When the pain had alleviated to the point that she could get dressed and go out more comfortably, the patient noted added relief from cognitive self-care with distraction. She reduced the intensity of her pain by exploring the city, going to eat with her husband and friends, and praying. She also limited the number of hours per day of her missionary work.

After a month of treatment, the patient noted up to 14 hours a day without pain, though she continued to note discomfort at night. She returned to her home at the conclusion of her mission with the plan to wean her medications over the next few weeks to months.

Fibromyalgia

An individual's description and self-report usually provides accurate, reliable, and sufficient evidence for the presence and intensity of pain.[1] The 2010 American College of Rheumatology (ACR) fibromyalgia diagnostic criteria were aimed at simplifying the diagnosis of fibromyalgia syndrome (FMS) and being suitable for use in primary care practice without requiring a tender point examination (Table 12.4). Another objective was to recognize the importance of the numerous non-pain symptoms of fibromyalgia.[35]

HISTORY

L.S. is a 68-year-old female with generalized body pains and fatigue. She was in a state of good health until she was diagnosed with breast cancer 15 years prior to her initial visit. She discontinued chemotherapy after surgery and radiation because she was unable to tolerate the side effects of the cancer medications. She was subsequently diagnosed with depression and treated with medications that caused weight gain. In addition to her depressed mood, she developed worsening generalized pain that was severe enough to prevent her from carrying a purse. With the progression of her pain and fatigue, she found her duties as director of sales and marketing progressively more difficult. At one point she could not understand the content of a proposal that she had previously

Table 12.4. American College of Rheumatology (ACR) 2010 Scoring and Diagnostic Criteria for Fibromyalgia

Scoring

A. Widespread Pain Index (WPI)
   1. Part 1: Total the number of areas of tenderness or pain (out of 19 possible)

B. Symptom Score (SS)
   1. Total the points from parts 2 and 3 (out of 12 possible)
   2. Part 2: Total the number of points from the 3 questions (assign 0–3 points for each of the 3 questions)
   3. Part 3: Assign 1 point for each of the 3 questions that are positive

Diagnosis

A. Criteria 1
   1. Widespread Pain Index (WPI): 7 of 19 and
   2. Symptom Score (SS): 5 of 12

B. Criteria 2
   1. Widespread Pain Index (WPI): 3-6 of 19 and
   2. Symptom Score (SS): 9 of 12

created. She compensated for her loss of words and inability to prioritize tasks for some time, though her employer eventually terminated her from her job.

L.S. was eventually diagnosed with fibromyalgia when her symptoms reached the point that she could "barely get out of bed, barely do much at all." She related, "When I was diagnosed with fibromyalgia, I asked, what is it? And I was told things about it—pain and fatigue and things like that. I was asked what could be done about it. I was told nothing could be done about it."

In addition to her history of breast cancer with ongoing left arm lymphedema treated with a compression sleeve, she had received therapy from a psychologist for posttraumatic disorder (PTSD) over the years. She also noted other functional symptoms: irritable bowel syndrome that began after a duodenal ulcer in her 20s; temporomandibular joint pain after multiple dental procedures; migraine, which had improved after menopause; and interstitial cystitis, which interfered with her sleep.[36] Medications for her pain and other conditions were an opioid, a benzodiazepine, and a selective serotonin reuptake inhibitor.

The patient described her pain as generalized, constant, and severe. She attributed her pain condition to cumulative stress from her health issues and psychological stress from family dynamics. The pain limited her ability to go grocery shopping and clean her apartment.

L.S. described her mood as depressed. She "did not feel herself" with the weight gain and her diminished cognitive function and inability to work. She reported that spirituality, inner strength from previous life experiences, and her problem-solving skills were resources to help her cope with her pain. She had hope that she could find a way to improve her health.

L.S. lived with her grown son and described their relationship as strained. She did not smoke or drink. She described herself as spiritual and not affiliated with organized religion.

PHYSICAL EXAMINATION

On physical examination, 18/18 tender points were noted as described by the ACR's 1990 Criteria for the Classification of Fibromyalgia.[37] The results of the neurological and musculoskeletal examination were otherwise normal.

ASSESSMENT

The findings of the history and physical examination were diagnostic of fibromyalgia. In addition to widespread pain, L.S. demonstrated the non-pain symptoms of the condition such as perceived cognitive impairment, fatigue, and sleep disturbance.[35]

TREATMENT APPROACH

In a discussion of lifestyle interventions, the patient began to reframe her relationship with family to focus on positive aspects and to manage challenging interactions. She built exercise tolerance by walking with the assistance of a wagon around a nearby grocery store until she was able to take walks in a park.

In addition to her self-care, the patient also opted to begin treatment with trigger point injections. She considered medical cannabis for her PTSD and chronic pain symptoms, though she was discouraged by the certification and procurement process. As her condition improved, L.S. was able to cut the dosage of her pain medications. She moved into her own apartment and established boundaries of her caretaking of others so she could focus on her healing. She began to reconnect with her artistic interests and proceeded to write two books of her poetry. She became active in movement therapies such as tai chi and yoga. Her condition ultimately improved to the point that she participated in ballroom dance instruction, demonstrating turns and dips as one of the most proficient students in the class.

Cancer-Related Pain

Pain syndromes are common in patients with cancer. Pain may occur as a direct consequence of the disease or of its treatment, though in the outpatient setting, patients with cancer may present with pain not related to their disease.[38] Myofascial pain syndromes may occur in 44% of patients following breast cancer surgery and are common following neck dissection in management of head and neck cancers as well as after thoracotomy.[22–24]

HISTORY

D.W. is a 75-year-old female with a diagnosis of multiple myeloma and with multiple pain symptoms. She was diagnosed with multiple myeloma that was incidentally discovered during a workup for pleurisy. Starting 3 years prior to her diagnosis of cancer, the patient had an episode of low back pain after cumulative events including pericarditis and, a few months later, an international flight. At that time, she was evaluated by a neurologist and neurosurgeon and diagnosed with degenerative changes. Electromyography (EMG) reportedly was suggestive of nerve conduction abnormalities. She declined NSAIDs and opioids because of her concern for side effects.

Along with self-care that included swimming a mile per day, she got relief of her low back pain as well as subsequent flares of low back pain and neck pain with trigger point injections and acupuncture. At the time of her cancer diagnosis, a scan by her oncologist demonstrated multiple myeloma activity in the ribs and femur. She was successfully treated for multiple myeloma. Cancer medications were subsequently discontinued for 2 years until chemotherapy was resumed because of laboratory abnormalities and associated rib and lower extremity pain.

D.W. had multiple pain symptoms. She described her cancer-related rib and lower extremity pain as burning, 1 to 2/10 intensity, primarily at night. She used distraction provided by her daily activities to get relief from her pain. Her intermittent neck and low back pain was 3 to 4/10 intensity. She noted a flare of her muscular pain symptoms related to cycles of her ongoing chemotherapy. During flares, her neck and low back pain worsened with walking uphill and kicking during swimming. Her pain did not limit her activity but interfered with her quality of life.

D.W. lived with her husband. She was a retired nurse and health counselor. She attended church every week and was involved in the church community. She also found comfort by participating in a multiple myeloma group as well as a group of swimmers. She relaxed with a "meditation" that she performed while she focused on her breathing during swimming. Her interests were travel, gardening, playing bridge, yoga, and Pilates.

ASSESSMENT

This patient described multiple pain symptoms, some of them cancer-related and some of them not directly related to her cancer or treatment. When evaluating a patient with cancer presenting for pain symptoms, a thorough examination of the muscular system may help the patient get some relief and improve quality of life while continuing aggressive cancer surveillance and management.

TREATMENT APPROACH

D.W. noted relief of her pain to the point that she was fully active. She got relief from her cancer-related bone pain with acetaminophen before bed. She maintained optimal health with exercise, a "raw" diet, and social support. She managed her flares of neck and low back pain with trigger point and acupuncture treatments. She got relief of pain symptoms and stress with reflexology as well. D.W. described herself as optimistic and fully active without any physical limitations.

REFERENCES

1. AGS Panel on Persistent Pain in Older Persons. The management of persistent pain in older persons. *J Am Geriatr Soc.* 2002;50(6 suppl):S205–S224.
2. Makris UE, Abrams RC, Gurland B, Reid MC. Management of persistent pain in the older patient: A clinical review. *JAMA.* 2014;312(8):825–37.
3. Davis M, Srivastava M. Demographics, assessment, and management of pain in the elderly. *Drugs Aging.* 2003;20(1):23–57.
4. American Geriatrics Society Panel on Pharmacological Management of Persistent Pain in Older Persons. Pharmacological management of persistent pain in older persons. *J Am Geriatr Soc.* 2009;57(8):1331–1346.
5. Goldman L, Schafer AI, eds. *Goldman's Cecil Medicine*, 25th ed. United States: Elsevier Saunders; 2016:129–130.

6. Cochrane Musculoskeletal. [Cited August 1, 2016.] Available from http://musculoskeletal.cochrane.org/search/reviews/knee%20osteoarthritis

7. Exercise prescription for older adults with osteoarthritis pain: Consensus practice recommendations. *J Am Geriatr Soc.* 2001;49:808–823.

8. Kaye AD, Baluch A, Scott JT. Pain management in the elderly population: A review. *The Ochsner Journal.* 2010;10(3):179–187.

9. Report of the Task Force on Research Standards for Chronic Low-Back Pain, Submitted to the NIH Pain Consortium Executive Committee, November 18, 2013.

10. Chou R. Low back pain. *Ann Intern Med.* 2014;160(11): ITC6-1–ITC6-13.

11. Kraus H. Prevention of low back pain. *J Occup Med.* 1967;9(11):555–559.

12. Kraus H, Nagler W, Melleby A. An evaluation of an exercise program for back pain. *Am Fam Physician.* 1983; 28:153–158.

13. Kraus H, Marcus NJ. The reintroduction of an exercise program to directly treat low back pain of muscular origin. *J Back Musculoskelet Rehabil.* 1997;(8)2:95–107.

14. Marcus N, Ough J. Muscle pain treatment. In: Deer TR, Leong MS, Ray AL, eds. *Treatment of Chronic Pain by Integrative Approaches: The American Academy of Pain Medicine Textbook on Patient Management.* New York: Springer; 2015:25–41.

15. Sherman KJ, Cherkin DC, Wellman RD, et al. A randomized trial comparing yoga, stretching, and a self-care book for chronic low back pain. *Arch Intern Med.* 2011;171(22):2019–2026.

16. Cherkin DC, Sherman KJ, Balderson BH, et al. Effect of mindfulness-based stress reduction vs cognitive behavioral therapy or usual care on back pain and functional limitations in adults with chronic low back pain: a randomized clinical trial. *JAMA.* 2016;315(12):1240–1249.

17. Mehling WE, Ugalde V, Goldberg H. Musculoskeletal disorders. In: Jacobs BP, Gundling K. *The ACP Evidence-Based Guide to Complementary and Alternative Medicine.* Philadelphia: American College of Physicians Press; 2009:289–325.

18. Castaldo M, Ge HY, Chiarotto A, Villafane JH, Arendt-Nielsen L. Myofascial trigger points in patients with whiplash-associated disorders and mechanical neck pain. *Pain Med.* 2014 May;15(5):842–849.

19. Ashina S, Bendtsen L, Lyngberg AC, Lipton RB, Hajiyeva N, Jensen R. Prevalence of neck pain in migraine and tension-type headache: A population study. *Cephalalgia.* 2015 Mar 26;35(3):211–219.

20. Fernández-de-Las-Peñas C, Galán-Del-Río F, Alonso-Blanco C, Jiménez-García R, Arendt-Nielsen L, Svensson P. Referred pain from muscle trigger points in the masticatory and neck-shoulder musculature in women with temporomandibular disorders. *J Pain.* 2010 Dec;11(12):1295–1304.

21. Cakit BD, Taskin S, Nacir B, Unlu I, Genc H, Erdem HR. Comorbidity of fibromyalgia and cervical myofascial pain syndrome. *Clin Rheumatol.* 2010 Apr;29(4):405–411.

22. Torres Lacomba M, Mayoral del Moral O, Coperias Zazo JL, Gerwin RD, Goñi AZ. Incidence of myofascial pain syndrome in breast cancer surgery: a prospective study. *Clin J Pain.* 2010 May;26(4):320–325.

23. Cardoso LR, Rizzo CC, de Oliveira CZ, Dos Santos CR, Carvalho AL. Myofascial pain syndrome after head and neck cancer treatment: Prevalence, risk factors, and influence on quality of life. *Head Neck.* 2015 Dec;37(12):1733–1737.

24. Hamada H, Moriwaki K, Shiroyama K, Tanaka H, Kawamoto M, Yuge O. Myofascial pain in patients with postthoracotomy pain syndrome. *Reg Anesth Pain Med.* 2000;25:302–305.

25. Travell JG, Simons DG. *Myofascial Pain and Dysfunction: The Trigger Point Manual.* Baltimore: Williams & Wilkins; 1983.

26. Centers for Medicare & Medicaid Services, Local Coverage Determination for Trigger Point Injections. [Cited June 17, 2016.] Available from https://www.cms. gov/medicare-coverage-database/search/search-results.aspx?CoverageSelection= Both&ArticleType=All&PolicyType=Final&s=All&KeyWord=trigger+point&Key WordLookUp=Title&KeyWordSearchType=And&FriendlyError=NoLCDIDVersi on&bc=gAAAAAAAAAAAA%3d%3d&=&

27. Chiarotto A, Clijsen R, Fernandez-de-Las-Penas C, Barbero M. The prevalence of myofascial trigger points in spinal disorders: A systematic review and meta-analysis. *Arch Phys Med Rehabil.* 2015 Oct. 14. pii: S0003-9993(15)01242-3.

28. McEwen BS1, Wingfield JC. The concept of allostasis in biology and biomedicine. *Horm Behav.* 2003 Jan;43(1):2–15.

29. Lederman RJ. Performing arts medicine. *N Engl J Med.* 1989 Jan 26;320(4):246–248.

30. MacPherson H, Tilbrook H, Richmond S, et al. Alexander Technique lessons or acupuncture sessions for persons with chronic neck pain: A randomized trial. *Ann Intern Med.* 2015;163:653–662

31. *Feldenkrais: Awareness Through Movement.* New York: Harper & Row; 1972.

32. Han T, Bai J, Liu W, Hu Y. A systematic review and meta-analysis of α-lipoic acid in the treatment of diabetic peripheral neuropathy. *Eur J Endocrinol.* 2012;167(4):465–471.

33. Ang CD, Alviar MJM, Dans AL, et al. Vitamin B for treating peripheral neuropathy. *Cochrane Database of Systematic Reviews* 2008, Issue 3. Art. No.: CD004573. DOI:10.1002/14651858.CD004573.pub3

34. Li S, Li Q, Li Y, et al. Acetyl-L-carnitine in the treatment of peripheral neuropathic pain: A systematic review and meta-analysis of randomized controlled trials. *PLoS ONE.* 2015;10(3):e0119479. doi:10.1371/journal.pone.0119479.

35. Wolfe F, Clauw D, Fitzcharles M, et al. The American College of Rheumatology preliminary diagnostic criteria for fibromyalgia and measurement of symptom severity for arthritis. *Care Res.* 2010;62(5):600–610.

36. Aaron LA, Buchwald D. A review of the evidence for overlap among unexplained clinical conditions. *Ann Intern Med.* 2001;134:868–881.

37. Wolfe F, Smythe H, Yunus M, et al. The American College of Rheumatology 1990 Criteria for the Classification of Fibromyalgia: Report of the multicenter criteria committee. *Arthritis Rheum.* 1990;33:160–172.

38. Cleeland CS, Gonin R, Hatfield AK, et al. Pain and its treatment in outpatients with metastatic cancer. *N Engl J Med.* 1994;330:592–559.

13

Cardiovascular Disease

MARA CAROLINE, RYAN BRADLEY,
AND MIMI GUARNERI

Case Study

An 81-year-old man presents to the office complaining of shortness of breath that has been progressing over the past several weeks. He has a history of hypertension, dyslipidemia, atrial fibrillation, and depression. He is taking 12 medications. His wife used to manage his medications, but she passed away 4 months ago and he is having trouble keeping them organized. He states the dyspnea occurs primarily while watching television, eating dinner, and going to sleep at night. Sometimes he also experiences palpitations during the night. He is able to perform activity without dyspnea; however, since his atorvastatin dose was increased to 40 mg he has felt physically limited due to leg cramping. On reviewing his dietary habits you discover that he is eating mainly frozen and instant meals and drinks two glasses of wine with dinner each night. During your visit, you bring up the issue of loneliness and depression and discuss strategies by which he can build social connections. He has always loved dogs, so you suggest that he get one. His medication list is reviewed and unnecessary drugs, including pantoprazole, are discontinued. Atorvastatin is switched to low-dose rosuvastatin, and you recommend magnesium 800 mg daily and coenzyme Q10 200 mg daily. You also discuss reducing his alcohol intake. An echocardiogram and an event monitor reveal frequent premature atrial complexes and normal cardiac function.

At his next visit he reports that his dyspnea has improved significantly and he is also sleeping better. His leg cramps have resolved and he is enjoying taking his dog for two long walks each day. Additionally, he looks forward to having dinner with his daughter three days per week. He is planning on joining a local cooking club so that he can prepare meals for his daughter.

Introduction

The older population in the United States is rising exponentially, with an expected doubling of the population over the age of 65 by the year 2050 from 46 million to 88 million.[1] The effects of aging influence the cardiomyocytes, vascular endothelial cells, and pacemaker cells, leading to changes in diastolic function, perfusion, vascular stiffening, and arrhythmia. Thus, cardiovascular disease (CVD) is endemic in the elderly population, and this subset of the population makes up the majority of visits to cardiologists.

Treating the aging population presents several specific challenges. Compared to the general population, they often have greater comorbidities, as well as physical and cognitive disabilities, which can be easily aggravated by many medications and therapies. They are also prescribed more medications, putting them at increased risk of adverse drug–drug and drug–disease reactions. The risk for adverse drug reactions is further increased by unpredictable drug absorption, metabolism, and elimination. Adding another challenge is the psychosocial context in which many geriatric patients live; they often lack social support and may experience loneliness, depression, and anxiety. These psychosocial factors not only impact the patient generally, and influence important treatment considerations like medication adherence, but are also associated with an increased risk of CVD and worse outcomes if it already exists.[2,3]

In addition to their different physiology and psychology, older adults also have different values, often prioritizing non-mortality objectives such as symptom relief, quality of life, functional capacity, reduced hospitalizations, and independence. On top of all of these issues, the elderly population, especially those who are most frail, are also extremely underrepresented in clinical trials,[4,5] leaving us with vague guidelines and little formal direction to address the unique needs of this population.

As caregivers for older patients we cannot base treatment purely on guidelines or age; rather, we must learn to reconcile physiological and biological age in the context of each patient's individual circumstances and goals. Cardiovascular care for seniors should begin with a comprehensive assessment of each individual's circumstances, including functional capacity, cognition, medications, psychosocial and cognitive health, social support, spiritual preferences, nutritional status, and goals of care.

Primary Prevention

DIET

According to the World Health Organization, physical inactivity and low intake of fruit and vegetables are two of the most significant modifiable risk factors of ischemic heart disease and are estimated to cause 22% and 31% of ischemic heart disease worldwide, respectively.[6] The main emphasis is on replacing saturated and trans fats with polyunsaturated fats, adding fish and plant-based omega-3-fatty acids, and reducing refined carbohydrates in favor of plant-based whole foods, including fruits, vegetables, nuts, beans, seeds, and whole grains, with minimal intake of meats and full-fat dairy products.

The PREDIMED study[7] was a primary prevention trial conducted in 7,447 elderly individuals with risk factors for cardiovascular disease. They were randomized to either a Mediterranean diet supplemented with olive oil, a Mediterranean diet supplemented with nuts, or a control diet and were followed for a median of 4.8 years. The researchers found a 30% relative risk reduction in the primary endpoint of myocardial infarction, stroke, and death from cardiovascular causes, though this outcome was primarily driven by a reduction in the rates of cerebrovascular accident (CVA). A meta-analysis looking at the relationship between a Mediterranean diet and healthy aging in the elderly population suggested that this diet not only lowers the incidence of acute myocardial infarction and cardiovascular mortality but also modifies risk factors for CVD, including lipoprotein levels, endothelial vasodilation, insulin resistance, and antioxidant capacity.[8] The nutrients provided in the Mediterranean diet are likely essential and possibly work synergistically to mediate positive changes in pathways of blood lipids, insulin sensitivity, resistance to oxidation, inflammation, and vasoreactivity.[9] In addition, the Mediterranean diet not only prevents the onset of events but may also temper the severity of the disease once it appears.[8,10]

STRESS MANAGEMENT

The connection between psychosocial stress and CVD is well established. Most physicians are accustomed to focusing on the biomedical causes of disease and have neither the time to recognize the psychosocial determinants of CVD nor the training to identify them as a key factor in the primary and secondary prevention of heart disease. INTERHEART, a large international case-control study, took a leap toward increasing awareness of the impact of stress on cardiovascular disease.[11] In this study, all patients admitted to the cardiac service for a first myocardial infarction (MI) were screened for common risk factors such as smoking, hypertension, diabetes, elevated apolipoprotein B levels, and waist circumference. They were also screened for psychosocial stress, including depression, the perception of lack of control of their surroundings, and several other factors. The researchers found that increased stress was responsible for over 30% of population-attributable risk for first MI, more than smoking or hypertension alone.

Classically, we recognize stress as a function of work life, family/children, divorce, and financial strain. However, the precipitants of stress evolve with age, and those triggers that are more common in the elderly, such as worry, loneliness, and depression, are often under-recognized. The worries of the elderly are also different, with more emphasis on their deteriorating functional capacity, physical resiliency, and memory changes, which are often a significant source of stress. The stress response may be heightened in situations where patients have the experience of little or no control, and elderly patients are often dependent on others due to physical or other limitations.

The Normative Aging Study is an ongoing longitudinal study that began in 1963 to follow healthy men in an effort to better characterize the determinants of healthy aging. In addition to looking at biomedical factors, the researchers also examined psychosocial components such as the patient's subjective perception of health, outlook, and social connectedness in relation to the development of disease. They found that higher reported levels of worry (especially about social isolation) were associated with a two- to three-fold increased risk of developing coronary heart disease (CHD) compared to those with lower reported levels.[12–14] Another prospective cohort study followed 5,000 patients over the age of 65 who did not have CVD. These patients provided information about their depressive status annually. The researchers found that among elderly Americans, depression is an independent risk factor for the development of coronary disease and total mortality, with the highest risk seen among participants with the highest cumulative mean depression scores.[15]

Research on social isolation and loneliness as risk factors is more subjective. A recent systematic review of prospective longitudinal studies found that a background of poor social relationships is associated with an 29% increase in the risk of CHD and a 31% increased risk of stroke, suggesting that these issues may be an important target in preventing cardiovascular morbidity.[16,17]

Stress is an inherent and necessary part of life; however, chronic maladaptation to stress is a common and modifiable risk factor for CHD events, especially among older adults, who commonly have under-recognized psychosocial stress. Therefore, we need to focus on interventions that enable them to handle stress more effectively, thus making them more resilient. Integrative medicine offers a wealth of resources that are effective for building resiliency by providing patients with simple, life-long survival tools for dealing with stress, many of which can be easily taught and used as needed for self-treatment.

The simplest intervention is to increase social support, which does not require training or organized participation. Popular ways of increasing social connectedness include volunteerism, an activity that has been linked to less depression and anxiety, as well as pet ownership, a non-human form of social support that has been associated with reductions in depression, cardiovascular risk, and mortality. Social support and pet ownership are significant predictors of survival post-MI, independent of other psychosocial and physiological factors,[18] and have been shown to improve outcomes in patients with depression and CVD.[19]

Many other nonpharmacological tools aim to trigger the "relaxation response," which is the physiological opposite of the sympathetic, catecholamine-driven, fight-or-flight response. This response is very powerful and is associated with physiological changes such as decreased blood pressure, heart rate, and respiratory rate, and an increase in heart rate variability, which is a healthy pattern.[20] Numerous mind–body practices are available to provide tools for managing daily stressors. Please see Chapter 9 for specific mind–body practices.

EXERCISE

Age-related changes lead to a reduced maximum heart rate and reduced stroke volume reserve as well as central arterial stiffening, increased left ventricular mass, and impaired diastolic filling. Exercise may attenuate some of these changes.[21] The protective benefits of exercise in the elderly with known CVD are also clear. In fact, the evidence supports the fact that the elderly may actually have a relatively greater response to exercise compared to younger patients given their relatively diminished baseline capacity.[22-24] Williams et al.[25] looked at the benefits of a 12-week standardized exercise training in elderly patients versus younger patients early after MI or coronary artery bypass grafting (CABG). Though their absolute physical capacity was lower than younger patients, elderly patients experienced the same magnitude of improvement in functional capacity, maximal heart rate, and reduction in body fat.

In addition to improvements in cardiovascular health seen with exercise, other physical and psychological benefits have been seen, including improved neuromuscular function and balance, mood, independence, and self-esteem. A cohort of 458 consecutive elderly (>65) and younger patients post-MI and CABG were enrolled in a cardiac rehabilitation program that included 36 educational and exercise sessions over a 3- to 4-month period. Not surprisingly, they found that elderly and young patients alike experienced significant improvements in functional capacity (43% vs. 32% increase) and reductions in body mass index (BMI) and body fat as well as modest improvements in HDL and the LDL/HDL ratio. The researchers also administered validated questionnaires to a subset of 151 patients to assess psychosocial characteristics and quality of life parameters and found statistically significant improvement in behavioral characteristics, including anxiety and depression, as well as in quality-of-life parameters, including energy, pain, function, and total quality of life, to a similar degree in both the elderly and young groups.[26]

Despite clear benefits in exercise capacity as well as in reducing disability and mortality, cardiac rehabilitation programs are extremely underutilized in the elderly population, with less than 20% of those eligible using these services.[27-29] Cardiac rehabilitation programs can reduce mortality, improve quality of life, and increase functional capacity in elderly patients with heart disease without any adverse effects. In addition, exercise mitigates important risk factors for progression of disease, including hypertension, obesity, insulin resistance, and psychosocial stress. It may also play a role in reducing inflammation, which is a risk factor for the development and progression of many chronic diseases;[30] it also reduces cognitive decline and depression and prolongs autonomy.[31] Of course, recommendations need to be responsible and individualized, especially in the very elderly or those with significant comorbidities. Cardiac rehabilitation centers provide a safe exercise environment and a venue for socialization and group support.[32]

LDL MANAGEMENT

Beyond diet and exercise, the next most important step is to optimize LDL using pharmaceutical therapy, such as statins, or non-prescription alternatives. The most reliable non-prescription therapies for LDL lowering include red yeast rice, niacin, soluble fiber, plant stanols/sterols, and soy.

Red rice yeast is the original source of lovastatin and remains available as a complex dietary supplement. Typical red rice yeast doses range from 1,200 to 3,600 mg/day, and red rice yeast is typically tolerated even when statin drugs are not, especially at lower doses. Notably, red rice yeast will still reduce CoQ10 concentrations and can cause myalgias and abnormal results on liver function tests. However, these side effects are less frequent compared to statins.[33-35]

Extended-release niacin has potent LDL-lowering and HDL-raising effects. Typical doses are 500 to 1,500 mg/day. Non-flush niacin is ineffective for LDL lowering, and niacin flushing may result in reflexive endothelial vasodilation, improving its cardiovascular effects. Admittedly, the flushing is often intolerable to patients, and in the elderly care must be given not to induce hypotension. Pretreatment with aspirin 30 minutes before dosing may reduce flushing.[36]

Soluble fiber reduces the intestinal absorption and hepatic synthesis of cholesterol, and 1 g daily can reduce LDL by 2.2 mg/dl.[37]

Plants contain *phytosterols* and *stanols*, which reduce intestinal absorption of cholesterol by competing with other sources of cholesterol. Clinical research supports an effective dose of 1,800 mg/day.[38]

NUTRITIONAL IMPLICATIONS
OF CARDIOVASCULAR MEDICATIONS

Vitamins, minerals, amino acids, and essential fatty acids are required by all cells in the body, and proper nutrition is essential for the prevention and management of CVD.[39–41] Micronutrient deficiencies are of particular concern in the elderly population for several reasons. First, foods that are richest in nutrients tend to be unprocessed, predominantly fruits, vegetables, and whole grains, while many older adults rely heavily on processed foods due to changes in taste preferences, difficulties with chewing or digestion, or inaccessibility. Nutrient depletion can impact the progression of CVD as well as contribute to overall worsening health and debilitating symptoms. Additionally, medication-induced deficiency is under-recognized and common. There are many mechanisms whereby this may happen, including increased excretion (as occurs in the case of water-soluble vitamins in patients taking diuretics), decreased absorption due to binding or increasing stomach pH (as occurs with proton pump inhibitors and H2 blockers), and blocking nutrient production (as occurs with statin-induced depletion of coenzyme Q10).

It is important to recognize common presenting symptoms of nutrient losses associated with common cardiovascular drugs in order to identify a symptom as due to illness, a medication side effect, or nutrient depletion. Knowledge of the relationship between modern drug therapy and natural medicine can improve quality of life by making it possible to treat symptoms of nutrient deficiency by supplementing with the deficient essential vitamins and minerals. The following is a review of common cardiovascular drug-induced nutrient deficiencies, including strategies for recognition and treatment.

Magnesium

In 2009, the World Health Organization reported that 75% of Americans consumed less magnesium than needed.[42] Additionally, the elderly exhibit increased renal excretion of magnesium as well as a decreased capacity of the bones to store and release magnesium.[43] Hypomagnesemia is associated with an increased incidence of hypertension, CHD, and diabetes.[44-46] Of note, serum magnesium levels do not accurately reflect total body magnesium as the majority is located intracellularly, with small quantities being drawn extracellularly to maintain serum levels. Symptoms of deficiency include muscle cramps/spasm, arrhythmia, constipation, osteoporosis, weakness, fatigue, insomnia, restless leg syndrome, irritability, anxiety, insulin resistance, depression, high blood pressure, and headache. Magnesium-rich foods include dark leafy greens; tree nuts and peanuts; seeds; oily fish; beans, lentils, legumes, and whole grains; avocado, yogurt, bananas, and dried fruit; dark chocolate; and molasses. Common forms for supplementation include magnesium aspartate, citrate, glycinate, or amino acid chelate, 400 to 800 mg/day. Cutaneous preparations are available in the form of creams and Epsom salt baths. Caution should be used when treating patients with renal impairment.

Coenzyme Q10 (Ubiquinone)

Coenzyme Q10 is a fat-soluble compound whose most important role is as a coenzyme in the electron transport chain. Natural synthesis of coenzyme Q10 is impaired in a dose-related fashion by statin drugs via inhibition of HMG-CoA-reductase, which blocks the synthesis of mevalonic acid, a precursor of coenzyme Q-10. Levels of CoQ10 are also decreased in older patients, including those with heart failure, where CoQ10 concentrations correlate with severity and are an independent predictor of mortality.[47] Given the safety of this substance, a case can be made to supplement most elderly patients, especially those with heart failure.[48,49] Symptoms of CoQ10 deficiency are myalgia/arthralgias, rhabdomyolysis, cardiomyopathy, hypertension, angina, stroke, arrhythmias, fatigue, leg weakness, loss of cognitive function, gingivitis, and a weakened immune system. A solubilized preparation is administered at up to 300 mg/day.

Folic Acid and Vitamin B12

Both are water-soluble vitamins and are often described together due to their joint role as co-factors for homocysteine remethylation. Deficiencies are common in the elderly population due to poor intake, deficiency in intrinsic factor, low stomach acid, or alcoholism. Several prospective studies, including a subset of the Framingham Heart Study, have found an inverse relation between folic acid levels and cardiovascular morbidity and mortality.[50] This relationship has been described both via homocysteine lowering and non-homocysteine-related mechanisms, including through its role as an antioxidant. Vitamin B12 deficiency should always be considered when starting folic acid supplementation due to the concern that folic acid may mask the clinical diagnosis of B12 deficiency (via anemia) and allow silent progression of neurological deterioration. Despite recent interest in the relationship among folate, B12, and methylene-tetrahydrofolate reductase (MTHFR) polymorphisms, "methylated" forms of folate and/or B12 must be recommended with caution due to recognition of "hypermethylation" syndromes secondary to methylated folate, which have been observed to be associated with severe clinical anxiety and panic attacks. Symptoms of B12 deficiency include elevated homocysteine levels, depression, anemia, fatigue, peripheral neuropathy, and breast and colon cancer. B12-rich foods include fish, shellfish, meat, eggs, and dairy. B12 supplementation is typically recommended as sublingual or intramuscular, with typical doses of 500 to 1,500 mcg/day. Folate-rich foods include green leafy vegetables, artificially fortified cereals, and grains. Folate supplementation is 400 to 800 mg/day.

Vitamin D

Vitamin D is a fat-soluble vitamin that functions as a hormone with receptors located in almost every tissue of the body. Vitamin D is integral to maintaining cardiovascular health, with receptors located in cardiomyocytes, endothelial cells, and nearly all immune cells. Low levels have also been implicated as a cause of hypertension, endothelial dysfunction, heart failure, and insulin resistance.[51,52] The main source of vitamin D is via skin synthesis from precursors when the skin is exposed to ultraviolet light, though skin synthesis is reduced with advanced age. Low levels have been linked with all-cause and cardiovascular mortality.[53] The recent VINDICATE study found that in patients with chronic systolic heart failure and vitamin D deficiency (levels <20 ng/ml), daily supplementation with 4,000 IU of vitamin D3 was associated with significant improvement in ejection fraction as well as reversal of remodeling (reduction in LVEDD and LVESD) and was also safe and well tolerated.[54] Symptoms of vitamin D deficiency include osteoporosis, increased risk of bony fracture, depression, hormonal imbalances, muscular weakness, hypertension, autoimmune disease, diabetes, and decreased immunity.

Foods rich in vitamin D include fish, eggs, fortified milk, and cod-liver oil. Supplementation of vitamin D3 should be titrated based on serum concentration of 25-hydroxycholecalciferol, but typical doses range from 2,000 to 10,000 IU of vitamin D3 per day. Optimal serum concentrations of 25-hydroxycholecalciferol have not been established.

Potassium

Potassium is the most abundant electrolyte in the body and is necessary for healthy cardiovascular function, including systolic blood pressure reduction,[55] as well as for proper nervous system function, muscle contraction, and digestion. Like magnesium, the highest concentrations of potassium are intracellular, with active transport occurring to maintain serum levels. Not only is the average intake of 45 mEq/day much less than the recommended 650 mEq/day, but many medications deplete potassium stores. All patients taking loop diuretics should be on potassium repletion barring a contraindication. Additionally, magnesium status should be assessed in patients with hypokalemia, because this makes it refractory to treatment as hypomagnesemia increases distal tubule potassium wasting.[56] Symptoms of potassium deficiency include irregular heartbeat, poor reflexes, muscle weakness, fatigue, thirst, confusion, constipation, dizziness, and nervousness. Potassium-rich foods include fruits and vegetables (especially parsley, potatoes, bananas, avocados, and dried apricots), nuts, soybeans, bran, chocolate, and salt substitutes. Potassium supplementation can be up to 80 mEq/day with a goal serum level of approximately 4 to 5 mEq/L.

In many cardiovascular diseases, modern drugs mediate improvements in symptoms and mortality, but possibly at the expense of important micronutrients. A desire to reconcile the need for drug therapy with these associated potential micronutrient depletions raises the question as to the value of empirical micronutrient supplementation to mitigate this impact. Two significant studies have examined this concept in the heart failure population. Witte et al.[57] conducted a small study of 30 heart failure patients with a mean age of 75.4 years and an ejection fraction of less than 35% on optimal medical therapy; they were randomized to capsules containing high-dose micronutrients (calcium, magnesium, zinc, copper, selenium, vitamin A, thiamine, riboflavin, vitamin B6, folate, vitamin B12, vitamin C, vitamin E, vitamin D, and coenzyme Q10) versus placebo for 9 months. The researchers found that patients in the active group experienced a statistically significant reduction in left ventricle volume as well as an increase in ejection fraction by 5.3 ± 1.4%, whereas no change in these parameters was seen in the placebo group. The active group also showed a significant improvement in breathlessness, sleep quality, concentration, and overall quality of life. There were no adverse effects reported.

McKeag et al.[58] conducted a larger study looking at the impact of micronutrient supplementation on left ventricular ejection fraction, but these patients had milder heart failure and were younger than those studied by Witte et al. They did not show any difference in the primary endpoint of mean left ventricular ejection fraction or in secondary endpoints of 6-minute walk distance and markers of inflammation. However, the intervention involved lower doses of B vitamins, vitamin C, and vitamin E, and did not include coenzyme Q10, a supplement that has been shown to reduce symptoms and mortality.[59]

Thus, there is not definitive evidence for improving outcomes with micronutrient supplementation. Yet, potential micronutrient depletions are real, especially in the elderly, and possible side effects of these deficiencies lead to clinically important presentations that can overlap with other diagnoses. Thus a decision should be individualized on the basis of risk factors, with the highest risk occurring in the elderly population and possibly in the heart failure population.

Integrative Approaches to Common Cardiovascular Conditions in the Elderly

ATRIAL FIBRILLATION

Atrial fibrillation (AF) is a supraventricular tachycardia defined by irregular atrial activity with variable symptomatic and hemodynamic consequences. It is the most common arrhythmia in the geriatric population. Approximately 9% of individuals over the age of 80 are affected, and the prevalence is expected to at least double by the year 2050. The anticipated rise is due in large part to the increasing geriatric population.[60,61] Additionally, the prevalence is highest in those with underlying CVD, especially in those with congestive heart failure, valvular disease, hypertension, and left atrial enlargement.[62-64] AF is a common reason for hospitalization in the elderly and thus constitutes a significant socioeconomic burden.[65] Given the associated risk of stroke, which increases linearly with age, it is also a significant source of morbidity and mortality.[66]

The management of AF in the geriatric population demands a highly individualized approach. Because elderly patients may be more susceptible to treatment side effects and toxicities, it is important to first define the impact of AF on the patient's quality of life and to understand the patient's goals of care in order to develop an appropriate strategy. As a rule, if the patient is tolerating the rhythm and is not in danger, then it is most prudent to start with simpler interventions before initiating invasive strategies.

After ensuring patient safety and understanding the patient's experience with AF, the most important next step is to investigate potential underlying causes and triggers. Often overlooked causes include sleep apnea, hypertension, hyperthyroidism, obesity, dietary factors such as alcohol use, and inflammation. A detailed history of when symptoms occur may elucidate a trigger that can be corrected without medications.

Patients with AF are at increased risk of stroke and are generally risk stratified based on the CHADSvasc score.[67] Although patients with a score of zero may not require anticoagulation, all patients in the geriatric age bracket are by definition at least at moderate risk, and this risk increases linearly with age. Therefore, unless patients have a clear contraindication to anticoagulation, a novel oral anticoagulant rather than warfarin, due to bleeding risks and management challenges during dietary changes, should be initiated. In studies including geriatric patients, aspirin alone has been shown to be less effective than warfarin at preventing stroke without any reduction in bleeding risk in this population;[68] therefore, aspirin is not a "safe" alternative.

Supplements

Magnesium has been shown to have numerous electrophysiological and anti-arrhythmic properties. Based on Framingham data, hypomagnesemia is frequently unrecognized and may be associated with the development of AF.[69] In fact, the ARIC study, which included 14,290 men and women, found that lower serum magnesium levels were correlated with a higher risk of AF.[70] However, there are no firm data that magnesium supplementation prevents the development of AF in patients without heart disease. However, given the existing data and the safety of magnesium supplementation, it is reasonable to use this supplement in patients with AF.

Hypokalemia has been implicated in many different rhythm disturbances. Patients taking potassium-depleting medications, such as diuretics, should be repleted. Any patient taking magnesium repletion should also be repleted with potassium to maintain serum levels above 4 mEq/L. As with magnesium, caution is advised in patients with abnormal kidney function.

Botanicals

Botanicals that have been used to treat AF include motherwort (*Leonurus cardiacus*), raspberry leaf, Khella (*Ammi visnaga*), hawthorn berry (*Crataegus officianalis*), and *Rhodiola rosea*. However, there are no randomized clinical trials to support their general use at this time.

Dietary Factors

Dehydration can be a trigger for AF, so maintaining adequate water intake is important. Consider the addition of electrolytes, especially in the setting of sweating, exercise, and extreme heat.

Moderate to heavy alcohol consumption is associated with a significantly increased risk of AF; the association between light drinking and AF is unclear.[71,72] The mechanism has not been fully elucidated.

Caffeine and dark chocolate are stimulants that activate the sympathetic nervous system. There is no clear evidence that they cause AF, but a trial of elimination is worthwhile. especially if the history suggests these substances as a potential trigger. Other potential stimulants include guarani, ginseng, gotu cola, and yohimbe.

Fluctuations in blood sugar can be a trigger for AF due to secondary influences on endothelial function. Glycemic variability can be reduced by encouraging adherence to a Mediterranean diet, choosing whole grains, high-fiber vegetables, and other plant-based foods.

Mind–Body Approaches

The YOGA My Heart Study showed that twice-weekly yoga sessions for 3 months in patients with paroxysmal AF reduced symptoms, arrhythmia burden, and associated anxiety and depression, and improved many quality-of-life parameters.[73]

Acupuncture may be comparable to antiarrhythmic drugs in preventing recurrences after cardioversion. A small study looked at 80 patients with AF after electrical cardioversion. The researchers compared 26 patients who were taking amiodarone versus 10 weeks of weekly acupuncture, sham acupuncture, or control and found that the rates of recurrence were similar in the amiodarone group and the acupuncture group but were significantly higher in the sham and control groups.[74]

Depression and anxiety can be triggered by AF, and they may in turn perpetuate the process. At the very least, recognizing and treating these common comorbidities will improve quality of life.[75]

CONGESTIVE HEART FAILURE

Heart failure is a clinical syndrome that is a consequence of impaired ventricular filling or ejection of blood. It is a multifactorial process and is a common endpoint of many common diseases encountered in the geriatric population, such as ischemic heart disease, hypertension, obesity, sleep apnea, and cardiotoxic drugs (chemotherapeutic agents). The incidence increases with age, with more than 80 per 1,000 individuals over the age of 85 years affected. Despite significant advances in this field, particularly in terms of drugs and devices, the mortality remains high, at approximately 50% at 5 years. The goal of the cardiologist is to recognize these antecedent factors early and implement interventions to prevent the development of heart failure.

The basic pathophysiology of heart failure involves myocardial injury ultimately leading to insufficient blood flow. In addition to neurohormonal, inflammatory, and oxidative mechanisms, an under-recognized mechanism is impaired myocardial energy production. Under normal circumstances, ATP production keeps pace with demand; however, in the case of the increasing energy demands in heart failure, ATP levels decline. In really desperate circumstances, ADP can be utilized as energy, which results in the loss of these essential phosphate donors, and de novo synthesis of ATP becomes more energy consuming than salvage. This process may be accelerated in the elderly as older age has been correlated with lower levels of myocardial ATP.[76]

Many current therapies address the hemodynamic and neurohormonal abnormalities, but no medications address the delicate metabolic needs of the failing heart. Metabolic therapy is an emerging strategy whereby a natural substance normally found in the body is administered with the goal of enhancing a metabolic reaction within a cell. These substances can be given to replace a component that is deficient for any reason (due to, e.g., aging, malabsorption, drug-induced depletion) or can be used in high amounts with the intention of inducing an enzymatic reaction in the desired direction (or simply not limiting the reaction by supplying lots of precursors!). In this way, metabolic therapy is somewhat opposite of a conventional drug aimed at blocking, rather than supporting, a process.[77]

Dietary supplements and natural products with existing evidence for heart failure include the following.

Levels of coenzyme Q10 (ubiquinone) are decreased in patients with heart failure, and low concentrations correlate with severity and are an independent predictor of mortality.[47,78] However, many studies investigating CoQ10 supplementation in heart failure have yielded mixed results and have been limited by small numbers and absence of modern therapies. In a 2013 meta-analysis of 13 randomized placebo-controlled trials of CoQ10 supplementation reporting the ejection fraction or New York Heart Association (NYHA) functional class as a primary outcome, supplementation resulted in a significant increase in ejection fraction of 3.67% and a nonsignificant improvement in NYHA functional classification.[79] However, the Q-SYMBIO trial, a recent randomized controlled trial, provides good evidence upon which to supplement CoQ10 in heart failure. In this trial, 420 patients with moderate to severe heart failure were randomized to CoQ10 100 mg three times a day versus placebo in addition to standard therapy. The researchers found that at the 2-year long-term endpoint, the treatment group showed significantly lower all-cause and cardiovascular mortality and fewer heart failure hospitalizations. They also found significant improvements in NYHA functional classification.[48] Current literature suggests that CoQ10 is relatively safe, with few drug interactions and no major adverse effects. Minor side effects that have been reported include gastrointestinal upset and possible rash;[59] it unknown if these effects are from CoQ10 per se or the supplement matrix material. The recommended supplementation dose for heart failure is 100 mg three times daily of a solubilized preparation.

Magnesium is used to correct low levels that are often associated with poor diet as well as to mitigate the effects of magnesium-wasting drugs, most notably diuretics (Table 13.1). Low magnesium status (along with high urine magnesium) has been found in heart failure patients with complex ventricular arrhythmias. In a double-blind placebo-controlled study of patients with systolic heart failure with an ejection fraction of less than 40% and NYHA II–IV classification, intravenous administration of 8 g magnesium sulfate resulted in a significant decrease in the number of ventricular ectopic beats and episodes of non-sustained ventricular tachycardia.[80] Spironolactone has been shown to reduce arrhythmia in heart failure, possibly due to lower sodium-dependent erythrocyte magnesium efflux and higher erythrocyte magnesium concentration.[81] Further research to elucidate the myriad effects of magnesium are necessary, but there are enough data to support its safety and utility at this time. The major limiting side effect of magnesium is loose stool, so the dose should be titrated to avoid this. Caution should be used when treating patients with renal impairment. Supplementation dosing was described in the preceding sections.

D-ribose is a pentose monosaccharide necessary for the salvage and de novo synthesis of ATP. In a small randomized, double-blind, placebo-controlled trial patients were supplemented with D-ribose or placebo for 3 weeks, followed by a washout period, and then crossed over to the other treatment. D-ribose improved diastolic functional parameters based on echocardiography as well as quality-of-life parameters.[82] Most recently, a retrospective trial of 366 patients who underwent off-pump CABG showed that those who received

Table 13.1. Common Drug-Induced Nutrient Depletions

Common Drug	Associated Nutrient Depletion
Beta blockers	CoQ10, melatonin
Cardiac glycosides	Calcium, magnesium, phosphorous, thiamine
Thiazide diuretics	CoQ10, magnesium, phosphorous, potassium, sodium, zinc
Loop diuretics	Calcium, magnesium, potassium, sodium, thiamine, vitamin B6, vitamin C, zinc
Potassium-sparing diuretics	Calcium, folic acid, zinc
Angiotensin-converting enzyme inhibitors	Zinc, sodium
Angiotensin receptor blockers	Zinc
Calcium channel blockers	Melatonin
HMG-CoA reductase inhibitors	CoQ10, vitamin E, vitamin D, carnitine, omega-3-fatty acids, zinc, selenium, copper, testosterone
Bile acid sequestrates	Vitamin A, calcium, folic acid, iron, magnesium, phosphorous, vitamin B12, vitamin D, vitamin E, vitamin K, zinc
Colestipol	Vitamin A, folic acid, iron, vitamin B12, vitamin E, CoQ10
Fibrates	Vitamin E, CoQ10, vitamin D, DHEA
Ezetimibe	Vitamin D
Aspirin	Folic acid, iron, potassium, sodium
Nonsteroidal anti-inflammatories	Folic acid, melatonin, sodium, zinc
Acetaminophen	Glutamate, cysteine
Biguanides (metformin)	CoQ10, folic acid, vitamin B12
Proton pump inhibitors	Calcium, folic acid, iron, sodium, vitamin C, vitamin D, vitamin B12, magnesium
H2 blockers	Calcium, folic acid, iron, vitamin B12, vitamin D, zinc

From reference 41.

preoperative D-ribose supplementation had greater improvement in post-revascularization cardiac index than those who did not, with no significant adverse outcomes.[83] These data support the possible benefit of supplementing with D-ribose, but larger randomized clinical trials are warranted. Rare adverse effects have been described in secondary sources, including diarrhea, nausea, hypoglycemia, hyperuricemia, and headache. The supplementation dose for heart failure is 5 to 15 g/day in divided doses. Patients should avoid using individual doses greater than 10 g due to gastrointestinal side effects. D-ribose may cause hypoglycemia.

L-carnitine (proprionyl L-carnitine) participates in cellular energy production, specifically in the transport of long-chain fatty acids from the cytosol to the mitochondria where beta-oxidation and ATP production occurs. Rizos et al.[84] found that long-term supplementation of L-carnitine (2 g/day) in addition to usual care in patients with NYHA class III–IV dilated cardiomyopathy improved mortality compared to placebo. Most recently, a 2013 Mayo Clinic meta-analysis examined 13 trials (N = 3,629) of L-carnitine. They found that L-carnitine was associated with a significant reduction in all-cause mortality, ventricular arrhythmias, and angina in the setting of acute MI. There was no difference in incidence of heart failure or re-infarction.[85] There are no known adverse effects, although there has been concern that L-carnitine metabolizes into trimethylamine N-oxide (TMAO), a metabolic product of L-carnitine by select gut microbes; TMAO concentrations have been associated with higher cardiovascular events and mortality.[86,87] Whether this is a reflection on the safety of carnitine or the importance of treating suboptimal gut flora remains in discussion. The recommended dose is 1 to 3 g/day.

As noted earlier in the chapter, the recent VINDICATE study found that in patients with chronic systolic heart failure and vitamin D deficiency (levels <20 ng/mL), daily supplementation with 4,000 IU vitamin D3 was associated with significant improvement in ejection fraction as well as in reverse remodeling (reduction in LVEDD and LVESD) and was also safe and well tolerated.[54] The ongoing EVITA trial[88] is enrolling 400 patients ages 18 to 80 with NYHA functional class II or greater to investigate whether vitamin D supplementation reduces mortality in end-stage CHF patients. Supplementation recommendations were described earlier in the chapter.

In 2008 the GISSI-HF, a randomized, double-blind, placebo-controlled trial including nearly 7,000 patients with NYHA class II–IV heart failure irrespective of ejection fraction, demonstrated a mortality benefit of supplementing 1 g/day of omega-3 fatty acid in addition to usual care.[89] Gastrointestinal distress, the most frequent complaint, occurred in 3% of each group. The recommended supplementation dose is 1 to 3 g/day, depending on serum status and dietary intake of fish.

Subclinical thiamine deficiency is not uncommon in heart failure patients, who are often receiving diuretic therapy.[90] Small studies suggest that supplementation with thiamine is associated with an improvement in left ventricular function, though larger clinical trials are necessary to further elucidate the potential benefit.

Hawthorn (*Crataegus* species) is a traditional herbal medicine for cardiac health and contains numerous constituents with cardiovascular effects, including positive inotropic, negative chronotropic, vasodilatory, antiarrhythmic, and antioxidant properties as well as angiotensin-converting enzyme inhibition.[91] The leaves and flowers contain oligomeric procyandins (antioxidants) and quercitin (anti-inflammatory), which are thought to mediate these effects. The berries have been used as well but are thought to be less potent due to a lesser concentration of oligomeric procyandins. Hawthorn has been shown to be superior to placebo in two meta-analyses that included randomized, double-blind, placebo-controlled trials using hawthorn as adjunctive therapy in patients with class I–III heart failure.[92,93] Both studies concluded that there was a significant increase in maximum workload as well as significantly improved symptoms of shortness of breath and fatigue in the hawthorn group. The SPICE trial[94] was a randomized, double-blind, placebo-controlled trial that found no mortality benefit of hawthorn versus placebo in addition to standard therapy; however, this trial did establish the safety in addition to standard therapy. Potential adverse effects that have been described include dizziness, nausea, gastrointestinal complaints, headache, palpitations, rash, and hypotension. Hawthorne is safe and well tolerated at doses from 160 to 1,800 mg/day.

Dietary inorganic nitrates such as beetroot (as opposed to organic nitrates such as nitroglycerine), which are reduced to nitric oxide in the body, have been shown to have beneficial vascular effects; in particular they significantly reduce blood pressure.[95] They also have been shown to improve exercise tolerance in heart failure patients. A recent study including 20 elderly patients with heart failure with reduced ejection fraction found that 1 week of supplementation with beetroot significantly improved aerobic exercise endurance while also reducing blood pressure.[96] The preferred method of supplementation is unclear, though it is available as a juice as well as in a lozenge form.

A summary of natural agents for heart failure is as follows:

- Coenzyme Q10: 100–200 mg three times daily
- Omega-3 fatty acids: 1–3 g/day
- Magnesium: 400–800 mg/day
- Vitamin D3: Replace based on serum status
- L-carnitine: 1–3 g/day
- D-ribose: 5–15 g/day (see text for cautions)
- Hawthorn: 160–1,800 mg/day as a standardized leaf, flower, and berry product
- Beetroot juice

REFERENCES

1. U.S. Census Bureau. 2014 National Population Projections. https://www.census.gov/population/projections/data/national/2014/publications.html. Accessed January 3, 2017.
2. Barefoot JC, Schroll M. Symptoms of depression, acute myocardial infarction, and total mortality in a community sample. *Circulation*. 1996;93(11):1976–1980.
3. Brown JM, Stewart JC, Stump TE, Callahan CM. Risk of coronary heart disease events over 15 years among older adults with depressive symptoms. *Am J Geriatr Psych*. 2011;19(8):721–729.
4. McLean AJ, Le Couture DG. Aging biology and geriatric clinical pharmacology. *Pharmacy Rev*. 2004; 56:163–184.
5. Forman DE, Rich MW, Alexander KP, et al. Cardiac care for older adults: time for a new paradigm. *J Am Coll Cardiol*. 2011;57(18):1801–1810.
6. The World Health Report 2002: Reducing Risks, Promoting Healthy Life. http://www.who.int/whr/2002/en/WHO 2002 health report. Accessed October 1, 2016.
7. Ostrich R, Ros E, Salas-Savado J, et al. Primary prevention of cardiovascular disease with a Mediterranean diet. *N Engl J Med*. 2013;368(14):1279–1290.
8. Roman B, Carta L, Angel M, Serra-Majem L. Effectiveness of the Mediterranean diet in the elderly. *Clinical Interventions in Aging*. 2008;3(1):97–109.
9. Jacobs DR, Gross MD, Tapsell LC. Food synergy: an operational concept for understanding nutrition *Am J Clin Nutr*. 2009;89(5):1543S–1548S.
10. Haynes SG, Feinleib M, Kannel WB. The relationship of psychosocial factors to coronary heart disease in the Framingham Study. III. Eight-year incidence of coronary heart disease. *Am J Epidemiol*. 1980 Jan;111(1):37–58.
11. Yusuf S, Hawken S, Ounpuu S. Effect of potentially modifiable risk factors associated with myocardial infarction in 52 countries (the INTERHEART study): Case-control study. *Lancet*. 2004;364:937–952.
12. Kawachi I, Sparrow D, Spiro A 3rd, et al. A prospective study of anger and coronary heart disease. The Normative Aging Study. *Circulation*. 1996;94(9):2090–2095.
13. Kubzansky LD, Kawachi I, Spiro A, et al. Is worrying bad for your heart? A prospective study of worry and coronary heart disease in the normative aging study. *Circulation*. 1997;95(4):818–824.
14. Sesso HD, Kawachi I, Vokonas PS, Sparrow D. Depression and the risk of coronary heart disease in the Normative Aging Study. *Am J Cardiol*. 1998;82(7):851–856.
15. Ariyo AA, Haan M, Tangen CM et al. Depressive symptoms and risks of coronary heart disease and mortality in elderly Americans. *Circulation*. 2000;102(15):1773–1779.
16. Perissinotto CM, Cenzer IS, Covinsky KE. Loneliness in older persons: A predictor of functional decline and death. *Arch Intern Med*. 2012;172(14):1078–1083.
17. Valtorta NK, Kanaan M, Gilbody S, Ronzi S, Hanratty B. Loneliness and social isolation as risk factors for coronary heart disease and stroke: Systematic review and meta-analysis of longitudinal observational studies. *Heart*. 2016;0:1–8.

18. Friedmann E, Thomas SA. Pet ownership, social support, and one-year survival after acute myocardial infarction in the Cardiac Arrhythmia Suppression Trial (CAST). *Am J Cardiol.* 1995;76(17):1213–1217.

19. Frasure-Smith N, Lesperance N, Talajic M. Depression and 18-month prognosis after myocardial infarction. *Circulation.* 1995;91:999–1005.

20. Dusek JA, Benson H. Mind-body medicine: A model of the comparative clinical impact of the acute stress and relaxation responses. *Minn Med.* 2009;92:47–50.

21. Forman D, Manning WJ, Hauser R, Gervino EV, Evan WJ, Wei JY. Enhanced left ventricular diastolic filling associated with long-term endurance training. *J Gerontol.* 1992;47(2):M56–M58.

22. Nakao M, Nomura S, Shinosawa T, et al. Clinical effects of blood pressure biofeedback treatment on hypertension by auto-shaping. *Psychosom Med.* 1997;59(3):331–338.

23. Nakao M, Yano E, Nomura S, Kuboki T. Blood pressure lowering effects of biofeedback treatment in hypertension: A meta-analysis of randomized controlled trials. *Hypertension Res.* 2003;26:37–46.

24. Yeh G, McCarthy EP, Wayne PM, et al. Tai chi exercise in patients with chronic heart failure: a randomized clinical trial. *Arch Intern Med.* 2011;171(8):750–757.

25. Williams MA, Maresh CM, Esterbrooks DJ, Harbrecht JJ, Sketch MH. Early exercise training in patients older than age 65 years compared with that in younger patients after acute myocardial infarction or coronary artery bypass grafting. *Am J Cardiol.* 1985;55(4):263–266.

26. Lavie CJ, Milani RV. Effects of cardiac rehabilitation programs on exercise capacity, coronary risk factors, behavioral characteristics, and quality of life in a large elderly cohort. *Am J Cardiol.* 1995;76:177–179.

27. Suaya JA, Shepard DS, Normand SL, Ades PA, Protass J, Season WB. Use of cardiac rehabilitation by Medicare beneficiaries after myocardial infarction or coronary bypass surgery. *Circulation.* 2007;116(15):1653–1662.

28. Suaya JA, Stason WB, Ades PA, Normand SL, Shepard DS. Cardiac rehabilitation and survival in older coronary patients. *J Am Coll Cardiol.* 2009;54(1):25–33.

29. Aragam KG, Dai D, Neely ML, et al. Gaps in referral to cardiac rehabilitation of patients undergoing percutaneous coronary intervention in the United States. *J Am Coll Cardiol.* 2015;65(19):2079–2088.

30. Hamer M, Batty SS, Shipley MJ, et al. Physical activity and inflammatory markers over 10 years: follow-up in men and women from the Whitehall II cohort study. *Circulation.* 2012 Aug 21;126(8):928–933.

31. Blumenthal JA, Babyak MA, Moore K, et al. Effects of exercise training on older patients with major depression. *Arch Intern Med.* 1999;159(19):2349–2356.

32. Becker DJ, Gordon RY, Halbert SC, et al. Red yeast rice for dyslipidemia in statin-intolerant patients. A randomized trial. *Ann Intern Med.* 2009;150(12):830–839.

33. Halbert SC, French B, Gordon RY, et al. Tolerability of red yeast rice (2,400 mg twice daily) versus pravastatin (20 mg twice daily) in patients with previous statin intolerance. *Am J Cardiol.* 2010;105:198–204.

34. Li Y, Jiang L, Jia Z, et al. A meta-analysis of red yeast rice: An effective and relatively safe alternative approach for dyslipidemia. *PLoS One.* 2014;9(6):e98611.

35. Menezes AR, Lavis CJ, Milani RV, Arena RA, Church TS. Cardiac rehabilitation and exercise therapy in the elderly: Should we invest in the aged? *J Geriatr Cardiol.* 2012;9(1):68–75.

36. Thakkar RB, Kashyap ML, Lewin AJ, Krause SL, Jiang P, Padley RJ. Acetylsalicylic acid reduces niacin extended-release-induced flushing in patients with dyslipidemia. *Am J Cardiovasc Drugs.* 2009;9(2):69–79.

37. Brown L, Rosner B, Willett WW, Sacks FM. Cholesterol-lowering effects of dietary fiber: A meta-analysis. *Am J Clin Nutr.* 1999;69:30–42.

38. Maki KC, Lawless AL, Reeves MS, Dicklin MR, Jenks BH, Shneyvas E, Brooks JR. Lipid-altering effects of a dietary supplement tablet containing free plant sterols and stanols in men and women with primary hypercholesterolaemia: A randomized, placebo-controlled crossover trial. *Int J Food Sci Nutr.* 2012 Jun;63(4):476–482. doi:10.3109/09637486.2011.636345. Epub 2011 Nov 17.

39. Bazzano LA, Serdula MK, Liu S. Dietary intake of fruits and vegetables and risk of cardiovascular disease 2003. *Curr Atheroscler Rep.* 2003;5(6):492–499.

40. Houston MC. Nutraceuticals, vitamins, antioxidants, and minerals in the prevention and treatment of hypertension 2005. *Prog Cardiovasc Dis.* 2005;47(6):396–449.

41. Sinatra ST, Houston MC. *Nutritional and Integrative Strategies in Cardiovascular Medicine.* 1st ed. Boca Raton, FL: CRC Press; 2015.

42. World Health Organization. *Calcium and Magnesium in Drinking Water: Public Health Significance.* Geneva, Switzerland: World Health Organization Press; 2009.

43. Barbagallo M, Belvedere M, Dominguez LJ. Magnesium homeostasis and aging. *Magnes Res.* 2009; 22:235–246.

44. Chiuve SE, Sun Q, Curhan GC, et al. Dietary and plasma magnesium and risk of coronary heart disease among women. *J Am Heart Assoc.* 2013;2:e000114.

45. Lopez-Ridaura R, Willett WC, Rimm EB, Liu S, Stampfer MJ, Manson JE, Hu FB. Magnesium intake and risk of type 2 diabetes in men and women. *Diabetes Care.* 2004;27:134–140

46. Del Gobbo LC, Imamura F, Wu JH, de Oliveira Otto MC, Chiuve SE, Mozaffarian D. Circulating and dietary magnesium and risk of cardiovascular disease: A systematic review and meta-analysis of prospective studies. *Am J Clin Nutr.* 2013;98(1):160–173.

47. Molyneux SL, Florkowski CM, George PM, et al. Coenzyme Q10: An independent predictor of mortality in chronic heart failure. *J Am Coll Cardiol.* 2008;52:1435–1441.

48. Mortensen SA, Rosenfeldt F, Kumar A. The effect of coenzyme Q10 on morbidity and mortality in chronic heart failure: Results from Q-SYMBIO: a randomized double-blind trial. *JACC Heart Failure.* 2014; 6:641–649.

49. Alehagen U, Johansson P, Bjornstedt M. Cardiovascular mortality and N-terminal-proBNP reduced after combined selenium and coenzyme Q10 supplementation: A 5-year prospective randomized double-blind placebo-controlled trial among elderly Swedish citizens. *Int J Cardiol.* 2013;167:1860–1866.

50. Selhub J, Jacques PF, Bostom AG, et al. Association between plasma homocysteine concentrations and extracranial carotid-artery stenosis. *N Engl J Med.* 1995;332:286–291.

51. Norman PE, Powell JT. Vitamin D and cardiovascular disease. *Circ Res.* 2014;114:379–393.

52. Kendrick J, Targher G, Smits G, Chonchol M. 25-Hydroxyvitamin D deficiency is independently associated with cardiovascular disease in the Third National Health and Nutrition Examination Survey. *Atherosclerosis.* 2009;205:255–260.

53. Dobnig H, Pilz S, Scharnagl H, et al. Independent association of low serum 25-hydroxyvitamin D and 1,25-dihydroxyvitamin D levels with all-cause and cardiovascular mortality. *Arch Intern Med.* 2008 Jun 23;168(12):1340–1349.

54. Witte KK, Byron R, Gierula J, et al. Effects of vitamin D on cardiac function in patients with chronic HF (VINDICATE study). *J Am Coll Cardiol.* 2016;67:2593–2603.

55. Gu D, He J, Wu X, Duan X, Whelton PK. Effect of potassium supplementation on blood pressure in Chinese: A randomized, placebo-controlled trial. *J Hypertens.* 2001 Jul;19(7):1325–1331.

56. Huang CL, Kuo E. Mechanisms of hypokalemia in magnesium deficiency. *J Am Soc Nephrol.* 2007;18:2649–2652.

57. Witte KK, Nikitin NP, Parker AC, et al. The effect of micronutrient supplementation on quality-of-life and left ventricular function in elderly patients with chronic heart failure. *Eur Heart J.* 2005;26:2238–2244.

58. McKeag NA, McKinley MC, Harbinson MT, et al. The effect of multiple micronutrient supplementation on left ventricular ejection fraction in patients with chronic stable heart failure: a randomized, placebo-controlled trial. *JACC Heart Failure.* 2014;2(3):308–317.

59. Sharma A, Fonarow GC, Butler J, Ezekowitz JA, Felker GM. Coenzyme Q10 and heart failure: A state-of-the-art review. *Circ Heart Fail.* 2016;9(4):e002639.

60. Aviles RJ, Martin DO, Apperson-Hansen C. Inflammation as a risk factor for atrial fibrillation. *Circulation.* 2003;108:3006–3010.

61. Go AS, Hylek EM, Phillips KA, et al. Prevalence of diagnosed atrial fibrillation in adults: national implications for rhythm management and stroke prevention: the anticoagulation and risk factors in atrial fibrillation (ATRIA) study. *JAMA.* 2001;285(18):2370–2375.

62. Andrade J, Khairy P, Dobrev D, Nattel S. The clinical profile and pathophysiology of atrial fibrillation. *Circ Res,* 2014;114:1453–1468.

63. Furberg CD, Psaty BM, Manolio TA, Gardin JM, Smith VE, Rautaharju PM. Prevalence of atrial fibrillation in elderly subjects (the Cardiovascular Health Study). *Am J Cardiol.* 1994;74:236–241.

64. Psaty BM, Manolo TAI, Kuller LH, et al. Incidence of and risk factors for atrial fibrillation in older adults. *Circulation.* 1997;96;114:1453–1468.

65. Kim MH, Johnston SS, Chu BC, Dalal MR, Schulman KL. Estimation of total incremental health care costs in patients with atrial fibrillation in the United States. *Circ Cardiovasc Qual Outcomes.* 2011;4(3):313–320.

66. Mozaffarian D, Benjamin EJ, Go AS, et al. Heart disease and stroke statistics—2015 update: a report from the American Heart Association. *Circulation.* 2015;131:e29–e322.

67. Zhu WG, Xiong QM, Hong K. Meta-analysis of CHADS2 versus CHADS2-VASc for predicting stroke and thromboembolism in atrial fibrillation patients independent of anticoagulation. *Tex Heart Inst J.* 2015;42:6–15.

68. Mant J, Hobbs FDR, Fletcher K, et al. Warfarin versus aspirin for stroke prevention in an elderly community population with atrial fibrillation (the Birmingham Atrial Fibrillation Treatment of the Aged Study, BAFTA): A randomised controlled trial. *Lancet.* 2007;370:493–503.

69. Khan AM, Lubitz SA, Sullivan LM, et al. Low serum magnesium and the development of atrial fibrillation in the community: The Framingham Heart Study. *Circulation.* 2013;127(1):33–38.

70. Misialek JR, Lopez FL, Lutsey PL, et al. Serum and dietary magnesium and incidence of atrial fibrillation in whites and in African Americans: Atherosclerosis Risk In Communities (ARIC) study. *Circ J.* 2013;77(2):323–329.

71. Diousse L, Levy D, Benjamin EJ. Long-term alcohol consumption and the risk of atrial fibrillation in the Framingham Study. *Am J Cardiol.* 2004;93:710–713.

72. Samokhvalov AV, Irving HM, Rehm J. Alcohol consumption as a risk factor for atrial fibrillation: a systematic review and meta-analysis. *Eur J Cardiovasc Prev Rehabil.* 2010;17:706–712.

73. Lakkireddy D, Atkins D, Pillarisetti J, et al. Effect of yoga on arrhythmia burden, anxiety, depression, and quality of life parameters in atrial fibrillation: The YOGA My Heart Study. *J Am Coll Cardiol.* 2013;61(11):1177–1182.

74. Lomuscio A, Belletti S, Bttezzati PM, Lombardi F. Efficacy of acupuncture in preventing atrial fibrillation recurrences after electrical cardioversion. *J Cardiovasc Electrophysiol.* 2011;22:241–247.

75. Patel D, McConkey ND, Sohaney R, McNeil A, Jedrzejczyk A, Armaganijgn L. A systematic review of depression and anxiety in patients with atrial fibrillation: The mind-heart link. *Cardiovasc Psychiatry Neurol.* 2013;2013:159850.

76. Schocke MF, Metzler B, Wolf C, et al. Impact of aging on cardiac high-energy phosphate metabolism determined by phosphorus-31 2-dimensional chemical shift imaging (31P 2D CSI). *Magn Reson Imaging.* 2003;21(5):553–559.

77. Hadj A, Pepe S, Rosenfeldt F. The clinical application of metabolic therapy for cardiovascular disease. *Heart Lung Circ.* 2007;16(Suppl 3):S56–S64.

78. Folkers K, Vadhanavikit S, Mortensen S. Biochemical rationale and myocardial tissue data on the effective therapy of cardiomyopathy with coenzyme Q10. *Proc Natl Acad Sci U S A.* 1985;82:901–904.

79. Fotino AD, Thompson-Paul AM, Bazzano LA. Effect of coenzyme Q10 supplementation on heart failure: a meta-analysis. *Am J Clin Nutr.* 2013;97:268–275.

80. Ceremuzynski K, Gebalska J, Wolk R, Makowska E. Hypomagnesemia in heart failure with ventricular arrhythmias. Beneficial effects of magnesium. *J Intern Med.* 2000;247:78–86.

81. Gao X, Peng L, Adhikari CM, Lin J, Zuo Z. Spironolactone reduced arrhythmia and maintained magnesium homeostasis in patients with congestive heart failure. *J Card Fail*. 2007;13(3):170–177.

82. Omran H, Illien S, MacCarter D, St Cyr J, Luderitz B. D-Ribose improves diastolic function and quality of life in congestive heart failure patients: a prospective feasibility study. *Eur J Heart Fail*. 2003 Oct;5(5):615–619.

83. Perkowski DJ, Wagner S, Schneider JR. A targeted metabolic protocol with D-ribose for off-pump coronary artery bypass procedures: A retrospective analysis. *Therapeutic Adv Cardiovasc Dis* 2011;5:185–192.

84. Rizos I. Three-year survival of patients with heart failure caused by dilated cardiomyopathy and L-carnitine administration. *Am Heart J*. 2000;139:S120–S123.

85. DiNicolantonia JJ, Lavie CJ, Fares H, Menezes AR, O'Keefe JH. L-carnitine in the secondary prevention of cardiovascular disease: systematic review and meta-analysis. *Mayo Clin Proc*. 2013;88:544–541.

86. Zhu W, Gregory JC, Org E, et al. Gut microbial metabolite TMAO enhances platelet hyperactivity and thrombosis risk. *Cell*. 2016;165:111–124.

87. Organ CL, Otsuka H, Bhushan S, et al. Choline diet and its gut microbe-derived metabolite, trimethylamine N-oxide, exacerbate pressure overload-induced heart failure. *Circ Heart Fail*. 2016;9(1):e002314.

88. ClinicalTrials.gov. Vitamin D and Mortality in Heart Failure (EVITA). http://clinicaltrials.gov/ct2/show/NCT01326650. Accessed September 27, 2016.

89. GISSI-HF Investigators. Effect of omega-3 polyunsaturated fatty acids in patients with chronic heart failure (the GISSI-HF trial): A randomized, double-blind, placebo-controlled trial. *Lancet*. 2008; 372:1223–1230.

90. Zenuk C, Healey J, Donnelly J, Vaillancourt R, Almalki Y, Smith S. Thiamine deficiency in congestive heart failure patients receiving long term furosemide therapy. *Can J Clin Pharmacol*. 2003;10:184–188.

91. Chang Q, Zuo Z, Harrison F, Chow MS. Hawthorn. *J Clin Pharmacol*. 2002;42(6);605–612.

92. Pittler MH, Schmidt K, Ernst E. Hawthorn extract for treating chronic heart failure: meta-analysis of randomized trials. *Am J Med*. 2003;114(8):665–674.

93. Pittler MH, Guo R, Ernst E. Hawthorn extract for treating chronic heart failure. *Cochrane Database Syst Rev*. 2008;1:CD005312.

94. Holubarsch CJ, Colucci WS, Meinertz T, Gaus W, Tendera M. The efficacy and safety of *Crataegus* extract WS 1442 in patients with heart failure: The SPICE trial. *Eur J Heart Fail*. 2008;10(12):1255–1263.

95. Kapil V, Khambata RS, Robertson A, Caulfield MJ, Ahluwalia A. Dietary nitrate provides sustained blood pressure lowering in hypertensive patients. *Hypertension*. 2014;65:320–327.

96. Eggebeen J, Kim-Shapiro DB, Haykowsky M, et al. One week of daily dosing with beetroot juice improves submaximal endurance and blood pressure in older patients with heart failure with preserved ejection fraction. *JACC Heart Failure*. 2016;4:428–437.

14

Endocrine Disorders: Integrative Treatments of Hypothyroidism, Diabetes, and Adrenal Dysfunction

JAMES YANG

The human body uses hormones, which are signaling molecules released into the blood, to control thousands of physiological processes. In this chapter we will focus on the physiology, evaluation, and treatment of the three common dysfunctions of hypothyroidism, adrenal dysfunction, and diabetes. These three hormone systems have such a broad and profound effect on so many essential functions that any approach to wellness of the geriatric patient should consider the function and optimization of these managers of the human body.

For many geriatric patients with common chronic symptoms such as feeling unwell, loss of vitality, worsening fatigue, increasing nonspecific pains, decreased cognitive function, decreased mood, and sleep disturbances, there are no clear diagnoses. Diagnoses like somatization, natural aging, and depression are often suggested. Without dismissing the difficulties of diagnosing geriatric mood disorders, the diagnosis of a psychiatric mood disorder for vague symptoms because the lab results are normal may lead to missing common, treatable endocrine conditions. Our perspective is that for many patients, decreased health and wellness is due to clinical and functional changes in hormones that control our very well-being.

There is significant cross-talk and interactions between the functions of the thyroid, hypothalamic–pituitary–adrenal (HPA) axis, and glucose dysregulation. While we do not have the space here to explore these interactions in detail, significant research has identified a network of relationships such as the links between hypothyroidism and the development of diabetes and diabetes complications,[1,2] HPA axis alterations and thyroid dysfunction,[3] and the effects of treating prediabetes on improving thyroid function.[4]

In recognizing the extensive overlap and influences between these three systems, we clinically use the approach of the Metabolic Code[5] to evaluate these three systems together as an interacting triad. By evaluating and treating dysfunctions of these three hormone systems concurrently, we improve our ability to address each part of the thyroid–adrenal–pancreas axis more effectively.

Hypothyroidism in the Geriatric Population

CASE STUDY

GK is a female in her 50s with a history of decades of chronic fatigue, cognitive complaints, and irritable mood. She had ordered her own workup, which initially showed a TSH of 8.06 with fT3 3.3 and fT4 1.15 with positive TPO and TG antibodies; her doctor then ordered an ultrasound, which was consistent with lymphocytic thyroiditis. Her lab results were significant for hyperlipidemia with a total cholesterol of 277 and a LDL of 214. She was referred to an endocrinologist and started on low-dose levothyroxine and noticed that within a month her chronic fatigue had lifted and she stated that she felt normal for the first time in over a decade. She again self-ordered lab studies 2 months later, which showed a TSH of 3.03, fT3 3.3, and fT4 1.44 with a spontaneous drop in her total cholesterol to 223 (a decrease of 54 points) and a LDL of 150 (a decrease of 64 points) without a change in diet. However, by the time she followed up with her endocrinologist at 4 months, she was feeling fatigued and unwell again. Her thyroid tests were normal with a TSH of 1.64, fT4 1.38, and fT3 3.4, but her cholesterol had crept back up to 265 and her LDL was 189.

INTRODUCTION AND EPIDEMIOLOGY

The thyroid is known as the master metabolic gland, and its role in controlling metabolism is well known. Most clinicians are aware of its role in regulating weight and body temperature, hair, skin, and nails, bowel motility, and mood. Less appreciated is its extensive role in almost every corner of our physiology. Hypothyroidism may decrease energy production through decreasing mitochondrial function; worsen neurological conditions including migraines, neuropathy, and dementia;[6] affect mood disorders through effects on neurotransmitter function, particularly through the serotonergic and dopaminergic pathways;[7,8] alter autonomic balance and precipitate dysautonomia;[9] cause hypogonadotropic hypogonadism with low testosterone;[10] worsen congestive heart failure through effects on diastolic[11] and systolic function;[12] and affect liver function and LDL receptors.[13] It can also play a role in fibromyalgia, muscle dysfunction, and widespread pain syndromes.[14]

Hypothyroidism in the geriatric population is common, with the American Thyroid Association noting that up to one in four patients in nursing homes may have undiagnosed hypothyroidism. The prevalence of hypothyroidism increases with age, with decreasing thyroid function and increasing thyroid stimulating hormone (TSH) so common that it is considered statistically normal in aging.[15] Moderate increases in TSH (above 2.5 and below 4.5) occur in 8.1% of the U.S. population overall but in 25.5% of people over 80 years of age without a diagnosis of thyroid disease.[15] Larger increases in the TSH (greater than the standard laboratory value of 4.5 mIU/liter limit) occur in 14.5% in this oldest category and are associated with positive thyroid antibodies in 40%.[15] While this increase is so common that some researchers have suggested using age-related reference ranges for the TSH, this increase in the TSH does not reflect simple aging, as in regions where iodine deficiency, but not autoimmune thyroid disease, is predominant, TSH tends to decrease with age.[16]

In geriatric medicine, treatment of subclinical and even clinical hypothyroidism has been conservative without frank symptoms. While significant research on possible benefits for cardiovascular disease, functional status, and cognitive functions has been conducted, the results of most research have been equivocal to date. Iatrogenic hyperthyroidism with increased risk of atrial fibrillation, angina, congestive heart failure, osteoporosis, dementia, and mood changes should be avoided through cautious case selection, treatment, and monitoring. In light of the unclear benefits of treating mild hypothyroidism, current guidelines recommend a patient-centered approach with a focus on symptoms. We agree overall with this approach, but we appreciate the difficulty in obtaining a sufficient review of patient-centered symptoms and thyroid-related comorbidities, differentiating hypothyroidism from normal aging, obtaining adequate laboratory testing, interpreting laboratory tests, and conducting a sufficient evaluation of the patient's condition to address the pros and cons of hypothyroid treatment.

SIGNS AND SYMPTOMS

A patient-centered approach to hypothyroidism begins with evaluating the patient for the signs and symptoms of hypothyroidism. In conducting

Table 14.1. Selected Symptoms of Hypothyroidism

Feeling more tired	Cognitive impairment	Dry skin	Puffy eyes
Change in functional status	Constipation	Feeling colder	Muscle cramps
Weaker muscles	Irritability	Change in social behavior	Increasing headaches
Confusion	Slowness	Depression or anxiety	Digestive complaints
Increased sleepiness	Weight gain	Increased shortness of breath	Dizziness

a history and physical, the patient-attributed significance of symptoms and disabilities is used to evaluate the patient for a syndrome consistent with clinical hypothyroidism. Table 14.1 lists a number of symptoms of hypothyroidism. Most patients with clinical hypothyroidism have only a limited number of classic symptoms, highlighting the fact that one or two significant symptoms, without a "hypothyroid syndrome," is the typical presentation of hypothyroidism.[17]

Of particular note is that the cognitive, memory, and affective symptoms of hypothyroidism are often particularly pronounced.[18] Thyroid hormone levels in the brain are maintained within a stable range, independently of their systemic levels, by the balance between the localized activity of type II deiodinase (D2), which converts T4 to T3, and type III deiodinase (D3), which catalyzes the inactivation of thyroid hormones. Cerebral concentrations of active T3 are inversely associated with increased D3 activity, and are lowest in the hippocampus and temporal cortex, suggesting that these areas of the brain may be particularly vulnerable to modest changes in thyroid hormone availability.[18] We therefore pay particular attention to symptoms of "brain fog," which include hippocampal deficits in attention, memory, and executive function as well as temporal lobe–associated affective symptoms of anxiety, depression, moodiness, and irritability.

The physical examination of a patient with suspected hypothyroidism includes evaluation of the following:

- Vital signs, including bradycardia, hypertension, low basal temperature
- Thyroid size and nodes
- Thin, dry, or brittle hair and dry skin
- Edema, often non-pitting (arms, legs, and/or hands)

- Delayed relaxation of deep tendon reflexes (Woltman's sign)
- Thinning of the outer third of the eyebrows
- Dark or puffy areas under eyes
- Thyroid ultrasound: In patients with high suspicion for hypothyroidism but negative antibodies, an ultrasound may still be strongly suggestive of Hashimoto's.

LABORATORY TESTS

Laboratory reference ranges for the TSH are based on population studies that define the bottom 2.5th percentile of the population as well as the 97.5th percentile as abnormal. This standard is based on statistical convention rather than on levels that have been shown to diagnose thyroid disease or correlate with pathology. TPO antibody prevalence progressively increases with a TSH level of more than 2 mIU/liter, with over 18% of the U.S. population without a thyroid diagnosis having thyroid antibodies.[16,19] Studies that attempt to define a normal TSH level based on the 97.5th percentile of the population have generally identified levels between 2.4 and 4.2 mIU/liter as being the upper limit, with some experts strongly advocating for a narrower reference range for the purpose of screening.[16,20] Current laboratory reference ranges, using wide reference ranges, are neither sensitive nor specific.

Current evidence is consistent that the pituitary TSH value is a personalized measure exhibiting a high degree of individuality, has poor correlation with thyroid hormones, undergoes significant circadian fluctuations, and is a clinically ambiguous measurement in the individual patient.[21] The variance of TSH in a population is greater than the intra-individual fluctuations, suggesting that thyroid dysfunction is best recognized by understanding that each person has a unique TSH set point and deviations from this set point suggest thyroid dysfunction, even if it is in the "normal" range.[22]

Functional changes in the thyroid set point are quite common and increase the complexity of identifying hypothyroidism. Current research has overturned the dogma of a static thyroid set point and supports the model that the hypothalamic–pituitary–thyroid (HPT) axis set point as well as peripheral thyroid hormone metabolism is flexible and dynamic and responds to environmental stimuli such as inflammation, stress, and food intake.[21,23] During food deprivation, stress, and inflammation, thyroid hormone serum concentrations decrease without a concomitant rise in TSH, reflecting a deviation from the expected feedback regulation in the HPT axis.[23]

Conditions associated with alterations in the HPT set point are common. The Centers for Disease Control and Prevention (CDC) reports that over 50% of the U.S. population has one or more chronic diseases, which are often associated with increased systemic inflammation, oxidative stress, and elevated C-reactive protein (CRP) levels. Included in this population are the 23.5 million Americans identified by the National Institute of Health who have autoimmune disease. Cytokines such as interleukin (IL)-1β, IL-6, and TNF-α are powerful suppressors of circulating T4 and T3 while suppressing the production of TSH.[24,25] These cytokines are highly correlated with clinical CRP testing and mediate their effects through increased oxidative stress. IL-6 increases cellular oxidative stress, suppressing intracellular D1- and D2-mediated T4-to-T3 conversion as well as increasing D3-mediated T3 and T4 inactivation, leading to cellular hypothyroidism.[25] Even common lifestyle exposures such as eating a high-fat fast-food diet allows clinically significant translocation of bacterial lipopolysaccharides (LPS), which depresses hypothalamic thyrotropin-releasing hormone (TRH) and can perpetuate chronic low-grade inflammation.[26] In depression, which affects 15.6 million Americans each year according to the CDC, abnormal TSH response to TRH stimulation occurs in approximately 25% to 30% of depressed patients.[7] Even hypothyroidism itself is associated with increased levels of CRP.[27]

The hypothalamic corticotrophin-releasing hormone, which is increased in acute stress, suppresses thyroid function by inhibiting the secretion of TRH and TSH, causing a mild form of functional central hypothyroidism.[28] Acute stress and chronic stress are common experiences in most of our lives, with approximately 25% of Americans reporting a recent experience of severe stress.[29] With chronic stress, chronic inflammation, and other sustained insults to the HPA axis, alterations in the thyroid set point may make the TSH measurement unreliable.[3]

For most patients, thyroid function tests provide useful guidance in evaluating and monitoring the thyroid. Broadening the testing to include not only thyroid function tests but also thyroid antibodies, measures of poor thyroid metabolism, and biomarkers of thyroid dependent processes improves our evaluation of global thyroid sufficiency.[25,30,31]

The following are thyroid tests to be completed for an initial evaluation:

- TSH
- Free T3 and free T4
- Reverse T3 (rT3): Actively blocks thyroid function; a measure of thyroid resistance, poor T4-to-T3 conversion under stress and illness, reduced cellular thyroid uptake[30]; inflammation/oxidative stress increases D3, which decreases T3 while inactivating T4 to rT3[25]

- Anti-thyroperoxidase (anti-TPO) and anti-thyroglobulin antibodies (anti-TG)

Supportive measures may also include the following:

- Decreased free T3 (or T3)/reverse T3 ratio: multifactorial "thyroid resistance," nonthyroidal illness physiology
- Decreased serum free T3/free T4 ratios: suggest decreased peripheral T4-to-T3 conversion; reference range is 0.27–0.37, with a median of 0.32[31]

Other supportive biomarkers of hypothyroidism include elevated lipids, measures of insulin resistance, elevated creatine kinase, low sex hormone binding globulin (SHBG), high homocysteine, elevated markers of oxidative stress, elevated liver enzymes, elevated serum creatinine, low basal temperature, and measured basal metabolic rate.

Diagnosing hypothyroidism requires combining the clinical evaluation of symptoms with a physical examination and then a review of direct and indirect markers of thyroid function and sufficiency. A review of the current research on thyroid testing suggests that thyroid function testing may be unreliable for a subgroup of patients. A patient-centered clinical evaluation is needed to determine the likelihood of thyroid disease.

INTEGRATIVE TREATMENT

For most patients, a comprehensive approach focusing on the patient's overall health and lifestyle factors is helpful for thyroid health. A review of factors important for optimizing a patient's thyroid health can found in *Stop the Thyroid Madness I and II*[32,33] and Izabella Wentz's *Hashimoto's Thyroiditis.*[34] We highlight a number of these considerations here.

Diet and Gluten

A healthy, whole-foods diet is the cornerstone of any approach to global wellness. An anti-inflammatory diet that improves insulin resistance addresses multiple mechanisms of decreased thyroid function. A nutrient-dense diet can help address occult deficiencies of nutrients essential for normal thyroid functioning. Specific measurement and/or repletion of vitamins A and D, selenium, and iron should be considered. Emphasis on organic foods mitigates the well-established effects of common pesticides and other environmental toxins on the thyroid.[35] Restriction of excess goitrogens may be considered, but most patients tolerate a moderate intake of cruciferous vegetables. Increased intake of soy protein mildly decreases thyroid function, but in patients with subclinical hypothyroidism, a threefold increase in the progression to overt hypothyroidism has been found.[36]

Gluten autoimmunity in Hashimoto's is common and prevalence studies suggest that 6.9% of patients have celiac antibodies.[37] Thyroid disease is frequently reversible in these patients with a gluten-free diet.[38] In people with known Hashimoto's hypothyroidism without celiac antibodies, the presence of celiac genetics (HLA) predicts the finding of intraepithelial lymphocytes in over 40% of patients with Hashimoto's, suggesting potential gluten sensitivity.[39] Current research suggests that in patients with a family history of celiac disease but negative lab results, the presence of celiac HLA markers and functional digestive symptoms predicts a 68% prevalence of intestinal anti-tissue transglutaminase 2 antibodies consistent with occult celiac disease.[40] The role of gluten in Hashimoto's thyroiditis is likely underestimated.

Stress and Sleep

Stress plays a significant role in thyroid function. As we have discussed, chronic HPA axis dysfunction leads to alterations in the HPT axis. Stress causes hypothyroid symptoms by disrupting the HPA axis, reduces the conversion of T4 to T3, increases reverse T3, promotes autoimmunity by weakening immune barriers, causes thyroid hormone resistance, and creates other interacting hormonal imbalances.[3] The role of even modest sleep restriction of 5.5 hours of sleep at night for 2 weeks leads to a decrease in T4 and TSH,[41] showing that common stressors quickly alter thyroid homeostasis.

Addressing Autoimmunity and Gut Health

While beyond the scope of this chapter, addressing thyroid autoimmunity using a comprehensive functional medicine and lifestyle approach should be considered, especially for patients with high residual symptoms despite normal thyroid function test results and high antibody titers. Elevated TPO antibodies, independently of thyroid function tests, are associated with increasing burdens of somatic symptoms, poor psychosocial wellness, obsessive–compulsive symptoms, and depression.[42]

Most functional medicine approaches to autoimmunity focus on strategies that address common dysfunctions of the intestinal mucosal barrier, which have been called the doorway to autoimmunity.[43] Morphological changes in gut epithelial cells, increased intestinal permeability, and intraepithelial lymphocyte infiltration have been demonstrated in patients with Hashimoto's thyroiditis,[44,45] suggesting a pathogenic role of the impaired gut barrier in the development of Hashimoto's thyroiditis. Studies have found that 73.3% of patients with euthyroid Hashimoto's disease have abnormal gut function with fructose or lactose malabsorption.[46] Intestinal dysbiosis negatively affects iodothyronines synthesis, metabolism, and catabolic pathways, triggers autoimmunity, and affects the thyroid hormone hepato-enteric cycle where thyroid hormones are recirculated back into the body.[47] Addressing potential celiac disease, an immunological cause of intestinal disruption, is an important part of this approach.

Exercise

The concept of thyroid resistance has been poorly researched and the role of exercise in improving thyroid resistance similarly to insulin resistance had limited evidence until recently. New research has identified the mechanisms whereby intracellular production of T3 via D2 enzymes is activated by exercise. In an animal model, 20 minutes on a treadmill increased D2 activity by almost threefold, with increased expression of key muscle mitochondrial enzymes suggestive of improved tissue thyroid activity.[48] This research supports the prescription of exercise as a nonpharmacological way of increasing cellular thyroid hormone signaling in the skeletal muscles.

Thyroid Hormone Replacement: Levothyroxine Versus Combination Treatment

Guidelines for the treatment of hypothyroidism by the American Thyroid Association and the American Society of Clinical Endocrinologists strongly recommend a T4-only approach to the treatment of hypothyroidism. Failure of this approach to improve symptoms in at least 15% of patients is well recognized, and current recommendations suggest that endocrinologists look for nonthyroidal causes for their symptoms. However, the biological basis for failure of treatment using levothyroxine has been established:

- Treatment with T4 leads to abnormally low levels of serum T3 with lower serum FT3/FT4 ratios in one-third of persons with hypothyroidism.[8,21,31,49]

- Treatment of T4 does not improve objective measures of tissue hypo-thyroidism and is associated with abnormal tissue T3 levels, abnormal tissue-specific markers of hypothyroidism, and residual hyperlipide-mia, all of which correct on combination treatment.[8]
- In normal physiology, the TSH vigorously defends the free T3 level, keeping it stable; T4-only treatment leads to an iatrogenic disjoint between TSH and T3.[21]
- T4 monotherapy itself is a cause for deiodinase inefficiency, and T4 dose escalation may not remedy T3 deficiency but could actually hinder its attainment.[21,50]
- Polymorphisms in deiodinase enzymes are found in 16% of the population and inhibit the activation of the inactive T4 hormone in the target tissues. These patients are more likely to fail conventional treatment and are more likely to respond to combination T3 and T4 treatment.[51]
- In autoimmune hypothyroidism, anti-type 2 iodothyronine deiodinase (D2) antibodies are found in 26% of patients; this may be one reason why problems with T4-to-T3 conversion are found in these patients.[52]
- T4-only treatment may be over-converted to reverse T3 due to chronic disease, elevated stress, and conditions associated with systemic inflammation.[25]

Given these scientific findings, some conventional thyroidologists, as cited earlier, and most of the integrative thyroid physician and patient community have embraced combination treatment as an important treatment option. A retrospective study of patients who remained symptomatic despite levothyroxine treatment showed a 78% response rate to combination treatment with Armour Thyroid.[53] In a recent randomized, double-blind, crossover study conducted by endocrinologists at the Walter Reed National Military Medical Center, 67% of participants had a clear preference after experiencing both desiccated (combination) thyroid and levothyroxine, with 72% of these patients preferring desiccated thyroid.[54]

Current combination treatment approaches include the use of branded, pharmaceutical desiccated thyroid such as WP Thyroid, NP Thyroid (Acella), Nature-Throid, and Armour; desiccated thyroid extract from a compounding pharmacy; or a combination of pharmaceutical T4 with T3. We generally prefer the use of desiccated thyroid medications, which are composed of a 4:1 ratio of T4 to T3.

FOLLOWING THE PATIENT

Re-evaluation of the patient in 4 to 6 weeks after starting thyroid replacement includes a comprehensive evaluation detailing thyroid symptoms and retesting thyroid function with at least a TSH, free T3, and free T4.[21] Previously abnormal test results such as a cholesterol panel, fasting glucose, or SHBG can be tracked to follow the response of thyroid-sensitive biomarkers. Titration of thyroid replacement takes into consideration the symptoms of the patient as well as lab results; clinically, we are trying to elucidate tissue and cellular thyroid adequacy. Often patients will improve with initial treatment, but with the resulting decrease in TSH, the endogenous output of thyroid hormone may decrease, reversing the previously achieved euthyroidism. Progressive titration of the dose to the patient's symptoms, with attention to optimizing all aspects of the thyroid lab results, is often needed.

Some patients with hypothyroidism may have residual symptoms of hypothyroidism despite achieving circulating levels of TSH and thyroid hormones within the normal range. In some patients, normalization of the TSH levels may still reflect hypothyroidism if there is a decreased set point of the HPT or a problem with intracellular deiodinase function. For patients on T4-only treatment, the hypothalamus is uniquely sensitive to T4 therapy, and this form of treatment may normalize the TSH despite residual hypothyroidism across multiple organs and other areas of the brain.[50,55] In some patients, increasing the thyroid dose using combination T4 and T3 with some suppression of the TSH may be needed to achieve brain and tissue thyroid sufficiency.

Treatment of patients to TSH levels lower than the lower limit of normal increases the risk of iatrogenic hyperthyroidism. We recommend gradual increases with regular monitoring to assess patient response and serum thyroid function tests. A broad-based integrative approach with attention to the whole thyroid–adrenal–pancreas triad and other factors that affect overall thyroid health may be needed to treat the hypothyroid patient with residual symptoms. Balancing the risks and benefits of treatment in the context of shared decision making with the patient is a tenet of patient-centered care.

Diabetes Mellitus

CASE STUDY

A 55-year-old male with a long history of diabetes and neuropathy treated with gabapentin and a tricyclic antidepressant presented as a new patient. He

Table 14.2. Case Example Lab Results

Time	Treatment	Weight (BMI)	Glycemic tests
Initial	Glyburide 5 mg started (previously not on medication)	176 lbs (26.7)	Nonfasting glucose 257 A1C 15.5%
38 days	Glyburide 5 mg	188 lbs (28.5)	Fasting glucose 92 A1c 10.2% (decrease of 5.3 in 1 month)
5 months	Glyburide 5 mg	205 lbs (31.1) (+29 lbs)	Nonfasting glucose 110 A1c 6.6% (decrease of 8.9)

admitted to noncompliance due to metformin-related digestive complaints. Initial testing showed hyperglycemia of 257 and an A1c of 15.5%. He was started on low-dose monotherapy and a low-carbohydrate whole-food diet (Table 14.2).

The low-carbohydrate diet led to immediate control of hyperglycemia despite minimal use of medication in this patient. This effect did not require weight loss or a change in insulin resistance. At the last visit, the patient was counseled to decrease calories and added oils, increase low-calorie plant-based foods, and increase exercise. Glyburide was changed to a dipeptidyl peptidase-4 inhibitor to avoid insulin-related weight gain.

INTRODUCTION AND EPIDEMIOLOGY

There is a pandemic of type 2 diabetes mellitus (DM) in the United States. A fourfold rise of diabetes since the 1980s has been documented by the CDC. This profound and recent increase is due to changes in our food, environment, and lifestyle that interact with our genetics. Every diabetic generation has an exponential increase in diabetes risk,[56] with earlier onset of diabetes attributed to a combination of in utero exposure, epigenetics, and the onset of diabetes in their parent(s). A 20-year-old born between 1930 and 1939 had only a 30.4% lifetime risk of diabetes.[57] In the same study, for the most recent measured cohort (those born between 1960 and 1969), the lifetime prevalence of developing DM was 54.8%.

The practice of geriatrics is associated with the dual burdens of late-stage diabetes and late-onset early DM. A disproportionate number of cases of advanced DM is found in geriatric practices, with often widely fluctuating hyper- and hypoglycemia. Studies have found that 46.6% of diabetic patients have an A1c of 7 or more.[58] Unfortunately for patients with advanced DM, conventional treatments that decrease the A1c to organ-preserving levels can lead to life-threatening hypoglycemia, which is not only associated with acute mental status changes, syncope, and falls but may also increase the risk of death.[59] Polypharmacy with multiple hypoglycemic agents and/or insulin is a particular burden in this population of patients, whose increasing physical and cognitive challenges make it increasingly difficult to self-manage their diabetes.

Prediabetic states, including insulin resistance and hyperinsulinemia without hyperglycemia, have been associated with significant morbidity and mortality.[60] Prediabetes and insulin resistance have been associated with decreased total cerebral brain volume, brain atrophy in Alzheimer's-associated regions, and cognitive dysfunction in multiple large studies.[61,62] "Idiopathic neuropathy" is associated with a 60% prevalence of prediabetes.[63] Insulin resistance and hyperinsulinemia induce glomerular hyperfiltration, increase renal vascular permeability, and induce low-grade inflammation and endothelial dysfunction.[64] While the results of research on cardiovascular disease are equivocal, as A1C levels increase from early prediabetes to levels greater than 6%, an increasing number of studies show an association with increased cardiovascular risk.[65]

PATHOPHYSIOLOGY

Insulin resistance is the underlying context of the development of type 2 diabetes. The CDC estimates that 86 million Americans, making up 35% of the U.S. population, have prediabetes, a hyperglycemic condition associated with maximal insulin resistance, 50% to 80% loss of beta-cell function, and an approximate 10% incidence of diabetic retinopathy.[66] Over-nutrition leads to ectopic storage of fat in the visceral organs that control glucose regulation. Levels of fasting glucose, a reflection of liver gluconeogenesis, become elevated with the development of hepatic insulin resistance due to fatty liver disease.[67,68] The ectopic storage of fat in the pancreas is associated with basal cell dysfunction with loss of first-phase insulin response, and is a major mediator in postprandial hyperglycemia, one of the earliest manifestations in diabetes.[67,69]

Hyperglycemia in type 2 DM is caused by impaired hepatic response to insulin in the basal and postprandial state, beta-cell dysfunction and loss, as well as impaired muscle glucose uptake after a meal. Not only is the acute insulin response blunted after a meal, but decreased insulin-stimulated glucose uptake leads to almost no muscle glycogen synthase activity, which is associated with saturated muscle glycogen storage compartments exacerbated by a sedentary lifestyle.[70] Postprandial glucose disposal in diabetics is almost completely reliant on liver glycogen storage, increasing the risk of fatty liver disease with chronic fuel surplus.[71]

Progression of DM is primarily due to progressive beta-cell dysfunction and failure. The role of early beta-cell dysfunction has been underappreciated; at the time of diagnosis, patients have lost 80% or more of their beta-cell function.[66] The hyperglycemia of an "early diagnosis" of DM is a manifestation of end-stage beta-cell failure, the result of a prolonged, silent process of progressive beta-cell dysfunction, inflammation, and destruction that begins as early as 12 years before disease onset.[72]

While we do not have the space to discuss the integrative network of pathophysiological abnormalities in DM, we will discuss therapeutics related to the emerging science showing diet and dietary compounds, chronic inflammation, gut microbiota, essential nutrients, environmental toxins, stress, and sleep dysfunction as important mediators of glucose intolerance.

LABORATORY EVALUATIONS

Integrative clinicians often utilize measures of insulin dysfunction beyond conventional tests of diabetes and prediabetes. While beta-cell dysfunction is a gradual, progressive process, the progression of hyperglycemia is not linear. Most people will maintain their fasting plasma glucose before showing a rapid rather than gradual onset of diabetes, which is due to the loss of the first-phase insulin response to elevated glucose.[72] The most important step in the early prevention of diabetes and the healing of metabolic dysfunction is to identify and address insulin resistance, the underlying cause of diabetes.

The use of the Homeostasis Model Assessment of Insulin Resistance (HOMA-IR) is the best-established clinical assessment of insulin resistance. HOMA-IR is calculated using lab testing after an 8-hour fast where insulin resistance = fasting serum insulin (μU/ml) × fasting plasma glucose (mmol l^{-1})/22.5. The optimal insulin resistance, based on normal subjects aged less than 35 years with normal weight, is 1. Values above 1 gradually increase the risk of insulin resistance, with data from the U.S. National Health and Nutrition Examination Survey (NHANES) suggesting a cutoff of 2.73 or more based on the 66th percentile.[73] A large study of nondiabetic individuals found that the best HOMA-IR cutoff levels ranged from 1.85 in men to 2.07 in women aged 50 years old, where the criteria were based on sensitivity to cardiometabolic risk.[73] HOMA-IR cutoff values vary by gender and age.

Clinically, the use of a fasting insulin or C-peptide measurement or fasting insulin-to-glucose ratio has been a common approach to identifying hyperinsulinemia and insulin resistance. For patients without a diagnosis of diabetes, a fasting insulin assessment may be as accurate at predicting insulin resistance as HOMA-IR.[74] Other biomarkers with consistent data showing association with metabolic syndrome and the risk of diabetes include low adiponectin,[75] elevated homocysteine, elevated uric acid, elevated triglycerides (and triglyceride:HDL ratio), and NMR lipoproteins. The use of anthropomorphic measures such as body mass index (BMI) and waist-to-hip ratio can be powerful predictors of insulin resistance. Using body measurements, the BMI strongly predicts whole-body insulin resistance, while the waist-to-hip ratio, a measure of central obesity, is the best predictor of hepatic insulin resistance.[76] Finally, a global pattern of a metabolic syndrome or the presence of an insulin-resistance–related condition, such as gout or polycystic ovarian syndrome, should increase the suspicion of insulin resistance.

TREATMENT

The presence of diabetes increases the risk of significant vascular events two- to four-fold, and medications do very little to decrease this risk. In fact, recent reviews current to 2015 reported that there was no evidence that medications for diabetes decrease the risk of heart and vascular disease,[77] until the 2015 FDA approval of empagliflozin for cardiovascular disease prevention. We favor medications that decrease excessive intake and storage of energy and/ or protect beta-cells including metformin, acarbose, sodium-glucose cotransporter-2 (SGLT2), and incretin-based therapies.

Diabetes is a progressive disease. For most diabetics, the A1c continues to increase by about 1% every 2 years despite treatment with most therapies.[72] Current evidence suggests that medications are not very effective at preventing and slowing down the underlying progression of DM.[65] Diet and lifestyle changes were superior to medications in the NIH Diabetes Prevention Program trial.[78]

Diet and Nutrition

The principles of intensive dietary therapy for DM overlap with the foundations of an approach for the prevention of heart disease. Strong evidence supports that adherence to a healthy diet pattern such as the Mediterranean diet or the Dietary Approaches to Stop Hypertension (DASH) diet improves cardiovascular risk factors and decreases the incidence of cardiovascular disease. Lifestyle approaches that effectively decrease hyperglycemia have pleotropic effects, including weight loss, decreasing inflammation and C-reactive protein, decreasing hypertension, improving hyperlipidemia, decreasing uric acid, decreasing homocysteine, and increasing adiponectin. Treating the metabolic syndrome and dysfunctional metabolome of type 2 diabetes primarily with targeted glucose-decreasing drugs fails to address the underlying disease process and the global metabolic risk.

Diabetes management that starts with a foundation of intensive diet and lifestyle management simplifies the management of hyperglycemia, decreases medication burden, and improves global cardiovascular risk factors. Patients are educated on a diet with an emphasis on vegetables and salads, seeds, nuts, berries, healthy fats, low-sugar fruits, and moderate amounts of protein and high-quality meats. Whole-food complex carbohydrates such as quinoa, legumes and beans, and sweet potatoes are introduced after hyperglycemia is controlled, and eaten as tolerated based on postprandial response. We educate patients on the importance of avoiding processed foods. Food choices and cooking methods that limit advanced glycation end-products have been shown to improve insulin resistance and reduce exposure to a significant mediator of diabetes complications.[79,80] Avoiding canned drinks, canned food, and frozen microwave meals helps limit bisphenol A (BPA) exposure, which has been linked to increased diabetes and obesity in the Endocrine Society's scientific statement on endocrine-disrupting chemicals.[81]

Low-carbohydrate diets quickly decrease exogenous glucose sources profoundly to levels well managed by residual pancreatic capacity. For immediate control of hyperglycemia, a low-carbohydrate diet and fasting are more powerful than oral medications. Significant evidence supports dietary carbohydrate restriction as the first approach to controlling diabetes.[82] For patients who are vegetarians or prefer a more plant-based diet, significant to profound improvements in hyperglycemia can be obtained with this approach.[83]

Reversing Diabetes

Recent studies by Dr. Roy Taylor elegantly show that diabetes is not only controllable but fundamentally reversible in the majority of type 2 diabetics. Using magnetic resonance imaging scans, he has shown that a low-calorie diet that decreases intrahepatic fat reverses insulin resistance in the liver, restoring basal euglycemia.[67] Perhaps more astounding is that a low-calorie diet also decreases intrapancreatic fat and restores beta-cell function, which was previously believed to have been lost through degenerative processes.[67,69] The reversal of diabetes with gastric bypass is established. A study comparing a very-low-calorie diet to Roux-en-Y gastric bypass showed equivalent improvement in weight loss, glucose tolerance tests, insulin sensitivity, acute insulin secretion after intravenous glucose, and beta-cell function within 21 days.[84]

Exercise and Sleep

Exercise reverses increases in insulin sensitivity for 24 to 48 hours.[70] After evaluation and clearance by a medical professional, a combination of resistance exercise and aerobic exercise three or four times a week for a total of at least 150 minutes a week is recommended. Sleep deprivation quickly increases insulin resistance. In fact, a single night of partial sleep deprivation increased insulin resistance and decreased glucose uptake by 25%.[85]

Supplements

Table 14.3 lists some of the most promising supplements for improving glycemic control and treating underlying processes associated with insulin resistance. For all herbal and supplementation regimens, we recommend checking liver enzyme levels for hepatic reactions. Use of existing combination formulas may improve patients' adherence and decrease cost.

Stress, Fatigue, and the HPA Axis

INTRODUCTION

We live in stressful times. The American Psychological Association conducts a yearly survey of stress in the United States, detailing the epidemic of stress and its correlates. In the latest report, the average American rates his or her stress as 5.1 on a 10-point scale, with 24% of adults reporting experiencing extreme stress (a rating of 8–10)[29]. Chronic discrimination, reported by 61%, and dealing with chronic disease, by 67%, joined the typical top stressors of money, work, and family responsibilities. A rising number of symptoms associated with worsening stress was reported, including problems with mental health in over 40%, poor sleep in 46%, and stress eating by 39%.[29]

The HPA axis is the central response center in managing emotional, physical, and physiological stressors. The HPA axis refers to the hierarchy of control of the adrenal glands. The hypothalamus's primary neuroendocrine function is creating releasing hormones that control the pituitary gland in the brain. In response, the pituitary, the "master gland," releases hormones that control the

Table 14.3. Supplements for Improving Glycemic Control and Treating Processes Associated with Insulin Resistance

Supplement	Dosing	Studies and effect
Berberine	500 mg, two or three times a day	A meta-analysis of 27 randomized controlled trials involving 2,569 subjects found berberine to be as effective as metformin and other oral hypoglycemics.[86,87]
Probiotics	Once a day	Meta-analysis shows significant effects in HOMA-IR, fasting blood glucose (FBG), and A1c.[88]
Gymnema sylvestre	200–1,000 mg/day	PPAR agonist; improves weight, decreases the required insulin dose, and lowers A1C; may also increase the number of beta cells in the pancreas[89]
Cassia Cinnamon	750 mg twice a day	Decreases fatty liver, insulin resistance, lipids, fasting blood sugars, and A1c[87,90]
CoQ10	75–300 mg twice a day or Ubiquinol 100–300 mg/day	Modest improvements in A1c and FBG; may prevent vascular complications secondary to associated oxidative stress[87]
L-carnitine	1–3 g/day in divided doses	Meta-analysis suggests improvement in FBG and lipids;[91] may improve fatty liver disease
Magnesium	500–1,000 mg/day	A recent meta-analysis found evidence for decreased insulin resistance as measured by HOMA-IR and decreased FBG.[92]
Chromium	200–400 mg/dly	An essential mineral needed for carbohydrate metabolism; a recent meta-analysis confirmed efficacy in decreasing A1c and FBG[93]
Mulberry extract	1 g before meals	Improvements in fasting glucose, A1c, and response to glucose challenge[87]
Aloe vera juice	15–30 ml juice two or three times a day	A meta-analysis concluded that aloe vera decreased FBG by 46.6 mg/dL and decreased A1c by 1.05%.[94]
Curcumin	1,500 mg to 6 g/day	Randomized controlled trial for prediabetic patients has shown prevention of diabetes; studies suggest improved B-cell function, decreased HOMA-IR, decreased diabetic nephropathy and retinopathy, and glycemic control.[87,95]

body's hormonal glands and organs, including the adrenals. In acute stressors, the well-described "fight or flight" response involves hypothalamic and pituitary activation that initiates an adrenal response with release of epinephrine, norepinephrine, cortisol, and DHEA.

Clinical medicine recognizes adrenal dysfunction and hypocortisolism at the extremes of glandular failure, such as with Addison's disease, a rare autoimmune condition. Current diagnostic criteria for adrenal disease define the disease at a stage that correlates with 90% or more of both adrenal cortices already destroyed and dysfunctional.[96] Diagnostic tests involving the administration of adrenocorticotropic hormone (ACTH) indicate disease only when there is a profound failure of the adrenal gland to produce cortisol. For comparison, if we defined hypothyroidism as a condition where infusions of TSH lead to decreased thyroid hormone production reflective of 10% or less of residual thyroid function, very few people would be diagnosed with thyroid dysfunction.

A quick search of Google Scholar for "HPA dysfunction" comes back with almost 50,000 published articles, with less than half of the studies relating to Addison's disease. Only by ignoring 50% of all research about abnormalities affecting the HPA axis can one conclude that this highly responsive, stress management hormone system is working without a glitch in 99.999% of people. We do agree with the Endocrine Society, however, that "adrenal fatigue is not a real medical condition," at least not a primary adrenal gland dysfunction. Leading integrative clinicians recognize that the use of the term "adrenal fatigue" is a simplified and perhaps inaccurate way of describing HPA axis dysregulation.[97] Given the incredible acute and chronic stress and chronic disease burden of our current population, the idea that this sensitive, overburdened hormone system never accumulates "wear and tear" and accumulated dysfunction throughout one's lifespan begs some amount of incredulity.

Thousands of scientific research studies have documented that significant changes in HPA regulation occur in the context of chronic, prolonged physical or emotional stress. Current published reviews describe functional adrenal dysfunction caused by conditions that can chronically activate the HPA axis, including major depression, anorexia nervosa, bulimia nervosa, alcoholism, diabetes mellitus, simple obesity, polycystic ovary syndrome, obstructive sleep apnea syndrome, panic disorder, generalized anxiety disorder, shift work, and end-stage renal disease.[98] The modern epidemics of inflammatory and autoimmune diseases has been related to impairments in HPA axis activity and associated hypocortisolism, or to peripheral glucocorticoid resistance in the context of chronic stress-induced hypercortisolism.[99] Common "functional" and psychological disorders including mood disorders, post-traumatic stress syndrome (PTSD), burnout, attention-deficit/hyperactivity disorder (ADHD), chronic fatigue syndrome, irritable bowel syndrome, and fibromyalgia have been linked to HPA axis abnormalities, highlighting the central role that this hormone system has in modulating disease and mediating symptoms of health and wellness.

Current neuroscience describes a complex model where cortisol, estrogen, DHEA, endocannabinoids, brain-derived neurotrophic factor (BDNF), glutamate, and a host of other mediators have profound effects on neuroplasticity.[100–102] Striking reversible changes with pruning of neuronal dendrites occur in laboratory animals with both acute and chronic stress.[100,101] The hippocampus, with elevated concentrations of glucocorticoid receptors, responds to persistent cortisol; hippocampal brain atrophy has been found in patients with Cushing's, women with chronic stress, and survivors of the 9/11 terrorist attack on the World Trade Center.[100,101] A blunted ACTH response may be due to downregulation of pituitary corticotrophin-releasing hormone receptors in functional hypercortisolemic states. The autonomic nervous system parallels and interacts with the HPA axis in chronic stress, and conditioned dysfunction can lead to persistence of increased catecholamines, elevated heart rate, decreased heart rate variability, and increased or reactive hypertension.[103] While the current science of HPA dysregulation is extremely multifaceted, the HPA dysfunction seen in the context of chronic stressors is primarily driven by adaptive neurological changes that affect central responses and regulation of the adrenal glands and other metabolic functions.

We believe that widespread HPA dysfunction in human health has been missed by conventional medicine due to its disease paradigm. A large body of research describing common dysfunctions of the HPA axis outnumber the rare failures of the adrenal system. The established concepts of "allostasis (active process of adaptation and maintaining homeostasis) and allostatic load (wear-and-tear produced by too much stress and a resulting unhealthy lifestyle)" describe the initially protective but eventually dysfunctional changes to the brain and body.[102] The significant burden of this condition has been missed even though the majority of consultations in primary care are for evaluation of symptoms and somatic syndromes that cannot be explained by current medical pathophysiology and respond poorly to current treatments.[104,105] Current research demonstrating widespread HPA axis abnormalities in dozens of common conditions suggest the importance that stress and HPA axis regulation have on our fundamental well-being.

EVALUATION AND LABORATORY MEASUREMENT

Most integrative clinicians evaluate HPA axis and adrenal dysfunction through a four-point salivary or urinary test. These tests report the diurnal pattern of cortisol output, which are often presented with measurements of secretory IgA and calculated estimates of total cortisol, DHEA-S, and the cortisol/DHEA-S ratio. Low-normal levels of serum AM cortisol, DHEA(S), and IgA can be supportive but are often insensitive when using conventional laboratory ranges.

The graph in Figure 14.1 shows the salivary cortisol test results of a previously healthy 55-year-old with no chronic diseases who presented with a history of persistent fatigue after an intensive period of prolonged work stress. Extensive evaluations by multiple physicians and subspecialists over 1 to 2 years were negative for an underlying etiology.

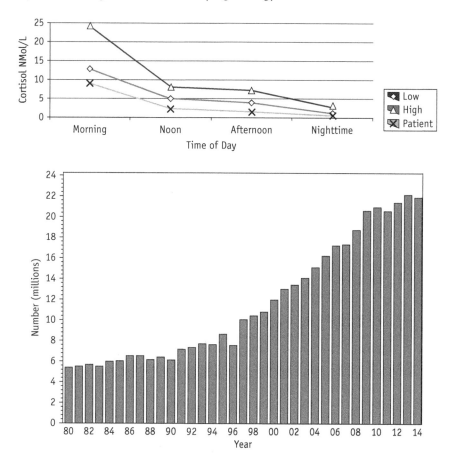

FIGURE 14.1. Adrenal Stress Index, Salivary Cortisol Test Result for the patient with chronic stress.

SYMPTOMS

Correlation of an abnormal cortisol test with symptoms of HPA axis dysfunction supports the clinical significance of laboratory abnormalities. Clinical experience highlights the common symptoms of persistent fatigue, unrefreshing sleep, increased energy at night often with insomnia, nocturnal awakening, night sweats, changes in mood (irritability, depression, or anxiety), and cognitive changes, often described as brain fog with memory or attention issues. Salty and/or sugary food cravings, recurrent lightheadedness with standing, insulin resistance or prediabetes, trouble losing weight, and low libido are common. Many patients have symptoms of hypoglycemia and often already snack or eat small meals throughout the day to avoid symptoms of irritability, weakness, lightheadedness, sweating, shaking, nausea, headaches, or heart palpitations.

TREATMENT

An integrative approach to HPA axis abnormalities starts with evaluation and interventions to correct four general categories of chronic HPA-axis stressors: mental and emotional stress, sleep disorders, metabolic and glycemic dysregulation, and chronic inflammation.[97]

Global Considerations: Addressing the Whole Person and Chronic Inflammation

Chronic health problems and systemic inflammation are mediators of chronic allostatic stress leading to dysfunction.[98,100] A comprehensive approach to improving a patient's physical health using conventional and integrative methods is important to create the context for an improved stress response. Functional medicine approaches that evaluate and treat causes of chronic inflammation and immune reactivity, including food intolerances, chronic infections, dysbiosis, digestive dysfunction, toxic load, obesity, and processed and reactive foods, should be considered.

Mind–Body and Sleep

Traditional relaxation practices of meditation, yoga, or mindfulness-based stress reduction training are proven approaches that address stress-related syndromes leading to chronic HPA axis dysfunction. We often utilize HeartMath, a convenient biofeedback training programs that allows patients to improve their stress response and increase heart rate variability, a measure of autonomic balance. Studies on participants using HeartMath have demonstrated decreases in cortisol by 23% while doubling the DHEA level.[106] Integrative therapies including acupuncture, massage, and Reiki can also be helpful adjuncts. Regular exercise is an important modality for improving multiple mediators of the stress response.

Evaluations and treatments for insomnia, nocturnal awakening, restless leg syndrome, sleep apnea, altered circadian rhythms, sleep deprivation, and poor sleep architecture are important considerations for improving HPA axis abnormality.

Psychological and Perceived Stress

The importance of a person's history of emotional and psychological stressors cannot be underestimated. An evaluation of significant life stressors, early childhood experiences, history of anxiety and depression, and recent physical or emotionally demanding periods in a person's life can help the clinician understand the impact of perceived stress. Addressing life stress often involves addressing a patient's lifestyle and changing his or her environment. Clinicians can help patients actively create a work–life balance, address family dynamics, engage in loving relationships and social support, and make lifestyle changes that support a healthy emotional balance. For some patients, referral to a skilled mental health clinician is often needed to address this mediator of HPA axis dysfunction.

Nutritional Considerations

The role of the HPA axis on stabilizing plasma glucose levels underlines the importance of stabilizing fluctuating glucose levels. In general, anti-inflammatory diets, which emphasize nutrient-dense foods, vegetables, and unprocessed "real foods," are the cornerstone of this approach. Recent evidence suggests that circadian timing of carbohydrates, with decreased amounts in the morning and modest amounts of whole-food carbohydrates toward the end of the day, may improve the HPA axis and adrenal response.[107]

Adaptogens and Selected Nutraceuticals

Adaptogens are widely used herbal and nutritional compounds that generally work on improving the resilience of the individual by decreasing the brain's response to stress. Commonly used supplements are listed in Table 14.4.

Table 14.4. Common Supplements

Supplement	Suggested dosing	Mechanisms, efficacy
Ashwagandha extract (providing at least 6 mg/day of withanolides)	300–500 mg, two or three times a day	Decreases excess cortisol, improves anxiety and the stress response
Rhodiola rosea (standardized extract containing 3% rosavins and/or 1% salidrosides)	170–680 mg/day, often divided into twice-a-day dosing	
Cordyceps	Dosing based on extract and preparation	Used as an adaptogen to improve energy and immune health
Maca powder	1 tablespoons once or twice a day	
Magnesium (as citrate, malate)	300–400 mg by mouth two or three times a day, or as Epsom salt bath	Decreases catecholamines, anxiety, and the cortisol response to stress
Acetyl-L carnitine	500–1,000 mg twice a day	Decreases excess glutamate signaling and prevents abnormal stress-induced neuroplasticity remodeling;[102] effective as an antidepressant[108]
The ginsengs: American ginseng, Asian ginseng (Panax), and Siberian ginseng	Dosing based on extract and preparation	Add-on therapy as a stimulating tonic for hypocortisolism
Curcumin extract[109]	500–1,000 mg twice a day	Broad effects on inflammation, immune modulation, neuroprotective, HPA axis
Licorice root		For significant hypocortisolism (see Guilliams[97] for dosing considerations)
Phosphytidylserine	200–600 mg/day	Decreases hypercortisolism, improves cognitive function
Vitamin and mineral support/B vitamins	Per label, generally multiple times a day	Recommended for all stress-related conditions[97]
DHEA and pregnenolone	See Guilliams[97] for dosing considerations.	

Conclusion

Abnormalities of the thyroid, insulin, and adrenal systems contribute to frank, debilitating disease as well as chronic feelings of low energy and decreased vitality. Current approaches to these conditions often address these overlapping systems separately, ignoring common interactions that drive widespread dysfunction across multiple "separate" hormone systems. Current guidelines for endocrine diseases lead to suboptimal treatment for a large percentage of patients. Conventional treatment of diabetes is not effective and is associated with a high residual risk of heart disease, widely fluctuating blood glucose, and iatrogenic, life-threatening hypoglycemia. Thyroid guidelines often dismiss patients' complaints and symptoms and misinterpret thyroid function tests due to an overreliance on the TSH.

Integrative medicine expands the evaluation of endocrine dysfunction through a person-centered approach to evaluating thyroid, adrenal, and blood sugar abnormalities. Treatments are safe and generally focus on common-sense interventions such as improving one's lifestyle through effective diet, exercise, and stress management. The role of thyroid hormone treatment, with an emphasis on the use of natural combination thyroid replacement, should be considered for patients with clinical hypothyroidism to alleviate symptoms and address conditions that affect their quality of life. Optimizing the thyroid, blood sugar, and stress response are cornerstones of healthy aging and are major determinants of a patient's sense of well-being.

REFERENCES

1. Brenta G. Why can insulin resistance be a natural consequence of thyroid dysfunction? *J Thyroid Res.* 2011;2011:e152850.
2. Han C, He X, Xia X, et al. Subclinical hypothyroidism and type 2 diabetes: A systematic review and meta-analysis. *PloS One.* 2015;10(8):e0135233.
3. Helmreich DL, Parfitt DB, Lu X-Y, Akil H, Watson SJ. Relation between the hypothalamic-pituitary-thyroid (HPT) axis and the hypothalamic-pituitary-adrenal (HPA) axis during repeated stress. *Neuroendocrinology.* 2005;81(3):183–192.
4. Karimifar M, Aminorroaya A, Amini M, et al. Effect of metformin on thyroid stimulating hormone and thyroid volume in patients with prediabetes: A randomized placebo-controlled clinical trial. *J Res Med Sci Off J Isfahan Univ Med Sci.* 2014;19(11):1019–1026.
5. LaValle J, Heyman A. et al. Metabolic Code. https://www.metaboliccode.com/.
6. Stasiolek M. Neurological symptoms and signs in thyroid disease. *Thyroid Res.* 2015;8(1):A25.
7. Bauer M, Goetz T, Glenn T, Whybrow PC. The thyroid-brain interaction in thyroid disorders and mood disorders. *J Neuroendocrinol.* 2008;20(10):1101–1114.

8. Gereben B, McAninch EA, Ribeiro MO, Bianco AC. Scope and limitations of iodo-thyronine deiodinases in hypothyroidism. *Nat Rev Endocrinol.* 2015;11(11):642–652.

9. Mahajan AS, Lal R, Dhanwal DK, Jain AK, Chowdhury V. Evaluation of autonomic functions in subclinical hypothyroid and hypothyroid patients. *Indian J Endocrinol Metab.* 2013;17(3):460–464.

10. Meikle AW. The interrelationships between thyroid dysfunction and hypogonadism in men and boys. *Thyroid.* 2004;14(suppl 1):17–25.

11. Masaki M, Komamura K, Goda A, et al. Elevated arterial stiffness and diastolic dysfunction in subclinical hypothyroidism. *Circ J Off J Jpn Circ Soc.* 2014;78(6):1494–1500.

12. Amin A, Chitsazan M, Taghavi S, Ardeshiri M. Effects of triiodothyronine replacement therapy in patients with chronic stable heart failure and low-triiodothyronine syndrome: A randomized, double-blind, placebo-controlled study. *ESC Heart Fail.* 2015;2(1):5–11.

13. Rizos C., Elisaf M., Liberopoulos E. Effects of thyroid dysfunction on lipid profile. *Open Cardiovasc Med J.* 2011;5:76–84.

14. Ahmad J, Tagoe CE. Fibromyalgia and chronic widespread pain in autoimmune thyroid disease. *Clin Rheumatol.* 2014;33(7):885–891.

15. Surks MI, Hollowell JG. Age-specific distribution of serum thyrotropin and anti-thyroid antibodies in the US population: Implications for the prevalence of subclinical hypothyroidism. *J Clin Endocrinol Metab.* 2007;92(12):4575–4582.

16. Spencer CA, Hollowell JG, Kazarosyan M, Braverman LE. National Health and Nutrition Examination Survey III thyroid-stimulating hormone (TSH)-thyroperoxidase antibody relationships demonstrate that TSH upper reference limits may be skewed by occult thyroid dysfunction. *J Clin Endocrinol Metab.* 2007;92(11):4236–4240.

17. Canaris GJ, Manowitz NR, Mayor G, Ridgway EC. The Colorado thyroid disease prevalence study. *Arch Intern Med.* 2000;160(4):526–534.

18. Menicucci D, Sebastiani L, Comparini A, et al. Minimal changes of thyroid axis activity influence brain functions in young females affected by subclinical hypothyroidism. *Arch Ital Biol.* 2013;151(1):1–10.

19. Hollowell JG, Staehling NW, Flanders WD, et al. Serum TSH, T(4), and thyroid antibodies in the United States population (1988 to 1994): National Health and Nutrition Examination Survey (NHANES III). *J Clin Endocrinol Metab.* 2002;87(2):489–499.

20. Wartofsky L, Dickey RA. The evidence for a narrower thyrotropin reference range is compelling. *J Clin Endocrinol Metab.* 2005;90(9):5483–5488.

21. Hoermann R, Midgley JEM, Larisch R, Dietrich JW. Homeostatic control of the thyroid-pituitary axis: Perspectives for diagnosis and treatment. *Front Endocrinol.* 2015;6:177.

22. Andersen S, Pedersen KM, Bruun NH, Laurberg P. Narrow individual variations in serum T(4) and T(3) in normal subjects: a clue to the understanding of subclinical thyroid disease. *J Clin Endocrinol Metab.* 2002;87(3):1068–1072.

23. Fliers E, Kalsbeek A, Boelen A. Beyond the fixed setpoint of the hypothalamus-pituitary-thyroid axis. *Eur J Endocrinol.* 2014;171(5):R197–R208.

24. De Groot LJ. Dangerous dogmas in medicine: The nonthyroidal illness syndrome. *J Clin Endocrinol Metab.* 1999;84(1):151–164.

25. Wajner SM, Goemann IM, Bueno AL, Larsen PR, Maia AL. IL-6 promotes non-thyroidal illness syndrome by blocking thyroxine activation while promoting thyroid hormone inactivation in human cells. *J Clin Invest.* 2011;121(5):1834–1845.

26. Vors C, Pineau G, Drai J, et al. Postprandial endotoxemia linked with chylomicrons and lipopolysaccharides handling in obese versus lean men: A lipid dose-effect trial. *J Clin Endocrinol Metab.* 2015;100(9):3427–3435.

27. Czarnywojtek A, Owecki M, Zgorzalewicz-Stachowiak M, et al. The role of serum C-reactive protein measured by high-sensitive method in thyroid disease. *Arch Immunol Ther Exp (Warsz).* 2014;62(6):501–509.

28. Tsigos C, Chrousos GP. Hypothalamic-pituitary-adrenal axis, neuroendocrine factors and stress. *J Psychosom Res.* 2002;53(4):865–871.

29. American Psychological Association. *Stress in America: The Impact of Discrimination. Stress in America Survey;* 2016.

30. Holtorf K. Thyroid hormone transport into cellular tissue. *J Restor Med.* 2014;3(1):53–68.

31. Gullo D, Latina A, Frasca F, Moli RL, Pellegriti G, Vigneri R. Levothyroxine monotherapy cannot guarantee euthyroidism in all athyreotic patients. *PLoS One.* 2011;6(8):e22552.

32. Bowthorpe JA. *Stop the Thyroid Madness: A Patient Revolution Against Decades of Inferior Treatment.* 2nd ed. Fredericksburg, TX: Laughing Grape Publishing; 2011.

33. Heyman A, Yang J. *Stop the Thyroid Madness II: How Thyroid Experts Are Challenging Ineffective Treatments and Improving the Lives of Patients.* Dolores, CO: Laughing Grape Publishing; 2014.

34. Wentz I. *Hashimoto's Thyroiditis: Lifestyle Interventions for Finding and Treating the Root Cause.* Lexington, KY: Wentz LLC; 2013.

35. Duntas LH, Stathatos N. Toxic chemicals and thyroid function: Hard facts and lateral thinking. *Rev Endocr Metab Disord.* 2015;16(4):311–318.

36. Sathyapalan T, Manuchehri AM, Thatcher NJ, et al. The effect of soy phytoestrogen supplementation on thyroid status and cardiovascular risk markers in patients with subclinical hypothyroidism: A randomized, double-blind, crossover study. *J Clin Endocrinol Metab.* 2011;96(5):1442–1449.

37. Marwaha RK, Garg MK, Tandon N, et al. Glutamic acid decarboxylase (anti-GAD) & tissue transglutaminase (anti-TTG) antibodies in patients with thyroid autoimmunity. *Indian J Med Res.* 2013;137(1):82–86.

38. Sategna-Guidetti C, Volta U, Ciacci C, et al. Prevalence of thyroid disorders in untreated adult celiac disease patients and effect of gluten withdrawal: An Italian multicenter study. *Am J Gastroenterol.* 2001;96(3):751–757.

39. Valentino R, Savastano S, Maglio M, et al. Markers of potential coeliac disease in patients with Hashimoto's thyroiditis. *Eur J Endocrinol.* 2002;146(4):479–483.

40. Not T, Ziberna F, Vatta S, et al. Cryptic genetic gluten intolerance revealed by intestinal antitransglutaminase antibodies and response to gluten-free diet. *Gut.* 2011;60(11):1487–1493.

41. Kessler L, Nedeltcheva A, Imperial J, Penev PD. Changes in serum TSH and free T4 during human sleep restriction. *Sleep*. 2010;33(8):1115–1118.

42. Müssig K, Künle A, Säuberlich A-L, et al. Thyroid peroxidase antibody positivity is associated with symptomatic distress in patients with Hashimoto's thyroiditis. *ResearchGate*. 2012;26(4):559–563.

43. Fasano A. Zonulin and its regulation of intestinal barrier function: The biological door to inflammation, autoimmunity, and cancer. *Physiol Rev.* 2011;91(1):151–175.

44. Cindoruk M, Tuncer C, Dursun A, et al. Increased colonic intraepithelial lymphocytes in patients with Hashimoto's thyroiditis. *J Clin Gastroenterol*. 2002;34(3):237–239.

45. Sasso FC, Carbonara O, Torella R, et al. Ultrastructural changes in enterocytes in subjects with Hashimoto's thyroiditis. *Gut*. 2004;53(12):1878–1880.

46. Heckl S, Reiners C, Buck AK, Schäfer A, Dick A, Scheurlen M. Evidence of impaired carbohydrate assimilation in euthyroid patients with Hashimoto's thyroiditis. *Eur J Clin Nutr*. 2016;70(2):222–228.

47. Virili C, Centanni M. Does microbiota composition affect thyroid homeostasis? *Endocrine*. 2015;49(3):583–587.

48. Bocco BMLC, Louzada RAN, Silvestre DHS, et al. Thyroid hormone activation by type 2 deiodinase mediates exercise-induced peroxisome proliferator-activated receptor-γ coactivator-1α expression in skeletal muscle. *J Physiol*. 2016;594(18):5255–5269.

49. Wiersinga WM. Paradigm shifts in thyroid hormone replacement therapies for hypothyroidism. *Nat Rev Endocrinol*. 2014;10(3):164–174.

50. Werneck de Castro JP, Fonseca TL, Ueta CB, et al. Differences in hypothalamic type 2 deiodinase ubiquitination explain localized sensitivity to thyroxine. *J Clin Invest*. 2015;125(2):769–781.

51. Panicker V, Saravanan P, Vaidya B, et al. Common variation in the DIO2 gene predicts baseline psychological well-being and response to combination thyroxine plus triiodothyronine therapy in hypothyroid patients. *J Clin Endocrinol Metab*. 2009;94(5):1623–1629.

52. Nakahara R, Tsunekawa K, Yabe S, et al. Association of antipituitary antibody and type 2 iodothyronine deiodinase antibody in patients with autoimmune thyroid disease. *Endocr J*. 2005;52(6):691–699.

53. Pepper, Gary, Casanova-Romero P. Conversion to Armour thyroid from levothyroxine improved patient satisfaction in the treatment of hypothyroidism. *J Endocrinol Diabetes Obes*. 2014;2(3):1055-.

54. Hoang TD, Olsen CH, Mai VQ, Clyde PW, Shakir MKM. Desiccated thyroid extract compared with levothyroxine in the treatment of hypothyroidism: A randomized, double-blind, crossover study. *J Clin Endocrinol Metab*. 2013;98(5):1982–1990.

55. McAninch EA, Bianco AC. New insights into the variable effectiveness of levothyroxine monotherapy for hypothyroidism. *Lancet Diabetes Endocrinol*. 2015;3(10):756–758.

56. Panikar VK, Joshi SR, Kakraniya P, Nasikkar N, Santavana C. Inter-generation comparison of type-2 diabetes in 73 Indian families. *J Assoc Physicians India*. 2008;56:601–604.

57. Preston S, Fishman E, Stokes A. Lifetime probability of developing diabetes in the United States. 14-4. *PSC Work Pap Ser WPS*. 2014;14(4).

58. Selvin E, Parrinello CM, Daya N, Bergenstal RM. Trends in insulin use and diabetes control in the U.S.: 1988-1994 and 1999-2012. *Diabetes Care*. 2016;39(3):e33–e35.

59. ACCORD Group. Effects of intensive glucose lowering in type 2 diabetes. *N Engl J Med*. 2008;358(24):2545–2559.

60. Cordain L, Eades MR, Eades MD. Hyperinsulinemic diseases of civilization: More than just Syndrome X. *Comp Biochem Physiol A Mol Integr Physiol*. 2003;136(1):95–112.

61. Tan ZS, Beiser AS, Fox CS, et al. Association of metabolic dysregulation with volumetric brain magnetic resonance imaging and cognitive markers of subclinical brain aging in middle-aged adults: The Framingham Offspring Study. *Diabetes Care*. 2011;34(8):1766–1770.

62. Willette AA, Xu G, Johnson SC, et al. Insulin resistance, brain atrophy, and cognitive performance in late middle-aged adults. *Diabetes Care*. 2013;36(2):443–449.

63. Papanas N, Vinik AI, Ziegler D. Neuropathy in prediabetes: Does the clock start ticking early? *Nat Rev Endocrinol*. 2011;7(11):682–690.

64. De Cosmo S, Menzaghi C, Prudente S, Trischitta V. Role of insulin resistance in kidney dysfunction: Insights into the mechanism and epidemiological evidence. *Nephrol Dial Transplant*. 2013;28(1):29–36.

65. Davidson MB, Kahn RA. A reappraisal of prediabetes. *J Clin Endocrinol Metab*. 2016;101(7):2628–2635.

66. DeFronzo RA. From the triumvirate to the ominous octet: A new paradigm for the treatment of type 2 diabetes mellitus. *Diabetes*. 2009;58(4):773–795.

67. Taylor R. Type 2 diabetes: Reversibility and etiology. *Diabetes Care*. 2013;36(4):1047–1055.

68. Shulman GI. Ectopic fat in insulin resistance, dyslipidemia, and cardiometabolic disease. *N Engl J Med*. 2014;371(12):1131–1141.

69. Steven S, Hollingsworth KG, Small PK, et al. Weight loss decreases excess pancreatic triacylglycerol specifically in type 2 diabetes. *Diabetes Care*. 2016;39(1):158–165.

70. Cartee GD. Mechanisms for greater insulin-stimulated glucose uptake in normal and insulin-resistant skeletal muscle after acute exercise. *Am J Physiol Endocrinol Metab*. 2015;309(12):E949–E959.

71. Macauley M, Smith FE, Thelwall PE, Hollingsworth KG, Taylor R. Diurnal variation in skeletal muscle and liver glycogen in humans with normal health and type 2 diabetes. *Clin Sci*. 2015;128(10):707–713.

72. Fonseca VA. Defining and characterizing the progression of type 2 diabetes. *Diabetes Care*. 2009;32(Suppl 2):S151–S156.

73. Gayoso-Diz P, Otero-González A, Rodriguez-Alvarez MX, et al. Insulin resistance (HOMA-IR) cut-off values and the metabolic syndrome in a general adult population: Effect of gender and age: EPIRCE cross-sectional study. *BMC Endocr Disord*. 2013;13:47.

74. Abbasi F, Okeke Q, Reaven GM. Evaluation of fasting plasma insulin concentration as an estimate of insulin action in nondiabetic individuals: Comparison with the homeostasis model assessment of insulin resistance (HOMA-IR). *Acta Diabetol*. 2014;51(2):193–197.

75. Li S, Shin HJ, Ding EL, van Dam RM. Adiponectin levels and risk of type 2 diabetes: A systematic review and meta-analysis. *JAMA*. 2009;302(2):179–188.

76. Ibarra-Reynoso L del R, Pisarchyk L, Pérez-Luque EL, Garay-Sevilla ME, Malacara JM. Whole-body and hepatic insulin resistance in obese children. *PloS One*. 2014;9(11):e113576.

77. Hirshberg B, Katz A. Insights from cardiovascular outcome trials with novel antidiabetes agents: What have we learned? An industry perspective. *Curr Diab Rep*. 2015;15(11):87.

78. Orchard TJ, Temprosa M, Goldberg R, et al. The effect of metformin and intensive lifestyle intervention on the metabolic syndrome: The Diabetes Prevention Program randomized trial. *Ann Intern Med*. 2005;142(8):611–619.

79. Ottum MS, Mistry AM. Advanced glycation end-products: Modifiable environmental factors profoundly mediate insulin resistance. *J Clin Biochem Nutr*. 2015;57(1):1–12.

80. Vlassara H, Striker GE. Advanced glycation endproducts in diabetes and diabetic complications. *Endocrinol Metab Clin North Am*. 2013;42(4):697–719.

81. Gore AC, Chappell VA, Fenton SE, et al. EDC-2: The Endocrine Society's Second Scientific Statement on Endocrine-Disrupting Chemicals. *Endocr Rev*. 2015;36(6):E1–E150.

82. Feinman RD, Pogozelski WK, Astrup A, et al. Dietary carbohydrate restriction as the first approach in diabetes management: Critical review and evidence base. *Nutr Burbank Los Angel Cty Calif*. 2015;31(1):1–13.

83. Barnard RJ, Massey MR, Cherny S, O'Brien LT, Pritikin N. Long-term use of a high-complex-carbohydrate, high-fiber, low-fat diet and exercise in the treatment of NIDDM patients. *Diabetes Care*. 1983;6(3):268–273.

84. Jackness C, Karmally W, Febres G, et al. Very low-calorie diet mimics the early beneficial effect of Roux-en-Y gastric bypass on insulin sensitivity and β-cell function in type 2 diabetic patients. *Diabetes*. 2013;62(9):3027–3032.

85. Donga E, van Dijk M, van Dijk JG, et al. A single night of partial sleep deprivation induces insulin resistance in multiple metabolic pathways in healthy subjects. *J Clin Endocrinol Metab*. 2010;95(6):2963–2968.

86. Lan J, Zhao Y, Dong F, et al. Meta-analysis of the effect and safety of berberine in the treatment of type 2 diabetes mellitus, hyperlipemia and hypertension. *J Ethnopharmacol*. 2015;161:69–81.

87. Shane-McWhorter L. Dietary supplements for diabetes are decidedly popular: Help your patients decide. *Diabetes Spectr*. 2013;26(4):259–266.

88. Kasińska MA, Drzewoski J. Effectiveness of probiotics in type 2 diabetes: A meta-analysis. *Pol Arch Med Wewn*. 2015;125(11):803–813.

89. Tiwari P, Ahmad K, Baig MH. *Gymnema sylvestre* for diabetes: From traditional herb to future's therapeutic. *Curr Pharm Des*. 2017;23(11):1667–1676.

90. Askari F, Rashidkhani B, Hekmatdoost A. Cinnamon may have therapeutic benefits on lipid profile, liver enzymes, insulin resistance, and high-sensitivity C-reactive protein in nonalcoholic fatty liver disease patients. *Nutr Res N Y N*. 2014;34(2):143–148.

91. Vidal-Casariego A, Burgos-Peláez R, Martínez-Faedo C, et al. Metabolic effects of L-carnitine on type 2 diabetes mellitus: Systematic review and meta-analysis. *Exp Clin Endocrinol Diabetes.* 2013;121(4):234–238.

92. Simental-Mendía LE, Sahebkar A, Rodríguez-Morán M, Guerrero-Romero F. A systematic review and meta-analysis of randomized controlled trials on the effects of magnesium supplementation on insulin sensitivity and glucose control. *Pharmacol Res.* 2016;111:272–282.

93. Suksomboon N, Poolsup N, Yuwanakorn A. Systematic review and meta-analysis of the efficacy and safety of chromium supplementation in diabetes. *J Clin Pharm Ther.* 2014;39(3):292–306.

94. Dick WR, Fletcher EA, Shah SA. Reduction of fasting blood glucose and hemoglobin A1c using oral aloe vera: A meta-analysis. *J Altern Complement Med N Y N.* 2016;22(6):450–457.

95. Rahimi HR, Mohammadpour AH, Dastani M, et al. The effect of nano-curcumin on HbA1c, fasting blood glucose, and lipid profile in diabetic subjects: A randomized clinical trial. *Avicenna J Phytomedicine.* 2016;6(5):567–577.

96. Griffling GT. Addison Disease. Emedicine Medscape. http://emedicine.medscape.com/article/116467. Updated Mar 23 2017.

97. Guilliams T. *The Role of Stress and the HPA Axis in Chronic Disease Management.* Point Institute; 2015.

98. Tirabassi G, Boscaro M, Arnaldi G. Harmful effects of functional hypercortisolism: A working hypothesis. *Endocrine.* 2014;46(3):370–386.

99. Silverman MN, Sternberg EM. Glucocorticoid regulation of inflammation and its functional correlates: From HPA axis to glucocorticoid receptor dysfunction. *Ann N Y Acad Sci.* 2012;1261:55–63.

100. McEwen BS, Gianaros PJ. Stress- and allostasis-induced brain plasticity. *Annu Rev Med.* 2011;62:431–445.

101. McEwen BS. Brain on stress: How the social environment gets under the skin. *Proc Natl Acad Sci.* 2012;109(Suppl 2):17180–17185.

102. McEwen BS, Bowles NP, Gray JD, et al. Mechanisms of stress in the brain. *Nat Neurosci.* 2015;18(10):1353–1363.

103. Ulrich-Lai YM, Herman JP. Neural regulation of endocrine and autonomic stress responses. *Nat Rev Neurosci.* 2009;10(6):397–409.

104. Kroenke K, Mangelsdorff AD. Common symptoms in ambulatory care: Incidence, evaluation, therapy, and outcome. *Am J Med.* 1989;86(3):262–266.

105. Edwards TM, Stern A, Clarke DD, Ivbijaro G, Kasney LM. The treatment of patients with medically unexplained symptoms in primary care: A review of the literature. *Ment Health Fam Med.* 2010;7(4):209–221.

106. McCraty R, Barrios-Choplin B, Rozman D, Atkinson M, Watkins AD. The impact of a new emotional self-management program on stress, emotions, heart rate variability, DHEA and cortisol. *Integr Physiol Behav Sci.* 1998;33(2):151–170.

107. Christianson NA, Perkins T, Audio T. *The Adrenal Reset Diet: Strategically Cycle Carbs and Proteins to Lose Weight, Balance Hormones, and Move From Stressed to Thriving.* Tantor Audio.

108. Wang S-M, Han C, Lee S-J, Patkar AA, Masand PS, Pae C-U. A review of current evidence for acetyl-L-carnitine in the treatment of depression. *J Psychiatr Res.* 2014;53:30–37.

109. Lopresti AL, Hood SD, Drummond PD. Multiple antidepressant potential modes of action of curcumin: A review of its anti-inflammatory, monoaminergic, antioxidant, immune-modulating and neuroprotective effects. *J Psychopharmacol.* 2012;26(12):1512–1524.

15

Osteoporosis

ANGELA J. SHEPHERD AND JULIET M. MCKEE

Epidemiology

Osteoporosis is a leading cause of mortality and morbidity worldwide. Women are affected more than men by 4:1 ratio.[1] Women and men who have osteoporosis experience hip fractures at a similar rate.[2] Men account for 30% of hip fractures and have worse in-hospital (2:1) and 1-year mortality rates (31% vs. 17%) after fracture than women.[3,4]

Pathophysiology

Peak bone mass is achieved during young adulthood and then is maintained by remodeling. Remodeling involves osteoblasts, which make bone, and osteoclasts, which break down bone. This remodeling is not completely effective, so adulthood is accompanied by a very slow decline in bone mass (loss of 0.7% per year). Men and women are affected equally by this age-related loss, and Caucasians are affected more than other race/ethnicities. In addition to age-related, low-turnover bone loss, women at menopause experience a high-turnover bone loss caused by estrogen deficiency. Interleukin-1 and interleukin-6 and tumor necrosis factor (TNF-α) are stimulators for osteoclastic activity, which outpaces the compensatory osteoblastic activity. This rapid-bone-loss phase may last 10 years and results in women experiencing osteoporotic fractures about a decade earlier than men.[5]

There are number of medications associated with increased bone loss. These are summarized in Table 15.1.

Table 15.1. Medications That Can Cause Bone Loss

Drug	Dosage/Duration	Comments
Glucocorticoids	7.5 mg/day orally for at least 3 months in 1 year	Creams and inhaled steroids implicated
Aromatase inhibitors (used in breast cancer therapy)	1–2 years	
Androgen deprivation therapy (used in prostate cancer therapy)	1 year	
Proton-pump inhibitors	Several years	May be related to decreased calcium absorption in stomach
Depo-Provera	Several years	Reversible upon discontinuation
Excess thyroid hormone replacement	Years	
Antiseizure and antidepressant medications (carbamazepine, phenytoin, selective serotonin reuptake inhibitors)	Years	
Diuretics (furosemide)		
Thiazolidinediones (used in diabetes mellitus treatment)	>4 years	
Antirejection/ immunosuppressive therapy (cyclosporine, tacrolimus; used after organ transplantation)		

From reference 6.

Testing and Diagnosis

FRAX (the World Health Organization's fracture risk assessment tool) is designed to be usable worldwide to assess future fracture risk in order to determine when it is appropriate to get a bone density test or begin treatment of osteoporosis. It estimates the 10-year risk of fracture based on age, sex, weight, height, previous fracture or parental fracture, current smoking, glucocorticoids, rheumatoid arthritis, secondary osteoporosis, alcohol (3+ units/day), and current bone mineral density if available. It is not necessary for patients who are already receiving treatment or who obviously need treatment due to history. It does not assess fall risk. It is available by computer calculation or by a printed "wheel" in areas of the world where computers are not feasible.[6]

Dual-energy x-ray absorptiometry (DEXA) is the standard of care for the diagnosis of osteoporosis (T-score ≤ –2.5). The U.S. Preventive Services Task Force (USPSTF) recommends screening with DEXA for all women age 65 years and up and for younger women who have a 10-year risk of 9.3% or more when calculated by the FRAX.[7]

Lifestyle

PHYSICAL ACTIVITY

There is agreement that regular weight-bearing and muscle-strengthening exercise is helpful to prevent falls and improve bone density.[8] Examples of weight-bearing activities include walking, jogging, dancing, housework, and tai chi. Examples of muscle-strengthening exercises include weight training, gardening, yoga, and Pilates. A meta-analysis of 18 studies evaluating the effect of exercise in postmenopausal women showed that walking increases bone mineral density at the hip, and aerobic, weight-bearing, and resistance exercises improved bone density at the spine. An interesting study evaluating serum trace mineral levels in response to aerobic activity found that aerobic activity was related to increased levels of calcium and manganese and decreased levels of copper and zinc. The researchers hypothesized that aerobic activity improves bone mineral density by regulating trace minerals.[9] Just 12 minutes of yoga daily can reverse osteoporotic bone loss.[10] A randomized controlled trial of women over 65 who were enrolled in a fitness program versus a control wellness program showed an improvement in bone density of the spine and femoral neck, decreased falls, and decreased overall need for health care.[11] In a 10-year prospective study, stronger back muscles were shown to reduce the risk of vertebral compression fractures.[12] Fall prevention is key to reducing fractures, and tai chi, a home safety evaluation, and gait evaluation/ training are good ways to help patients prevent falls.[13] Use of low-frequency vibratory plates has been shown in a randomized control trial to be effective in reducing the risk of fracture.[14] Plates for whole-body vibration are available commercially and can also be found in fitness facilities.

NUTRITION

Epidemiological studies have long noted differences in the incidence of osteoporosis based on nationality. These differences have been thought to be due to physical activity and diet.[13] A robust, long-term, observational study of dietary patterns in over 90,000 women ages 50 to 79 showed that following a Mediterranean diet was associated with decreased hip fractures. The Mediterranean diet includes plenty of vegetables, fruit, fish, nuts, whole grains, legumes, and monounsaturated fats such as olive oil and limited amounts of red and processed meats.

In the past, high intake of animal protein was thought to be associated with increased fracture rates and decreased bone density.[15,16] However, more recent data suggest that this effect is more likely to be due to inadequate calcium intake.[17,18] Diets rich in vegetables and fruit have been associated with increased peak bone mass and improved bone health in older patients.[19] The anti-inflammatory properties of the Mediterranean diet and other diets rich in vegetables and fruit and low in processed foods may account for the improvement in bone health with these diets.[20,21]

Consumption of soy from the diet and with supplements has been associated with increased bone density.[22,23] A pilot study comparing calcium bicarbonate supplementation with kefir (a fermented milk drink) showed short-term positive changes in bone-turnover markers such as serum osteocalcin and serum parathyroid hormone as well as increased bone mineral density as measured by DEXA.[24] Increased intake of fish was associated with a decreased risk of osteoporosis in Chinese women.[25] Another study found a lower incidence of osteoporosis in patients who had higher levels of monounsaturated fatty acids in their erythrocytes.[26] In aggregate, these studies suggest that eating a diet rich in vegetables, fruit, nuts, fish, and probiotics has a positive effect on bone density.

SUBSTANCE USE

Tobacco directly increases the risk for fracture in both men and women. After adjustments for bone density, body mass index (BMI), and age, current smokers' risk of hip fracture was 55% higher than that of non-smokers. A history of smoking was also associated with a higher risk of fracture, although the risk for former smokers was not as high as for current smokers.[13] The U.S. Surgeon General reported that smoking increased risk for both men and women.[27] For women, smoking cigarettes is an established risk factor for early menopause, which may contribute additional fracture risk for female smokers.[28]

Alcoholism is known to have negative effects on bone,[29] and heavy drinking is likely related to an increased risk of home-based falls.[30] Moderate alcohol use in women (two or less drinks/day) has been associated with higher bone density in some studies,[31,32] but it does not seem to lower fracture risk.[33,34] In summary, drinking less than two alcohol-containing beverages per day appears to cause no harm.

SUPPLEMENTS

Calcium is essential for healthy bones. When making recommendations about calcium supplementation, it is important to consider dietary calcium intake from both dairy and non-dairy sources. The Institute of Medicine has made recommendations on supplementation based on average intake for people over 50 (Table 15.2).[35]

Vitamin D is essential for calcium absorption and may also help to prevent falls in elderly patients by improving skeletal muscles and increasing strength and balance (see Table 15.2).[36] In an epidemiological multinational study, more than half of postmenopausal women with osteoporosis were found to have low serum vitamin D concentrations (<30 ng/mL).[37] Supplementation with 800 IU vitamin D is associated with a lower fracture risk.[38] Many recommend that supplementation of vitamin D be determined by serum levels and that different patients may require different amounts of supplementation to maintain appropriate serum levels (>30 ng/ml).

Adequate vitamin K intake is important for bone health. There are different forms of vitamin K. Vitamin K1 is available from food sources such as green leafy vegetables. Women who ate at least one serving of lettuce daily were found to have a 0.55 relative risk for hip fracture.[39] Vitamin K2 is not available from food sources and is mostly formed by gut flora. There are several forms of vitamin K2 and there has been recent interest in evaluating the efficacy of supplementing with vitamin K2. The most common forms are menoquinone 4 (MK4) and menoquinone 7 (MK7). Low-dose MK7 supplementation was found to improve osteocalcin carboxylation, but this study did not evaluate clinical outcomes.[40] One review evaluated the effect of vitamin K on bone metabolism and determined that the evidence supports supplementing 45 mg of MK4 for all postmenopausal women with osteoporosis.[41]

Vitamin C is essential for collagen formation; there are few studies, but some small epidemiological studies indicate that vitamin C intake and/or supplementation may be associated with improved bone density and decreased bone resorption.[42] It was previously thought that excess vitamin A intake was associated with an increased risk of hip fracture.[39] However, a more recent study of over 2,000 people who took large doses (25,000 IU/day) for several years showed no increased risk of fracture.[43]

Table 15.2. Dietary Reference Intakes for Calcium and Vitamin D

Age	Calcium and Vitamin D					
	Estimated Average Requirement (mg/day)	Recommended Dietary Allowance (mg/day)	Upper Level Intake (mg/day)	Estimated Average Requirement (IU/day)	Recommended Dietary Allowance (IU/day)	Upper Level Intake (IU/day)
51- to 70-year-old males	800	1,000	2,000	400	600	4,000
51- to 70-year-old females	1,000	1,200	2,000	400	600	4,000
>70 years old	1,000	1,200	2,000	400	800	4,000

Trace minerals are important for bone health. A study comparing concentrations of trace minerals in bone from patients with osteoporosis to patients with osteoarthritis found significantly decreased levels of Ca, Mg, and Zn in patients with osteoporosis.[9] Low serum levels of Cu, Zn, Fe, and Mg were associated with increased osteoporosis. The same study of 728 postmenopausal women found that serum levels of calcium, potassium, sodium, and phosphorus were not associated with decreased bone density.[44] A review of the literature reported that bone density is improved by Zn, Cu, Fl, Mg, Mn, Fe, and B and that deficiency of these elements can accelerate bone loss in elderly patients.[45]

BOTANICALS

Tea has many beneficial properties, including anti-inflammatory effects, and unlike coffee, it was not found to have an adverse effect on bones.[46] While compliance with the regimen may be a factor, one study did find that consumption of one cup of onion juice daily improved bone density.[47] Other botanicals that have been implicated in bone health include black cohosh, *Astragalus membranaceus*, walnut extract, and curcumin. However, data are limited and more research is needed to determine the optimal role of botanicals for bone health.

PRESCRIPTION MEDICATIONS

Pharmacological treatment should be considered for postmenopausal women and men 50 years of age and older if they are found to have the following:

1. Hip or vertebral fracture and osteopenic or osteoporotic range on bone density scan
2. T-score of –2.5 or less at hip or spine
3. T-score between –1 and –2.5 plus 10-year probability of hip fracture of at least 3% or 10-year probability of a major osteoporosis-related fracture of at least 20% based on ultrasound-based World Health Organization algorithm[13]

Table 15.3 lists drugs for osteoporosis that have been approved by the U.S. Food and Drug Administration.[48]

Table 15.3. Drugs Approved by U.S. Food and Drug Administration for the Treatment of Osteoporosis

Drug	Men	Women	Duration of Treatment (Years)
1. Aledronate	X		3–5
2. Risedronate	X		3–5
3. Ibandronate		X	3–5
4. Zoledronic acid	X		
5. Estrogen/hormone replacement therapy (HRT)			≤5
6. Raloxifene		X	
7. Tissue selective estrogen complex conjugated estrogen/bazedoxifene		X	No data
8. Teriparatide	X		1.5–2
9. Deonsumab	X		
10. Salmon calcitionin*		X	

* long term intake may increase risk of certain cancers.

Summary

1. Dietary interventions such as the Mediterranean diet and an anti-inflammatory diet help to improve bone density.
2. Exercise is key to improving bone health. Incorporation of weight-bearing exercise, muscle-strengthening exercise, and balance training help improve bone density and reduce the risk of fractures.
3. Fall prevention is accomplished by muscle strengthening, balance training, and maintaining a safe environment.
4. Avoid tobacco smoking and heavy drinking.
5. Supplement with at least 800 IU vitamin D3 daily—more if necessary to keep serum levels above 30 ng/mL.
6. Supplement with calcium citrate if dietary calcium intake is less than 1,000 mg.
7. Adequate intake of vitamins K and C is important to maintain bone mineral density.
8. More research is necessary to determine if botanicals can be of use clinically to improve bone mineral density.

REFERENCES

1. Yoon PW, Scheuner MT, Peterson-Oehlke KL, Gwinn M, Faucett A, Khoury MJ. Can family history be used as a tool for public health and preventive medicine? *Genet Med.* 2002;4(4):304–310.

2. Kanis JA, Oden A, Johnell O, Jonsson B, De Laet C, Dawson A. The burden of osteoporotic fractures: a method for setting intervention thresholds. *Osteoporosis International.* 2001;12(5):417–427.

3. Center JR, Nguyen TV, Schneider D, Sambrook PN, Eisman JA. Mortality after all major types of osteoporotic fracture in men and women: an observational study. *Lancet.* 1999;353(9156):878–882.

4. Forsen L, Søgaard AJ, Meyer HE, Edna TH, Kopjar B. Survival after hip fracture: short-and long-term excess mortality according to age and gender. *Osteoporosis International.* 1999;10(1):73–78.

5. Cosman F, de Beur SJ, LeBoff MS, et al. Clinician's guide to prevention and treatment of osteoporosis. *Osteoporosis International.* 2014;25(10):2359–2381.

6. Kanis JA, Hans D, Cooper C, et al. Interpretation and use of FRAX in clinical practice. *Osteoporosis International.* 2011;22(9):2395–2411.

7. Welcome to FRAX. 2016; http://www.shef.ac.uk/FRAX/.

8. Feskanich D, Willett W, Colditz G. Walking and leisure-time activity and risk of hip fracture in postmenopausal women. *JAMA.* 2002;288(18):2300–2306.

9. Karaaslan F, Mutlu M, Mermerkaya MU, Karaoğlu S, Saçmaci Ş, Kartal Ş. Comparison of bone tissue trace-element concentrations and mineral density in osteoporotic femoral neck fractures and osteoarthritis. *Clinical Interventions in Aging.* 2014;9:1375.

10. Lu Y-H, Rosner B, Chang G, Fishman LM. Twelve-minute daily yoga regimen reverses osteoporotic bone loss. *Topics in Geriatric Rehabilitation.* 2016; 32(2):81.

11. Kemmler W, von Stengel S, Engelke K, Häberle L, Kalender WA. Exercise effects on bone mineral density, falls, coronary risk factors, and health care costs in older women: The randomized controlled Senior Fitness and Prevention (SEFIP) study. *Arch Intern Med.* 2010;170(2):179–185.

12. Sinaki M, Itoi E, Wahner H, et al. Stronger back muscles reduce the incidence of vertebral fractures: A prospective 10-year follow-up of postmenopausal women. *Bone.* 2002;30(6):836–841.

13. Cosman F, De Beur S, LeBoff M, et al. Clinician's guide to prevention and treatment of osteoporosis. *Osteoporosis International.* 2014;25(10):2359–2381.

14. Gusi N, Raimundo A, Leal A. Low-frequency vibratory exercise reduces the risk of bone fracture more than walking: A randomized controlled trial. *BMC Musculoskeletal Disorders.* 2006;7(1):1.

15. Feskanich D, Willett WC, Stampfer MJ, Colditz GA. Protein consumption and bone fractures in women. *Am J Epidemiol.* 1996;143(5):472–479.

16. Weikert C, Walter D, Hoffmann K, Kroke A, Bergmann MM, Boeing H. The relation between dietary protein, calcium and bone health in women: Results from the EPIC-Potsdam cohort. *Annals of Nutrition and Metabolism.* 2005;49(5):312–318.

17. Calvez J, Poupin N, Chesneau C, Lassale C, Tomé D. Protein intake, calcium balance and health consequences. *Eur J Clinical Nutr.* 2012;66(3):281–295.

18. Misra D, Berry S, Broe K, et al. Does dietary protein reduce hip fracture risk in elders? The Framingham osteoporosis study. *Osteoporosis International.* 2011;22(1):345–349.

19. Lanham-New SA. Fruit and vegetables: The unexpected natural answer to the question of osteoporosis prevention? *Am J Clin Nutr.* 2006;83(6):1254–1255.

20. Ginaldi L, Di Benedetto MC, De Martinis M. Osteoporosis, inflammation and ageing. *Immunity & Ageing.* 2005;2(1):14.

21. Straub RH, Cutolo M, Pacifici R. Evolutionary medicine and bone loss in chronic inflammatory diseases—A theory of inflammation-related osteopenia. Paper presented at Seminars in Arthritis and Rheumatism, 2015.

22. Zhang X, Shu X-O, Li H, et al. Prospective cohort study of soy food consumption and risk of bone fracture among postmenopausal women. *Arch Intern Med.* 2005;165(16):1890–1895.

23. Wei P, Liu M, Chen Y, Chen D-C. Systematic review of soy isoflavone supplements on osteoporosis in women. *Asian Pacific J Tropical Med.* 2012;5(3):243–248.

24. Tu M-Y, Chen H-L, Tung Y-T, Kao C-C, Hu F-C, Chen C-M. Short-term effects of kefir-fermented milk consumption on bone mineral density and bone metabolism in a randomized clinical trial of osteoporotic patients. *PloS One.* 2015;10(12):e0144231.

25. Chen Y-m, Ho S, Lam S. Higher sea fish intake is associated with greater bone mass and lower osteoporosis risk in postmenopausal Chinese women. *Osteoporosis International.* 2010;21(6):939–946.

26. Moon H-J, Kim T-H, Byun D-W, Park Y. Positive correlation between erythrocyte levels of omega-3 polyunsaturated fatty acids and bone mass in postmenopausal Korean women with osteoporosis. *Ann Nutr Metab.* 2012;60(2):146–153.

27. Kanis JA, Johnell O, Oden A, et al. Smoking and fracture risk: A meta-analysis. *Osteoporosis International.* 2005;16(2):155–162.

28. Kim KH, Lee CM, Park SM, et al. Secondhand smoke exposure and osteoporosis in never-smoking postmenopausal women: The Fourth Korea National Health and Nutrition Examination Survey. *Osteoporosis International.* 2013;24(2):523–532.

29. Schapira D. Alcohol abuse and osteoporosis. Paper presented at Seminars in Arthritis and Rheumatism, 1990.

30. *Bone Health and Osteoporosis: A Report of the Surgeon General.* Rockville, MD: Office of the Surgeon General; 2004.

31. Felson DT, Zhang Y, Hannan MT, Kannel WB, Kiel DP. Alcohol intake and bone mineral density in elderly men and women: The Framingham Study. *Am J Epidemiol.* 1995;142(5):485–492.

32. Sampson HW. Alcohol and other factors affecting osteoporosis risk in women. *Alcohol Research and Health.* 2002;26(4):292–298.

33. Cummings SR, Nevitt MC, Browner WS, et al. Risk factors for hip fracture in white women. *N Engl J Med.* 1995;332(12):767–774.

34. Høidrup S, Grønbæk M, Gottschau A, Lauritzen JB, Schroll M. Alcohol intake, beverage preference, and risk of hip fracture in men and women. *Am J Epidemiol.* 1999;149(11):993–1001.

35. Institute of Medicine. DRI's for Calcium and Vitamin D. 2010; https://www. nationalacademies.org/hmd/Reports/2010/Dietary-Reference-Intakes-for-Calcium-and-Vitamin-D/DRI-Values.aspx. Accessed December 2016.

36. Shuler M, Franklin D, Schlierf T, Wingate M. Preventing falls with vitamin D. *W V Med J.* 2014 May-Jun;110(3):10–12.

37. Lips P, Hosking D, Lippuner K, et al. The prevalence of vitamin D inadequacy amongst women with osteoporosis: An international epidemiological investigation. *J Intern Med.* 2006;260(3):245–254.

38. Bischoff-Ferrari HA. Optimal serum 25-hydroxyvitamin D levels for multiple health outcomes. In: *Sunlight, Vitamin D and Skin Cancer.* Springer; 2014:500–525.

39. Feskanich D, Weber P, Willett WC, Rockett H, Booth SL, Colditz GA. Vitamin K intake and hip fractures in women: A prospective study. *Am J Clin Nutr.* 1999;69(1):74–79.

40. Inaba N, Sato T, Yamashita T. Low-dose daily intake of vitamin K2 (menaquinone-7) improves osteocalcin γ-carboxylation: A double-blind, randomized controlled trial. *J Nutr Sci Vitaminol.* 2015;61(6):471–480.

41. Villa JKD, Diaz MAN, Pizziolo VR, Martino HSD. Effect of vitamin K in bone metabolism and vascular calcification: A review of mechanisms of action and evidences. *Crit Rev Food Sci Nutrition.* 2016; doi:10.1080/10408398.2016.1211616.

42. Aghajanian P, Hall S, Wongworawat MD, Mohan S. The roles and mechanisms of actions of vitamin C in bone: New developments. *J Bone Mineral Res.* 2015;30(11):1945–1955.

43. Ambrosini G, Bremner A, Reid A, et al. No dose-dependent increase in fracture risk after long-term exposure to high doses of retinol or beta-carotene. *Osteoporosis Int.* 2013;24(4):1285–1293.

44. Okyay E, Ertugrul C, Acar B, Sisman AR, Onvural B, Ozaksoy D. Comparative evaluation of serum levels of main minerals and postmenopausal osteoporosis. *Maturitas.* 2013;76(4):320–325.

45. Zofková I, Nemcikova P, Matucha P. Trace elements and bone health. *Clin Chem Lab Med.* 2013;51(8):1555–1561.

46. Chen Z, Pettinger M, Ritenbaugh C, et al. Habitual tea consumption and risk of osteoporosis: A prospective study in the Women's Health Initiative observational cohort. *Am J Epidemiol.* 2003;158(8):772–781.

47. Law Y-Y, Chiu H-F, Lee H-H, Shen Y-C, Venkatakrishnan K, Wang C-K. Consumption of onion juice modulates oxidative stress and attenuates the risk of bone disorders in middle-aged and post-menopausal healthy subjects. *Food & Function.* 2016;7(2):902–912.

48. Sanders S, Geraci SA. Osteoporosis in postmenopausal women: Considerations in prevention and treatment. *South Med J.* 2013;106(12):698–706.

16

The Healthy Gut in Older Adults

VICTOR SIERPINA, KAREN WELCH, DIMPLE DESAI,
AND ANNA ROTKIEWICZ

Case Study

A 72-year-old woman presents with complaints of episodic lower abdominal pain accompanied by cramping and occasional gas. She reports infrequent bowel movements in the past 2 or 3 years, occasional blood on tissue paper after a hard stool, but no other symptoms such as weight loss. A colonoscopy last year was clear of pathology except for some moderate sigmoid diverticulosis and internal hemorrhoids. Past medical history includes treatment for hypertension with an angiotensin-converting enzyme inhibitor, osteoarthritis treated with a nonsteroidal anti-inflammatory, and stress incontinence treated with tolterodine and Kegel exercises. She has had several urinary tract infections treated with quinolones. Past surgical history includes hysterectomy and bilateral oophorectomy, appendectomy as a child, and a negative thyroid nodule biopsy. She is up to date on all immunizations and screening examinations.

Examination shows a well-developed female looking appropriate for stated age and in no distress. Findings are as follows:

- HEENT: normal including dentition.
- No carotid bruit
- Thyroid with several sub-centimeter nodules in each lobe
- Lungs are clear.
- Heart sounds RRR, no M/G/R
- Abdomen without masses, guarding rigidity, or tenderness. Normal bowel sounds.

- Pelvic exam shows moderate atrophic mucosal changes.
- Metabolic panel including liver functions, TSH, CBC, and UA are normal.

What are the best next recommendations?

Introduction

Gastrointestinal issues are among the most common problems in any primary care practice. These are increasingly prevalent with older adults, who present a unique set of issues related to the aging gut. An integrative physician attends to these issues by avoiding polypharmacy, reducing overuse of invasive procedures, and supporting quality of life. This chapter describes a variety of approaches that include functional medicine, lifestyle, mind–body, bioenergetics, botanical, herbal, and other measures to improve gut health.

Pathophysiology

Aging affects the gut from stem to stern.[1,2] In the mouth, gingivitis, poor dentition, decreased saliva formation, and appetite changes affect nutritional intake, inflammation, and appetite. Further downstream, esophageal and gastric motility, reflux, secretion of acid necessary for digestion, and gastric emptying are all affected by the aging process. These changes often result in the prescribing of medications such as proton-pump inhibitors (PPIs) that further reduce absorption of essential dietary components such as B12, vitamin D, calcium, and iron, and also alteration of gut microbiota.[3,4] Bisphosphonates, nonsteroidal anti-inflammatories (NSAIDs), and other medications frequently further alter esophageal and gastric function.[5] Hepatobiliary and pancreatic function may also decrease with age, affecting digestive and absorptive capacities as well as metabolism and clearance of drugs and toxins.[6] The slowing of motility may cause seemingly minor problems such as constipation or cause problems with abdominal pain, gas, diverticular disease, and hemorrhoids. Often this delay in gut transit time is due to decreased fluid intake, lowered fiber consumption, and loss of function in the myenteric plexus.[7]

The clinical challenges causes by these changes include sorting out serious and emergent problems such as ulcers, gastrointestinal bleeding, and colon cancer from benign and otherwise manageable conditions of the aging gut. Some specific physiological changes with gut aging are described in Figure 16.1.

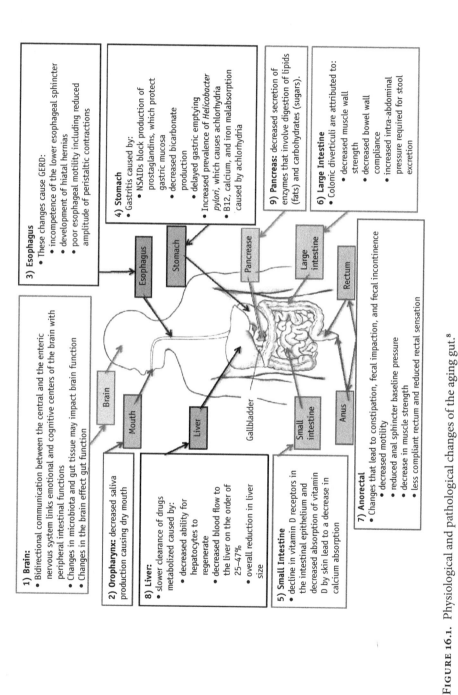

1) Brain:
- Bidirectional communication between the central and the enteric nervous system links emotional and cognitive centers of the brain with peripheral intestinal functions
- Changes in microbiota and gut tissue may impact brain function
- Changes in the brain effect gut function

2) Oropharynx: decreased saliva production causing dry mouth

8) Liver:
- slower clearance of drugs metabolized caused by:
  - decreased ability for hepatocytes to regenerate
  - decreased blood flow to the liver on the order of 25–47%
  - overall reduction in liver size

5) Small Intestine
- decline in vitamin D receptors in the intestinal epithelium and decreased absorption of vitamin D by skin lead to a decrease in calcium absorption

7) Anorectal
- Changes that lead to constipation, fecal impaction, and fecal incontinence
  - decreased motility
  - reduced anal sphincter baseline pressure
  - decrease in muscle strength
  - less compliant rectum and reduced rectal sensation

3) Esophagus
- These changes cause GERD:
  - incompetence of the lower esophageal sphincter
  - development of hiatal hernias
  - poor esophageal motility including reduced amplitude of peristaltic contractions

4) Stomach
- Gastritis caused by:
  - NSAIDs block production of prostaglandins, which protect gastric mucosa
  - decreased bicarbonate production
  - delayed gastric emptying
- Increased prevalence of *Helicobacter pylori*, which causes achlorhydria
- B12, calcium, and iron malabsorption caused by achlorhydria

9) Pancreas: decreased secretion of enzymes that involve digestion of lipids (fats) and carbohydrates (sugars).

6) Large Intestine
- Colonic diverticuli are attributed to:
  - decreased muscle wall strength
  - decreased bowel wall compliance
  - increased intra-abdominal pressure required for stool excretion

Brain

Mouth

Esophagus

Stomach

Pancrease

Liver

Gallbladder

Small intestine

Large intestine

Rectum

Anus

FIGURE 16.1. Physiological and pathological changes of the aging gut.[8]

Integrative Management

An integrative approach to the gastroenterological problems of the older adult is tempered by clinical reasoning and appreciation of well-evidenced standard-of-care approaches, and incorporates the broader range of considerations available to an integrative practitioner.

Some of these approaches are often not considered in standard gastrointestinal medical care. However, the advice of thoughtful clinicians that is available in popular and academic texts providing enormous information and practical clinical approaches is slowly percolating into conventional medical therapy.[9-14]

Functional Medicine and Gastrointestinal Health

A particular approach we have found highly useful in gastroenterological health is termed "functional medicine." This is an approach that goes beyond the "one disease, one drug" model to probe for underlying causes and to develop sustainable, effective treatments that are particularly useful in the aging gut. This approach is particularly useful in addressing patients with complex gastroenterological issues. Additional training and continuing medical education, including advanced training in functional gastroenterology, can be found at the Institute for Functional Medicine's website.[15]

Functional medicine is a systems biology approach arising from a foundational science basis in physiological mechanisms and biological processes. Its methodology helps assess, prevent, and treat complex chronic disorders by identifying core pathological processes and ameliorating dysfunction in the physiology and biochemistry. It recognizes that even with human genome mapping, the "one gene, one disease" model does not adequately explain all pathology. Interactions among lifestyle habits, nutrient insufficiencies, toxic exposures, psychosocial stressors, and single nucleotide polymorphisms (SNPs) help explain signs and symptoms of chronic diseases. This approach has led to the understanding that the epigenome is modifiable by our behavior and lifestyle, affecting protein expression in microbiome, nutrigenome, and metabolome.[16]

Systems biology–based medicine suggests that optimal nutrition is highly variable from person to person. Each patient has biochemical individuality, which has a major influence on individual need for nutrients as well as the clinical presentation of the nutrient insufficiency. Similar clinical presentations may include different underlying imbalances and triggers, and very different clinical presentation may share similar underlying pathogenic factors.

A tool for functional medicine evaluation of the patient's health is called the Functional Medicine Matrix. Functional medicine starts by considering antecedents, which are the elements from the past such as past medical history, mediators of current disorders, and trigger factors associated with appearance of current symptoms. It examines imbalances in the following areas:

1. *Assimilation and elimination*: digestion, absorption, microbiota, and respiration
2. *Biotransformation*: toxicity and detoxification
3. *Communication*: endocrine, neurotransmitter, and immune messengers and cognition
4. *Defense and repair*: immune system, inflammatory processes
5. *Energy*: energy regulation and mitochondrial dysfunction, oxidation–reduction imbalances
6. *Structural integrity*: from cellular membranes to the musculoskeletal system
7. *Transport*: cellular transport (of nutrients, hormones, cellular messengers), then lymphatic, microcirculation, and macrocirculation[17]

These are layered onto inquiry into mental, emotional, and spiritual factors. Additional information is sought regarding cognitive function, perceptual patterns, emotional regulation and resilience, history of psychological trauma, meaning and purpose in life, relationship to something greater than oneself, and current spiritual practices. Additionally, diet and hydration, sleep patterns and restoration techniques, relationships, exercise and movement, and financial status are all considered in this integrative and holistic approach.

Gastrointestinal function includes assimilation of food, digestion, absorption of nutrients and electrolytes, antigen–food interaction, and cross-talk between intestinal mucosa microbiota and epithelial-neuro-endocrine and immune cells. The first step in a functional medicine approach to any dysfunction is often gastrointestinal restoration. The model is a program started by Dr. Jeffrey Bland, today called the 5R Program: remove, replace, re-inoculate, repair and regenerate, rebalance and retain[18] (Table 16.1):

Table 16.1. The 5 Rs of Functional Medicine and Gut Health

Remove	Eliminate offending factors
Replace	Supply missing nutrients, micronutrients
Re-inoculate	Provide support for the microbiome
Repair and Regenerate	Help the gut to heal
Rebalance and Retain	Restore and support homeostasis

Remove: Evaluate for parasites, pathogenic bacteria, opportunistic organisms, overgrowth of yeast, toxins, food allergens and substances producing sensitivities and immune reactions starting with six most common (gluten [wheat], casein [milk], soy, egg, corn, yeast) and other frequent allergens such as peanuts and shellfish as well as moldy foods. Medications that damage the gastrointestinal tract (e.g., NSAIDs) need to be reviewed and possibly stopped and other techniques of pain control introduced.

Replace: Evaluate for decreased hydrochloric acid, digestive enzymes, and bile acids; if needed, replace any that are deficient.

Reinoculate: Add probiotics and prebiotics—*Lactobacillus acidophilus*, *Bifidobacterium lactis*, and *Streptococcus thermophilus* as well as *Lactobacillus rhamnosus* and many times *Saccharomyces boulardii*. Many fermented foods that are natural sources of these, such as yogurt, do not contain much diversity in species and have relatively low colony counts, so a therapeutic dose may require powdered or encapsulated delivery forms.

Repair and regenerate: Will include healing of the intestinal mucosal barrier. The intercellular tight junction is a multi-protein network where zonulin is a key physiological modulator of its integrity and is a biomarker of impaired gut barrier function. Antigens like gliadin from wheat gluten, in genetically predisposed individuals, can trigger opening of the epithelial T-junction through zonulin release for a much longer time than normal.[19]

Rebalance and Retain: Stress and psychological trauma play major roles in the function of the gastrointestinal tract. The gut–heart–brain axis needs to be healed through appropriate diet, exercise, restful sleep, stress management, and treatment of trauma. Dysregulation of the brain–gut axis increases intestinal permeability, visceral sensitivity, and alteration in gastrointestinal motility and leads to profound mast-cell activation, resulting in the release of many pro-inflammatory mediators. Stress increases membrane permeability and thus antigen presentation, resulting in inflammation and immune response activation.[20]

Functional and integrative medicine offers a range of diagnostic approaches to gastrointestinal disorders. In the following sections, we address some common gastrointestinal conditions that are important in older patients and provide a spectrum of choices to address them. Table 16.2 and Figure 16.2 provide useful guidance and a general approach.

Table 16.2. Overview of Conditions and Lifestyle/Functional, Mind–Body, Bioenergetic, Biomedical, and Biochemical Prevention

Condition	Lifestyle Functional Medicine Prevention	Mind–Body	Bioenergetics	Biomedical	Biochemical
Gastroesophageal Reflux	– Smaller meals – Avoid eating 2–3 hours before going to bed – Elevate head of bed or use wedge pillow – Avoid offending foods and beverages (alcohol, caffeine, fatty foods, spicy foods) and high intake of simple carbs and in some cases gluten – Weight management – Quit smoking – Drink 8–10 glasses of water daily	– Mindful eating to facilitate behavior change – Manage stress with psychotherapy, hypnotherapy, relaxation	– Acupuncture as adjunct for failed PPI	– Testing for *H. pylori* – Esophageal acid monitoring (pH monitor) – Endoscopy of esophagus and stomach (EGD) – Dilation of narrowed esophagus – Surgical repair of hiatal hernia	– Antacids – H2 blockers – PPIs Herbal supplements: – Aloe vera juice – DGL: 2–4 tablets (380 mg) before meals – Rice bran oil: 150 mg TID – Slippery elm: 2 Tbsp in water after meals and bedtime

(continued)

Table 16.2. Continued

Condition	Lifestyle Functional Medicine Prevention	Mind–Body	Bioenergetics	Biomedical	Biochemical
Gastritis/Ulcers	– Eat breakfast and regular meals – Avoid caffeine and alcohol – Avoid NSAIDs, steroids – Regular exercise – Adequate sleep	– Mindful eating to facilitate behavior change – Manage stress with psychotherapy, hypnotherapy, relaxation, trauma treatment – Vagal biofeedback for functional dyspepsia		– Testing for *H. pylori* – Endoscopy of esophagus and stomach (EGD) – Surgery for bleeding and scarring	– Antacids – H2 blockers – PPIs <u>Supplements:</u> – DGL: 2–4 tablets (380 mg) before meals – Mastic gum: 500 mg TID – Slippery elm: 2 Tbsp mixed in water after meals and at bedtime – Aloe vera juice: 1/2 cup TID – Cabbage juice: 1 glass BID – Chamomile tea: 3 cups daily – Turmeric: 600 mg 5 times daily – Vitamin C: 1,200–5,000 mg/day to suppress *H. pylori* (no more than 500 mg a dose, up to 4 weeks total) – Zinc: 30–50 mg/day as arginate or hydrate form for 3–6 weeks; supplement with at least 1–2 mg copper daily

Colon Cancer					
	– High-fiber, Mediterranean-type diet – Cruciferous vegetables (broccoli family) – At least 5–11 servings of fruits and vegetables daily – Avoid smoking – Avoid processed meats – Regular exercise – Maintain BMI < 30 – Maintain adequate vitamin D levels – Anti-inflammatories, including NSAIDs, aspirin, calcium, selenium, curcumin, and folate to reduce polyp formation	– Manage stress to facilitate reduction of stress-related behaviors that promote cancer and possibly to prevent metastasis – Manage stress to improve coping with cancer – Therapies include cognitive-behavioral therapy, guided meditation, progressive muscle relaxation, journaling, body scan	– Acupuncture for cancer pain, mood, sleep, neuropathy, and chemotherapy-related gastrointestinal distress – Self-administered acupressure for mood and nausea – Reiki as a safe and tolerable option for overall well-being	– Regular physical activity, either occupational or leisure time, is associated with protection from colorectal cancer – Screening for colorectal cancer using fecal occult blood testing annually, sigmoidoscopy every 5 years, or colonoscopy every 10 years in adults beginning at age 50 years and continuing until age 75 years. Screen earlier in patients with risk factors.	– Diet high in fruits and vegetables offers protection from colorectal cancer – Aspirin and NSAIDs Supplements: – Calcium and vitamin D – B6 – Caffeine: 3 cups daily – Garlic – Magnesium – Fish oil – Olive oil

– Glutamine: 1,600–3,000 mg in 3 or 4 divided doses for 4 weeks
– Fish oil and black currant oil: 1 g of each daily for 8 weeks for suppression of *H. pylori*

Table 16.2. Continued

Condition	Lifestyle Functional Medicine Prevention	Mind–Body	Bioenergetics	Biomedical	Biochemical
Constipation	– Adequate hydration – Fruits and vegetables, 5–11 servings daily – 30 g fiber daily – Regular exercise – Tea or coffee in moderation – Bowel-habit diary – Review medications that may be constipating	– Mindful eating for facilitating behavior change – Recto-anal neuromuscular training using biofeedback for pelvic floor dyssynergy	Acupuncture for stimulating gastrointestinal motility: Tianshu (ST25), Shangjuxu (ST37), Dachangshu (BL25), Zusanli (ST36), and Zhigou (TE6).	– Exclude medical and surgical conditions via history, physical exam, and, if needed x-rays, endoscopy, or other tests – Manual disimpaction – Surgery for neurological causes	Dietary changes: – Fiber and other bulk-forming agents such as psyllium, methylcellulose, or calcium polycarbophil; however, they may not be useful in slow-transit constipation. Laxatives: – Docusate, milk of magnesia: 1–2 Tbsp daily – Magnesium citrate: 350–500 mg/day in chelated form – Polyethylene glycol, sorbitol, lactulose, bisacodyl – Senna: tea with ½ tsp of senna in cup of water once or twice daily – Saline or mineral oil enema Supplements: – Aloe vera: short term use only (<1 week); ½ cup juice TID; 40–170 mg dehydrated juice in capsule

| Diarrhea | Handwashing, Care with food and water when traveling, Be cautious in use of antibiotics (C. difficile risk), Regular intake of fermented foods, yogurt, prebiotics, probiotics | Biofeedback for fecal incontinence | | Infectious diarrhea will need physician consultation and may need lab studies of stool | | Cascara: short term use only (<1 week); 250 mg BID or TID |

						– Cascara: short term use only (<1 week); 250 mg BID or TID
						– Vitamin C: 500–2,000 mg/day
						– Wheat or corn bran: 1 Tbsp daily
						– Probiotic *Bifidobacteria*: at least 4 billion units BID or TID

World Health Organization's rehydration formula:

3.5 g sodium chloride, 2.9 g trisodium citrate, or 2.5 g sodium bicarbonate, 1.5 g potassium chloride, 20 g glucose or 40 g sucrose. Solution prepared at home using ½ tsp salt, ½ tsp baking soda, 4 Tbsp sugar, and 1 L water.

Antimotility agents:

– Loperamide (Imodium): 4 mg to start and 2 mg after each unformed stool to a maximum of 16 mg/day for no more than 2 days

– Diphenoxylate (Lomotil): 4 mg up to QID daily for no more than 2 days*

Caution: Use either sparingly and avoid if fever or bloody diarrhea.

(continued)

Table 16.2. Continued

Condition	Lifestyle Functional Medicine Prevention	Mind–Body	Bioenergetics	Biomedical	Biochemical
					Antibiotics: - Ciprofloxacin, levofloxacin, trimethoprim/sulfamethoxazole, doxycycline, azithromycin, erythromycin, and vancomycin Anti-parasitics: Metronidazole Supplements: - Bilberry: capsules (240–600 mg/day); tincture (1–2 ml BID); juice (½ cup BID or TID) - Ginger: 500 mg BID or 1–2 cups ginger tea - Glutamine: 1,000–3,000 mg TID - Red raspberry, blackberry, or blueberry leaf: tea (1–2 tsp dried leaves in cup of boiling water); capsule (5–10 mg/day) - Slippery elm: tea (3 cups daily); capsule (500 mg/day for 3 days) - Avoid magnesium and vitamin C during diarrhea.

		– Probiotics: to re-establish bacterial balance, 3–6 capsules *Lactobacillus* and *Bifidobacteria* at least 4 billion units daily. – Bulk-forming agents: Kaopectate, Metamucil, and psyllium – Anti-inflammatory agents: Pepto-Bismol – Lactase (Lactaid) if dairy/lactose intolerance suspected (chronic diary)	Antibiotics: – Ciprofloxacin (Cipro): 500 mg BID – Metronidazole (Flagyl): 500 mg TID – Other options: amoxicillin-clavulanate, clindamycin, or moxifloxacin Supplements: – Rice bran oil: 100 mg TID for 3–6 weeks – Glutamine: up to 8 g/day in 3 or 4 divided doses – Slippery elm bark: 1 or 2 capsules TID or make a tea with 1 tsp in 2 cups of water	
Diverticulosis	– Maintain high fiber intake 25–30 g/day – Vegetarian diet – Maintain healthy weight – Regular exercise – Prevent constipation – May not be necessary to avoid seeds and nuts			

(continued)

Table 16.2. Continued

Condition	Lifestyle Functional Medicine Prevention	Mind–Body	Bioenergetics	Biomedical	Biochemical
					– Soluble fiber such as psyllium and ground flaxseed (2–3 Tbsp daily); high-fiber diet when acute condition subsides – Probiotics to prevent infection: *Acidophilus/Bifidobacteria*: 1 capsule BID for prevention or 2 capsules TID for flare-ups
Irritable Bowel Syndrome	– High-fiber diet, balancing soluble and insoluble fiber based on symptoms – Anti-inflammatory diet – Avoid NSAIDs and COX2 inhibitors – Regular intake of fermented foods, yogurt, prebiotics, probiotics – Consider food allergy, sensitivity (e.g., gluten, dairy) as contributing or exacerbating factors	– Mindful eating to facilitate behavior change – Maximize empathy and therapeutic alliance – Yoga is beneficial – Consider hypnotherapy – Cognitive-behavioral therapy for managing psychological triggers			– Dietary modifications: lactose, gluten, carbohydrates, food allergy, gas-producing foods – Fiber (insoluble vs. soluble): psyllium, wheat bran or polycarbophil, methylcellulose (trial of ½–1 Tbsp daily to start). Soluble fiber as flaxseed 2–3 Tbsp daily. Antispasmodics: – Dicyclomine (Bentyl): 20 mg up to QID – Hyoscyamine (Levsin): 0.125–0.25 mg TID or QID – Sustained-release hyoscyamine (Levbid): 0.375–0.75 mg q12h

– Reduce alcohol intake – Reduce caffeine intake – Regular exercise – Stress management			Antidepressants: – Amitriptyline, desimipramine, imipramine, and nortriptyline: Dosing is variable based on response and side effects. – Paroxetine: 20 mg/day – Fluoxetine: 20 mg/day – Sertraline: 100 mg/day Antidiarrheals: Loperamide (Imodium): 2–4 mg as needed not to exceed 16 mg/day Anxiolytics (for short-term use only): – Lorazepam (Ativan): 0.5–1 mg up to TID – Diazepam (Valium): 1–10 mg up to TID – Oxazepam (Serax): 10–30 mg TID Serotonin antagonists (for relief of abdominal pain and discomfort): – Ondansetron (Zofran): 4–8 mg once or twice daily – Granisetron (Granisol): 2 mg/day – Lubiprostone (Amitiza): 8 mcg BID for women >18 with constipation variety irritable bowel syndrome

(continued)

Table 16.2. Continued

Condition	Lifestyle Functional Medicine Prevention	Mind–Body	Bioenergetics	Biomedical	Biochemical
					Supplements: – Peppermint oil: 1 or 2 enteric-coated capsules TID – Caraway oil: enteric-coated volatile oil 0.05–0.2 ml TID; can be taken with peppermint oil – Fennel: 1 tsp with food – Ginger: 250–500 mg TID or QID – Chamomile: 1 cup of tea TID – Iberogast: 20 drops TID for 4 weeks – Rifaximin: 400 mg TID for 4 weeks – Probiotics: 25 billion units of *Bifidobacteria* and 25 billion units of *Lactobacillus* for 4–6 weeks, then 10 billion units daily
Inflammatory Bowel Disease	– Anti-inflammatory diet – Avoid NSAIDs and COX2 inhibitors – Regular intake of fermented foods, yogurt, prebiotics, probiotics	– Hypnosis as adjunct for remission – Relaxation and mindfulness for quality of life	– Acupuncture and moxibustion as adjunct	Specific therapy for Crohn's disease: – Mesalamine (Pentasa): 2 g/day with an increase to a maximum of 4.8 g/day – Sulfasalazine (Asacol): 2–4 g/day	Supplements: – Aloe: ½ cup TID – Rice bran oil: 100 mg TID for 3–6 weeks – Boswellia: 550 mg TID – Curcumin: 1 mg BID – Fish oil: 6 g/day, at least 3.2 g EPA and 2.2 g DHA

– Consider food allergy, sensitivity (e.g., gluten, dairy) as contributing or exacerbating factors – Reduce alcohol intake – Regular exercise – Stress management	– Mind–body interventions for coexisting anxiety and disease-related stress	– Prednisone: 40–60 mg/day for 10–14 days, then decrease – Budesonide (Entocort EC): 8 mg/day for 8 weeks, then decrease to 6 mg for up to 3 months – Immunosuppressant therapy such as infliximab, adalimumab, and certolizumab pegol – Immunomodulators such as azathioprine or 6-mercaptopurine – Antibiotics such as metronidazole or quinolones – Surgery: multiple types such as removal of sections of bowel, ileostomy, treatment of infection, strictures, and fistulas	– Glutamine: 1,600–3,000 mg/day divided in 3 or 4 doses – Wheat grass juice: 3.5 ounces daily for a month <u>Supplements to replace malabsorbed nutrients:</u> – Calcium: 1,200 mg/day – Magnesium: 350 mg/day – Iron: 300 mg/day – Selenium: 200 mcg/day – Zinc: 30 mg/day – Vitamin A: 5,000 IU/day – Vitamin B1: 50 mg/day – Vitamin B6: 50 mg/day – Folic acid: 400 mcg/day – Vitamin B12: 50 mcg/day – Vitamin D: 2,000 IU/day <u>Antioxidants:</u> – Beta carotenoids: 10,000 IU/day – Vitamin C: 250–500 mg/day – CoQ10: 50–100 mg/day <u>Probiotics (mixed species):</u> Start with 1 billion units TID and gradually increase over a month to 20–30 billion units daily. – *Saccharomyces boulardii* : 250 mg TID – Fecal transplant therapy

(continued)

Table 16.2. Continued

Condition	Lifestyle Functional Medicine Prevention	Mind–Body	Bioenergetics	Biomedical	Biochemical
				Specific therapy for ulcerative colitis: – Sulfasalazine (Azulfidine), mesalamine (Pentasa), Asacol, Lialda, Apriso, olsalazine (Dipentum), or balsalazide (Colazal): local application as enemas and suppositories for rectal or left-sided colon problems – Steroids: prednisone and budesonide as above for Crohn's disease – Immunosuppressive therapy such as infliximab, cyclosporine, methotrexate, azathioprine, and mercaptopurine – Nicotine patches – Surgery: colectomy and multiple variations with and without colostomy	

Hemorrhoids	– Maintain high fiber intake (25–30 g/day) – Adequate hydration – Use stool softeners if needed for constipation – Maintain a healthy weight – Using topical moisturized towelettes for anal hygiene to decrease irritation		– Lancing and draining of thrombosed hemorrhoids if <48 hours old – Minimally invasive surgical treatments: banding, coagulation, injection with sclerosing agent, cryotherapy – Hemorrhoidectomy with surgical scalpel, diathermy, laser, ultrasonic scalpel, or stapling for more extensive or severely prolapsed hemorrhoids – Colonoscopy for those over 40 with rectal bleeding to exclude other causes of gastrointestinal bleeding besides hemorrhoids, such as colon cancer and diverticulitis	– Conservative treatment with fiber and increased fluids – Application of topical hydrocortisone for up to a week with pain and itching Herbal supplements: – Horse chestnut: 300 mg BID or TID – Bioflavonoid complex: 1000 mg TID during flares – Butcher's broom: 100 mg TID – Application of topical gels or creams containing 2% aescin – Topical witch hazel – Soluble fiber such as psyllium or ground flaxseed, 2–3 Tbsp/day

Integrative Medicine Treatment Ladder:

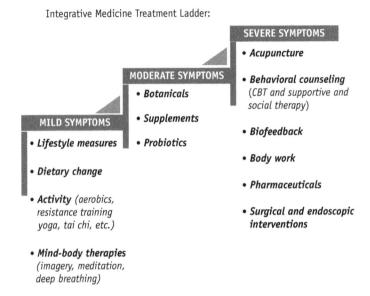

SEVERE SYMPTOMS

• *Acupuncture*

MODERATE SYMPTOMS

• *Botanicals*

• *Behavioral counseling*
  (*CBT and supportive and
  social therapy*)

MILD SYMPTOMS

• *Supplements*

• *Biofeedback*

• *Lifestyle measures*

• *Probiotics*

• *Body work*

• *Dietary change*

• *Pharmaceuticals*

• *Activity* (*aerobics,
  resistance training
  yoga, tai chi, etc.*)

• *Surgical and endoscopic
  interventions*

• *Mind-body therapies*
  (*imagery, meditation,
  deep breathing*)

FIGURE 16.2. Treatment Ladder.

Gastrointestinal Reflux Disease

LIFESTYLE INTERVENTIONS

Gastroesophageal reflux disease (GERD) is highly prevalent, affecting up to 8% of the adult population. It is a contributor to worsening asthma, laryngeal disease, increased risk of pneumonia, and premalignant Barrett's esophagus and increasingly to eosinophilic esophagitis. Weight loss is often important, as all clinicians have seen a person develop a new case of reflux or an exacerbation of symptoms following weight gain. This may be due to a hiatal hernia or just from the increased pressure of intra-abdominal fat on the stomach and lower esophageal sphincter. Caffeine, alcohol, highly spiced foods, chocolate, fatty foods, nicotine, and peppermint can all increase GERD, as can food sensitivities such as gluten. Avoiding a recumbent position within 2 hours of eating and elevating the head of the bed or using a wedge pillow can reduce symptoms.

Chronic GERD is often treated with PPIs, but these medications carry attendant risks on the cardiovascular, bone, nutritional, pneumonia, renal function, and gut bacterial health.[21,22] A trial taper from these useful but potentially harmful medications is recommended (Box 16.1).

Box 16.1. Weaning from PPIs

Weaning Protocol for Proton Pump Inhibitors (pantoprazole, omeprazole, etc.)

Skip dose every third day, substituting ranitidine 150 mg or famotidine 20 mg or other H2 blocker for 2 weeks.

If the patient tolerates this, skip every other day with substitution every other day for 2 weeks.

If this is tolerated, at the end of a month, switch entirely to ranitidine, famotidine, or other H2 blocker and keep pantoprazole or other PPI in reserve for flare-ups of heartburn.

May also consider DGL or aloe as an alternative to H2 blockers or to assist in the taper.

BIOENERGETICS

Acupuncture and electro-acupuncture have been shown to modulate acid secretion, gastrointestinal motility, neuro-hormone levels, and pain perception. A number of small studies have shown the efficacy of acupuncture alone or as combined therapy in the management of GERD.[23] Acupuncture may be particularly useful as an adjunct for patients who failed to respond to PPI therapy.

BIOMEDICAL

Testing for *Helicobacter pylori* should be performed if symptoms are not improving or are worsening with H2 blockers or PPIs; standard triple or quadruple therapy should be used if test results are positive. Surgical correction of a hiatal hernia can be done by itself or as part of the Nissen fundoplication procedure. In this procedure the upper part of the stomach is wrapped around the lower esophageal sphincter to strengthen the sphincter and prevent reflux and repair the hiatal hernia. Surgical dilation of a narrowed esophagus can be done as well.

BIOCHEMICAL

Herbal supplements used to alleviate symptoms are aloe vera juice, deglycyrrhizinated licorice (DGL), rice bran oil, or slippery elm. First-line therapy is usually with antacids such as over-the-counter aluminum/magnesium and calcium carbonate compounds. Typical H2 blockers are ranitidine, famotidine, and nizatidine. Cimetidine is not recommended in older patients because of its side-effect profile. PPIs such as omeprazole, pantoprazole, esomeprazole, and rabeprazole are usually very effective, but practitioners should be aware of the risks as mentioned earlier.

Gastritis/Ulcers

LIFESTYLE INTERVENTIONS

Adequate rest, regular exercise, eating breakfast and regular meals, and limiting caffeine and alcohol intake are all recommended measures to prevent or manage gastritis or ulcers.

MIND–BODY

Prior to the discovery of *H. pylori* as an etiology, mind and psychological influences were thought to have a significant effect on peptic ulcer disease (PUD). Since this discovery, such factors have been debated as being inconsequential or of only minimal influence. However, PUD is a multifactorial condition, with evidence supporting a role of stress in its development.[24-26] Psychodynamics play a role in the formation and exacerbation of idiopathic or non-ulcer (functional) dyspepsia as well.[27] Mind–body therapies combine well with anti-secretory therapy in PUD and can be valuable primary elements in the management of functional dyspepsia. Breathing exercises have been combined with vagal biofeedback with increased drinking capacity and improved quality of life in one randomized controlled trial of patients with functional dyspepsia.[28] Therapies for the management of dyspepsia include brief psychotherapy, hypnotherapy, and other stress and mood management modalities with varying evidence.[29,30] Mindful eating can be a useful tool to both address associated psychological stress and facilitate adoption of supportive behaviors such as limiting exacerbating substances, optimizing portions, and timing meals appropriately.[31]

BIOMEDICAL

Since the discovery of *H. pylori* infection as a proximal cause of gastritis and peptic ulcers, therapies have been directed toward eradication of this organism. Testing for *H. pylori* is indicated in situations where symptoms are not improving with H2 blockers or PPIs, and treatment of *H. pylori*–positive acute cases with PPIs and antibiotics is recommended. Perforated peptic ulcer is a surgical emergency and requires urgent surgical repair of the perforation by endoscopy to stop bleeding with cautery, injection, or clipping. In the older adult, gastropathy from NSAIDs is extremely common and is often a cause of potentially fatal gastrointestinal bleeding. Atrophic gastritis and use of PPIs and post–gastric bypass state can decrease absorption of iron, calcium, magnesium, B12, vitamin D, and other essential nutrients.

BIOCHEMICAL

Some patients wish to avoid pharmaceuticals or antibiotics. A broad variety of supplements are available to alleviate symptoms of gastritis or PUD. These alternatives can be tried in any order the patient and clinician agree is appropriate, depending on response, acuity, chronicity, cost, and convenience: DGL, mastic gum, slippery elm, aloe vera juice, cabbage juice, chamomile tea, turmeric, zinc arginate supplemented with 1 to 2 mg copper, glutamine, vitamin C, or fish oil and black currant oil for suppression of *H. pylori*.

Colon Cancer

LIFESTYLE INTERVENTIONS

Regular physical activity, either occupational or leisure time, is associated with protection from colorectal cancer. Nutrition offers the best-evidenced, safest approach to the prevention of colon cancer. Beyond regular colonoscopy screening, reducing risk involves incorporating a high-fiber, Mediterranean-type diet. Of particular potential benefit is the sulforaphane antioxidant in cruciferous vegetables such as broccoli, cauliflower, and Brussels sprouts. Sulforaphane has been demonstrated to reduce colorectal cancer risk by suppressing tumor formation in mice. Young broccoli sprouts are richer in the precursor glucoraphanin than more mature broccoli.[32] The National Cancer Institute recommends the consumption of five to nine servings of fruits and vegetable daily, though they do not address optimal intakes of crucifers. It seems prudent to include these cancer-fighting vegetables in the diet several times a week. Other factors in reducing risk include maintaining adequate vitamin D levels,[33] weight reduction, and regular exercise. Processed meats and red meats in general increase the risk of colorectal cancer. Anti-inflammatories,

including NSAIDs, as well as supplements such as calcium, selenium, curcumin, and folate reduce polyp formation.

MIND–BODY

Mind–body therapies can be useful in mitigating behavioral contributors to
colon cancer, preventing cancer progression, and coping with cancer. Behaviors
that contribute to colon cancer, including excess alcohol consumption, smoking, and overeating, are often coping strategies for stress and thereby can be
decreased by employing mind–body therapies for stress management such as
meditation, imagery, hypnosis, mindfulness, journaling, cognitive-behavioral
therapy, yoga, tai chi, and creative arts therapies. Chronic stress plays a role in
cancer progression including metastasis, making mind–body therapies potential tools for prevention.[34] Mind–body therapies are additionally useful for
acute stress associated with cancer workup, diagnosis, and treatment.

BIOENERGETICS

Bioenergetic therapies such as acupuncture, reiki, and healing touch are used
by and large for symptom management and supporting overall well-being.
Acupuncture is being offered by many cancer centers as management for cancer pain, mood and sleep problems, and chemotherapy-related gastrointestinal distress and peripheral neuropathy.[35,36] Acupressure points can be taught
to patients for self-treatment and have demonstrated efficacy for modulating
nausea and mood.[37]

Healing touch and reiki have demonstrated efficacy in some studies in
improvement of cancer-related pain, fatigue, and mood disturbance; more
studies are needed to clarify conflicting data.[38,39] Healing touch and reiki offer
a distinct advantage in their high safety profile. These energetic therapies are
good options for patients who desire this type of therapy, are informed of the
evidence, and have the means.

BIOMEDICAL

Screening for colorectal cancer involves fecal occult blood testing annually,
sigmoidoscopy every 5 years, or colonoscopy every 10 years in adults beginning at age 50 and continuing until age 75. Screening can be done earlier in
patients with risk factors.

BIOCHEMICAL

A diet high in fruits and vegetables is protective in colorectal cancer. Common herbal supplements that are protective and ought to be considered are calcium and vitamin D, B6, three cups of caffeine daily, garlic daily, magnesium, fish oil, or olive oil. These can be used individually but are synergistic, so a blended combination is likely to be most helpful.

Constipation

LIFESTYLE INTERVENTIONS

While constipation may seem like more of a nuisance than a disease, it is perennially one of the most common complaints in the older adult. Changes in fiber intake due to dentition problems, the constipating effects of many medications, changes in gut motility and myenteric plexus enervation, and disturbance of muscular coordination all are factors in causing constipation. Avoiding dependence on laxatives, enemas, and stool softeners is a worthwhile goal but not always an attainable one. Often overlooked, however, are basics such as adequate hydration, sufficient intake of fruits and vegetables and other sources of high fiber in the diet, and regular physical exercise. Tea or coffee in moderation can offer gentle stimulation. A bowel-habit diary can be useful and reassuring, particularly for those with high anxiety about not having adequate stooling patterns. Often reassurance is all that is necessary that a daily bowel movement may no longer be necessary in the aging gut and that bowel habits change over time. Of course, medical or surgical causes must be considered and excluded. Constipation can contribute to other conditions such as hemorrhoids, diverticulosis, and even hernias. While constipation has been feared to increase the risk of colorectal cancer, prospective cross-sectional surveys and cohort studies demonstrate that there is no increase in prevalence of colorectal cancer in individuals with constipation.[40,41]

MIND–BODY

Mindfulness can be used to foster attentiveness to body signals and empower patients to consume in a way that supports normal bowel function. Intra-anal biofeedback has been successfully applied in cases of constipation secondary to pelvic floor dyssynergia, with five biofeedback sessions proving more effective than continuous polyethylene glycol, and benefits lasting 2 years.[42]

Whether this finding can be reproduced and whether the technique can be successfully applied more broadly to functional defecation disorder is being investigated.[43,44]

BIOENERGETICS

Acupuncture has been shown to be effective for management of functional constipation. Many protocols have been used, and in a 2015 review of 17 articles, the top five acupoints used for stimulating gastrointestinal motility were Tianshu (ST25), Shangjuxu (ST37), Dachangshu (BL25), Susanli (ST36), and Zhigou (TE6).[45] In one multicenter randomized controlled trial, deep and shallow needling at Tianshu (ST25) was compared to lactulose, with all groups demonstrating efficacy; interestingly, the acupuncture group had a reduced need for emergency medication and showed longer-lasting improvements in spontaneous bowel movements as measured at 8 and 16 weeks after treatment.[46]

BIOMEDICAL

The first step in treatment is to exclude medical and surgical conditions that can cause constipation via history, physical examination, and if needed x-rays, endoscopy, or other tests. Bowel obstruction or partial ileus from metabolic factors such as low potassium levels or hypothyroidism must be excluded. If relief cannot be obtained by saline or mineral oil enema, manual disimpaction is sometimes required. Surgery is only rarely indicated for neurological causes of constipation.

BIOCHEMICAL

Adding fiber and other bulk-forming agents such as psyllium, methylcellulose, or calcium polycarbophil may not be as useful in slow-transit constipation. The dosing for soluble fiber such as psyllium or ground flaxseed is 1 to 3 tablespoons daily. In our experience, ground flaxseed is effective when other bulk-forming agents have been ineffective. Common laxatives are docusate, 1 to 2 tablespoons of milk of magnesia daily, 350 to 500 mg of magnesium citrate a day in chelated form, polyethylene glycol, sorbitol, lactulose, bisacodyl, or senna tea in a cup of water once or twice daily (may double if needed to obtain soft stool).

Herbal supplements include aloe vera, which can be taken as a half-cup of juice three times daily or in capsule form, cascara, vitamin C, or wheat or corn bran. Several studies have examined the role of various species and doses of probiotic for constipation. We recommend at least 4 billion colony-forming units (CFUs) of *Bifidobacteria* two or three times daily. Probiotics may improve whole gut transit time, stool frequency, and stool consistency; one study showed beneficial effects of *Bifidobacterium lactis* in particular and other studies suggested use of *Lactobacillus reuteri*.[47–49]

Diarrhea

LIFESTYLE INTERVENTIONS

Infections are leading causes of diarrhea, so regular handwashing, attention to food and water sources, particularly while traveling, and minimizing antibiotic use are vital strategies. Maintaining adequate hydration is critical in an older adult as orthostatic hypotension is often preexisting and balance and stability issues are aggravated by dehydration. Fluid replacement may be complicated at times by compromised renal or cardiac function, reduced baseline intravascular volume, and a decreased thirst drive. Be aware of the paradox of overflow diarrhea around an impacted stool; by managing constipation, one can help prevent this kind of diarrhea.

MIND–BODY

Diarrhea may lead to fecal incontinence. A 2008 review in *Nature* concluded that randomized controlled trials suggest that biofeedback combining strength training and sensory discrimination training is effective in approximately 75% of patients with fecal incontinence and is more effective than placebo. However, interestingly, verbal feedback provided by a therapist during digital examination may be equally effective.[50]

BIOCHEMICAL

First-line therapy is rehydration, such as the World Health Organization's rehydration formula. Rehydration solution can be prepared at home using a half-teaspoon of salt, a half-teaspoon of baking soda, 4 tablespoons of sugar, and 1 liter of water.

Herbal supplements that may be useful for diarrhea are bilberry capsules, bilberry tincture or bilberry juice, ginger or ginger tea, glutamine, red raspberry, blackberry, or blueberry teas or capsules, and slippery elm tea capsule. Avoid oral magnesium and vitamin C as they can worsen diarrhea. Probiotics can be used to re-establish bacterial balance and to shorten acute diarrheal episodes. Mixed probiotics such as *Lactobacillus* and *Bifidobacteria*, at least 4 to 20 billion units daily, are likely to be helpful. *S. boulardii* has been specifically helpful in *Clostridium difficile* diarrhea. Bulk-forming agents such as Kaopectate, Metamucil, and psyllium are worthwhile. Lactase (Lactaid) can considered if dairy/lactose intolerance is suspected as a cause of diarrhea.

A Cochrane review found moderate-quality evidence that probiotics are both safe and effective for preventing *C. difficile*-associated diarrhea.[51,52] Despite many studies, additional research is needed for the use of probiotics in specific gut conditions in terms of dosing, timing, and species selection. In general, choosing a mix of species, refrigerated forms, and multi-billion-unit dosing is most rational and evidenced.

A commonly used anti-inflammatory agent is Pepto-Bismol. Antimotility agents include loperamide or diphenoxylate. Antibiotics that can be useful are ciprofloxacin, levofloxacin, trimethoprim/sulfamethoxazole, doxycycline, azithromycin, erythromycin, and vancomycin. Metronidazole is an anti-parasitic that can be useful in diarrhea from *C. difficile*, diverticulitis, and colitis. Antibiotics can also cause diarrhea, and diarrhea is the most common adverse effect of treatment with antibiotics, so they should be used cautiously (see Chapter 17). Probiotics can be used to prevent this complication, to re-establish bacterial balance, and to shorten acute diarrheal episodes.

Diverticular Disease

LIFESTYLE INTERVENTIONS

The most important lifelong habit to prevent diverticular disease is maintaining a high-fiber diet. Recommended fiber levels are around 25 to 40 grams for adults, but this goal is often not achieved in the standard American diet, with its high-carbohydrate and refined and processed foods that have milled away the healthy, high-fiber bran layer from whole grains. Eating less than the recommended 5 to 11 servings of fruits and vegetables contributes to an increased risk of diverticulosis. Once diverticulosis is established, a balance of roughage and high levels of soluble and insoluble fiber is important as some patients find that certain vegetables or fruits actually irritate their bowel. Keep diet prescriptions patient-centered by listening to patients' histories of their tolerance or intolerance of certain foods. In general, however, maintaining a high intake with supplemental bulk-forming agents (see the biochemical section below) is the best bet. Avoiding seeds and nuts, long a gospel recommendation of diverticulosis management, has not been found to be evidence-based.[53] In general, if certain seeds and nuts are tolerated, we encourage them because of their other health benefits, including for cardiac health,[54] as they include fiber, unsaturated and omega-3 fats, selenium, and vitamin E. If they cause irritation, we advise abstaining and finding other high-fiber substitutes. Individualization can be the most useful strategy. In addition to fiber, adequate fluids are essential to preventing constipation.

BIOCHEMICAL

Herbal supplements useful in diverticulosis are rice bran oil, glutamine, and slippery elm bark capsules or tea. Soluble fiber such as psyllium and ground flaxseed can also be used.

During the acute phase of diverticulitis infection, use a clear liquid diet for 3 days. Resume a high-fiber diet when the acute condition subsides. Probiotics, such as *Acidophilus* and *Bifidobacteria*, are used to prevent infection. If antibiotics are given, 20 to 30 billion units of probiotics, taken at least 2 hours away from antibiotics and continued for up to 4 weeks, is a common strategy used by many experienced integrative practitioners.[55]

Antibiotics are recommended when bacterial infection is suspected. Common useful agents are ciprofloxacin, metronidazole, amoxicillin–clavulanate, clindamycin, and moxifloxacin.

Irritable Bowel Syndrome and Inflammatory Bowel Disease

LIFESTYLE INTERVENTIONS

These conditions are generally diagnosed earlier in life, so symptoms in the older adult should occasion a vigorous gastrointestinal workup. An anti-inflammatory diet is a worthwhile approach to prevention and management of both conditions (see Chapter 2). Intake of fermented foods and probiotics can serve a useful role, and consideration of the contribution of food allergy is recommended. If possible, avoid NSAIDs and COX2 inhibitor drugs, which are commonly given in older adults for rheumatologic and pain conditions, because they can clearly aggravate the gut, leading to exacerbation of bleeding, inflammation, and other symptoms. Minimizing alcohol intake can be helpful. Consultation with a dietician may be useful in difficult cases.

Perceived stress is a predictor for flares in inflammatory bowel disease, and most patients see stress as a disease modifier, with an even greater number of patients indicating the belief that their ability to cope with stress impacts the disease course.[56] Indeed, one study demonstrated altered expression of genes for both of these conditions with NF-κB as a target molecule using a relaxation-based mind–body intervention; these results paved the way for future research.[57] Studies looking at the effect of hypnosis on the use of medications for ulcerative colitis as well as relaxation and mindfulness on quality of life in patients with inflammatory bowel disease are encouraging, and there are some intriguing studies examining the possibility of mind–body approaches to prevent flares; however, much remains to be known.[56] Patients who report high psychological stress are likely to benefit from mind–body interventions for the primary purpose of stress management and overall wellness.

Stress has been noted as a causative factor in irritable bowel syndrome, and these patients report higher levels of perceived stress than the general population.[58] One can imagine the complex interplay of perceived stress in the brain leading to altered gut function by way of the brain–gut axis, and conversely stimulation of visceral pain receptors leading to increased perceived stress.[59] Hypnotherapy has been used with success, decreasing symptoms of irritable bowel syndrome and distress, with a 2007 Cochrane review underscoring the need for more research.[60,61] Cognitive-behavioral therapy has demonstrated efficacy in improving severity scale scores in patients with irritable bowel syndrome as well as quality of life.[62] Mindfulness-based stress reduction is in the early stages of investigation for use in irritable bowel syndrome.[63] Yoga is proving useful in managing irritable bowel syndrome, with a 2016 systematic review reporting that it had significant benefits on bowel symptoms, severity, anxiety, and quality of life.[64] The patient–provider relationship is an important component in irritable bowel syndrome and was studied in a 2008 randomized controlled trial published in *BMJ* in which placebo augmented with warmth, attention, and confidence in the patient–provider relationship produced greater improvement in measures of global improvement, symptoms, and quality of life at 3 and 6 weeks than placebo alone.[65] The authors concluded that "factors contributing to the placebo effect can be progressively combined in a manner resembling a graded dose escalation of component parts . . . the patient–practitioner relationship is the most robust component."

To decrease symptoms of irritable bowel syndrome, trials of dietary modifications can be used to decrease lactose, gluten, carbohydrates, food allergy, or gas-producing foods. A comprehensive elimination diet is often an effective diagnostic and therapeutic approach. It helps to identify foods that precipitate symptoms and those that are well tolerated. This approach involves a 2- to 3-week trial of a hypoallergenic diet followed by a re-introduction of a food group two or three times daily for 2 to 3 days while noting any recurrence of gastrointestinal symptoms. Allergy testing may be helpful as well.

Fiber is a key component to treatment of irritable bowel syndrome, and both insoluble and soluble intake should be assessed. Insoluble fiber includes psyllium, polycarbophil, or methycellulose. Soluble fiber to always consider is exemplified by ground flaxseed or wheat bran. Discussion with the patient regarding his or her past experience with different fiber types, raw versus cooked vegetables, and selected fruits allows for a nuanced, personalized dietary plan. Keep in mind that not all fiber is equal. The so-called FODMAP diet has been proposed for relief of irritable bowel syndrome.[66]

BIOENERGETICS

Acupuncture and moxibustion are being studied as potential management tools for both Crohn's disease and ulcerative colitis with some success and little to no side effects.[67–69]

BIOCHEMICAL

Herbal supplements used for IBS symptom relief and their antispasmodic effects are enteric- coated capsules of peppermint oil, enteric-coated volatile caraway oil (which can be taken with peppermint oil), fennel, ginger, chamomile tea, and Iberogast. A 4-week course of rifaximin is used to manage proven or suspected small bowel bacterial overgrowth. See more on this in chapter 17, Common Geriatric Infections. Probiotics can also be considered and may be helpful. Dosing recommendations are 25 to 100 billion units of *Bifidobacteria* or *Lactobacillus*, with or without other species, for 4 to 6 weeks, then 10 to 30 billion units daily for maintenance. Some cases will improve dramatically. If symptoms worsen or do not improve after a month, decrease to maintenance doses or discontinue probiotics.[70]

Herbal supplements used for relief of IBD are aloe, rice bran oil, boswellia, curcumin, fish oil, glutamine, and wheat grass juice. Supplements are usually needed to replace malabsorbed nutrients such as calcium, magnesium, iron, zinc, vitamin A, vitamins B1, B6, and B12, folic acid, and vitamin D. Antioxidants to offer are beta carotenoids, vitamin C, and CoQ10. Probiotics (mixed species) can be used by starting with 1 billion units three times daily and gradually increasing the dose over a month to 20 to 30 billion units daily.

The literature supports much higher doses such as VSL, which provides 500 billion units, or probiotics, or even as high as 3 trillion units of mixed probiotics in selected cases. *S. boulardii* may be particularly useful.[71]

BIOMEDICAL

Prescription antispasmodics such as dicyclomine or hyoscyamine may be useful. Antidepressants such as amitriptyline, desimipramine, imipramine, and nortriptyline can also be helpful. Other antidepressants that are worth a trial due to their effects on the richly represented serotonin receptors in the gut include paroxetine, fluoxetine, and sertraline. They also help manage the commonly coexisting affective disorders seen with irritable bowel syndrome.

Antidiarrheals like loperamide can be useful for short-term use. Anxiolytics such as clonazepam, lorazepam, diazepam, or oxazepam may be included in an integrative treatment plan. Consider serotonin antagonists such as ondansetron, granisetron, or lubiprostone for relief of abdominal pain and discomfort in the constipation variant of irritable IBS.

Specific therapies for Crohn's disease and ulcerative colitis are listed in Table 16.2 and are available in standard medical texts.

Hemorrhoids

LIFESTYLE INTERVENTIONS

Reducing the risk of hemorrhoids includes maintaining a healthy weight, avoiding straining at stool, and avoiding sitting or standing for prolonged periods of time. Those whose occupation requires prolonged sitting, such as truck and bus drivers, are at higher risk. Regular exercise can be helpful. Genetic factors seem to play a role in both hemorrhoids and varicose veins, and pregnancy increases risk. Chronic constipation is controversial as a cause of hemorrhoids, though it can definitely aggravate existing cases.

BIOMEDICAL

Rectal hygiene should include use of wipes moisturized with witch hazel or other emollients that can be more soothing than standard toilet tissue. Applying topical steroid cream after bowel movements can significantly reduce itching, burning, and irritation.

Further methods of treatment include lancing and draining of thrombosed hemorrhoids if less than 48 hours old. Minimally invasive surgical treatments include banding, coagulation, injection with sclerosing agents, and cryo-therapy. Hemorrhoidectomy approaches include surgical scalpel, diathermy, laser, ultrasonic scalpel, or stapling for more extensive or severely prolapsed hemorrhoids. Colonoscopy is recommended for those over 40 with rectal bleeding to exclude other causes of gastrointestinal bleeding besides hemor-rhoids, such as colon cancer and diverticulitis.

BIOCHEMICAL

Conservative treatment usually involves fiber intake and increased fluids. Topical hydrocortisone can be applied for up to a week for pain and itching. Common herbal supplements are horse chestnut bioflavonoid complex dur-ing flares, butcher's broom, application of topical gels or creams containing 2% aescin, or topical witch hazel. Soluble fiber such as psyllium or ground flaxseed can also be used to maintain soft stools to prevent irritating inflamed hemorrhoids.

Case Follow-up and Summary

This 72-year-old female is suffering from chronic constipation, a likely con-tributor to her internal hemorrhoids and diverticulosis. With her recent colonoscopy and lack of red flags we can feel safe in proceeding with con-servative interventions. First-line interventions would include adequate oral hydration, increased intake of fibrous plants, and if necessary supple-mentation with a gentle fiber such as methylcellulose or ground flaxseed. Considering her prior treatment with antibiotics and changes in gut flora that occur with low intake of plants, the patient may benefit from probiotic supplementation and increased intake of probiotic and prebiotic foods. She would benefit from a holiday from or permanent cessation of NSAIDs. She may want to combine these interventions with acupuncture. Gentle move-ment and stress reduction with a practice such as yoga may be therapeutic for both the condition and any disease-related anxiety. In case of an inad-equate response, the patient may need further workup and, if appropriate, consideration for biofeedback. As with any patient encounter, providing empathy and cultivating a robust healing relationship can lead to better outcomes.

This case illustrates some general core principles of integrative medicine applied to gastroenterology in the aging gut and in a more general sense. These are as follows:

1. Assess the patient for acute or life-threatening conditions and treat them appropriately. If these are not present, then utilize steps 2 through 4.
2. Use a stepped-care approach moving from low-intensity, safe measures to those that are gradually more intense.
3. Apply a shared model of decision making with the patient, including him or her in appropriate choices and selection of level and intensity of therapy.
4. Continue to reassess the patient and provide follow-up, discarding ineffective therapies and adding additional integrative methods as appropriate.

Key Web Resources

1. Natural Medicines Comprehensive Database: http://naturaldatabase. therapeuticresearch.com/home
2. UpToDate: http://www.uptodate.com/contents/search
3. University of Wisconsin Integrative Medicine: http://www.uwhealth. org/alternative-medicine/health-professionals/11434
4. Institute for Functional Medicine: https://www.functionalmedicine. org/files/library/Intro_Functional_Medicine.pdf
5. Stop, Breathe, and Think: http://www.stopbreathethink.org
6. Self Compassion: www.selfcompassion.org
7. Dr. Andrew Weil's website: http://www.drweil.com

REFERENCES

1. Morley JE. The aging gut: Physiology. *Clin Geriatr Med.* 2007;23(4):757–767.
2. Salles N. Basic mechanisms of the aging gastrointestinal tract. *Dig Dis.* 2007;25(2):112–117.
3. Wood RJ, Serfaty-Lacrosniere C. Gastric acidity, atrophic gastritis, and calcium absorption. *Nutr Rev.* 1992;50(2):33–40.
4. Marcus DL, Freedman ML. Clinical disorders of iron metabolism in the elderly. *Clin Geriatr Med.* 1985;1(4):729–745.
5. Fligiel SE, Relan NK, Dutta S, Tureaud J, Hatfield J, Majumdar AP. Aging diminishes gastric mucosal regeneration: Relationship to tyrosine kinases. *Lab Invest.* 1994;70(5):764–774.

6. Turnheim K. When drug therapy gets old: Pharmacokinetics and pharmacodynamics in the elderly. *Exp Gerontol.* 2003;38(8):843–853.
7. Hall KE, Proctor DD, Fisher L, Rose S. American Gastroenterological Association future trends committee report: Effects of aging of the population on gastroenterology practice, education, and research. *Gastroenterology.* 2005;129(4):1305–1338.
8. National Institute of Diabetes and Digestive and Kidney Diseases. The digestive system and how it works. https://catalog.niddk.nih.gov/imagelibrary/detail.cfm?id=1473. Accessed June 8, 2016.
9. Mullin GE. *Integrative Gastroenterology.* New York: Oxford University Press; 2011.
10. Mullin GE. *The Gut Balance Revolution.* New York: Rodale Press; 2015.
11. Lipski E. *Digestive Wellness: Strengthen the Immune System and Prevent Disease Through Healthy Digestion.* New York: McGraw-Hill; 2005.
12. Blaser MJ. *Missing Microbes: How the Overuse of Antibiotics Is Fueling Our Modern Plagues.* New York: Henry Holt and Company; 2014.
13. Nichols TW, Faass N. *Optimal Digestive Health: A Complete Guide.* Rochester, VT: Healing Arts Press; 2005.
14. Sierpina V. *The Healthy Gut Workbook: Whole-Body Healing for Heartburn, Ulcers, Constipation, IBS, Diverticulosis, and More.* Oakland, CA: New Harbinger Publications; 2010.
15. Institute for Functional Medicine. 2016; https://www.functionalmedicine.org/. Accessed June 8, 2016.
16. Fitzgerald K. A case report of a 53-year-old female with rheumatoid arthritis and osteoporosis: Focus on lab testing and CAM therapies. *Altern Med Rev.* 2011;16(3):250–263.
17. Jones DS. *Textbook of Functional Medicine.* Gig Harbor, WA: Institute for Functional Medicine; 2010.
18. Bland JS. *The Disease Delusion.* New York: Harper-Collins; 2014.
19. Fasano A. Zonulin, regulation of tight junctions, and autoimmune diseases. *Ann N Y Acad Sci.* 2012;1258:25–33.
20. Konturek PC, Brzozowski T, Konturek SJ. Stress and the gut: Pathophysiology, clinical consequences, diagnostic approach and treatment options. *J Physiol Pharmacol.* 2011;62(6):591–599.
21. Wolfe MM. Overview and comparison of the proton pump inhibitors for the treatment of acid-related disorders. In: Post TW, ed. *UpToDate.* Waltham, MA; 2016.
22. Gulmez SE, Holm A, Frederiksen H, Jensen TG, Pedersen C, Hallas J. Use of proton pump inhibitors and the risk of community-acquired pneumonia: A population-based case-control study. *Arch Intern Med.* 2007;167(9):950–955.
23. Maradey-Romero C, Kale H, Fass R. Nonmedical therapeutic strategies for nonerosive reflux disease. *J Clin Gastroenterol.* 2014;48(7):584–589.
24. Levenstein S. The very model of a modern etiology: A biopsychosocial view of peptic ulcer. *Psychosom Med.* 2000;62(2):176–185.
25. Overmier JB, Murison R. Restoring psychology's role in peptic ulcer. *Appl Psychol Health Well Being.* 2013;5(1):5–27.

26. Levenstein S, Ackerman S, Kiecolt-Glaser JK, Dubois A. Stress and peptic ulcer disease. *JAMA*. 1999;281(1):10–11.

27. Talley NJ, Ford AC. Functional dyspepsia. *N Engl J Med*. 2015;373(19):1853–1863.

28. Hjelland IE, Svebak S, Berstad A, Flatabo G, Hausken T. Breathing exercises with vagal biofeedback may benefit patients with functional dyspepsia. *Scand J Gastroenterol*. 2007;42(9):1054–1062.

29. Hamilton J, Guthrie E, Creed F, et al. A randomized controlled trial of psychotherapy in patients with chronic functional dyspepsia. *Gastroenterology*. 2000;119(3):661–669.

30. Calvert EL, Houghton LA, Cooper P, Morris J, Whorwell PJ. Long-term improvement in functional dyspepsia using hypnotherapy. *Gastroenterology*. 2002;123(6):1778–1785.

31. Center for Mindful Eating. 2016; http://thecenterformindfuleating.org/. Accessed June 8, 2016.

32. Prochaska HJ, Santamaria AB, Talalay P. Rapid detection of inducers of enzymes that protect against carcinogens. *Proc Natl Acad Sci USA*. 1992;89(6):2394–2398.

33. Gorham ED, Garland CF, Garland FC, et al. Optimal vitamin D status for colorectal cancer prevention: A quantitative meta-analysis. *Am J Prev Med*. 2007;32(3):210–216.

34. Moreno-Smith M, Lutgendorf SK, Sood AK. Impact of stress on cancer metastasis. *Future Oncol*. 2010;6(12):1863–1881.

35. Sellick SM, Zaza C. Critical review of 5 nonpharmacologic strategies for managing cancer pain. *Cancer Prev Control*. 1998;2(1):7–14.

36. Ezzo JM, Richardson MA, Vickers A, et al. Acupuncture-point stimulation for chemotherapy-induced nausea or vomiting. *Cochrane Database Syst Rev*. 2006;2.

37. Hmwe NT, Subramanian P, Tan LP, Chong WK. The effects of acupressure on depression, anxiety and stress in patients with hemodialysis: A randomized controlled trial. *Int J Nurs Stud*. 2015;52(2):509–518.

38. Post-White J, Kinney ME, Savik K, Gau JB, Wilcox C, Lerner I. Therapeutic massage and healing touch improve symptoms in cancer. *Integr Cancer Ther*. 2003;2(4):332–344.

39. Thrane S, Cohen SM. Effect of Reiki therapy on pain and anxiety in adults: An in-depth literature review of randomized trials with effect size calculations. *Pain Management Nursing*. 2014;15(4):897–908.

40. Power AM, Talley NJ, Ford AC. Association between constipation and colorectal cancer: Systematic review and meta-analysis of observational studies. *Am J Gastroenterol*. 2013;108(6):894–903; quiz 904.

41. Citronberg J, Kantor ED, Potter JD, White E. A prospective study of the effect of bowel movement frequency, constipation, and laxative use on colorectal cancer risk. *Am J Gastroenterol*. 2014;109(10):1640–1649.

42. Chiarioni G, Whitehead WE, Pezza V, Morelli A, Bassotti G. Biofeedback is superior to laxatives for normal transit constipation due to pelvic floor dyssynergia. *Gastroenterology*. 2006;130(3):657–664.

43. Frizelle F, Barclay M. Constipation in adults. *BMJ Clin Evid*. 2007;2007.

44. Rao SS, Bharucha AE, Chiarioni G, et al. Functional anorectal disorders. *Gastroenterology.* 2016. doi:10.1053/j.gastro.2016.02.009 [Epub ahead of print].

45. Wang X, Yin J. Complementary and alternative therapies for chronic constipation. *Evid Based Complement Alternat Med.* 2015;2015:396396.

46. Wu J, Liu B, Li N, et al. Effect and safety of deep needling and shallow needling for functional constipation: A multicenter, randomized controlled trial. *Medicine (Baltimore).* 2014;93(28):e284.

47. Dimidi E, Christodoulides S, Fragkos KC, Scott SM, Whelan K. The effect of probiotics on functional constipation in adults: a systematic review and meta-analysis of randomized controlled trials. *Am J Clin Nutr.* 2014;100(4):1075–1084.

48. Chmielewska A, Szajewska H. Systematic review of randomised controlled trials: Probiotics for functional constipation. *World J Gastroenterol.* 2010;16(1):69–75.

49. Ojetti V, Ianiro G, Tortora A, et al. The effect of *Lactobacillus reuteri* supplementation in adults with chronic functional constipation: A randomized, Double-blind, placebo-controlled trial. *J Gastrointest Liver Dis.* 2014;23(4):387–391.

50. Chiarioni G, Whitehead WE. The role of biofeedback in the treatment of gastrointestinal disorders. *Nat Clin Pract Gastroenterol Hepatol.* 2008;5(7):371–382.

51. Goldenberg JZ, Ma SS, Saxton JD, et al. Probiotics for the prevention of *Clostridium difficile*-associated diarrhea in adults and children. *Cochrane Database Syst Rev.* 2013(5):Cd006095.

52. Szajewska H, Kolodziej M. Systematic review with meta-analysis: *Saccharomyces boulardii* in the prevention of antibiotic-associated diarrhoea. *Aliment Pharmacol Ther.* 2015;42(7):793–801.

53. Strate LL, Liu YL, Syngal S, Aldoori WH, Giovannucci EL. Nut, corn, and popcorn consumption and the incidence of diverticular disease. *JAMA.* 2008;300(8):907–914.

54. Kelly JH, Jr., Sabate J. Nuts and coronary heart disease: An epidemiological perspective. *Br J Nutr.* 2006;96(Suppl 2):S61–S67.

55. Brown DJ, Leyer G, Lipski E, Sierpina VS, Kiefer D. Nature supplements: An evidence-based update. Scripps Natural Supplements Conference; January 16–18, 2015; San Diego, CA.

56. Langhorst J, Wulfert H, Lauche R, et al. Systematic review of complementary and alternative medicine treatments in inflammatory bowel diseases. *J Crohns Colitis.* 2015;9(1):86–106.

57. Kuo B, Bhasin M, Jacquart J, et al. Genomic and clinical effects associated with a relaxation response mind-body intervention in patients with irritable bowel syndrome and inflammatory bowel disease. *PLoS One.* 2015;10(4):e0123861.

58. Murray CD, Flynn J, Ratcliffe L, Jacyna MR, Kamm MA, Emmanuel AV. Effect of acute physical and psychological stress on gut autonomic innervation in irritable bowel syndrome. *Gastroenterology.* 2004;127(6):1695–1703.

59. Mayer EA, Tillisch K. The brain-gut axis in abdominal pain syndromes. *Annu Rev Med.* 2011;62:381–396.

60. Webb AN, Kukuruzovic RH, Catto-Smith AG, Sawyer SM. Hypnotherapy for treatment of irritable bowel syndrome. *Cochrane Database Syst Rev.* 2007;4(4).

61. Kearney DJ, Brown-Chang J. Complementary and alternative medicine for IBS in adults: Mind–body interventions. *Nat Clin Pract Gastroenterol Hepatol.* 2008;5(11):624–636.

62. Altayar O, Sharma V, Prokop LJ, Sood A, Murad MH. Psychological therapies in patients with irritable bowel syndrome: A systematic review and meta-analysis of randomized controlled trials. *Gastroenterol Res Pract.* 2015;2015:549308.

63. Zernicke KA, Campbell TS, Blustein PK, et al. Mindfulness-based stress reduction for the treatment of irritable bowel syndrome symptoms: A randomized wait-list controlled trial. *Int J Behav Med.* 2013;20(3):385–396.

64. Schumann D, Anheyer D, Lauche R, Dobos G, Langhorst J, Cramer H. Effect of yoga in the therapy of irritable bowel syndrome: A systematic review. *Clin Gastroenterol Hepatol.* 2016;14(12):1720–1731.

65. Kaptchuk TJ, Kelley JM, Conboy LA, et al. Components of placebo effect: Randomised controlled trial in patients with irritable bowel syndrome. *BMJ.* 2008;336(7651):999–1003.

66. Gibson PR, Shepherd SJ. Evidence-based dietary management of functional gastrointestinal symptoms: The FODMAP approach. *J Gastroenterol Hepatol.*25(2):252–258.

67. Joos S, Brinkhaus B, Maluche C, et al. Acupuncture and moxibustion in the treatment of active Crohn's disease: A randomized controlled study. *Digestion.* 2004;69(3):131–139.

68. Joos S, Wildau N, Kohnen R, et al. Acupuncture and moxibustion in the treatment of ulcerative colitis: A randomized controlled study. *Scand J Gastroenterol.* 2006;41(9):1056–1063.

69. Bao CH, Zhao JM, Liu HR, et al. Randomized controlled trial: Moxibustion and acupuncture for the treatment of Crohn's disease. *World J Gastroenterol.* 2014;20(31):11000–11011.

70. Ford AC, Ford AC, Quigley EMM, Lacy BE, Lembo AJ. Efficacy of prebiotics, probiotics, and synbiotics in irritable bowel syndrome and chronic idiopathic constipation: Systematic review and meta-analysis. *Am J Gastroenterol.*109(10):1547–1561.

71. Mallon P, McKay D, Kirk S, Gardiner K. Probiotics for induction of remission in ulcerative colitis. *Cochrane Database Syst Rev.* 2007(4):Cd005573.

17

Common Geriatric Infections

CHRISTINA PRATHER, MARIATU KOROMA-NELSON, AND MIKHAIL KOGAN

Case Study

A 74-year-old wheelchair-bound woman living in the community presents for evaluation of recurrent urinary tract infections (UTIs). History is notable for prior stroke, hypertension, and diabetes. She is dependent for bathing and food setup and is occasionally incontinent of urine. She lives with her daughter and participates in activities at an adult day center weekly, including art and music therapy as well as occasional physical and occupational therapy. Prior treatment for confirmed positive UTIs on urine culture included recurrent antibiotic use with oral agents such as Augmentin, ciprofloxacin, and cefpodoxime. Therapy was initiated with 1 scoop of D-mannose powder twice daily, delivering 4 g of D-mannose per day, and one 500-mg capsule of cranberry concentrate twice daily. For the following 3 years she did not have a confirmed UTI.

Incidence and Mortality of Infection in the Elderly

Immunosenescence and resultant impaired immune function lead to both increased risk and incidence of infection in the elderly. Additionally, older adults with infection have increased mortality; this observation persists across the spectrum of disease.[1] For example, the incidence of *Clostridium difficile* colitis is among the highest in the very elderly and is also associated with increased mortality rates.[2,3] Elders with chronic infections are at risk for frequent emergency room visits and hospitalizations. Additionally, sequelae of frequent infections include increased health care utilization, potentially increasing the risk for iatrogenic consequences as well as resultant physical decompensation from infection and expenditure of remaining physiological reserve.

Derangements of the Immune System in Aging

Aging is associated with a natural decline in immune functioning that is termed immunosenescence.[4] This occurs in each of the two core components of immunity: innate and adaptive immunity. Innate immunity occurs immediately. It is stimulated when circulating innate immune cells recognize a problem and initiate an immediate pathway response. Natural killer cells are a core component of innate immunity. They originate from common lymphoid tissue and stimulate the destruction of virus-infected cells or tumors cells in response to stimulatory cytokines. Response to stimulatory cytokines by natural killer cells is impaired in older individuals, resulting in suboptimal performance of this core component of innate immunity.[5] Adaptive immunity occurs later and relies on the coordination and expansion of targeted adaptive immune cells in response to a specific trigger. Adaptive immunity is compromised in aging due to impaired activation and decreased production and proliferation of T and B lymphocytes, which are the core component of this immune cascade.[6] Table 17.1 summarizes these changes in core immune system components and associated clinical implications.

Optimizing Immune Function

Physical activity and nutrition can improve immune function. Regular exercise in older adults improves Th1/Th2 cytokine balance, reduces levels of pro-inflammatory cytokines, and positively changes naïve/memory cell ratios. Moderate exercise, defined as 5 days weekly for 6 months, improved CD28 expression on T cells and improved Th1/Th2 balance.[7] Traditional Chinese practices blending martial arts, meditation, and relaxation, like qi gong and tai chi, may also improve immune-related responses. Participation in qi gong and tai chi resulted in improved antibody titers following vaccination with influenza and varicella zoster.[8,9] A recent meta-analysis demonstrated that in addition to tai chi, mind–body therapies such as yoga and meditation improve the immune system by decreasing systemic inflammation and improve response to vaccinations.[10] Nutrition interventions also correlate with improved overall immunity and Th1/Th2 balance in older

Table 17.1. Clinical Implications of Age-Associated Changes to
Core Adaptive Immune System Components

Immune System Component	Age-Associated Changes	Clinical Implications
T cells	Decrease in naïve T cells narrowing the T-cell receptor repertoire Imbalance between Th1 and Th2 responses Increased sensitivity to CD95-mediated apoptosis Decreased ratio of CD8+ CD28+ / CD28—T cells Decrease in IL-2 Decreased number of memory B cells and naïve T cells	Decreased response to immune stimulation leading to impaired vaccination response Decreased response to immune stimulation leading to increased infection risk Increased predisposition to cancer Increased risk of reactivation of chronic infections
B cells	No change in the total number of B cells Production of lower-affinity antibodies Reduced number of specific antibodies, increased number of nonspecific antibodies due to downregulation of the enzymes involved in differentiating B cells to have more specific actions B-cell clonal expansions, appearance of monoclonal antibodies	Increased risk for autoimmune disease Impaired responses to fight infection and cancer cells Decreased response to immune stimulation leading to impaired vaccination response Increased potential for late-life B-cell lymphomas

Source: National Institute of Allergy and Infectious Disease.

adults. Zinc, probiotics, vitamin D, and vitamin E play an important role in immune function.[11]

Gastrointestinal System

Gut microbiota produce an extremely diverse metabolic stock through anaerobic fermentation of exogenous undigested dietary components and generation of endogenous compounds by microorganisms and the host. The single layer of epithelial cells that makes up the mucosal interface between the host and microorganisms allows microbial metabolic products to gain access to and interact with host cells, influencing immune responses and disease risk. This area is of major clinical and research interest.[12] The system can be influenced through the use of probiotics and prebiotics, as well as by fasting and other holistic approaches. Refer to Chapter 16 for additional information.

PROBIOTICS AND PREBIOTICS

Probiotics contain active bacteria that interfere with toxin and cell-binding sites, improving function of the mucosal barrier, intestinal microflora, and gut-associated lymphoid tissue. Prebiotics influence the gut immune system via stimulation of microbial metabolism. Both appear to lower inflammation and allergies.[13]

Food-based examples of probiotics include active culture yogurt, kefir, kombucha, sauerkraut, and others. Refer to Chapters 2 and 16 for additional information. Many probiotic supplements exist, some refrigerated and some not. Practitioners should be familiar with several products that patients can obtain quickly to avoid a critical time delay to treatment.

DISEASES SPECIFIC TO THE GASTROINTESTINAL SYSTEM

C. difficile–*Associated Diarrhea*

C. difficile is one of the myriad of bacteria in naturally occurring gut flora. With antibiotic use, isolation of *C. difficile* from the originally complex gut microbiome occurs and can result in pathological *C. difficile*–associated diarrhea (CDAD). Recent data suggest that most cases of CDAD do not occur in hospitals, but rather in the community or long-term care facilities.[14] Additionally, adults presenting with CDAD from long-term care may have more severe disease due to the limited diversity of their microbiome resulting from frequent antibiotic use.[15] The standard treatment for CDAD is oral metronidazole. For severe or refractory disease, oral vancomycin with or without intravenous metronidazole is used respectively. Recently, refractory and recurrent cases of CDAD have increasingly become a public health concern.[16] Fecal transplantation has been increasingly available at major medical centers and has good efficacy in decreasing the rate of recurrent CDAD,[17,18] despite lack of regulation by the U.S. Food and Drug Administration (FDA).[19]

The integrative approach to CDAD is based on preventive strategies. In addition to minimizing the use of antibiotics when possible, optimizing the diversity of intestinal microflora appears to be the key. Adding oral probiotics from foods or supplements and eating foods rich in prebiotics are the foundation of prevention. Many positive trials and several meta-analyses

> **Box 17.1. "The Hand That Writes for Antibiotics Must Write for Probiotics"**
>
> Strong evidence exists to recommend probiotic supplementation at the time of or before starting any antibiotics course to decrease risk of CDAD. The authors recommend prescribing products where one dose contains at least 10 billion colony-forming units ([CFUs], a standard measure of probiotic potency) of mixed strains to include *S. boulardii*, *Lactobacillus*, and *Bifidobacterium*. Top products routinely have 25 billion or more CFUs containing at least eight bacterial strains per dose, administered once or twice daily.

conclusively demonstrated that prescribing probiotics at the time of or just before administering antibiotics is essential for decreasing the risk of CDAD (Box 17.1).[20,21]

In addition to beneficial bacterial species, the beneficial yeast *Saccharomyces boulardii* also decreases the risk of CDAD.[22] While some experts recommend combined use of the probiotics *S. boulardii*, *Lactobacillus*, and *Bifidobacterium* at 200 billion CFU daily, the best dose and formulation of probiotics remains to be unclear. The authors recommend using broad-spectrum probiotics of a variety of different species, often 9 or 10 or even more, and ideally also include *S. boulardii*, with a minimum of 10 billion CFU once or twice daily.

Viral Gastroenteritis

Viral gastroenteritis is generally a self-limited, brief illness characterized by nausea, abdominal cramping, vomiting, and watery diarrhea. Evaluation should include a comprehensive exposure history, including risk of foodborne illness and recent travel. Assessment should include an abdominal examination to identify rebound, guarding, or rigidity, or signs of complications or severe dehydration, both indications for hospitalization. Treatment is primarily based on symptom control with an emphasis on maintaining hydration and subsequently restoring nutrition. The mainstay of treatment is oral rehydration therapy or intravenous resuscitation, depending on availability and severity of illness. Of note, antidiarrheal agents affecting gut motility are not recommended.

Probiotics have demonstrated a good effect in shortening the duration of diarrhea and reducing stool frequency in the setting of viral gastroenteritis. Well-studied agents that are recommended include *S. boulardii*, *Lactobacillus*, and *Bifidobacterium*.[23] Preferred products would also include *S. boulardii*.

Traveler's Diarrhea

Taking *S. boulardii* and other probiotics during traveling can reduce the risk of developing traveler's diarrhea.[22,23] This is important since many older people enjoy travel. The authors recommend nonrefrigerated probiotics to all geriatric patients traveling to areas with food safety concerns. Most probiotics require refrigeration but many do not. Providers should familiarize themselves with both types so they can use them in different scenarios.

Small Intestinal Bacterial Overgrowth

Small intestinal bacterial overgrowth (SIBO) is a condition of excessive colonization of the small intestine by bacteria. It can be associated with mucosal inflammation and nutrient malabsorption and may have systemic pro-inflammatory effects resulting from pro-inflammatory cytokines stimulated by toxic agents produced by bacteria. Symptoms include bloating, abdominal discomfort, diarrhea, dyspepsia, and, in severe cases, weight loss and malnutrition.[24] SIBO may be misdiagnosed as irritable bowel syndrome (IBS), and diagnosis must rely on specialized breath tests.[25] A detailed review of functional tests used in the diagnosis of SIBO is covered in Chapter 25. SIBO may be more common in elders with lactose malabsorption.[26]

Treatment of SIBO is multifactorial and includes elimination of bacterial overgrowth, treatment of underlying disease, and nutritional support. Elimination of bacteria occurs via dietary changes and administration of oral antibiotic medications or herbs for 4 weeks.[27] The most commonly used antibiotic, rifaximin, is typically dosed at 550 mg twice daily or 200 mg two tablets TID. This regimen rarely fails, but when it does, combination with clindamycin 300 mg TID, metronidazole 250 mg TID, or neomycin 500 mg TID is generally effective.[27] A number of herbal mixed products in capsules or tinctures are on the market, but they are not covered by insurance plans. Patients who fail to respond to an herbal regimen often respond to rifaximin. Using herbs in combination with diet seems to be most reasonable first-line approach for mild cases of disease without evidence of malnutrition.

The Low-Fermentable Oligosaccharide Disaccharide Monosaccharide and Polyol Diet (FODMAP) has been rapidly gaining ground as a mainstay of treatment for mild cases of SIBO and IBS. It is suspected that IBS patients who respond to FODMAP actually have undiagnosed SIBO. Use of this diet is based on the elimination of foods with highly fermented carbohydrates that are poorly absorbed and drive increased intestinal permeability.[28] Implementation of the low FODMAP diet consists of eliminating foods high in FODMAPs for

6 to 8 weeks followed by gradual reintroduction of foods high in fermentable carbohydrates to determine individual tolerance to specific FODMAPs.[28] Recommended patient resources on the FODMAP diet are Gerald Mullin, MD's book *The Gut Balance Revolution: Boost Your Metabolism, Restore Your Inner Ecology, and Lose the Weight for Good!* and the website http://www.ibsgroup.org/brochures/fodmap-intolerances.pdf.

Nutritional support is important for all patients with SIBO. Deficiencies of calcium, magnesium, iron, vitamins D and B12, and fat-soluble vitamins should be assessed and repleted as appropriate.[24] Prolonged attention is necessary in severe cases when mucosal damage is severe and may be persistent. Use of probiotics as treatment for SIBO is controversial, although it is logical to support healthy gut microbial diversity after SIBO resolves.[29]

Skin

The skin serves multiple functions in the role of mitigating infection. It provides a barrier, resisting bacterial and fungal invasion, and initiates an immune response against penetrating foreign bodies. Repair of wounds and lacerations is important for maintaining integrity to minimize infection risk. While the quality of wound repair is not impaired in aging, the healing process is delayed and can result in increased infection risk.[30]

This section lists several natural products to treat a variety of commonly encountered skin wounds and infections. For additional information regarding nutritional support for pressure ulcers refer to Chapter 24.

Aloe is derived from aloe vera, a cactus-like, succulent plant that grows native in many tropical climates. Aloe may help in the healing of abrasions and burns,[31] but the data on wound healing are lacking.[32] Of note, aloe may be helpful for other skin conditions such as herpes infections and psoriasis.[33]

Bromelain (pineapple extract) is a protein-digesting enzyme that demonstrates in vitro and in vivo fibrinolytic, anti-edematous, antithrombotic, and anti-inflammatory activities. Its active enzyme, escharase, is beneficial for debridement of necrotic tissue and acceleration of healing. Additionally, it has anti-inflammatory properties that help with wound healing. Use is generally topical for treatment of wounds and burns using 35% bromelain in a lipid base.[34]

Melaleuca alternifolia (tea tree oil) has been used medicinally for centuries by the aboriginal people of Australia. Its mechanism of action is primarily antimicrobial and anti-inflammatory. Today, tea tree oil is used to treat a number of conditions, including acne, athlete's foot, nail fungus, wounds, infections, lice, oral candidiasis (thrush), cold sores, dandruff, and skin lesions.

Some small clinical studies have shown positive results for treating athlete's foot, nail fungus, dandruff, and acne. Use is primarily topical as it can be toxic if ingested; it is available in a standard oil called TTO (Oil of *Melaleuca*—terpinen-4-ol type), which is regulated by international standards. It is important that the oil be stored in a cool, dry, dark location as light, heat, exposure to air, and moisture all affect its stability.[35]

Hypericum perforatum (St. John's wort) contributes to wound healing through mediation of a faster inflammatory response and better wound healing. It has a longstanding history of topical use in the form of oil or tincture for treatment of minor wounds and burns, abrasions, ulcers, psoriasis, atopic dermatitis, and herpes simplex.[36] While safe for topical use, oral intake of St. John's wort is strongly discouraged in the geriatric population due to a high risk of medication interactions.[37]

Calendula officinalis (calendula or marigold), similar to aloe, tea tree oil, and St. John's wort, has been used topically for centuries. Calendula has anti-inflammatory and mild antimicrobial properties. The German Commission E approves topical use of calendula for poorly healing wounds and any inflammatory skin conditions.[38] Despite nearly universal European use, the actual randomized data for use of calendula are very limited and evidence for its efficacy in wound healing is weak.[39]

The use of topical *virgin coconut oil* is well received by patients and is often recommended as supportive therapy for mild skin infections such as tinea. While no clinical studies have demonstrated efficacy for this very cheap, safe, and rather pleasant therapy, coconut oil has clear antibacterial and antifungal properties and in vitro has been shown to be comparable to antifungal medications.[40,41] The authors frequently recommend applying topical food-grade coconut oil two or three times a day as supportive treatment for mild skin irritations. This method could be a good alternative for some extremely sensitive patients as long as they are not allergic to coconuts.

Topical *propolis* is made by honeybees to seal and sterilize parts of a hive. It has been used traditionally as a natural antiseptic. In the authors' experience, a liquid propolis tincture mixed with fractionated coconut oil or high-grade filtered honey at a 1:4 ratio is an effective antibiotic cream alternative for minor skin wound infections. One of the important advantages is that propolis has a surprisingly wide range of effectiveness against bacterial, fungal, and viral infections.[42] In addition, oral propolis was shown to effectively boost the immune system.[43] Resistance to propolis has not been documented and growing evidence indicates that it may be effective in clinical settings, at least for chronic wounds.[44]

Topical *MediHoney*, a variant of Manuka honey based on the *Leptospermum* plant (a type of myrtle native to New Zealand), has been approved by the FDA for the treatment of chronic wounds. The approval was based on a number of studies showing strong antibacterial properties and good efficacy in healing of chronic wounds.[45-47] MediHoney also appears to be effective at preventing different types of skin infections, such as at a site of hemodialysis catheter insertion and at skin damage sites.[48,49] It is available in a variety of forms, including creams, gels, and impregnated dressings. While the authors are happy to see this natural product turned into a medication, there is a lack of precise understanding as to whether MediHoney's effectiveness is linked specifically to the *Leptospermum* plant or is simply due to the fact that it is very high in propolis concentration. If the latter is correct, utilizing a dilution of pure propolis tincture into coconut oil or high-grade liquid honey should have similar efficacy and would be much less expensive.

Genitourinary System

Aging results in multiple changes to the genitourinary system and pelvic floor, resulting in increased frequency of urinary tract infections (UTIs) in many older adults. In women, vaginal epithelial atrophy associated with postmenopausal hormonal changes and weakening of the pelvic floor play a role in permitting bacterial translocation and impaired bladder emptying. In men, increased prostate volume due to benign prostatic hypertrophy or prostate cancer can also increase the risk of UTIs. In addition to maintaining good hydration and avoiding the use of mucous membrane irritants, several natural products have been researched as means to prevent UTIs.

D-mannose is a naturally occurring sugar found in some fruits and berries, including cranberries. It has a number of important metabolic functions and, similarly to the active ingredient in cranberry, it blocks bacterial adhesion to the bladder wall. In a randomized clinical trial of 308 women with a history of recurrent UTI, participants were given 2 g D-mannose daily or nitrofurantoin for 6 months after initial antibiotic treatment of acute cystitis. D-mannose powder significantly reduced the risk of recurrent UTI and was non-inferior to the nitrofurantoin group. D-mannose is slightly sweet, does not contribute to sugar or caloric load, and is very well tolerated, although occasionally some patients may get diarrhea. In addition, the authors often recommend doses above 2 g/day and in divided doses. D-mannose should be diluted in a cup of water, so this can also promote better hydration, which is often needed for geriatric patients. While doses as high as 4 to 6 g/day can be considered for therapeutic use for acute UTI in early phases, this is not supported by evidence and carries a higher risk of bloating and diarrhea.

Use of *cranberry extract* has been classically associated with UTI prevention. The amount of D-mannose in cranberries is too low for this to be the

> **Box 17.2. Combination of Cranberry and D-Mannose for UTI**
>
> Given the favorable safety profile, once- or twice-daily use of a commercially available mix of D-mannose and cranberry extract with a ratio of 2 gm to 1 gm is recommended as a preventive strategy for patients with frequent UTIs.

source of its efficacy. Cranberries contain proanthocyanidins that block the adhesion of some types of *Escherichia coli* to uroepithelial cells.[50] Hence, one would expect that only *E. coli*–positive UTI prophylaxis would make sense. The literature overall is not robust for cranberry use for UTI prevention. A recent large randomized controlled trial comprising nearly 1,000 patients conducted in long-term care facilities demonstrated modest (26%) risk reduction of UTI in patients taking cranberry capsules.[51] Given its low risk and high potential quality-of-life benefit, regular use is endorsed and implemented by the authors. It is best not to use cranberry juice, however, given its high sugar concentration. Cranberry extracts are readily available in the form of capsules or tablets. The ideal dose is unclear, especially given the variability of products on the market.

While no studies have investigated the combination of D-mannose and cranberry extract, it appears to be the logical next research step. Given the favorable safety profile and existing evidence, the authors utilize a commercially available mix of powdered D-mannose and cranberry extract at a ratio of 2 grams to 1 gram, twice daily, taken with a glass of water (Box 17.2).

Respiratory System

COMMON UPPER RESPIRATORY INFECTION

The most commonly encountered infectious disease of the pulmonary system is the upper respiratory infection (URI) or a similar viral infection with a varying presentation such as bronchitis. Symptoms are well known to most people and classically include nasal drainage and congestion, sore throat, sinus pressure, sneezing, and cough. Reactive airways may result in a prolonged cough or predominant cough in the symptom complex, resulting in a condition more characteristic of bronchitis than the common cold as generally experienced. Notably, cough can last for several days or weeks, prompting inquiries for antibiotic use, which is inappropriate for these viral infections.

Due to the aging process, changes in the lungs contribute to an increased incidence of pulmonary infections, and an increased risk of mortality from them, in the elderly.[52] In addition to having impaired physiological mechanisms to overcome infection, the pro-inflammatory response can precipitate asthma or an exacerbation of chronic obstructive pulmonary disease, the latter a commonly encountered comorbidity for older adults who are hospitalized or acutely ill with pneumonia or a viral URI.[53]

Treatment of viral URI is predominantly symptomatic. There is no cure for the common cold and for each of the following treatment options discussed, only modest symptomatic benefit is reported in the supporting literature.

Botanicals

Andrographis paniculata, from the ayurvedic tradition, is commonly used to treat or prevent the common cold. A systematic review of seven double-blinded randomized controlled trials with nearly 1,000 total subjects supports that *A. paniculata* is superior to placebo in alleviating symptoms of the common cold or uncomplicated URI.[54] This herb is generally well tolerated but at high doses can cause transient elevation of liver enzymes. The dose is one 300-mg tablet four times daily taken for several days at the onset of symptoms.

Several species of *Echinacea* have been discussed in the treatment of the common cold, including *angustifolia, purpurea*, and *pallida*. There is extensive research on the role of *Echinacea* in symptom management for respiratory illness, and despite many studies demonstrating trends toward positive outcomes, there are a roughly equal number of trials refuting its efficacy.[55] The best-studied type of echinacea is *E. purpurea*. Recommended doses are 50 to 1,000 mg of standardized extract or 1 to 3 ml of tincture in divided doses daily. Side effects are mild and uncommon.

Sambucus canadensis (elderberry) is a tree native to Europe, Asia, Africa, and some areas in the United States. It is traditionally used to treat pain, swelling, infections, cough, and skin conditions. An in vitro study show that the flavonoids in elderberry bind to and deactivate flu viruses.[56] Small studies show that elderberry may shorten the length of flu symptoms.[57] Elderberry usually comes as sweet syrup and with short use, side effects are not known.

Allium sativum L. (garlic) is used in many medical conditions due to its antioxidant, antiplatelet, antihypertensive, antihyperlipidemic, chemotherapeutic, and antimicrobial properties.[58] Its organosulfur compound, allicin, contributes to its antimicrobial and antifungal properties. Use of high-dose allicin extract (180 mg/day) for 12 weeks during the winter months in one study resulted in 64% fewer colds, and symptom duration was reduced by 70%.[59] However, a Cochrane review concluded that the evidence is insufficient, as only one study ended up meeting the selection criteria.[60] There is a theoretical risk of bleeding for patients on antiplatelet therapy, but this is probably unlikely with typical food-based intake.

Ginseng stimulates antibodies, natural killer cell activity, and production of cytokines, lymphocytes, and T-helper cells to combat infection.[61] Multiple randomized studies demonstrated a preventive effect and shortening of duration of cold symptoms. A systematic review of a number of studies concluded that North American ginseng is effective in preventing colds.[62,63] Ginseng is well tolerated with minimal side effects, although it notably can cause insomnia, which is already a common complaint of many older adults, as well as tachycardia and palpitations, which may preclude its use in this population. Dosage is suggested at 100 to 200 mg/day.

Pelargonium sidoides (Umckaloabo) is an herbal extract available in both tablet and liquid forms. Scientific evidence for its use is limited. There have been Cochrane reviews on this topic, most recently in 2013, concluding that it has possible efficacy although most studies were of poor methodology.[64,65] Clinical trials used a dose of 30 drops three times daily of 11% aqueous ethoanolic extract equivalent to 8 g of extracted plant material or a highly concentrated tincture dosed at 1 ml two to four times a day. Side effects are uncommon and mild.

Nutritional Supplements

Polyunsaturated fatty acids (PUFA), including eicosapentaenoic acid (EPA), docosahexaenoic acid (DHA) and alpha-linolenic acid, have anti-inflammatory properties that have been effective in the treatment of infectious diseases. EPA and DHA are found in fish oil and cod liver oil. Alpha-linolenic acids are found in flaxseed oil, walnuts, peanuts, and spinach. In animal studies, there was a significant decrease in pneumonia symptoms and bacterial burden with dietary supplementation of omega-3 PUFA (flaxseed oil and Fish Oil) compared to control.[11]

Vitamins C and D have long played a role in the treatment of respiratory infections. Vitamin D has a historical role for use in URI as well as tuberculosis. It has been shown that individuals receiving vitamin D 1,000 to 2,000 IU daily have a reduced risk of URI, including pneumonia and sinusitis.[66] Vitamin C in particular has been extensively studied, specifically for its role in prevention and treatment of URI. A 2013 Cochrane review concluded "given the consistent effect of vitamin C on the duration and severity of colds in the regular supplementation studies, and the low cost and safety, it may be worthwhile for common cold patients to test on an individual basis whether therapeutic vitamin C is beneficial for them."[67]

Trials use daily doses of 1 to 8 g. Doses of more than 5 g/day may cause diarrhea and should be taken with caution.

High-dose intravenous use of vitamin C (IVC), 25 to 200 g/infusion, has been used in many integrative medicine clinics for a variety of infections, but few clinical trials have been performed. IVC triggers production of low-dose hydrogen peroxide, which is toxic to many infectious organisms. Pilot studies show possible effectiveness in treating sepsis,[68] Epstein-Barr virus infections,[69] and shingles.[70] High-dose IVC appears to be remarkably safe, but it is not routinely covered by insurance and is costly.[71] Most patients getting IVC receive it for cancer. This topic is beyond the scope of this chapter; see Chapter 21 for additional information.

Zinc, like vitamin C, has a long history of use for treatment of cold symptoms. A 2011 Cochrane review concluded that zinc does shorten the length and decreases the severity of cold symptoms if administered within 24 hours from the onset of symptoms.[72] Zinc lozenges, 13 to 23 mg, used every 2 hours or oral elemental zinc gluconate, 9 to 24 mg every 2 hours, may reduce symptom severity and duration of symptoms. Use of nasal zinc is essentially contraindicated after the nasal formulation, Zicam, was removed from the market by the FDA due to loss of smell resulting from use. In two small randomized controlled trials, the combination of zinc 10 mg and vitamin C 1,000 mg daily showed synergistic effect.[73] The authors routinely recommend this low-cost and safe approach to elderly patients.

Probiotics

The use of probiotics in the prevention and treatment of pulmonary illness, including the common cold, is inconsistent. A recent meta-analysis showed modest risk reduction.[74] Given the high safety profile, it may be a reasonable idea to recommend an oral course of probiotics for patients with a history of frequent colds.

SINUSITIS

Chronic sinusitis is a very common condition in older adults, affecting nearly 15% of the population, with a slightly higher incidence in women.[75] The mucous lining of the nasal passages and sinuses represents a continuation of the respiratory epithelium and serves to filter, humidify, and regulate the temperature of air entering the body. It is a vital component of the immune system and a first line of defense against pathogens, including viruses, bacteria, pollen, pollutants, smoke, dust, and other potentially harmful particles. Chronic inflammation of this mucous membrane drives the underlying process of chronic sinusitis. Identifying potential irritants may be a therapeutic target for many patients. An additional population of patients worth mentioning are those with chronic sinusitis who have concurrent fungal growth in the nasal mucosa. A prominent study from the Mayo Clinic showed that of 210 patients with chronic sinusitis, 96% had concurrent fungal infection.[76] A comprehensive review of the pathophysiology of the disease and epidemiological risk factors is beyond the scope of this text, but it is worth noting that an additional contribution to acute and chronic sinusitis in the elderly results from weakening of the nasal cartilage and resultant narrowing of the nasal passage, according to the American Academy of Otolaryngology—Head and Neck Surgery.

Treatment of chronic sinusitis through the integrative approach includes adherence to several components of therapy: treating and preventing infections and colds; practicing nasal hygiene; eating an anti-inflammatory and hypoallergenic diet; improving indoor air quality; treating yeast overgrowth or fungal sinusitis; detoxification; strengthening and restoring immune system balance; and tissue healing through mental, emotional, spiritual, and social health factors.[77]

For acute and even chronic sinusitis, a trial of intranasal steroids is an acceptable strategy.[78] Prescribing oral antibiotics should be limited, however, to bacterial or fungal infections, which are much less common. Most often antibiotics are overprescribed due to patient demands. When a patient is suspected to have bacterial sinusitis or natural methods do not work and a patient insists on the use of antibiotics, the authors often recommend compounded nasal sprays that include antibiotic/antifungal medication(s) combined with quercetin and/or steroids. This helps to deliver local treatment, minimizing generalized negative effects of oral antibiotics on gut microbial flora. Contacting local compounding pharmacies to learn about available formulations is a good starting place.

Garlic is highly effective in treatment of sinusitis given its antibacterial, antiviral, and antifungal properties when taken at therapeutic doses. A recommended dose for a sinus infection is Allimed, two capsules three times daily for 10 days, or Allimax, five capsules three times daily for 10 days. For treating colds and preventing sinus infections, the recommended dose is, at the first sign of a cold, Allimed, two capsules (or Allimax, five capsules) three times daily for 2 to 3 days; after symptoms subside, continue one capsule of Allimed (or Allimax two capsules) twice daily for 2 to 3 days.[77]

Grape seed extract is used for its antioxidant, anti-inflammatory, and antihistamine effects. The recommended dose is 300 mg/day on an empty stomach.[77]

Nasal saline irrigation may improve symptoms of URI as well as acute and chronic sinusitis. Irrigation is typically performed with a warm salt-water solution multiple times daily for the first several days of symptoms. Proper cleaning of the irrigation equipment is necessary to avoid the risk of serious infections.

Dietary modification that optimizes immune function should be maintained. Sugar, dairy, wheat, gn-based carbohydrates, alcohol, and caffeine should be avoided due to their weakening effects on immunity or pro-inflammatory response to intake. Anti-inflammatory and elimination diets are reviewed in Chapter 2.

Candida-Related Illnesses

Candida can colonize any body cavity that is open to the external environment, including nasal passages, sinuses, the gastrointestinal tract, and the vagina. It is also a common skin colonizer and thus is a frequent source of infection. Most of the time *Candida* colonization does not represent a significant clinical problem, but in patients with a weakened immune system and dysbiosis, *Candida* overgrowth can occur, resulting in systemic symptoms such as headaches, fatigue, anxiety, chronic sinusitis, and skin rashes. Diagnosing *Candida* overgrowth can be difficult. Cultures are considered the gold standard but may not be easily obtainable due to location or limitations related to sample collection. Commonly available *Candida* serum antibodies are not diagnostic and should not be used routinely. Many integrative and functional medicine practitioners pursue diagnosis through use of specialized functional stool tests that are described in detail in Chapter 25. An alternative method used by many integrative medicine providers is the Candida Questionnaire. This method is simple, and although strong evidence supporting its use is lacking, it may be one of the best diagnostic tools. The questionnaire can be found at http://yeastconnection.com/pdf/yeastfullsurv.pdf

Treatment for *Candida* overgrowth always starts with diet changes. Most patients respond well to implementation of an anti-*Candida* diet. The most important part of this diet is complete avoidance of all sugars and rapidly metabolized simple carbohydrates (e.g., breads, potatoes). Please see Chapter 2 for details on this diet.

In addition to dietary modifications, several herbal and antifungal medications are available for use in a variety of formulations. The duration of treatment is typically several weeks to months. Garlic (*Allium sativum*), berberine from Oregon grape root, or other botanicals such as milk thistle, sage, thyme, and lemon balm can be used.[79] Fluconazole and other systemic anti-fungals should be used with caution due to possible liver toxicity. Nystatin is the preferred medication for *Candida* overgrowth due to lack of intestinal absorption.

Antibiotic Stewardship

The authors seek to reinforce the importance of antibiotic stewardship in clinical practice. The increasing incidence of inappropriate antibiotic use is associated with increased bacterial resistance but also can lead to adverse drug events and undesirable outcomes, especially in older adults. According to the Centers for Disease Control and Prevention (CDC), close to 50% of antibiotic prescriptions are inappropriate and contribute to unnecessary hospitalization, morbidity, and mortality. The book *Missing Microbes: How the Overuse of Antibiotics Is Fueling Our Modern Plagues* by Dr. Blaser provides an excellent review of this topic for consumers and clinicians alike.[80]

Key Web Resources

National Institute of Allergy and Infectious Disease (https://www.niaid.nih.gov/): federally funded program with main focus on "Leading research to understand, treat, and prevent infectious, immunologic, and allergic diseases"

Candida Questionnaire: http://yeastconnection.com/pdf/yeastfullsurv.pdf

FODMAP diet brochure: http://www.ibsgroup.org/brochures/fodmap-intolerances.pdf

REFERENCES

1. Heppner HJ, Cornel S, Peter W, Philipp B, Katrin S. Infections in the elderly. *Crit Care Clin.* 2013;29(3):757–774. doi:10.1016/j.ccc.2013.03.016.
2. Rupnik M, Wilcox MH, Gerding DN. *Clostridium difficile* infection: New developments in epidemiology and pathogenesis. *Nat Rev Microbiol.* 2009;7(7):526–536. doi:10.1038/nrmicro2164.
3. Zilberberg MD, Shorr AF, Micek ST, Doherty J, Kollef MH. *Clostridium difficile*-associated disease and mortality among the elderly critically ill. *Crit Care Med.* 2009;37(9):2583–2589. doi:10.1097/CCM.0b013e3181ab8388.

4. Denkinger MD, Leins H, Schirmbeck R, Florian MC, Geiger H. HSC aging and senescent immune remodeling. *Trends Immunol.* 2015;36(12):815–824. doi:10.1016/j.it.2015.10.008.

5. Gomez CR, Gomez CR, Boehmer ED, Boehmer ED, Kovacs EJ, Kovacs EJ. The aging innate immune system. *Curr Opin Immunol.* 2005;17(5):457–462. doi:10.1016/j.coi.2005.07.013.

6. Weng N. Aging of the immune system: How much can the adaptive immune system adapt? *Immunity.* 2006;24(5):495–499. doi:10.1016/j.immuni.2006.05.001.

7. Senchina DS, Kohut ML. Immunological outcomes of exercise in older adults. *Clin Interv Aging.* 2007;2(1):3–16. doi:10.2147/ciia.2007.2.1.3.

8. Irwin MR, Pike JL, Cole JC, Oxman MN. Effects of a behavioral intervention, tai chi chih, on varicella-zoster virus specific immunity and health functioning in older adults. *Psychosom Med.* 2003;65(5):824–830. http://www.psychosomaticmedicine.org/cgi/content/abstract/65/5/824.

9. Yang Y, Verkuilen J, Rosengren KS, et al. Effects of a Taiji and Qigong intervention on the antibody response to influenza vaccine in older adults. *Am J Chin Med.* 2007;35(4):597–607. doi:10.1142/S0192415X07005090.

10. Morgan N, Irwin MR, Chung M, Wang C. The effects of mind-body therapies on the immune system: Meta-analysis. *PLoS One.* 2014;9(7). doi:10.1371/journal.pone.0100903.

11. Pae M, Meydani SN, Wu D. The role of nutrition in enhancing immunity in aging. *Aging Dis.* 2012;3(1):91–129. doi:10.1007/978-94-017-9331-5.

12. Rooks MG, Garrett WS. Gut microbiota, metabolites and host immunity. *Nat Rev Immunol.* 2016;16(6):341–352. doi:10.1038/nri.2016.42.

13. Gourbeyre P, Denery S, Bodinier M. Probiotics, prebiotics, and synbiotics: Impact on the gut immune system and allergic reactions. *J Leukoc Biol.* 2011;89(5):685–695. doi:10.1189/jlb.1109753.

14. Garg S, Mirza YR, Girotra M, et al. Epidemiology of *Clostridium difficile*-associated disease (CDAD): A shift from hospital-acquired infection to long-term care facility-based infection. *Dig Dis Sci.* 2013;58(12):3407–3412. doi:10.1007/s10620-013-2848-x.

15. Makris AT, Gelone S. *Clostridium difficile* in the long-term care setting. *J Am Med Dir Assoc.* 2007;8(5):290–299. doi:10.1016/j.jamda.2007.01.098.

16. Stepan C, Surawicz CM. Treatment strategies for recurrent and refractory *Clostridium difficile*-associated diarrhea. *Expert Rev Gastroenterol Hepatol.* 2007;1(2):295–305. doi:10.1586/17474124.1.2.295.

17. Youngster I, Sauk J, Pindar C, et al. Fecal microbiota transplant for relapsing *Clostridium difficile* infection using a frozen inoculum from unrelated donors: A randomized, open-label, controlled pilot study. *Clin Infect Dis.* 2014;58(11):1515–1522. doi:10.1093/cid/ciu135.

18. Jorup-Rönström C, Håkanson A, Sandell S, et al. Fecal transplant against relapsing *Clostridium difficile*-associated diarrhea in 32 patients. *Scand J Gastroenterol.* 2012;47:548–552. doi:10.3109/00365521.2012.672587.

19. Vyas D, Aekka A, Vyas A. Fecal transplant policy and legislation. *World J Gastroenterol.* 2015;21(1):6–11. doi:10.3748/wjg.v21.i1.6.

20. Lau CS, Chamberlain RS. Probiotics are effective at preventing *Clostridium difficile*-associated diarrhea: A systematic review and meta-analysis. *Int J Gen Med.* 2016;9:27–37. doi:10.2147/IJGM.S98280.

21. Pattani R, Palda VA, Hwang SW, Shah PS. Probiotics for the prevention of antibiotic-associated diarrhea and *Clostridium difficile* infection among hospitalized patients: Systematic review and meta-analysis. *Open Med.* 2013;7(2).

22. McFarland LV. Systematic review and meta-analysis of *Saccharomyces boulardii* in adult patients. *World J Gastroenterol.* 2010;16(18):2202–2222. doi:10.3748/wjg.v16.i18.2202.

23. Allen SJ, Martinez EG, Gregorio GV, Dans LF. Probiotics for treating acute infectious diarrhoea. *Cochrane Database Syst Rev.* 2010;(11):CD003048. doi:10.1002/14651858.CD003048.pub3.

24. Bures J, Cyrany J, Kohoutova D, et al. Small intestinal bacterial overgrowth syndrome. *World J Gastroenterol.* 2010;16(24):2978–2990. doi:10.3748/wjg.v16.i24.2978.

25. Shah ED, Basseri RJ, Chong K, Pimentel M. Abnormal breath testing in IBS: A meta-analysis. *Dig Dis Sci.* 2010;55(9):2441–2449. doi:10.1007/s10620-010-1276-4.

26. Almeida JA, Kim R, Stoita A, McIver CJ, Kurtovic J, Riordan SM. Lactose malabsorption in the elderly: role of small intestinal bacterial overgrowth. *Scand J Gastroenterol.* 2008;43(2):146–154. doi:10.1080/00365520701676617.

27. Chedid V, Dhalla S, Clarke JO, et al. Herbal therapy is equivalent to rifaximin for the treatment of small intestinal bacterial overgrowth. *Glob Adv Heal Med.* 2014;3(3):16–24. doi:10.7453/gahmj.2014.019.

28. Digestive Health Center. The Low FODMAP Diet (FODMAP = Fermentable Oligo-Di-Monosaccharides and Polyols). *Stanford Hosp Clin.* 2012;2012(1):1–3. doi:10.5867/medwave.2006.10.1013.

29. Quigley EMM, Quera R. Small intestinal bacterial overgrowth: Roles of antibiotics, prebiotics, and probiotics. *Gastroenterology.* 2006;130:S78–S90. doi:10.1053/j.gastro.2005.11.046.

30. Gerstein AD, Phillips TJ, Rogers GS, Gilchrest BA. Wound healing and aging. *Dermatol Clin.* 1993;11(4):749–757. doi:10.1111/1523-1747.ep12532775.

31. Maenthaisong R, Chaiyakunapruk N, Niruntraporn S, Kongkaew C. The efficacy of aloe vera used for burn wound healing: A systematic review. *Burns.* 2007;33(6):713–718. doi:10.1016/j.burns.2006.10.384.

32. Dat AD, Poon F, Pham KBT, Doust J. Aloe vera for treating acute and chronic wounds. *Cochrane Database Syst Rev.* 2012;2(2):CD008762. doi:10.1002/14651858.CD008762.pub2.

33. Vogler BK, Ernst E. Aloe vera: A systematic review of its clinical effectiveness. *Br J Gen Pract.* 1999;49(447):823–828.

34. Pavan R, Jain S, Shraddha, Kumar A. Properties and therapeutic application of bromelain: A review. *Biotechnol Res Int.* 2012;2012:976203. doi:10.1155/2012/976203.

35. Carson CF, Hammer KA, Riley TV. *Melaleuca alternifolia* (tea tree) oil: A review of antimicrobial and other medicinal properties. *Clin Microbiol Rev.* 2006;19(1):50–62. doi:10.1128/CMR.19.1.50-62.2006.

36. Wölfle U, Seelinger G, Schempp CM. Topical application of St John's wort (Hypericum perforatum). *Planta Med.* 2014;80(2-3):109–120. doi:10.1055/s-0033-1351019.

37. Borrelli F, Izzo A. Herb–drug interactions with St. John's wort (*Hypericum perforatum*): An update on clinical observations. *AAPS J.* 2009;11(4):710–727. doi:10.1208/s12248-009-9146-8.

38. Braun L. Calendula (*Calendula officinalis*). *J Complement Med.* 2005;4(6):78–81. http://search.informit.com.au.ezproxy.endeavour.edu.au/documentSummary;dn=088804148229746;res=IELHEA.

39. Leach MJ. Calendula officinalis and wound healing: A systematic review. *Wounds A Compend Clin Res Pract.* 2008;20(8):236–243. http://search.ebscohost.com/login.aspx?direct=true&db=jlh&AN=105660747&site=ehost-live.

40. DebMandal M, Mandal S. Coconut (*Cocos nucifera* L.: Arecaceae): In health promotion and disease prevention. *Asian Pac J Trop Med.* 2011;4(3):241–247. doi:10.1016/S1995-7645(11)60078-3.

41. Ogbolu D, Oni A, Daini O, Oloko A. In vitro antimicrobial properties of coconut oil on *Candida* species in Ibadan, Nigeria. *J Med Food.* 2007;10(2):384–387. doi:10.1089/jmf.2006.1209.

42. Toreti VC, Sato HH, Pastore GM, Park YK. Recent progress of propolis for its biological and chemical compositions and its botanical origin. *Evidence Based Complement Altern Med.* 2013;2013. doi:10.1155/2013/697390.

43. Sforcin JM. Propolis and the immune system: A review. *J Ethnopharmacol.* 2007;113(1):1–14. doi:10.1016/j.jep.2007.05.012.

44. Kucharzewski M, Kózka M, Urbanek T. Topical treatment of nonhealing venous leg ulcer with propolis ointment. *Evidence Based Complement Altern Med.* 2013;2013. doi:10.1155/2013/254017.

45. Biglari B, vd Linden PH, Simon A, Aytac S, Gerner HJ, Moghaddam A. Use of MediHoney as a non-surgical therapy for chronic pressure ulcers in patients with spinal cord injury. *Spinal Cord.* 2012;50(2):165–169. doi:10.1038/sc.2011.87.

46. Robson V, Dodd S, Thomas S. Standardized antibacterial honey (Medihoney) with standard therapy in wound care: Randomized clinical trial. *J Adv Nurs.* 2009;65(3):565–575. doi:10.1111/j.1365-2648.2008.04923.x.

47. George NM, Cutting KF. Antibacterial honey (Medihoney™): in-vitro activity against clinical isolates of MRSA, VRE, and other multiresistant gram-negative organisms including *Pseudomonas aeruginosa*. *Wounds A Compend Clin Res Pract.* 2007;19(9):231–236.

48. Greenwood M, Handsaker J. Honey and Medihoney barrier cream: Their role in protecting and repairing skin. *Br J Community Nurs.* 2012;17(12 Suppl.):S32–S37. doi:10.1111/j.1468-2494.

49. Van Biesen W, Jorres A. Medihoney: Let nature do the work? *Lancet Infect Dis.* 2014;14(1):2–3. doi:10.1016/S1473-3099(13)70284-6.

50. Howell AB, Reed JD, Krueger CG, Winterbottom R, Cunningham DG, Leahy M. A-type cranberry proanthocyanidins and uropathogenic bacterial

anti-adhesion activity. *Phytochemistry*. 2005;66(18 Spec. Iss.):2281–2291. doi:10.1016/j.phytochem.2005.05.022.

51. Caljouw MAA, Van Den Hout WB, Putter H, Achterberg WP, Cools HJM, Gussekloo J. Effectiveness of cranberry capsules to prevent urinary tract infections in vulnerable older persons: A double-blind randomized placebo-controlled trial in long-term care facilities. *J Am Geriatr Soc*. 2014;62(1):103–110. doi:10.1111/jgs.12593.

52. Louie JK, Yagi S, Nelson FA, et al. Rhinovirus outbreak in a long term care facility for elderly persons associated with unusually high mortality. *Clin Infect Dis*. 2005;41(2):262–265. doi:10.1086/430915.

53. Gern JE, Busse WW. The role of viral infections in the natural history of asthma. *J Allergy Clin Immunol*. 2000;106(2):201–212. doi:10.1067/mai.2000.108604.

54. Coon JT, Ernst E. *Andrographis paniculata* in the treatment of upper respiratory tract infections: A systematic review of safety and efficacy. *Planta Med*. 2004;70(4):293–298. doi:10.1055/s-2004-818938.

55. Karsch-Volk M, Barrett B, Kiefer D, Bauer R, Ardjomand-Woelkart K, Linde K. Echinacea for preventing and treating the common cold (Review). *Cochrane Libr*. 2014;(2):1–72.

56. Roschek B, Fink RC, McMichael MD, Li D, Alberte RS. Elderberry flavonoids bind to and prevent H1N1 infection in vitro. *Phytochemistry*. 2009;70(10):1255–1261. doi:10.1016/j.phytochem.2009.06.003.

57. Zakay-Rones Z, Thom E, Wollan T, Wadstein J. Randomized study of the efficacy and safety of oral elderberry extract in the treatment of influenza A and B virus infections. *J Int Med Res*. 2004;32:132–140. doi:10.1177/147323000403200205.

58. Bayan L, Koulivand PH, Gorji A. Garlic: A review of potential therapeutic effects. *Avicenna J Phytomedicine*. 2014;4(1):1–14.

59. Josling P. Preventing the common cold with a garlic supplement: a double-blind, placebo-controlled survey. *Adv Ther*. 2001;18(4):189–193. doi:10.1007/BF02850113.

60. Lissiman E, Bhasale AL, Cohen M. Garlic for the common cold. *Cochrane Database Syst Rev*. 2009;(3). doi:10.1002/14651858.CD006206.pub2.

61. Kiefer D, Pantuso T. *Panax ginseng*. Am Fam Physician. 2003;68(8):1539–1542.

62. McElhaney JE, Gravenstein S, Cole SK, et al. A placebo-controlled trial of a proprietary extract of North American ginseng (CVT-E002) to prevent acute respiratory illness in institutionalized older adults. *J Am Geriatr Soc*. 2004;52(1):13–19. doi:10.1111/j.1532-5415.2004.52004.x.

63. Kuhle S, Seida JK, Durec T. North American (*Panax quinquefolius*) and Asian ginseng (*Panax ginseng*) preparations for prevention of the common cold in healthy adults: A systematic review. *Evidence Based Complement Altern Med*. 2011;2011. doi:10.1093/ecam/nep068.

64. Timmer A, Günther J, Rücker G, Motschall E, Antes G, Kern WV. Pelargonium sidoides extract for acute respiratory tract infections. *Cochrane Database Syst Rev*. 2008;(3). doi:10.1002/14651858.CD006323.pub2.

65. Timmer A, Günther J, Motschall E, Rücker G, Antes G, Kern WV. *Pelargonium sidoides* extract for treating acute respiratory tract infections. *Cochrane Database Syst Rev*. 2013;10(10):1–93. doi:10.1002/14651858.CD006323.pub3.

66. Zittermann A, Pilz S, Hoffmann H, März W. Vitamin D and airway infections: A European perspective. *Eur J Med Res.* 2016;21:14. doi:10.1186/s40001-016-0208-y.

67. Hemila H, Chalker E. Vitamin C for preventing and treating the common cold. *Cochrane Database Syst Rev.* 2013;1:Cd000980. doi:10.1002/14651858.CD000980. pub4.

68. Fowler AA, Syed AA, Knowlson S, et al. Phase I safety trial of intravenous ascorbic acid in patients with severe sepsis. *J Transl Med.* 2014;12:32.

69. Mikirova N, Hunninghake R. Effect of high-dose vitamin C on Epstein-Barr viral infection. *Med Sci Monit.* 2014;20:725–732. doi:10.12659/MSM.890423.

70. Schencking M, Vollbracht C, Weiss G, et al. Intravenous vitamin C in the treatment of shingles: Results of a multicenter prospective cohort study. *Med Sci Monit.* 2012;18(4):CR215–24.

71. Padayatty SJ, Sun AY, Chen Q, Espey MG, Drisko J, Levine M. Vitamin C: Intravenous use by complementary and alternative medicine practitioners and adverse effects. *PLoS One.* 2010;5(7). doi:10.1371/journal.pone.0011414.

72. Singh M, Das RR. Zinc for the common cold (Review). *Cochrane Database Syst Rev.* 2011;(2):1–71. doi:10.1002/14651858.CD001364.pub3.

73. Maggini S, Beveridge S, Suter M. A combination of high-dose vitamin C plus zinc for the common cold. *J Int Med Res.* 2012;40(401):28–42. doi:10.1177/14732300204000104.

74. Kang E-J, Kim SY, Hwang I-H, Ji Y-J. The effect of probiotics on prevention of common cold: a meta-analysis of randomized controlled trial studies. *Korean J Fam Med.* 2013;34(1):2–10. doi:10.4082/kjfm.2013.34.1.2.

75. Kaliner MA, Osguthorpe JD, Fireman P, et al. Sinusitis: Bench to bedside. Current findings, future directions. *Otolaryngol Head Neck Surg.* 1997;116(6 Pt 2):S1–S20.

76. Ponikau JU, Sherris DA, Kern EB, et al. The diagnosis and incidence of allergic fungal sinusitis. *Mayo Clin Proc.* 1999;74(9):877–884. doi:10.4065/74.9.877.

77. Ivker RS, Silvers WS, Anderson RA. Clinical observations and seven-and-one-half-year follow-up of patients using an integrative holistic approach for treating chronic sinusitis. *Altern Ther Health Med.* 2009;15(1):36–43.

78. Hayward G, Heneghan C, Perera R, Thompson M. Intranasal corticosteroids in management of acute sinusitis: A systematic review and meta-analysis. *Ann Fam Med.* 2012;10(3):241–249. doi:10.1370/afm.1338.

79. Kogan M, Castillo CC, Barber MS. Chronic rhinosinusitis and irritable bowel syndrome: A case report. *Integr Med (Encinitas).* 2016;15(3):44–54.

80. Blaser MJ. *Missing Microbes: How the Overuse of Antibiotics Is Fueling Our Modern Plagues.* New York: Henry Holt Co LLC; 2014;35(9):261.

18

Integrated Approaches to Treating Lung Diseases in the Geriatric Population

SEEMA RAO

Case Study

Mary, a youthful and active 65-year-old, worked as an executive manager at a prominent firm. She lived a very productive life, which was interrupted by a hospitalization for asthma. After her discharge from the hospital Mary came to us for a follow-up appointment. Mary was very upset with her diagnosis of asthma as she never had any history of asthma as a child or a teenager. She never smoked in her life. Mary had a history of allergy to cats but insisted that she had had no close contact with cats for many years. Mary loved nature and liked to take long walks. For 2 to 3 months before her admission to the hospital, she started experiencing tightness of the chest and shortness of breath that interfered with her walks. Mary attributed that to her work stress and fatigue. Fifteen to 20 days before her admission to the hospital, she developed a dry cough that was aggravated by speaking and exhaling. Prior to her hospitalization, Mary went on a hiking trip with her friends. After that trip, her shortness of breath and tightness of the chest increased and she was not able to breathe.

A thorough history was taken and a physical examination was performed. The patient has no history of allergies, no history of GERD or heartburn, had been taking hormone replacement therapy for 5 years, and experienced job stress as an executive. Physical examination showed tightness of her bilateral rhomboid muscles and tenderness of the thenar eminence (lung acupuncture point 9), right > left. Pulmonary function test showed that FEV1 was 59% predicted. After bronchodilator treatment it improved to 102%. The patient was treated on the same visit with acupuncture that brought immediate relief to her feeling of tightness in the chest.

The patient was recommended to hold hormone replacement therapy, was prescribed fish oil and vitamin C 1,500 mg/day, and hops liquid extract 0.5 ml three times a day. She was advised to increase the amount and number of fresh fruits and vegetables in her diet. Breathing exercises were prescribed. The patient was encouraged to keep a diary for peak flow meter readings to encourage her to be a partner in disease management.

The patient followed up for acupuncture visits. She stopped coughing and did not experience shortness of breath and chest tightness after two treatments. She was gradually able to return to her previous life with more enthusiasm and functionality. She was encouraged to participate in mindfulness meditation so that she could enjoy working without being part of the stress that comes with the process.

Introduction

The prevalence of pulmonary diseases such as chronic obstructive pulmonary disease (COPD) increases with age, and with the projected increase in the geriatric population in the next decades, it is likely that more geriatric patients will be developing pulmonary complaints in the future.[1] The trajectory of pulmonary diseases in the elderly is chronic, remitting and relapsing, and tenuous in course, and in turn it affects the functional status of the elderly patient. Pulmonary diseases have a negative impact on morbidity and mortality and quality of life in older patients with uncontrolled and untreated pulmonary symptoms.[2] Holistic integrative approaches, as an adjunct to standard of care, could be useful in improving quality of life and functionality in the elderly population.[3]

Figure 18.1 shows changes that occur in the aging lung.

Asthma

Asthma in older adults affects quality of life and results in a higher hospitalization rate and mortality.[17] After childhood the prevalence of asthma has a second peak, affecting 4% to 8% of the population above the age of 65 years.[18] This population accounts for more than 50% of total asthma fatalities annually.[19] In common clinical practice, asthma in the elderly is either underdiagnosed and undertreated, or overdiagnosed and mistreated.[17]

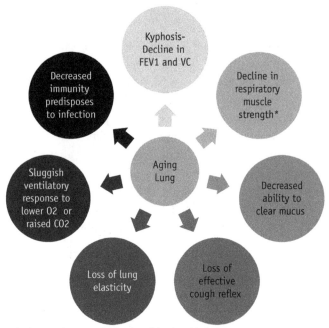

*Diaphragmatic strength is reduced in the elderly by 25%.

FIGURE 18.1. Structural and functional changes in the respiratory system due to aging.[4–16]

Neutrophil-predominant inflammation increases with age and is generally more severe and difficult to control.[20] Asthma in the elderly population is often non-atopic and more severe; it mainly affects females[21] and is associated with a faster decline in lung function and a low remission rate.[22] Although atopy is considered to be less common in older adults, sensitization to cat allergen[23] and household dust mites[24] has been associated with late-onset asthma. Sensitization to mold and cockroaches can increase the prevalence of asthma in the elderly.[25] Mycotoxin-producing species of mold include *Fusarium, Trichoderma*, and *Stachybotrys atra*. Many of the reported symptoms due to mold allergy are subjective and difficult to quantify, and symptoms have been associated with moisture damage and moldy buildings.[26]

It can be nearly impossible to distinguish asthma from COPD in many patients.[27] Reduction in the patient's usual activity may be an early warning sign that deserves further evaluation before the subjective sensation of dyspnea occurs. The use of the 6-minute walk test has been shown to be helpful to determine functional capacity.[27]

The traditional threshold of forced expiratory volume in 1 second (FEV1)/ forced vital capacity (FVC) of 70% used in a younger population may be a

normal finding in the elderly population. A significant reduction in FEV1 predicts increased mortality.[27]

Risk factors are as follows:

- Active and passive cigarette smoking[28]
- Hormone replacement therapy[28]
- Use of ASA, nonsteroidal anti-inflammatory drugs (NSAIDs),
  angiotensin-converting enzyme (ACE) inhibitors and beta-blockers,
  including topical preparations.[26] Use of paracetamol is a putative risk
  factor for the development of asthma. Glutathione depletion in the
  airways and increased oxidative stress may be the mechanism underlying the link between paracetamol use and asthma development.[28]
- The occurrence of acute lower respiratory infections is strongly associated with the risk of new adult-onset asthma.[28]
- Obesity[28]
- Stress[28]
- Gastroesophageal reflux disease (GERD) commonly coexists with
  asthma and can exacerbate symptoms.[28]

Elderly patients tend to have more than one pulmonary disease, which
further complicates the diagnosis and management of asthma. Several problems unique to elderly asthmatic patients are particularly challenging. These
include delayed appearance of symptoms, the presence of multiple comorbidities, dementia, poor eyesight, noncompliance, lack of social and family support, inability to distinguish asthma from other medical conditions such as
COPD, polypharmacy, difficulties with inhaler techniques, lack of treatment
response or poorer response to drugs such as beta agonists, and physiological changes in the respiratory and immune systems.[27] A multidisciplinary
approach is required for better management.

Chronic Obstructive Pulmonary Disease

The prevalence of COPD in individuals 65 years of age and older was recently
estimated to be 14.2% (11–18%) compared with 9.9% (8.2–11.8%) in those 40
years or older.[29] COPD is the third leading cause of death in the United States,
behind cancer and heart disease.[29,30] The number of women dying from COPD
has exceeded the number in men since 1999, and the hospital discharge rate
for COPD has been higher in women than in men since 1993.[30] Pooled analyses of prevalence studies show a stepwise rise in the prevalence of COPD with
advancing age.[31] Asthma/COPD overlap syndrome (ACOS), a condition in

which a person has the clinical features of both asthma and COPD, is common in elderly asthmatic people with a history of smoking or long-term asthma. ACOS is estimated to be present in 15% to 45% of patients with obstructive airway disease, and the prevalence increases with age.[25]

Older people with COPD often have sarcopenia of respiratory and larger muscle groups, malnutrition, and deconditioning.[32] Skeletal muscle wasting is associated with a poor prognosis. Malnutrition, which may be found in up to 30% of patients with advanced COPD, is an independent risk factor for mortality and increased hospitalization risk.[33] Chronic systemic inflammation in COPD may be partly responsible for conditions such as muscle wasting, heart disease, and osteoporosis.[33] The GOLD staging system might misclassify up to 28% of elderly patients as having "moderate" COPD by not accounting for age-related changes.[32] Use of a fixed FEV1/FVC ratio of 0.7 may result in overdiagnosis of COPD.[33]

Anemia due to malnutrition in the elderly can worsen dyspnea.[32] Depression, anxiety, chronic pain, and social isolation can worsen the subjective experience of dyspnea.[32] Outdoor air pollution increases rates of acute exacerbations in the elderly and increases the rate of emergency room visits.[33]

Polypharmacy due to comorbid conditions can be a problem when dealing with COPD in the elderly. For example, antihypertensives and antidepressants can cause postural hypotension and interfere with aerobic activity; corticosteroids may cause muscle weakness; and opioids and benzodiazepines may reduce ventilatory drive.[33]

Chronic Dyspnea

Dyspnea is common in the elderly and should not be considered an inevitable consequence of aging. Older people are less sensitive to hypercapnia and hypoxia and therefore may become breathless later in the course of the disease.[34]

Clinically significant dyspnea is often underreported, unrecognized, and undertreated in older adults. Common pulmonary disorders are frequently overlooked as contributors to dyspnea in older patients, and dyspnea is often ascribed to multiple etiologies such as medical comorbidities and deconditioning. The prevalence of chronic dyspnea could be as high as 36% in the elderly. About 60% of those presenting with dyspnea are aged 65 years and up; women suffer more strongly from dyspnea than men; and in 70% of these patients, the origin is either cardiac or pulmonary.[35-37] Dyspnea is an independent risk factor for mortality after adjustment for age, gender, and underlying diseases.[2]

Common causes of dyspnea in the elderly are as follows:[34,38,39]

- Respiratory: asthma, chronic bronchitis, COPD, emphysema, interstitial lung disease, pneumonia, malignancy, effusion

- Cardiovascular: heart failure, elevated pulmonary venous pressure, congenital heart disease, atrial fibrillation
- GERD
- Deconditioning
- Kyphoscoliosis
- Ascites, obesity
- Anemia
- Anxiety, depression

Correctly identifying the cause will determine the treatment and plan of action.

Table 18.1 describes some common pharmaceuticals used to treat lung diseases.

Integrative Approaches to Treating Lung Disease

ENVIRONMENT

Taking a detailed history of allergy to mold, cats, and dust mites is advised. Mold toxicity and allergy are especially challenging for patients living in suboptimal housing. Patients could undergo RAST testing and hypersensitivity skin testing; if the results are positive, patients are encouraged to avoid exposures.[42] Pillows and mattresses should be enclosed in airtight polyurethane covers. Patients should avoid down or foam pillows and down jackets. Bedrooms should be frequently cleaned with a vacuum that has a high-efficiency particulate air (HEPA) filter.[43] Removing pets from the home and eliminating exposure to tobacco smoke may help.

NUTRITION

There is considerable evidence to suggest that a high intake of fruits and vegetables is favorable for all life stages of asthma and COPD and decreases the risk of exacerbation.[44,45] In COPD patients, lung function improved with a diet high in fruits and vegetables. Increased intake of fruits and vegetables may be protective against COPD development and decline of lung function.[44,45]

Persons with a higher intake of polyunsaturated fatty acids (i.e., omega-6 fatty acids) have been found to have a higher prevalence of asthma, eczema, and allergic rhinitis. It is recommended to increase intake of omega-3 fatty

Table 18.1. Pharmaceuticals

Drug Class	Drugs	Adverse Events	Comments
Short-acting inhaled beta-2 agonists (SABAs)	Albuterol, levabuterol, fevalbuterol	Palpitations, tremors, nervousness, hypertension, angina	Used as needed for mild and intermittent symptoms. SABAs are mainstay of treatment in elderly with asthma. Patients who use more than twice a week need to return to clinic for re-evaluation of suboptimal asthma control.
Long-acting inhaled beta-2 agonists (LABAs)	Salmeterol, vilanterol, indacaterol, formoterol	Headache, throat irritation, nasal congestion, dysarrhythmia, association with risk of asthma-related deaths	Preferred in patients with persistent symptoms. Responsiveness to beta-2 agonists decreased with age. Incidence of dysarrhythmia can be as high as 65%, especially with history of myocardial infarction. Incidence of hypokalemia increases in patients taking insulin or diuretics.
Inhaled anticholinergics	Ipratropium, tiotropium	Xerostomia, dyspepsia, insomnia, urinary hesitancy	Bronchodilator response to anticholinergics is less age-dependent. They are ideal alternative rescue agents for asthma. Anticholinergics should not be used for maintenance therapy similar to beta-2 agonists because their bronchodilator capability is limited, especially in patients with $FEV_1 < 60\%$ predicted.
Inhaled corticosteroids	Budesonide, fluticasone, mometasone, beclomethasone	Upper respiratory infection, rhinitis, cough, oral candidiasis	There is generalized under-usage of inhaled corticosteroids in the elderly. Clinicians should initiate treatment with inhaled corticosteroids at the earliest opportunity.
Oral corticosteroids	Prednisone	Adrenal suppression, glaucoma, osteoporosis, diabetes mellitus, hypertension	Long-term glucocorticoid use can decrease morbidity and mortality in asthma. However, their oral use has been associated with an increased risk of vertebral fractures (increased by 56%).

Data from references 40 and 41.

acids by eating cold-water fish (e.g., sardines, herring, salmon) and reduce intake of omega-6 fatty acids by eliminating vegetable oils and instead using olive oils. Omega-3 fatty acids can be anti-inflammatory agents and may counter the airway inflammation seen in COPD.[46,47] Higher fish intake is associated with a lower risk for COPD.[46,47] Omega-3 polyunsaturated fatty acids are found largely in oily fish and to a lesser extent in flaxseed, walnuts, soybeans, and canola oil.

The risk of COPD and decline in lung function may be lower in people consuming more soybean products, including soy foods such as tofu and bean sprouts.[48,49] Increased soy consumption was associated with a decreased risk of COPD and breathlessness.[48,49] Flavonoids from soy foods might act as anti-inflammatory agents in the lung. Eating a diet rich in soy, possibly due to consumption of isoflavones, may reduce the incidence of chronic respiratory symptoms.[49]

Cured meats such as sausage, ham, bologna, bacon, and hot dogs contain high levels of nitrites, which are added to prevent rancidity and bacterial growth and enhance the meat's pink color. Just like cigarette smoking and air pollution, nitrites generate molecules known as reactive oxygen and nitrogen species that have been linked to COPD.[50]

WEIGHT TRAINING, MOTOR AND RESPIRATORY PHYSIOTHERAPY

Patients with a chronic lung disease such as emphysema or bronchitis can strengthen their arms and legs with resistance training, and this strength may help them perform everyday tasks more easily.[51] A number of studies have demonstrated that exercise programs and motor and respiratory physiotherapy improve aerobic capacity, breathing pattern, muscle strength, and quality of life in senior citizens.[52] Exercise programs tailored for asthmatic patients have a positive effect both on physical, physiological, and psychological parameters and on social and personal relationships.[53]

Breathing exercises can improve patient-reported outcomes, and increased respiratory muscle strength may be associated with greater ability to deal with an asthma crisis.[54] Breathing exercises should be offered to all asthma (and COPD) patients. A specific form of breathing exercise known as the Butyeko breathing technique can help asthma by decreasing the respiratory rate and allowing the carbon dioxide concentration in the lung and blood to rise, causing bronchodilatation, or may help by improving the biomechanics of breathing.[55] In a randomized controlled trial, the Butyeko technique reduced inhaled corticosteroid use[55] (https://www.youtube.com/watch?v=e2UDtUQcn8g, www.butyeko.com).

WEIGHT LOSS

Among people with COPD, usually emphysema, a low fat-free body mass index (BMI) appears to be associated with greater mortality.[56] There is a clear association between decreasing BMI and mortality both in the general population and in those with COPD. Therefore, nutritional support, including consultation with a nutritionist, is advised to maintain BMI.

YOGA

A recent meta-analysis suggests that yoga training that lasts from 12 weeks to 9 months has a positive effect on lung function and exercise capacity and could be used as an adjunct pulmonary rehabilitation program for COPD patients. Yoga training aids in toning up general body systems, increasing respiratory stamina, relaxing chest muscles, expanding the lungs, raising energy levels, and calming the body. Yoga improves blood circulation and increases the strength of respiratory muscles. Yoga training also helps patients to breathe more deeply by using the shoulder, thoracic, and abdominal muscles efficiently.[57,58]

Yogic breathing exercises improve diffusion capacity. They are beneficial to COPD patients and can be used as an adjunct therapy with conventional medical therapy. The exercises help open blocked airways caused by bronchitis or emphysema.[59]

Recommended yoga exercises are as follows:[60]

Daily pranayama (breathing exercises): Bhastrika: 5 minutes; Anulom vilom: 15 minutes; Kapalbhati: 10 minutes; Bhramari: 5 times
Daily asanas (postures): Surya Namaskar: 3 to 10 times, 3 repeats; Tadasana: 3 times; Sukhasana: 3 times; Paschimotanasana: 3 times; Shavasana: 10 minutes

For specific yoga and pranayama techniques see www.yogicwayoflife.com.

Per yogic tradition, "prana" is the life force that permeates all living things and in fact all matter, and "yama" means roughly to extend or to lengthen. Thus, pranayama involves extending and lengthening the breath and life force. It was this understanding of the close relationship between breath and consciousness that led to the invention of the various techniques of breath control, or pranayama. A Cochrane review of breathing exercises that included studies on yoga and diaphragmatic breathing showed improved functional exercise capacity in people with COPD as compared to no intervention.[61] For an explanation of pranayama technique, see http://www.onemedical.com/blog/

live-well/breathing-pranayama-techniques/ and http://www.yogicwayoflife.
com/?s=pranayama.

Breathing more than 15 times in a minute is a stress signal. Abdominal breathing is also known as diaphragmatic breathing. When the diaphragm contracts, it produces a negative pressure within the thoracic cage and pulls blood into the chest, increasing venous return to the heart. Diaphragmatic contractions during deep breathing enhance lymphatic flow.[62] We have twice the amount of lymphatic fluid in our body as we do blood. Deep breathing can help to get lymph flowing properly so the body can work more efficiently. Abdominal breathing can also decrease anxiety and depression by helping the mind–body to relax and reconnect.

ACUPUNCTURE

Although there are conflicting results from controlled trials in treating bronchial asthma with acupuncture, the majority of the reports suggest that acupuncture is effective.[63-65] A recent systematic review and meta-analysis of eight randomized controlled trials showed that acupuncture was effective in in improving FEV1 and FEV1/vital capacity significantly.[66] Acupuncture may also provide symptomatic improvement in late stages of bronchial asthma, where there are complications of disabling breathlessness due to impaired lung function.[67] While bronchial asthma cannot be cured by acupuncture, it may be relieved substantially, with success rates of 60% to 70%.[68] Acupuncture has a limited role in acute asthma, but it may serve as a prophylactic measure over the long term. Controlled trials have shown that acupuncture brings about modest improvement in objective parameters, with significant subjective improvement, including improved peak flow; less coughing, wheezing, and dyspnea; and fewer nocturnal awakening episodes.[69] Corticosteroid-dependent bronchial asthma may better respond to acupuncture: the dose of corticosteroids can gradually be decreased during the first weeks of acupuncture treatment.[70] In patients with dyspnea and shortness of breath, acupuncture resulted in marked improvement in subjective feelings of breathlessness, relaxation, and anxiety even in patients resistant to other treatments, including opioids, steroids, nebulizers, and oxygen.[67,71] Acupressure point stimulation can also help to relieve dyspnea in COPD patients.[67,71]

BOTANICALS

Table 18.2 describes botanicals that can be used in treatment.

Table 18.2. Botanicals

Botanical	Dose	Precautions	Comments
Boswellia serrata	300 mg of standardized extract TID	May increase the effect of zafrilukast or montelukast. Efficacy of NSAIDs, warfarin, and sedatives may be reduced. Can cause epigastric pain, heartburn, nausea, and diarrhea.	Patients taking boswellia had fewer exacerbations and improved lung function.[72] Boswellia is poorly absorbed; formulations such as RadoQOL* (Thorne Research) combine boswellia with a phytosome for enhanced absorption.
Coleus forskohlii	50 mg BID or TID of a standardized extract (18% forskolin) or 10-mg dose via an inhaler device	Avoid in patients with diabetes or thyroid condition; can interact with warfarin. Forskolin lowers blood pressure and can interact with antihypertensives such as calcium-channel blockers.	Preliminary results show that inhaled forskolin powder can relieve symptoms of asthma,[73,74] but more research is required.
Ma Huang	See precautions and comments.	Complications, including death, have been reported when Ma Huang is taken in high doses or with caffeine-containing products.[75] Death has been reported with even one use of the product.	Also known as Chinese ephedra. Not recommended for use because of potentially dangerous side effects and U.S. Food and Drug Administration warning.[76,77]
Licorice (*Glycyrrhiza glabra*)[78–80]	Licorice tincture 2–5 ml TID	Side effects are minimal if prolonged use is avoided. Long-term use can cause headache, hypertension, dizziness, edema, and other signs of aldosteronism (through the binding of mineralocorticoids). Licorice may also cause low serum potassium and should be avoided in patients taking cardiac glycosides, blood pressure medications, corticosteroids, diuretics, or monoamine oxidase inhibitors.	Efficacy is due to its inflammatory effect and enhancement of endogenous steroids. The active ingredient is glycyrrhizin or glycyrrhizic acid. Licorice is also thought to be an expectorant, aiding in the expulsion of mucus from the bronchial passages, as well as a demulcent, which can be soothing to irritated airways and bronchioles.

Pycnogenol (*Pinus pinaster*)	30–100 mg/day	DO NOT use pycnogenol if you have diabetes or take medication for high blood pressure. If you take blood thinners, such as warfarin (Coumadin), or aspirin, taking pycnogenol may increase your risk of bleeding.	A 2002 review of studies on a standardized extract of pycnogenol suggests that it may reduce symptoms and improve lung function in people with asthma.[81]
Saiboku-to	Taken as tea BID or TID	Saiboku-to contains several herbs, including Asian ginseng (*Panax ginseng*), Chinese skullcap (*Baikal scutellaria*), licorice (*Glycyrrhiza glabra*), ginger (*Zingiber officinale*), black cumin, chamomile, cinnamon, cloves, rosemary, sage, thyme, and spearmint. These herbs can interact with other medications.	In three preliminary studies, a traditional Japanese herbal mixture called Saiboku-to has helped reduce airway activity and allowed study participants to reduce doses of corticosteroids, thus allowing better asthma control.[82] Saiboku-to has shown anti-inflammatory effects by blocking 5 lipooxygenase and inhibiting PAF.[83]
Eucalyptus	3–10 drops as needed, added to water for steam inhalation	Do not take eucalyptus oil by mouth.	*Eucalyptus globulus*, when used either as cough drops or by inhalation, can help to loosen phlegm. Concomitant therapy with cineole (active ingredient in eucalyptus oil) reduces exacerbations[84] as well as dyspnea and improves lung function and health status. It is sometimes combined with an extract from pine called essential oil monoterpenes.
Ginseng	200–400 mg once daily of a standardized extract containing 2–3% total ginsenosides	Ginseng lowers blood sugar, increases levels of free warfarin, can cause insomnia and arrhythmia.	*Panax ginseng* may help COPD patients improve exercise tolerance and pulmonary function.[85]

Fennel (*Foeniculum vulgaris*) is useful for stimulating ciliary motility and reducing congestion, bronchitis, and cough due to the presence of cineole and anetol, which are expectorants and break up phlegm.[86,87] Osha root (*Ligusticum porteri*), indigenous to North America in the area of the Rocky Mountains, contains camphor and other beneficial oils that act as expectorants and make breathing easier.[86,87] Elecampane (*Inula helenium*), also known as horse heal and marchalan, has been used traditionally as a remedy for chronic bronchitis and asthma and to relieve cough.[88,89] Mullein (*Verbascum thapsus*) has a long history of relieving coughs and has been claimed to have a soothing effect on bronchioles; it is an expectorant.[90] Marshmallow (*Althaea officinalis*) is commonly used to ease sore throats and dry coughs.[91] Marshmallow leaves and roots have antitussive and mucilaginous properties.[92]

SUPPLEMENTS

Table 18.3 describes supplements that can be used in treatment.

BIOMECHANICAL APPROACHES

Clinical trials investigating the effect of massage in the elderly are lacking. However, in other age groups, daily massage was shown to improve airway caliber and control of asthma.[100] Referral to an experienced massage therapist is worth a try. Reflexology points can be massaged once a day by the patient or a family member or friend. Osteopathic manipulation and chiropractic adjustments have been shown to help patients with pulmonary diseases, especially breathing difficulties.[101–103] Osteopathic manipulative treatments such as "doming" (https://www.youtube.com/watch?v=Hqpejuh8Bxs) and the "rib raising technique" (https://www.youtube.com/watch?v=A4lW9K7v5TA) can be useful adjunctive tools to improve breathing. Doming of the thoracic diaphragm involves doming the muscle to relieve hypertonicity associated with a flattened or dysfunctional state; the rib raising technique augments lymphatic flow by improving respiratory excursion and reducing sympathetic outflow.[104]

Well-controlled studies are generally lacking in the elderly. A systematic review of manual therapies that included chiropractic therapy, osteopathic therapy, and other physical therapies concluded that current evidence is insufficient to support or refute the use of manual therapies in patients with asthma.[105]

Table 18.3. Supplements

Supplement	Dose	Precautions	Comments
Vitamin C[93]	Not recommended		Insufficient evidence to recommend vitamin C for asthma or COPD. Low levels of vitamin C were associated with more wheezing, phlegm production, and dyspnea. No studies showed benefit of vitamin C supplementation in improving symptoms, decreasing hospitalization, or improving pulmonary function.
Vitamin D[94]		Range of safe dose of vitamin D is not known to prevent upper respiratory tract infection. Vitamin D levels should be maintained within normal levels.	Lower level of vitamin D levels were shown to be inversely associated with recent upper respiratory infections, which are a common trigger for acute asthma. Taking supplemental vitamin D to help prevent upper respiratory tract infections could help decrease asthma exacerbation.
Vitamin B6[95]	The recommended dose range is 50–100 mg/day.	Avoid doses >500 mg/day and prolonged use; associated with peripheral neuropathy.	In a double-blind randomized study, vitamin B6 was shown to improve peak flow rates in a group of adults with severe asthma. In patients with low serum pyridoxine (vitamin B6) levels, supplementation helped decrease episodes of wheezing. Lowering of serum vitamin B6 levels may be a side effect of common asthma medications.
Vitamin E[96]	The recommended dose is 400 units/day of mixed tocopherols.	The risk of all-cause mortality may be increased with prolonged use of doses >400 units/day.	Intake of vitamin E is recommended in the diet or through supplementation because patients who have a high antioxidant intake have fewer pulmonary problems. Poorly controlled asthma has been shown to be associated with low vitamin E levels.

(continued)

Table 18.3. Continued

Supplement	Dose	Precautions	Comments
Magnesium[97,98]	The dose is 200–400 mg/day.	Oral magnesium can cause diarrhea. Magnesium gluconate and magnesium glycinate are the forms least likely to cause diarrhea.	People who have asthma often have low levels of magnesium. Intravenous magnesium is now commonly used for serious asthma symptoms (status asthmaticus). In adults, magnesium was shown to decrease symptoms but not to improve pulmonary function in one study and to have no benefit in another. In a more recent study of 55 adults taking 340 mg of magnesium a day for 6 months, objective measurements of lung function, including bronchial reactivity to methacholine and peak flow measurements, improved, as did subjective measures of asthma control and quality of life.
Fish oil[46,47]	500-mg capsule BID or TID	See text.	Benefit may not be evident for months
N-acetylcysteine (NAC)[99]	600–1,200 mg/day	Contraindicated in patients taking nitroglycerin. NAC can interact with warfarin, and patients with asthma have reported bronchospasms.	NAC is a modified form of cysteine, an amino acid. NAC is an antioxidant; it reduces the risk of exacerbations and improves symptoms in patients with chronic bronchitis.

MIND–BODY THERAPIES

Mind–body techniques include relaxation therapy, hypnosis, biofeedback, and guided imagery. The theory behind these therapies is to decrease the inflammation that is often triggered by emotions via the autonomic nervous system. Different types of cognitive-behavioral therapies may decrease the symptoms, the inflammatory response of airway cells, and medication use.[106,107]

Hypnosis has been shown to be effective in patients with an emotional component to their disease and can improve pulmonary function, decrease medication use, and improve symptoms in asthma. Guided imagery, a form of self-hypnosis, can be effective in patients with an active imagination; however, in the elderly this can be a difficult process to successfully implement.

Breathing retraining in combination with coping strategies may reduce breathlessness and improve functional capacity. Modalities that improve function such as walking also enhance quality of life.[71]

TAI CHI QI GONG

Efficient, intentional, and mindful breathing is a key element of tai chi. A fundamental component of tai chi is the deliberate attention to bodily sensation, movement, breath, and emotion, which fosters acute self-awareness, both physically and emotionally. Tai chi may help increase muscle strength and endurance, decrease chest wall stiffness, and deepen and slow the respiratory rate, thereby increasing gas exchange efficiency.[108] Mindfulness training, which is part of tai chi, can impact interoceptive awareness of key COPD symptoms, which may lead to better symptom management.[109-111] A meta-analysis showed that tai chi qi gong (TCQ) had significant effects on 6-minute walk distance, FEV1, predicted FEV1 percentage, and the St. George's Respiratory Questionnaire score; however, caution is needed to draw a firm conclusion because of the low methodological quality of the included trials.[112] A small Thai trial investigating the effect of TCQ training in COPD showed that it improved both functional and maximum exercise capacities in COPD as a result of decreased dynamic hyperinflation, and also improved respiratory muscle strength and quality of life.[113]

For a demonstration of tai chi breathing exercises, visit https://www.youtube.com/watch?v=DZRiHDrhJZY&index=4&list=PLvwvv4bKx3QojLqopkT3-xGbSXbhng8Yw.

OPTIMIZING THE GASTROINTESTINAL MICROBIOME

The microbiome is the total collection of microbiota that reside within humans or on their skin surface. The microbiota is defined as all microorganisms that inhabit a particular site or place (e.g., the gastrointestinal tract, skin, or airways)[114] Bacteria coexist with fungi and viruses in these locations.

Commensal organisms like *Lactobacillus* and *Prevotella* spp. may regulate inflammatory responses of the lungs induced by possible pathogenic organisms and protect the lung against inflammatory and oxidative stress. There is increased expression of *Firmicute* and *Proteobacteria* phylum (*Haemophilus, Moraxella,* and *Neisseria* spp.) in the lungs of patients with COPD and asthma.[114] There is substantial overlap between microorganisms in the oral cavity and lungs that may be related to micro-aspirations, which occur in nearly all individuals during sleep.[115] Due to impairment of mucociliary function in COPD, pooling of mucus and mucous plugging can occur, entrapping the aspirated bacteria and causing them to grow and accumulate in this new ecosystem.[116,117] There is some evidence that the response of the lung could be altered by gut microbiota. Animals treated with antibiotics demonstrated deficiencies in the regulatory T-cell response to influenza[118] and hyperreponsiveness to ovalbumin in the lung.[119] Babies delivered vaginally harbor a microbiota (gut, oral cavity, nasopharynx, skin) in which *Lactobacillus* predominates; in contrast, babies born via cesarean section harbored a microbiota that was similar to that found on the mother's skin, where *Staphylococcus* and *Acinetobacter* were much more common colonizers.[120] Epidemiological studies have shown that babies born by cesarean section have a significantly higher risk of asthma than babies delivered vaginally.[121] Environmental exposures shape the composition of gut microbiota, which in turn shapes the immune function. Differences in immune function shape the nature and intensity of responsiveness to allergens and viruses encountered.[122] The role of orally administered probiotics for asthma and COPD is not clear. The few clinical trials of orally administered probiotics for respiratory diseases are small and isolated but suggest benefit in prevention of ventilator-associated pneumonia (40% vs. 19% in mechanically ventilated patients), upper respiratory tract infection, and cystic fibrosis exacerbations.[123,124] In none of the studies is it known whether the benefit was conveyed via direct alteration of the lung microbiota or indirectly via gut-mucosa–mediated effects on systemic immunity.[123]

REFERENCES

1. Trends in COPD (Chronic Bronchitis and Emphysema): Morbidity and Mortality. American Lung Association Epidemiology and Statistics Unit Research and Health Education Division, March 2013.

2. Akgün KM, Crothers K, Pisani M. Epidemiology and management of common pulmonary diseases in older persons. *J Gerontol A Biol Sci Med Sci.* 2012;67A(3):276–291.

3. Bellia V, Incalzi RA. Introduction. In Bellia V, Incalzi RA, ed. *Respiratory Diseases in the Elderly.* Sheffield, UK: European Respiratory Society; 2009:ix.

4. Sharma G, Goodwin J. Effect of aging on respiratory system physiology and immunology. *Clin Interv Aging.* 2006;1(3):253–260.

5. Crapo RO, Morris AH, Gardner RM. Reference spirometric values using techniques and equipment that meets ATS recommendations. *Am Rev Respir Dis.* 1981;123:659–64.

6. Enright PL, Kronmal RA, Higgens M, Schenker M, Haponik EF. Spirometry reference values for women and men 65 to 85 years of age. Cardiovascular Health Study. *Am Rev Respir Dis.* 1993;147:125–33.

7. Enright PL, Kronmal RA, Manolio TA, Schenker MB, Hyatt RE. Respiratory muscle strength in the elderly. Correlates and reference values. Cardiovascular Health Study Research Group. *Am J Respir Crit Care Med.* 1994 Feb;149(2 Pt 1):430-8.

8. Feldman RD, Limbird LE, Nadeau J, Robertson D, Wood AJ. Alterations in leukocyte β-adrenergic affinity with aging. A potential explanation of altered β-adrenergic sensitivity in the elderly. *N Engl J Med.* 1984;310:815–19

9. Gillooly M, Lamb D. Airspace size in lungs of lifelong non-smokers: Effect of age and sex. *Thorax.* 1993;48:39–43.

10. Hopp RJ, Bewtra A, Nair NM, Townley RG. The effect of age on methacholine response. *J Allergy Clin Immunol.* 1985;76:609–13.

11. Janssens JP, Pache JC, Nicod LP. Physiological changes in respiratory function associated with aging. *Eur Respir J.* 1999;13:197–205.

12. Kelly FJ, Dunster C, Mudway I. Air pollution and the elderly: Oxidant/antioxidant issues with consideration. *Eur Respir J Suppl.* 2003;40:70–75s.

13. Stupka JE, Mortensen EM, Anzueto A, Restrepo MI. Community-acquired pneumonia in elderly patients. *Aging Health.* 2009;5(6):763–774. doi:10.2217/ahe.09.74.

14. Kronenberg RS, Drage CW. Attenuation of the ventilatory and heart rate responses to hypoxia and hypercapnia with aging in normal men. *J Clin Invest.* 1973;52(8):1812–1819.

15. Lowery EM, Brubaker AL, Kuhlmann E, Kovacs EJ. The aging lung. *Clin Interv Aging.* 2013;8:1489–96.

16. Pawelec G. Immunosenescence comes of age. Symposium on Aging Research in Immunology: The Impact of Genomics. *EMBO Reports.* 2007;8(3):220–223.

17. Tzortzaki EG, Proklou A, Siafakas NM. Asthma in the elderly: Can we distinguish it from COPD? *J Allergy.* 2011;2011:843543. doi: 10.1155/2011/843543.

18. Kitch BT, Levy BD, Fanta CH. Late-onset asthma: Epidemiology, diagnosis and treatment. *Drugs Aging.* 2000 Nov;17(5):385–97.

19. Trends in asthma morbidity and mortality. American Lung Association Epidemiology and Statistics Unit Research and Health Education Division, September 2012. http://www.lung.org/assets/documents/research/asthma-trend-report.pdf

20. Gillman A, Douglass JA. Asthma in the elderly. *Asia Pac Allergy.* 2012;2:101–108.

21. Rackemann FM. Intrinsic asthma. *J Allergy.* 1940;11:147.
22. de Marco R, Locatelli F, Cerveri I, Bugiani M, Marinoni A, Giammanco G; Italian Study on Asthma in Young Adults study group. Incidence and remission of asthma: A retrospective study on the natural history of asthma in Italy. *J Allergy Clin Immunol.* 2002; 110: 228–235.
23. Litonjua AA, Sparrow D, Weiss ST, O'Connor CT, Long AA, Ohman JL. Sensitization to cat allergen is associated with asthma in older men and predicts new-onset airway hyperresponsiveness. *Am J Respir Crit Care Med.* 1997;156:23–27.
24. Ariano R, Panzani RC, Augeri C. Late-onset asthma clinical and immunological data: Importance of allergy. *J Invest Allergol Clin Immunol.* 1998;8:35–41.
25. Ozturk AB, Iliaz S. Challenges in the management of severe allergic asthma in the elderly. *J Asthma Allergy.* 2016;9:55–63.
26. Boulet LP, Becker A, Bérubé D, Beveridge R, Ernst P. Canadian Asthma Consensus Report, 1999. Canadian Asthma Consensus Group. CMAJ. 1999 Nov 30;161(11 Suppl):S1–61.
27. Madeo J, Li M, Frieri M. Asthma in the geriatric population. *Allergy Asthma Proc.* 2013;34:427–433.
28. de Nijs SB, Venekamp LN, Bel EH. Adult-onset asthma: Is it really different? *Eur Respir Rev.* 2013 Mar 1;22(127):44–52.
29. Halbert RJ, Natoli JL, Gano A, Badamgarav E, Buist AS, Mannino DM. Global burden of COPD: Systematic review and meta-analysis. *Eur Respir J.* 2006;28:523–532.
30. Trends in COPD (Chronic Bronchitis and Emphysema): Morbidity and Mortality. American Lung Association Epidemiology and Statistics Unit Research and Health Education Division, March 2013. http://www.lung.org/assets/documents/research/copd-trend-report.pdf
31. Chronic Respiratory Diseases. Chronic Obstructive Pulmonary Disease. World Health Organization. Statistical Dataset. Geneva, Switzerland: World Health Organization; 2000 3-1-2009 Available at: http://www.who.int/respiratory/copd/burden/en/index.html
32. Fried TR, Vaz Fragoso CA, Rabow MW. Caring for the older person with chronic obstructive pulmonary disease. *JAMA.* 2012;308(12):1254–1263.
33. Nazir SA, Erbland ML. Chronic obstructive pulmonary disease: An update on diagnosis and management issues in older adults. *Drugs Aging.* 2009; 26(10):813–831.
34. Poole PJ. Breathlessness in older people. *NZ Med J.* 1999;112:450–453.
35. Ahmed T, Steward TA, O'Mahoney MS. Dyspnoea and mortality in older people in the community: A 10-year follow-up. *Age Ageing.* 2012;41:545–549.
36. Charles J, Ng A, Britt H. Presentations of shortness of breath in Australian general practice. *Aust Fam Physician.* 2005 Jul;34(7):520–521.
37. Hayen A, Herigstad M, Pattinson KTS. Understanding dyspnea as a complex individual experience. *Maturitas.* 2013;76(1):45–50.
38. Bull A. Primary care of chronic dyspnea in adults. *Nurse Practitioner.* 2014;39(8):34–40.
39. Chotirmall SH, Watts M, Branagan P, Donegan CF, Moore A, McElvaney NG. Diagnosis and management of asthma in older adults. *J Am Geriatr Soc.* 2009 May;57(5):901–909.

40. Qaseem A, Wilt TJ, Weinberger SE, et al. Diagnosis and management of stable chronic obstructive pulmonary disease: A clinical practice guideline update from the American College of Physicians, American College of Chest Physicians, American Thoracic Society, and European Respiratory Society. *Ann Intern Med.* 2011 Aug 2;155(3):179–191.
41. Barnes PJ. Pulmonary pharmacology. In: Brunton LL, Chabner BA, Knollman BC, ed. *Pharmacological Basis of Therapeutics*, 12th ed. New York: McGraw Hill; 2011:1031–1066.
42. Mathur SK. Allergy and asthma in the elderly. *Seminars in Respiratory and Critical Care Medicine.* 2010;31(5):587–595.
43. Marks JD. Asthma. In: Rakel D, ed. *Integrative medicine*, 3rd ed. Philadelphia, PA: Elsevier; 2012:258–267.
44. Berthon BS, Wood LG. Nutrition and respiratory health—feature review. *Nutrients.* 2015;7(3):1618–1643.
45. Shaheen SO, Jameson KA, Syddall HE, et al. Cohort Study Group. The relationship of dietary patterns with adult lung function and COPD. *Eur Respir J.* 2010;36:277–284.
46. Berthon BS, Wood LG. Nutrition and respiratory health—feature review. *Nutrients.* 2015;7(3):1618–1643.
47. Varraso R, Barr RG, Willett WC, Speizer FE, Camargo CA Jr. Fish intake and risk of chronic obstructive pulmonary disease in 2 large US cohorts. Higher fish intake is associated with a lower risk for COPD. *Am J Clin Nutr.* 2015;101(2):354–361.
48. Hirayama F, Lee AH, Binns CW, et al. Soy consumption and risk of COPD and respiratory symptoms: A case-control study in Japan. *Respir Res.* 2009 Jun 26;10:56.
49. Butler LM, Koh W, Lee H, Yu MC, London SJ. Dietary fiber and reduced cough with phlegm. A cohort study in Singapore. *Am J Respir Crit Care Med.* 2004;170:279–287.
50. Varraso R, Jiang R, Barr RG, Willett WC, Camargo CA. Prospective study of cured meats consumption and risk of chronic obstructive pulmonary disease in men. *Am J Epidemiol.* 2007 Dec 15;166(12):1438–1445.
51. O'Shea SD, Taylor NF, Paratz JD. Progressive resistance exercise improves muscle strength and may improve elements of performance of daily activities for people with COPD: A systematic review. *Chest.* 2009 Nov;136(5):1269–1283.
52. American College of Sports Medicine. Physical activity programs and behaviour counseling in older adult populations. *Med Sci Sports Exerc.* 2004;36:1997–2003.
53. Ram FSP, Wellington SR, Barnes NC. Inspiratory muscle training for asthma. *Cochrane Database Syst Rev.* 2003;(4):CD003792.
54. Gomieiro LTY, Nascimento A, Tanno LK, Agondi R, Kalil J, Giavina-Bianchi P. Respiratory exercise program for elderly individuals with asthma. *Clinics.* 2011;66(7):1165–1169.
55. Courtney R, Cohen M. Investigating the claims of Konstantin Buteyko, M.D., Ph.D: the relationship of breath holding time to end tidal CO_2 and other proposed measures of dysfunctional breathing. *J Altern Complement Med.* 2008;14:115–123.
56. Yamauchi Y, Hasegawa W, Yasunaga H. Association between body mass index and in-hospital mortality in elderly patients with chronic obstructive pulmonary disease in Japan. *Int J Chron Obstruct Pulmon Dis.* 2014; 9: 1337–1346.

57. Pumar MI, Gray CR, Walsh JR, Yang IA, Rolls TA, Ward DL. Anxiety and depression—Important psychological comorbidities of COPD. *J Thorac Dis.* 2014;6(11):1615–1631.

58. Liu X-C, Pan L, Hu Q, Dong W-P, Yan J-H, Dong L. Effects of yoga training in patients with chronic obstructive pulmonary disease: A systematic review and meta-analysis. *J Thorac Dis.* 2014;6(6):795–802.

59. Soni R, Munish K, Singh K, Singh S. Study of the effect of yoga training on diffusion capacity in chronic obstructive pulmonary disease patients: A controlled trial. *International Journal of Yoga.* 2012;5(2):123–127.

60. http://www.yogicwayoflife.com/?s=pranayama (Accessed 8/21/2016)

61. Holland AE, Hill CJ, Jones AY, McDonald CF. Breathing exercises for chronic obstructive pulmonary disease. *Cochrane Database Syst Rev.* 2012, Issue 10. Art. No.: CD008250.

62. Bordoni B, Zanier E. Anatomic connections of the diaphragm: Influence of respiration on the body system. *Journal of Multidisciplinary Healthcare.* 2013;6:281–291.

63. McCarney RW, Brinkhaus B, Lasserson TJ, Linde K. Acupuncture for chronic asthma. *Cochrane Database System Rev.* 1999, Issue 1. Art. No.: CD000008.

64. Fung KP, Chow OK, So SY. Attenuation of exercise-induced asthma by acupuncture. *Lancet.* 1986 Dec 20–27;2(8521-22):1419–1422.

65. Acupuncture: Review and analysis of reports on controlled clinical trials. WHO Consultation on Acupuncture held in Cervia, Italy, 1996. http://apps.who.int/medicinedocs/pdf/s4926e/s4926e.pdf.

66. Su L, Meng L, Chen R, Wu W, Peng B, Man L. Acupoint application for asthma therapy in adults: A systematic review and meta-analysis of randomized controlled trials. *Forsch Komplementmed.* 2016;23(1):16–21.

67. Jobst K, Chen JH, McPherson K, et al. Controlled trial of acupuncture for disabling breathlessness. *Lancet.* 1986 Dec 20–27;2(8521-22):1416–1419.

68. Joshi YM. Acupuncture in bronchial asthma. *J Assoc Physicians India.* 1992 May;40(5):327–331.

69. Pai HJ, Azevedo RS, Braga AL, **et al.** A randomized, controlled, crossover study in patients with mild and moderate asthma undergoing treatment with traditional Chinese acupuncture. *Clinics.* 2015 Oct;70(10):663–669.

70. Batra YK. Acupuncture in corticosteroid-dependent asthmatics. *Am J Acupunct.* 1986;14(3):261–264.

71. Pan CX, Morrison RS, Ness J, Fugh-Berman A, Leipzig RM. Complementary and alternative medicine in the management of pain, dyspnea, and nausea and vomiting near the end of life. A systematic review. *J Pain Symptom Manage.* 2000 Nov;20(5):374–387.

72. Gupta I, Gupta V, Parihar A, et al. Effects of *Boswellia serrata* gum resin in patients with bronchial asthma: Results of a double-blind, placebo-controlled, 6-week clinical study. *Eur J Med Res.* 1998 Nov 17;3(11):511–514.

73. González-Sánchez R, Trujillo X, Trujillo-Hernández B, Vásquez C, Huerta M, Elizalde A. Forskolin versus sodium cromoglycate for prevention of asthma attacks: a single-blinded clinical trial. *J Int Med Res.* 2006;34(2):200–207.

74. Alasbahi RH, Melzig MF. *Plectranthus barbatus*: A review of phytochemistry, ethnobotanical uses and pharmacology—part 2. *Planta Med.* 2010;76(8):753–765.

75. Hallas J, Bjerrum L, Stovring H, Andersen M. Use of a prescribed ephedrine/caffeine combination and the risk of serious cardiovascular events: a registry-based case-crossover study. *Am J Epidemiol.* 2008;168(8):966–973.

76. Food and Drug Administration. Consumer Alert: FDA plans regulation prohibiting sale of ephedra-containing dietary supplements and advises consumers to stop using these products. December 30, 2003.

77. Cohen PA, Ernst E. Safety of herbal supplements: A guide for cardiologists. *Cardiovasc Ther.* 2010;28(4):246–253.

78. Fiore C, Eisenhut M, Ragazzi E, Zanchin G, Armanini D. A history of the therapeutic use of liquorice in Europe. *J Ethnopharmacol.* 2005;99(3):317–324.

79. Ruetzler K, Fleck M, Nabecker S, et al. A randomized, double-blind comparison of licorice versus sugar-water gargle for the prevention of postoperative sore throat and post-extubation coughing. *Anesth Analg.* 2013;117(3):614–621.

80. Shibata S. A drug over the millennia: Pharmacognosy, chemistry, and pharmacology of licorice. *Yakugaku Zasshi.* 2000;120(10):849–862.

81. Schoonees A, Visser J, Musekiwa A, Volmink J. Pycnogenol (extract of French maritime pine bark) for the treatment of chronic disorders. *Cochrane Database Syst Rev.* 2012 Apr 18;4:CD008294.

82. Homma M, Oka K, Kobayashi H, et al. Impact of free magnolol excretions in asthmatic patients who responded well to saiboku-to, a Chinese herbal medicine. *J Pharm Pharmacol/* 1993 Sep;45(9):844–846.

83. Shindo K, Koide K, Fukumura M. Enhancement of leukotriene B4 release in stimulated asthmatic neutrophils by platelet activating factor. *Thorax.* 1997;52(12):1024–9.

84. Worth H, Schacher C, Dethlefsen U. Concomitant therapy with Cineole (Eucalyptole) reduces exacerbations in COPD: A placebo-controlled double-blind trial. *Respir Res.* 2009 Jul 22;10:69. doi: 10.1186/1465-9921-10-69.

85. Gross D, Shenkman Z, Bleiberg B, Dayan M, Gittelson M, Efrat R. Ginseng improves pulmonary functions and exercise capacity in patients with COPD. *Monaldi Arch Chest Dis.* 2002 Oct-Dec;57(5-6):242–246.

86. Sinclair S. Chinese herbs: A clinical review of *Astragalus, Ligusticum,* and *Schizandrae. Alternative Medicine Review.* 1998;3(5):338–344.

87. Badgujar SB, Patel VV, Bandivdekar AH. *Foeniculum vulgare* Mill: A review of its botany, phytochemistry, pharmacology, contemporary application, and toxicology. *BioMed Research International.* 2014;2014:842674. doi:10.1155/2014/842674.88. Leung AY, Foster S. *Encyclopedia of Common Natural Ingredients Used in Food, Drugs, and Cosmetics.* New York: John Wiley & Sons, 1996:222–224.

89. Hoffman D. *The Herbal Handbook: A User's Guide to Medical Herbalism.* Rochester, VT: Healing Arts Press; 1988:67.

90. Turker AU, Gurel E. Common mullein (*Verbascum thapsus* L.): Recent advances in research. *Phytother Res.* 2005 Sep;19(9):733–9.

91. Bone K. Marshmallow soothes cough. *Br J Phytother.* 1993/1994;3:93.

92. Büechi S, Vögelin R, von Eiff MM, Ramos M, Melzer J. Open trial to assess aspects of safety and efficacy of a combined herbal cough syrup with ivy and thyme. *Forsch Komplementarmed Klass Naturheilkd.* 2005 Dec;12(6):328–332.

93. Kaur B, Rowe B, Arnold E. Vitamin C supplementation for asthma. *Cochrane Database Syst Rev.* (1)2009.

94. Ginde A, Mansbach J, Camargo C. Association between serum 25-hydroxyvitamin D level and upper respiratory tract infection in the Third National Health and Nutrition Examination Survey. *Arch Intern Med.* 2009;169:384–390.

95. Collipp PJ, Goldzier S, Weiss N, et al.: Pyridoxine treatment of childhood bronchial asthma. *Ann Allergy.* 1975;35:93–97.

96. Bakkeheim E, Mowinckel P, Carlsen K, et al. Altered oxidative state in schoolchildren with asthma and allergic rhinitis. *Pediatr Allergy Immunol.* 2011;22:178–185.

97. Hill J, Micklewright A, Lewis S, et al. Investigation of the effect of short-term change in dietary magnesium intake in asthma. *Eur Respir J.* 1997;10:2225–2228.

98. Kazaks A, Uriu-Adams J, Albertson T, et al. Effect of magnesium supplementation on measures of airway resistance and subjective assessment of asthma control and quality of life in men and women with mild to moderate asthma: a randomized placebo controlled trial. *J Asthma.* 2010;47:83–92.

99. Cazzola M, Calzetta L, Page C, Jardim J, Chuchalin AG, Rogliani P, Matera MG. Influence of N-acetylcysteine on chronic bronchitis or COPD exacerbations: a meta-analysis. *Eur Respir Rev.* 2015 Sep;24(137):451–461.

100. Field T, Henteleff T, Hernandez-Reif M, et al. Children with asthma have improved pulmonary functions after massage therapy. *J Pediatr.* 1998;132:854–858.

101. Paul FA, Buser BR. Osteopathic manipulative treatment applications for the emergency department patient. *J Am Osteopath Assoc.* 1996;96:403–409.

102. Guiney PA, Chou R, Vianna A, et al. Effects of osteopathic manipulative treatment on pediatric patients with asthma: A randomized controlled trial. *J Am Osteopath Assoc.* 2005;105:7–12.

103. Rowane WA, Rowane MP. An osteopathic approach to asthma. *J Am Osteopath Assoc.* 2005;99:259–264.

104. Yao S, Hassani J, Gagne M, George G, Gilliar W. Osteopathic manipulative treatment as a useful adjunctive tool for pneumonia. *J Vis Exp.* 2014 May 6;(87).

105. Hondras MA, Linde K, Jones AP. Manual therapy for asthma. *Cochrane Database Syst Rev.* 2005(2); CD001002.

106. Vazquez MI, Buceta JM. Psychological treatment of asthma: effectiveness of a self-management program with and without relaxation training. *J Asthma.* 1993;30:171–183.

107. Ewer TC, Stewart DE. Improvement in bronchial hyper-responsiveness in patients with moderate asthma after treatment with a hypnotic technique: A randomized controlled trial. *BMJ.* 1986;293:1129–1132.

108. Yeh GY, Wayne PM, Litrownik D, Roberts DH, Davis RB, Moy ML. Tai chi mind-body exercise in patients with COPD: Study protocol for a randomized controlled trial. Trials. 2014 Aug 28;15:337.

109. Pbert L, Madison JM, Druker S, Olendzki N, Magner R, Reed G, Allison J, Carmody J. Effect of mindfulness training on asthma quality of life and lung function: A randomised controlled trial. *Thorax.* 2012;67:769–776.

110. Daubenmier J, Sze J, Kerr CE, Kemeny ME, Mehling W. Follow your breath: Respiratory interoceptive accuracy in experienced meditators. *Psychophysiology.* 2013;50:777–789.

111. Young EC, Brammer C, Owen E, Brown N, Lowe J, Johnson C, Calam R, Jones S, Woodcock A, Smith JA. The effect of mindfulness meditation on cough reflex sensitivity. *Thorax.* 2009;64:993–998.

112. Ding M, Zhang W, Li K, Chen X. Effectiveness of *T'ai Chi* and *Qigong* on chronic obstructive pulmonary disease: A systematic review and meta-analysis. *J Altern Comp Med.* 2014;20(2):79–86.

113. Kiatboonsri S, Amornputtisathaporn N, Siriket S, Boonsarngsuk V, Kiatboonsri C. Tai chi qigong exercise training in COPD. *Chest.* 2007;132(4, MeetingAbstracts):535a.

114. Sze MA, Hogg JC, Sin DD. Bacterial microbiome of lungs in COPD. *Int J COPD.* 2014;9:229–238.

115. Gleeson K, Eggli DF, Maxwell SL. Quantitative aspiration during sleep in normal subjects. *Chest.* 1997;111(5):1266–1272.

116. Smaldone GC, Foster WM, O'Riordan TG, Messina MS, Perry RJ, Langenback EG. Regional impairment of mucociliary clearance in chronic obstructive pulmonary disease. *Chest.* 1993;103(5):1390–1396.

117. Fanta CH. Clinical aspects of mucus and mucous plugging in asthma. *J Asthma.* 1985;22(6):295–301.

118. Ichinohe T, Pang IK, Kumamoto Y, et al. Microbiota regulates immune defense against respiratory tract influenza A virus infection. *Proc Natl Acad Sci U S A.* 2011;108(13):5354–5359.

119. Russell SL, Gold MJ, Hartmann M, et al. Early life antibiotic-driven changes in microbiota enhance susceptibility to allergic asthma. *EMBO Rep.* 2012; 13(5):440–447.

120. Dominguez-Bello MG, Costello EK, Contreras M, et al. Delivery mode shapes the acquisition and structure of the initial microbiota across multiple body habitats in newborns. Proc Natl Acad Sci U S A. 2010;107(26):11971–11975.

121. Renz-Polster H, David MR, Buist AS, et al. Caesarean section delivery and the risk of allergic disorders in childhood. *Clin Exp Allergy.* 2005;35(11):1466–1472.

122. Huang YJ, Boushey HA. The microbiome in asthma. *J Allergy Clin Immunol.* 2015;135(1):25–30.

123. Dickson RP, Erb-Downward JR, Huffnagle GB. The role of the bacterial microbiome in lung disease. *Exp Rev Resp Med.* 2013;7(3):245–257.

124. Morrow LE, Kollef MH, Casale TB. Probiotic prophylaxis of ventilator-associated pneumonia: A blinded, randomized, controlled trial. *Am J Respir Crit Care Med.* 2010;182(8):1058–1064.

19

Integrative Geriatric Psychiatry

RONALD GLICK, MARIE ANNE GEBARA, AND ERIC LENZE

Case Study

M rs. Smith is a 68-year-old married retired female who presented 1 year ago after involvement in an intensive outpatient program and completion of 65 sessions of electroconvulsive treatment for bipolar depression. She continued with prominent depressive symptoms, social withdrawal, and tearfulness despite treatment with four pharmacological agents. She also endorsed prominent anxiety and somatization with a gastrointestinal focus. There had been a question of cognitive impairment on prior testing, and it was unclear if this represented mild cognitive impairment or was a function of her mood disturbance. Depressive symptoms began 23 years prior, concurrent with perimenopause, but became more prominent over the prior 2 years.

Lab testing revealed low normal DHEA-S at 37.7, borderline elevated homocysteine of 13, and markedly elevated whole blood histamine, suggesting undermethylation. She was started on DHEA, 5 mg in the morning, which was increased to 10 mg daily in 1 week. She did not tolerate methionine initially, given increased gastrointestinal complaints, but this was added in later. She was also prescribed SAM-e 400 mg daily, B vitamins excluding folate, antioxidants, and zinc.

Within 1 month, she reported that her mood and energy were somewhat improved and she was no longer tearful throughout the day. In subsequent months, she described further improvement and has been going out for lunch with friends and family, which she had not done in over 1 year. Homocysteine went up to 17 and subsequently normalized after the addition of trimethyl-glycine and removal of SAM-e. DHEA-S was above the age-related norms on 15 mg/day and the dosage was decreased to 10 mg. One year out from the initial consultation, she and her husband note that her mood and anxiety continue to be moderately improved. Concerns regarding concentration and memory, noted previously, are no longer apparent.

The onset of symptoms at midlife without other specific provocation suggested a hormonal trigger. DHEA supplementation was a reasonable consideration given this history and the low-normal DHEA-S concentration. The rapid response was likely due to DHEA. It was a challenge treating undermethylation in the face of elevated homocysteine. This treatment likely contributed to further improvement of depression and anxiety. The continuation of L-methionine without SAM-e may be adequate for addressing undermethylation. This case highlights the potential of a broader model to address treatment resistance.

Introduction

Two converging forces have led to the growth of integrative psychiatry and mental health: the limitations of our standard approaches and the potential benefits of the expanding array of complementary approaches available. Traditional approaches, including psychopharmacology and standardized psychotherapeutic approaches such as cognitive-behavioral therapy (CBT), are often helpful, but not every patient benefits, with about half showing partial or minimal response. Moreover, many cannot tolerate, do not prefer, or do not have access to these traditional treatments. Making an integrative approach compelling is the inclusion of a range of complementary modalities such as mind–body therapies and nutritional approaches, which have the potential to be of benefit by themselves and to enhance other treatments.

In geriatric psychiatry, the stakes are high as mental illnesses such as depression are disabling, accelerate cognitive decline, and lead to premature mortality.[1] Medical comorbidities and chronic pain issues contribute to the impairment related to mental health disorders such as depression.

Integrative medicine, by its nature, is inclusive of traditional approaches. In this spirit, we provide a discussion of common psychiatric disorders seen in older adults and a description of traditional treatments (antidepressants and psychotherapy). Our focus is on the two most prevalent conditions, major depressive disorder and generalized anxiety disorder. In the second section we discuss approaches that fall under the heading of complementary and integrative interventions.

Late-Life Anxiety and Depression

Late-life depression and anxiety disorders are common but not inevitable with available preventive and treatment options. Improving both quality of life and function is the main treatment goal, with improved cognitive function and prevention of cognitive and health declines as potential secondary benefits of good treatment. Maintenance treatment is essential in relapse prevention, as these are chronic illnesses in most cases.

Clinical depression entails lack of interest and pleasure as well as persistent feelings of sadness most of the day for nearly every day. In the community, up to 4% of older adults have major depressive disorder (MDD) and 15% have clinically significant symptoms of depression.[2] Factors associated with improved outcomes in depression in late life include employment and absence of substance use disorders.[3] Risk factors include disability, poor health and new medical illness, and female gender.[4] Psychosocial risk factors such as death of a spouse or social isolation also contribute to morbidity.[5]

Anxiety disorders comprise worry, fear, or stress far in excess of what would be expected of a situation. They include generalized anxiety disorder (GAD), posttraumatic stress disorder, phobias (e.g., social phobia, agoraphobia), and panic disorder. Approximately 7% of older adults have anxiety disorders.[6] This may occur partly due to the increased stressors related to medical illnesses in later life.[7-9] Risk factors for anxiety disorders include female gender, early life stress, and chronic disability of the patient or spouse.

A key part of assessment and management relates to the clinician's role in maximizing protective factors and mitigating risk factors involved in the incidence and progression of depression and anxiety disorders (Box 19.1).[2,5,10,11]

Box 19.1. Risk Factors and Protective Factors for Depression and Anxiety Disorders in Older Adults

Risk Factors	Protective Factors
Social isolation	Social support
Functional limitation	Religious or spiritual practice
Medical illnesses	Physical activity
Cognitive decline	Cognitive stimulation
Lower income Grief/bereavement	Coping skills/life experiences
	Optimism and mastery

(Adapted from Fiske et al., 2009[10])

PRESENTATION

Older adults may have a harder time articulating concerns in the affective arena, and they are more likely to present with other symptoms. Anxiety disorders often manifest with cognitive concerns or somatic symptoms such as sleep disturbance, gastrointestinal problems, and muscle tension. Depressed older adults may also have a somatic focus, with common complaints including fatigue and apathy rather than low mood. Key symptoms can be elucidated by screening for MDD and GAD symptoms, following DSM-5 symptomatology.[12]

For a diagnosis of MDD, patients should have five or more of the following symptoms for at least 2 weeks:

Mood: sad, depressed, empty
Interest: diminished interest or pleasure in most activities
Guilt: feelings of excessive or inappropriate guilt or worthlessness
Sleep: insomnia or hypersomnia
Energy: fatigue, loss of energy
Concentration: inability to think, indecisiveness or poor memory
Appetite: low appetite and/or weight loss or weight gain (5% of body
    weight)
Psychomotor: retardation or agitation, can be subjective or objective
Suicide: thoughts of death; in more severe cases, suicidal ideation, plan,
    and intent

For a diagnosis of GAD, patients have symptoms more days than not in the past 6 months, including the following:

Worry: excessive or unreasonable
Control: difficulty controlling the worry
Physical signs: three or more: restless or feeling on edge, easily fatigued,
    difficulty concentrating, irritability, muscle tension, sleep disturbance
Distress: causing social impairment or change in lifestyle and decrease
    in activities

EVALUATION

Since suicide occurs most commonly in depressed patients, providers must screen for suicidal ideation and assess for suicide risk.[2,13] It is important to question the patient about active suicidal ideation, type, frequency, plan, and suicidal intentions as well as reasons for living.[14,15] As with depression and anxiety in general, with any clinically significant distress, it is important to assess risk and protective factors for suicide. Risk factors include older age, being a white male, prior attempt, family history of suicide, history of violence and impulsivity,[16,17] cognitive impairment, medical illness,[18] substance abuse, hopelessness, access to firearms, social isolation, and lack of social support.[19-22] With any concern of thoughts of death or suicidal ideation expressed, a key discussion centers around identification of firearms in the home and recommendation for removal and safe storage.

MANAGEMENT AND TREATMENT

The combination of psychotherapy with pharmacotherapy may be more effective than either intervention alone. However, maximizing the desirable effects of treatment may be best and most cost-effectively obtained by a sequential rather than simultaneous application of therapies. In anxiety disorders, for example, one may start with a course of pharmacotherapy followed by CBT. Similarly, if a patient is experiencing an anergic depression, a first step may be medication, accompanied by concrete guidelines to slightly increase activity. Electroconvulsive therapy is an effective option in resistant and severe cases of depression. Transcranial magnetic stimulation is another option for treatment-resistant depression, but at this time, cost and lack of insurance coverage are limitations.

Managing depression and anxiety disorders in older adults can be as simple as "ABCDEF": *A*ssessment, *B*enzodiazepine avoidance, *C*lose follow-up, *D*ose, *E*ducation, and *F*irst-line treatment:

A. *Assessment*: Older adults have varied presentations of depression and anxiety. Medical conditions must be ruled out, as they may be confounders of psychiatric symptoms. A basic workup includes screening for thyroid disease, vitamins B12 and D deficiency, electrolyte disturbances, or other general medical conditions that may mimic or exacerbate psychiatric illnesses. Providers should assess cognitive function, as delirium and dementia may contribute to mood problems. It is essential to review the patient's medications as anticholinergics and sedatives may cause depressive or anxiety symptoms and cognitive impairment. Screening should include a severity measure, such as the PHQ-9 or CESD, and medical comorbidities need to be factored in.

B. *Benzodiazepine avoidance*: Benzodiazepines may be beneficial when used in low doses over a short period (up to 6–8 weeks) for acute anxiety management. However, they have a poorer risk/benefit ratio in older adults given the potential to contribute to cognitive impairment and fall risk.

C. *Close follow-up:* Once treatment is initiated, close follow-up is important. Periodic contact with providers can help prevent early discontinuation of medication and allow treatment to be modified according to side effects or lack of efficacy.

D. *Dose:* The mantra is "start low, go slow, but go." Once initial treatment has been started and is tolerated, follow-up every 4 to 6 weeks can clarify the benefits and side effects prior to titration. If a maximum tolerated dose has not achieved remission, then augmentation or switch should be considered. Another important point relating to medication dose is maintenance; generally, "the dose that gets you well, keeps you well." Patients are discouraged from discontinuing medications; continuing medications reduces the relapse risk by 50% or more in late-life depression and anxiety disorders.

E. *Education:* Psychoeducation can instill hope and reassure patients that they have a manageable condition. Providers should address the stigma of psychiatric illness, clarifying any misconceptions that the patient or family might have about disorders or medication. Other considerations include cessation or minimization of alcohol consumption and increased physical activity.

F. *First-line treatment:* First-line treatment options include selective serotonin reuptake inhibitors (SSRIs), serotonin-norepinephrine reuptake inhibitors (SNRIs), and CBT. The selection process should involve the patient's preference, the physician's preference and expertise, and the availability of expert providers.

Psychotherapy

The qualities of a successful geriatric psychotherapist include flexibility of approach and experience and interest in geriatric mental health; this orientation is more important than the provider's specific training or discipline. Common approaches are CBT, interpersonal therapy, and mindfulness-based therapies. CBT is effective in the treatment of both depression and anxiety disorders in older adults, assuming that they are both motivated and cognitively intact.

Psychotherapists working in geriatrics draw from a wide range of approaches. Psychology and behavioral medicine practitioners have been practicing what has come to be known as mind–body medicine for several decades. These approaches are particularly helpful for the management of psychosocial stressors, chronic pain, and other general health conditions. Beyond the evidence-based therapies listed earlier, psychotherapists may engage patients in specific therapeutic approaches that may have salient benefit for older adults:

- Eye Movement Desensitization and Reprocessing (EMDR): This is a form of psychotherapy that uses visual, tactile, or auditory stimulation, from side to side, to facilitate the emotional processing of traumatic experiences. This is an effective treatment for posttraumatic stress disorders.[23] Additionally, older adults are likely to have had an accumulation of smaller traumatic events. To the extent that such experiences have an impact on mood, anxiety, sleep, and other health issues, EMDR may provide benefit and "cut to the chase" more quickly than traditional talk therapies.
- Narrative medicine and journaling: Anyone who has spent time with older relatives or neighbors can be transported by their tales and experiences. Is this "telling" of value to the individual? Narrative medicine is seen as a way to engage individuals in a therapeutic activity by relaying their stories, either verbally or in writing.[24]
- Directive activities: Erik Erikson described eight psychosocial phases that are a part of human experience and development.[25] The eighth phase is "ego integrity versus despair." The challenges at this stage may be more existential, and coping with losses, both external and to the person, is part of the task. A psychotherapist can help such a person find activities that he or she finds meaningful and that will restore a sense of productivity, contribution, or purpose.

Other therapeutic approaches include supportive therapy, problem-solving therapy, guided self-help, and instruction on relaxation techniques.

Provision of supportive measures is not the sole purview of licensed psychotherapists. A primary care provider is often in the best position to offer psychotherapeutic assistance to patients because they have an established relationship, they have frequent contact, and there is commonly a high level of trust. It is unlikely that primary care providers would be trained in or have time to carry out a full course of a formalized therapy such as CBT, but time-limited techniques may include bibliotherapy; instruction on sleep hygiene; instruction on basic relaxation techniques; referral to supportive resources through the internet, audiotapes, or community programs; counseling regarding reduction or cessation of alcohol use; exercise recommendations; and recommendations to increase overall activity, particularly social activities.

Pharmacotherapy

SSRIs are a reasonable choice for both MDD and GAD. Bupropion, given its favorable side-effect profile, is a reasonable first choice for depression, but not anxiety disorders. If a medication is not tolerated, the patient is typically switched to another class, such as the SNRIs. Options for lack of efficacy include change of class, adding a second medication from another class, and adding an adjunctive agent such as a second-generation antipsychotic (SGA) or a mood stabilizer.[26]

Some drugs for the treatment of anxiety and depression are more challenging to use in older adults, mainly due to their side-effect profiles. Such agents include tricyclic antidepressants (TCAs), monoamine oxidase inhibitors (MAOIs), lithium, and SGAs,[27] as well as the previously mentioned concerns about benzodiazepines and other sedatives. However, few drugs should be eliminated altogether from consideration for elders.[28] Since no medication has been demonstrated as superior in efficacy for depression, the medication choice in elderly should be based on the side-effect profile and minimizing risks. The common comorbidity of pain and depression may guide medication choice. TCAs, particularly amitriptyline and nortriptyline, have potent analgesia, but anticholinergic and antihistaminic effects may be limiting for older patients. Of the SNRIs, duloxetine has been best studied, but venlafaxine appears to have a reasonable analgesic effect as well.[29]

Table 19.1 gives information about antidepressants.

Complementary and Integrative Approaches

Which approaches or therapies do we consider to be complementary? As our evidence increases, the future will bring us to only one form of medicine. For this discussion, we include three areas: mind–body interventions, nutritional supplements, and spirituality/spiritual practice. While healthy nutrition is essential for mental health, we review some aspects within the discussion of specific supplements and refer the reader to Chapter 2 for further consideration.

Within this spectrum, a number of approaches can be employed to enhance mood, energy, sleep, and stress and anxiety management. Some measures are symptom or disorder specific such as melatonin for sleep disturbance. Others provide benefits across a wider spectrum, such as mindfulness-based interventions. In addition to ameliorating specific symptoms or mood-related problems, benefits may extend to other areas of health, including the potential to decrease pain and enhance cognitive function.

Table 19.1. Antidepressants

Class	Drug	Initial dose	Target dose	Side effects/considerations
Selective serotonin reuptake inhibitors (SSRI)	Escitalopram	5 mg	10–20 mg	L-isomer of citalopram
	Citalopram	10 mg	20–40 mg	U.S. Food and Drug Administration recommends not to exceed 20 mg in older adults because of QTc prolongation.
	Sertraline	25–50 mg	50–200 mg	
	Paroxetine	10–20 mg	20–40 mg	Less favorable because of anticholinergic effects and drug interactions
	Fluoxetine	10–20 mg	20–40 mg	Less favorable because of drug interactions and long half-life
Serotonin–norepinephrine reuptake inhibitors (SNRI)	Venlafaxine ER	37.5–75 mg	150–300 mg	Once-daily "ER" version favored over older multiple-daily-dosing version
	Duloxetine	30 mg	60–120 mg	CYP2D6 inhibitor
	Desvenlafaxine	50 mg	50–100 mg	Active metabolite of venlafaxine
	Milnacipran	12.5 mg	100 mg	Twice-daily dosing (50 mg BID)
Serotonin agonists	Mirtazapine	7.5–15 mg	30–45 mg	Side effects significant for sedation and increased appetite
	Vortioxetine	5–10 mg	5–20 mg	Mild pro-cognitive benefits, generally well tolerated
	Vilazodone	10 mg	20–40 mg	Has SSRI and serotonin 1A partial agonist properties. Nausea is common side effect.
Norepinephrine and dopamine reuptake inhibitor	Bupropion XL	150 mg	300–450 mg	Use in AM, may cause anxiety or agitation. Also used for smoking cessation. Once-daily "XL" version generally preferred to multiple daily dosing.
Tricyclic antidepressants (TCAs)	Nortriptyline	10–25 mg	50–100 mg	Anticholinergic, antihistaminic side effects, cardiac risk
	Desipramine	50 mg	100–200 mg	Anticholinergic, antihistaminic side effects, cardiac risk

MIND–BODY AND MOVEMENT-BASED INTERVENTIONS

In medicine, as in integrative health, we commonly discuss the "big three" areas of lifestyle with our patients: diet, exercise, and stress management. When we ask, "How do you manage stress?" responses vary from a blank stare to "I used to" . . . go to the gym, walk, do yoga. Why do we want our patients to engage in a mind–body practice? Considerations include the following:

- Stressors, such as financial difficulties, losses, and health problems, are common.
- As we age, measures of autonomic function, such as heart rate variability (HRV), move from parasympathetic toward sympathetic predominance.[30]
- Stress, anxiety, and depression are associated with a higher risk of health problems and add to the morbidity of these health conditions.[31]
- Mind–body approaches have potential benefit for mood,[32] anxiety, sleep, health conditions, and other measures of health and immune status.

These approaches are discussed in Chapters 6 and 9. More important than the specific practice is encouraging our patients to participate in a regular self-care practice.

What constitutes mind–body approaches? Broadly, this includes any activity that an individual engages in on a regular basis that has a beneficial effect on stress response and resilience. This definition would extend to aerobic exercise and spiritual practice; pragmatically, if our patients are engaging in those activities, it bodes well for their health and ability to cope with stress. These activities share with common mind–body practices a beneficial effect on autonomic functioning, immunity, and general health.[33,34] For the purpose of this discussion, we will focus on self-management or self-care practices, which an individual may engage in independently or as part of a group activity. This includes yoga, tai chi, and meditation, including Mindfulness-Based Stress Reduction (MBSR) and related approaches.

Studies of yoga have shown that it enhances clinical outcomes such as perceived stress, mood, sleep, health status, well-being, and quality of life.[35,36] It improves sleep quality among older adults.[36-38] A meta-analysis showed that yoga offers significant benefit for depression.[39] Yoga produces favorable changes in biological measures, including humoral and cardiac measures of autonomic stress response, beta endorphins, and inflammatory and anti-inflammatory cytokines.[35,40-420]

Studies of tai chi and qi gong have shown a shift in the autonomic balance toward a parasympathetic response;[43,44] improvement in psychoneuroimmunological measures, including augmentation of response to varicella and influenza vaccination, reduction in interleukin-6 and NF-κB, and decreased cortisol;[45-48] improvement in mood, perceived stress, and anxiety ratings;[49,50] and improved response and remission for older adults with treatment-resistant depression.[51]

Studies of MBSR, other mindfulness practices, and meditation have shown benefit for management of anxiety disorders and depression;[52] favorable autonomic and immune effects;[53-56] a beneficial effect on health and aging for individuals experiencing caregiver burden;[57] improvement for individuals with fibromyalgia, fatigue, or irritable bowel syndrome;[58] improvement in impaired memory performance for individuals with anxiety or depression;[59] and enhanced telomerase activity.[60]

NUTRITIONAL SUPPLEMENTS

There are three scenarios in which we utilize nutritional supplementation in psychiatric practice. The first reflects the roots of Western medicine, similar to employing natural agents such as foxglove or rauwolfia. In this case, we follow a biomedical model, prescribing agent A to treat condition B. The second area involves the use of high-dose multivitamin and mineral preparations. The final approach follows whole-systems models.

Prescribing Supplements Within a Biomedical Model

Agents may be used for a single indication, as with S-adenosyl methionine (SAM-e) for depression, or with broader effects on multiple psychiatric disorders, as with fish oil. As with psychopharmacology, one is vigilant about the potential for drug–drug interactions and adverse effects. Another challenge for clinicians in recommending supplements is to gain sufficient knowledge about high-quality supplements. In identifying such manufacturers, one looks for quality indications such as US Pharmacopeia (USP) and Good Manufacturing Practices (GMP). Having undergone assay by an independent laboratory increases confidence in a product's purity, quality, and freedom from toxic agents or contaminants.

Following is a short list of agents to consider, with a brief discussion of each (Table 19.2). Absent from this list is hypericum (St. John's wort). Given issues with hepatic enzyme induction, we find its use in geriatrics limited. However,

Table 19.2. Prescribing Supplements Within a Biomedical Model

Agent	Indication	Dosage	Common adverse events	Comments
Fish oil	Depression Bipolar disorder	1,000–2,000 mg/d	Belching, dyspepsia, bruising	Use high-EPA preparations.
Melatonin-SR Melatonin-IR	Insomnia-sleep continuity disturbance Sleep-onset insomnia	3–6 mg at HS 3–6 mg at HS	Limited Limited	
SAM-e	Depression	400–800 mg once or twice a day	Limited	Take at least 10 minutes before eating.
Inositol	Anxiety	2–4 g in water TID	Cramping and diarrhea	May use at a lower dose in capsule form prn
DHEA	Depression/ Fatigue	5–25 mg/day for women 10–50 mg/day for men	Irritability, anxiety, hirsutism	Potential risk for hormone-sensitive tumors
L-Methylfolate	Depression/ Fatigue	800 μg/d to 15 mg/d	Rare if starting with low dose	

as in the above discussion of pharmacotherapy, individual considerations may be a factor.

Fish Oil

Omega-3 fatty acids associated with fish and fish oil can help in the treatment of depression[61] and mood stabilization in bipolar disorder.[62] Consuming fish once or twice weekly not only provides omega-3s but enhances other vitamins, mineral, and fats; fish is also a good source of protein. Small, wild nonpredatory fish are recommended to avoid gradual mercury accumulation.

David Servan Schreiber eloquently describes the change in brain chemistry as a function of the shift in omega-6 to omega-3 balance over time.[63] In prehistoric times, the ratio of omega-6 to omega-3 in our diet was estimated to be 1 to 1. At the turn of the century (1900's) the Western diet shifted to a ratio of 4 to 1. Given changes in our food chain such as grain feeding of livestock, as well as the shift from a plant- to an animal-based diet, by the year 2000 this had quintupled to 20 to 1. As our brains are heavily lipid-based, this change has a dramatic impact on cell membrane permeability, neuronal conduction, and brain activity. This impact is brought home when one looks at the prevalence of psychiatric disorders in various cultures: the prevalence closely tracks the changes from a traditional to a Western diet. Fish consumption has been inversely association with depression.[64] Additionally, this may be a contributing factor to the increased prevalence and earlier onset of conditions such as bipolar disorder over the last several decades. The anti-inflammatory effect of omega-3 fatty acids may be a potential mechanism of action, given our recent knowledge of inflammation as a core concomitant of depression.[65]

Fish oil is among the most commonly used nutritional supplements, and it has potential benefit for cardiac health as well as mood. Higher-quality preparations are derived from cold-water fish and are filtered to minimize exposure to mercury and other potential toxins. The two active components are eicosapentaenoic acid (EPA) and docosahexaenoic acid (DHA). Dosage is typically from 1,000 to 2,000 mg/day with preparations high in EPA.[66] Commercial fish oil commonly has an EPA/DHA ratio of 1.5 to 1, which is used for medical indications such as treating elevated triglyceride levels. For mental health disorders, including depression and bipolar disorder, EPA appears to be the key ingredient, and ratios between 3.5 to 1 and 7 to 1 are preferable. A study is under way in Australia and New Zealand to test the potential benefit of omega-3 supplementation for older adults with subthreshold depression on mood and neurobiological outcomes.[67]

Fish oil is generally well tolerated. The most common complaint is mild dyspepsia, along with a fishy taste. When used at a dose of 2,000 mg/day, platelet inhibition can be seen, and older adults may be sensitive to bleeding or bruising even at lower doses. This is a particular concern as many seniors are prescribed low-dose aspirin or may be taking NSAIDs for pain.

Melatonin

As we age, the pineal gland decreases its secretion of melatonin, which partially explains the common decrease in sleep duration among older adults. We are flooded by light, electronic devices, and electromagnetic stimulation, which impact further on melatonin production. Melatonin is rapidly metabolized; consequently, exogenously administered melatonin is helpful for sleep-onset disturbance but less so for sleep maintenance problems, which are pervasive. While most pharmacies carry only immediate-release melatonin, a number of manufacturers produce a sustained-release (SR) form, which is found commonly as 2 or 3 mg. The average adult dosage is between 3 and 6 mg, taken at hour of sleep, although doses as low as 2 mg showed benefit for insomnia in middle-aged and older adults.[68] For concurrent sleep-onset delay, 3 to 6 mg of the immediate-release formula can be taken at the same time. While adverse effects are limited, we recommend dosing on the lower side for older adults. As this is an endogenous compound, side effects are rare; for that same reason, it is less likely to produce rebound when used intermittently, as seen with pharmaceutical agents. In the psychiatry consultation-liaison world, we have shifted away from other sedating medications to the use of melatonin for regulation of the sleep cycle in older adults in a medical setting such as the intensive care unit, particularly for those at risk for delirium.[69]

S-Adenosyl Methionine (SAM-e)

SAM-e (pronounced "Sammy") promotes methylation, is an integral part of B-vitamin metabolism, and stimulates serotonin and norepinephrine production and activity. Some studies have found comparable effects to the TCAs, although a Cochrane review found lack of convincing evidence of efficacy for depression.[70] When used as an adjunct to SSRIs, as compared to placebo, twice the remission and response rate was seen with SAM-e at doses of 800 to 1,600 mg/day.[71] The main limitation is cost, which can be several dollars per day. SAM-e has minimal adverse effects, but as with combined pharmaceutical agents, when taken with an antidepressant it can precipitate mania. The full dose is 1,600 mg/day, but given costs, it is commonly dosed between 400 and 800 mg/day. It should be taken on an empty stomach to facilitate absorption and it should be refrigerated to prevent degradation.

Inositol

Myoinositol (inositol) is a six-carbon ring isomer of glucose that is naturally occurring in the body and is involved with cell signaling, enhancing serotonin and norepinephrine pathways. It has prominent anxiolytic effects, with benefit for panic disorder, obsessive-compulsive disorder, and posttraumatic stress disorder.[72,73] It lacks the sedation commonly associated with pharmacological agents such as benzodiazepines. The full adult dose is 12 g/day divided into three doses, and studies have supported the efficacy and tolerability of up to 18 g/day. For individuals taking this on an intermittent basis and at a lower dose, it is given as 500- or 650-mg capsules, one or two capsules three times a day as needed. For those taking the full dose, it is provided as a powder, both for ease of administration as well as cost. As a sugar, it is readily dissolved in water and quite palatable. One can start with 2 g in water three times a day; the dose can be increased as tolerated, typically in 1 week, to 4 g three times a day. The main side effects are gastrointestinal, with cramping and diarrhea. Approximately 10% of patients cannot tolerate even a low dose; for another 10%, gastrointestinal symptoms limit dosage, with the majority tolerating this well. While primarily utilized for the management of anxiety disorders, it has benefit for depression as well.

Dehydroepiandrosterone (DHEA)

DHEA is produced jointly by the gonads and adrenal gland, and in late life production can drop to a fraction of the level in a healthy young adult.[74] In addition to age, production is lowered by stress, chronic disease, immunosuppressant medications, and cholesterol-blocking agents. It is a neurohormone, with both production and activity in the brain.

DHEA is a mother hormone, giving rise to estrogen and testosterone. The same cautions and risks are present as with other hormone replacement therapy. Especially when given at higher doses, downstream hormone levels may increase, with the potential to promote hormone-sensitive tumors. A history of or risk factors for breast or prostate cancer would be a relative contraindication for use of this agent. On the positive side, in the case of a hormonal trigger for fatigue and depression, such as menopause, DHEA can be of significant benefit. This has the advantage of targeting a physiological change that occurs with aging.

Screening for deficiency is done through testing of DHEA-sulfate (DHEA-S), the more stable form of the hormone. Lower levels of DHEA-S may correlate with depressed mood in postmenopausal women.[75] The literature does not provide guidelines as to what specific blood level warrants treatment, although one trial used a threshold of less than 100 µg/dl for males and less than 60 µg/dl for women.[76]

Trials have shown benefit of DHEA when used as monotherapy or for augmentation of treatment of depression, with subjects experiencing cognitive enhancement as well.[76–80] Dosages range from 30 to 500 mg/day. There is a fine line between correcting a deficiency state and "messing with Mother Nature," and a pragmatic approach does not try to raise levels to what are seen in young adulthood.

DHEA is available over the counter, commonly as 25- or 50-mg tablets. These doses are suited to this agent's use as an anabolic agent for athletes, who may take this in doses of 200 to 500 mg/day. Erring on the side of caution, we start at 5 mg/day in women and 10 mg/day in men. Although doses may go higher in specific circumstances, we commonly titrate to 25 mg/day in women and 50 mg/day in men. With a low initial dosage, slow titration, and a low ceiling dose, side effects are infrequent and generally mild. Activation can occur, particularly when the levels have been quite suppressed, resulting in irritability or insomnia. Androgenic effects include hirsutism and acne.

In addition to clinical effects, it is important to assess endocrine response. While one cannot eliminate the risk of this contributing to hormone-sensitive tumors, we recommend close monitoring. Following up on DHEA-S level ensures that one does not overshoot the physiological range. For women, we verify that the estradiol level stays below the age-related or postmenopausal cutoff. Although screening guidelines have changed for mammography, we recommend yearly mammogram and gynecological checks for women taking any form of hormone replacement. For men, we monitor prostate-specific antigen and free testosterone levels and encourage a regular digital examination.

Methylfolate

Folate deficiency is one of the most common nutritional deficiencies in the world. It is associated with neuropsychiatric disorders, including depression. Diets that are rich in leafy green vegetables provide folate or folic acid (vitamin B_9). The Western diet has incorporated folate by fortification of grains, which has been a requirement in the United States since 1998.[81] Folate is inactivated by cooling and processing food. Low levels of folate are associated with depression and dementia. Methylfolate supplementation can be effective, by itself or as an adjunctive therapy with psychotropic drugs,[82] for the reduction of depressive symptoms in individuals with low or normal folate levels, for bipolar disorder,[83] with comorbid alcoholism and improvement of cognitive function in older adults with folate deficiency.[84]

Folic acid in pill form undergoes four methylation steps to form L-5 methyltetrahydrofolate or methylfolate. The last step is mediated by the enzyme methylenetetrahydrofolate reductase (MTHFR). There are multiple single nucleotide polymorphisms (SNPs), with two prevalent variants, C677T and A1298C. The C667T variant, when homozygous, is associated with health conditions including hypercoagulability, conferring risk for stroke, recurrent miscarriage, migraines, and depression. MTHFR variants likely contribute to other conditions such as fatigue and fibromyalgia.

Why do we care about methylation? There has been increasing attention to this area as it affects metabolism on a cellular level throughout our body, it is involved in turning on and off genetic expression, and it plays a key role in the synthesis of monoamines.

Independent of the discussion of MTHFR, both folic acid and methylfolate have been used in the treatment of depression. While methylfolate is an over-the-counter agent, it is available in pharmacological strength by prescription as Deplin, in 7.5- and 15-mg doses. In studies, the 15-mg dose, but not 7.5 mg, significantly reduces depressive symptoms and induces remission. Fifteen milligrams of methylfolate rather than placebo, when added to an SSRI, doubles the rate of response and confers a four times greater likelihood of remission.[85] In a follow-up to the studies by the Harvard group, 70% of subjects who were considered nonresponders during the acute trial showed a response during a 12-month open extension with 15 mg of methylfolate.[86] Sixty-one percent of that original group of nonresponders experienced complete remission of symptoms. An additional report analyzed biological factors that correlated with response to methylfolate; among them, being homozygous for C677T predicted response.[87] Another trial found that methylfolate compared favorably to SGAs, both in terms of cost and response rates as an augmentation strategy for depression.[88] High doses of methylfolate should be used with caution to avoid hypermethylation syndrome, clinically manifested as irritability, anxiety, insomnia, nausea, and other symptoms.

Multivitamin and Mineral Preparations

Vitamins and minerals are essential for numerous metabolic pathways, act as cofactors for enzyme activity, and have an impact on the functioning of every cell in our bodies, including the central nervous system. Although a Western diet is not lacking in calories, it is often deficient in nutritional quality. Soil may be depleted of essential minerals and "vitamin-enriched" foods may not contain the same high-quality nutrients found in nature. Additionally, a number of factors may affect the status of essential nutrients, such as proton-pump inhibitors affecting vitamin B12 and iron absorption. Consequently, one would expect to see beneficial effects of vitamins, minerals, and antioxidants. Typically, research has failed to find a direct benefit of single nutrients when taken in pill form; in fact, at times adverse effects have been found. Vitamin E supplementation can increase the risk of prostate cancer,[89] and questions have been raised regarding calcium and cardiovascular risk.[90] Conversely, nutrients such as antioxidants, when ingested in the original foods found in nature, do in fact promote health.

If we do not see health effects of individual micronutrients, why would we expect combinations to be of greater benefit, particularly in a mental health setting? Proponents suggest several reasons:

- Nutritional deficiencies are common, with potential impact on central nervous system function.
- Given the frequency of deficiencies, the beneficial effect of one agent (e.g., one member of the B vitamin family) may be obscured by deficiencies of its siblings (e.g., use of folate with concurrent B6 deficiency).
- There are multiple forms of many micronutrients, and the ones tested may not be the most biologically active or may have deleterious effects.
- In older adults, micronutrient status is more likely to be affected by inadequate nutrition or impaired absorption of essential nutrients due to medications, gastrointestinal issues, or medical comorbidities.

Two Canadian companies have developed products that provide up to several times the recommended dietary allowance of over 30 essential vitamins and minerals (EMPowerplus® and Daily Essential Nutrients®). The manufacturers caution that this higher level of supplementation can increase sensitivity to psychotropic agents, necessitating significant dosage reduction. This has been studied in children with attention-deficit/hyperactivity disorder and in children and adults with depression and bipolar disorder. One geriatric study found that inpatients provided with supplementation showed improved mood, regardless of whether or not they were depressed at baseline,[91] and a second study found benefit of supplementation on depression in a nursing home setting.[92]

Whole-Systems Approaches

The National Center for Complementary and Integrative Health has used this term to describe culturally based healing systems, such as traditional Chinese medicine.[93] Each system includes a conceptualization of what promotes health or causes disease, a method of diagnosis, and treatments that ameliorate the underlying pathology within that system. Two whole-systems approaches are described here: the Walsh-Pfeiffer approach is focused on psychiatric disorders, and Functional Medicine has wider applications in general and geriatric medicine. These systems share an understanding of cellular metabolism, epigenetics, and neurochemistry with Western medicine. It is difficult to study complex interventions within our gold standard of double-blind placebo-controlled trials. Given the plausibility of these systems and empirical results in practice, they are embraced by early adopters, including integrative health practitioners, but are not widely accepted in allopathic medicine.

The Walsh/Pfeiffer Protocol

Carl Pfeiffer MD, PhD, was one of the fathers of the field of orthomolecular psychiatry, with particular interests in bipolar disorder and schizophrenia. One of the early observations, the mauve color of schizophrenic patients' urine when left overnight in a cold laboratory, led to the discovery of kryptopyrroles, a porphyrin metabolite.[94] Treatment with niacin, vitamin B6, and zinc resulted in resolution of the mauve factor and clinical improvement. William Walsh PhD, with formal training in chemistry, has advanced Dr. Pfeiffer's work on the description and management of five common metabolic problems: undermethylation, overmethylation, copper toxicity, zinc deficiency, and pyroluria.[95,96] All of these are over-represented among patients with psychiatric disorders; are epigenetically determined; contribute to neurochemical abnormalities, which may cut across specific psychiatric disorders; are associated with specific mental health, physical health, or constitutional symptoms; can be identified through laboratory testing; and are likely to respond to specific nutrient therapies. With this approach, if a response to supplementation is seen in 2 to 4 months, patients can review options with their treating psychiatrist or physician. This may lead to more complete remission of symptoms and a decrease in the psychotropic regimen, potentially with a corresponding decrease in adverse effects.

This protocol has pertinence for geriatric psychiatry in several regards: often, psychiatric disorders have their genesis earlier in life, making it plausible that they are driven by genetically based metabolic problems; given loss, health issues, and other disease manifestations, psychiatric disorders readily treated early in life may become resistant to treatment, necessitating adjunctive therapies; and constitutionally, older adults are more sensitive to the side effects of medications, limiting the strategies used in younger adults of higher doses and polypharmacy.

Functional Medicine

This approach seeks to answer the question "Why do we see a greater prevalence of chronic and disabling health conditions that defy standard treatments in Western societies?"[97] We are increasingly suffering from disorders such as arthritis, irritable bowel syndrome, fibromyalgia, fatigue, and migraines. From a mental health standpoint, depression, anxiety, and insomnia have become more prevalent and are commonly resistant to traditional pharmacological approaches. Often, our patients have a combination of mental and physical health conditions. Allopathic medicine directs specific pharmacological or surgical interventions to each disease. Within Functional Medicine, the specific disease may be incidental and the underlying pathophysiology may cut across conditions. There may be a cascade of events within this system leading to ripples of changes and health issues, with each compounding the others. Problem areas within this system include abnormal gut microbiome, impaired gut wall integrity, food allergies and intolerances, nutritional deficiencies, impaired detoxification pathways, hormonal dysfunction and deficiencies, impairment in energy production, inflammation and oxidative stress, and psychological stress.

Diagnosis is based on history, physical examination findings, and the judicious use of specialized testing as noted in Chapter 25. Treatment commonly begins with dietary changes, often an elimination diet, given how common dietary intolerance is. Rounding out treatment is directed use of nutritional supplements and modification of lifestyle factors.

Spiritual Practice
As noted in Chapter 9, spiritual practice is an important part of our existence and a potential area to connect with patients to enhance general and mental health. Spirituality and religious practice have been linked to better health outcomes in general, such as lower morbidity and mortality.[98] The benefit of spirituality and religion extends to mental health, with spiritual practice varying inversely with the prevalence of mental disorders, including depression,[99,100] suicidality,[101] and substance use.[102] Spiritual and religious practices have also been found to slow the progression of Alzheimer's disease.[103] It is proposed that the benefit of spiritual and religious practice on mental health comes from several mechanisms that include the ability to cope with stress,[104] thereby increasing positive emotions, giving meaning to difficult circumstances, and offering a subjective sense of control.[105]

Particularly at times of health challenges, our patients are interested in discussing spirituality, but it is not commonly addressed in a mainstream medical setting. Puchalski describes a simple assessment to open the door to a dialogue with our patients, the FICA Spiritual History Tool.[106]

It is important for the clinician to understand a patient's meaning of religion or spirituality so that it can be incorporated in assessment and treatment, given the beneficial effects of religion and spirituality in various types of mental illness, including mood and psychotic disorders.[107,108]

Conclusions

Mental health difficulties in older adults are common, interfere with daily functioning and quality of life, and have an impact on general health status, with the potential to hasten cognitive decline. Adverse effects from medications and treatment resistance are common. The use of complementary and integrative approaches can enhance treatment response. The greatest impact commonly comes from lifestyle-oriented approaches, with counseling directed toward diet, exercise, and stress management. Mind–body approaches can enhance mood, quality of life, and general health. Spirituality and spiritual practice is often neglected and provides another window to enhance coping. The judicious use of nutritional supplements has great potential to treat problems such as depression, anxiety disorders, and insomnia, and more research on the use of these agents with older adults is needed.

REFERENCES

1. Christensen GT, Maartensson S, Osler M. The association between depression and mortality: A comparison of survey- and register-based measures of depression. *J Affect Disord.* 2016;210:111–114.

2. Blazer DG. Depression in late life: Review and commentary. *J Gerontol A Biol Sci Med Sci.* 2003;58(3):249–265.

3. Cole MG, Bellavance F, Mansour A. Prognosis of depression in elderly community and primary care populations: A systematic review and meta-analysis. *Am J Psychiatry.* 1999;156(8):1182–1189.

4. Cole MG, Dendukuri N. Risk factors for depression among elderly community subjects: A systematic review and meta-analysis. *Am J Psychiatry.* 2003;160(6):1147–1156.

5. Bruce ML. Psychosocial risk factors for depressive disorders in late life. *Biol Psychiatry.* 2002;52(3):175–184.

6. Gum AM, King-Kallimanis B, Kohn R. Prevalence of mood, anxiety, and substance-abuse disorders for older Americans in the national comorbidity survey-replication. *Am J Geriatr Psychiatry.* 2009;17(9):769–781.

7. Chou KL, Mackenzie CS, Liang K, Sareen J. Three-year incidence and predictors of first-onset of DSM-IV mood, anxiety, and substance use disorders in older adults: Results from Wave 2 of the National Epidemiologic Survey on Alcohol and Related Conditions. *J Clin Psychiatry.* 2011;72(2):144–155.

8. Lenze EJ, Mulsant BH, Mohlman J, et al. Generalized anxiety disorder in late life: Lifetime course and comorbidity with major depressive disorder. *Am J Geriatr Psychiatry.* 2005;13(1):77–80.

9. Sheikh JI, Swales PJ, Carlson EB, Lindley SE. Aging and panic disorder: Phenomenology, comorbidity, and risk factors. *Am J Geriatr Psychiatry.* 2004;12(1):102–109.

10. Fiske A, Wetherell JL, Gatz M. Depression in older adults. *Ann Rev Clin Psychol.* 2009;5:363–389.

11. Krishnan KR. Biological risk factors in late life depression. *Biol Psychiatry.* 2002;52(3):185–192.

12. American Psychiatric Association. *The Diagnostic and Statistical Manual of Mental Disorders: DSM-5.* Washington, DC: American Psychiatric Publishing; 2013.

13. Conwell Y, Duberstein PR, Cox C, Herrmann JH, Forbes NT, Caine ED. Relationships of age and axis I diagnoses in victims of completed suicide: A psychological autopsy study. *Am J Psychiatry.* 1996;153(8):1001–1008.

14. Raue PJ, Brown EL, Meyers BS, Schulberg HC, Bruce ML. Does every allusion to possible suicide require the same response? *J Fam Pract.* 2006;55(7):605–612.

15. Raue PJ, Ghesquiere AR, Bruce ML. Suicide risk in primary care: Identification and management in older adults. *Curr Psychiatry Rep.* 2014;16(9):466.

16. Conner KR, Conwell Y, Duberstein PR, Eberly S. Aggression in suicide among adults age 50 and over. *Am J Geriatr Psychiatry.* 2004;12(1):37–42.

17. McGirr A, Alda M, Seguin M, Cabot S, Lesage A, Turecki G. Familial aggregation of suicide explained by cluster B traits: A three-group family study of suicide controlling for major depressive disorder. *Am J Psychiatry.* 2009;166(10):1124–1134.

18. Waern M, Rubenowitz E, Runeson B, Skoog I, Wilhelmson K, Allebeck P. Burden of illness and suicide in elderly people: Case-control study. *BMJ (Clinical research ed).* 2002;324(7350):1355.

19. Duberstein PR, Conwell Y, Conner KR, Eberly S, Evinger JS, Caine ED. Poor social integration and suicide: Fact or artifact? A case-control study. *Psychol Med.* 2004;34(7):1331–1337.

20. Holt-Lunstad J, Smith TB, Layton JB. Social relationships and mortality risk: A meta-analytic review. *PLoS Med.* 2010;7(7):e1000316.

21. Nock MK, Borges G, Bromet EJ, Cha CB, Kessler RC, Lee S. Suicide and suicidal behavior. *Epidemiol Rev.* 2008;30:133–154.

22. Rubenowitz E, Waern M, Wilhelmson K, Allebeck P. Life events and psychosocial factors in elderly suicides—a case-control study. *Psychol Med.* 2001;31(7):1193–1202.

23. Chen L, Zhang G, Hu M, Liang X. Eye movement desensitization and reprocessing versus cognitive-behavioral therapy for adult posttraumatic stress disorder: Systematic review and meta-analysis. *J Nervous Mental Dis.* 2015;203(6):443–451.

24. Cenci C. Narrative medicine and the personalisation of treatment for elderly patients. *Eur J Intern Med.* 2016;32:22–25.

25. Erkison EH, Erkison JM. *The Life Cycle Completed.* New York: W. W. Norton; 1997.

26. Gaynes BN, Warden D, Trivedi MH, Wisniewski SR, Fava M, Rush AJ. What did STAR*D teach us? Results from a large-scale, practical, clinical trial for patients with depression. *Psychiatr Serv.* 2009;60(11):1439–1445.

27. Lenze EJ, Mulsant BH, Blumberger DM, et al. Efficacy, safety, and tolerability of augmentation pharmacotherapy with aripiprazole for treatment-resistant depression in late life: A randomised, double-blind, placebo-controlled trial. *Lancet.* 2015;386(10011):2404–2412.

28. Katona C, Hansen T, Olsen CK. A randomized, double-blind, placebo-controlled, duloxetine-referenced, fixed-dose study comparing the efficacy and safety of Lu AA21004 in elderly patients with major depressive disorder. *Int Clin Psychopharmacol.* 2012;27(4):215–223.

29. Bril V, England JD, Franklin GM, et al. Evidence-based guideline: Treatment of painful diabetic neuropathy—report of the American Association of Neuromuscular and Electrodiagnostic Medicine, the American Academy of Neurology, and the American Academy of Physical Medicine & Rehabilitation. *Muscle Nerve.* 2011;43(6):910–917.

30. Jandackova VK, Scholes S, Britton A, Steptoe A. Are changes in heart rate variability in middle-aged and older people normative or caused by pathological conditions? Findings from a large population-based longitudinal cohort study. *J Am Heart Assoc.* 2016;5(2).

31. Slavich GM. Life stress and health: A review of conceptual issues and recent findings. *Teaching of Psychology.* 2016;43(4):346–355.

32. D'Silva S, Poscablo C, Habousha R, Kogan M, Kligler B. Mind-body medicine therapies for a range of depression severity: A systematic review. *Psychosomatics.* 2012;53(5):407–423.

33. Kurita A, Takase B, Shinagawa N, et al. Spiritual activation in very elderly individuals assessed as heart rate variability and plasma IL/10/IL-6 ratios. *Int Heart J.* 2011;52(5):299–303.

34. Soares-Miranda L, Sattelmair J, Chaves P, et al. Physical activity and heart rate variability in older adults: The Cardiovascular Health Study. *Circulation.* 2014;129(21):2100–2110.

35. Huang FJ, Chien DK, Chung UL. Effects of Hatha yoga on stress in middle-aged women. *J Nurs Res.* 2013;21(1):59–66.

36. Halpern J, Cohen M, Kennedy G, Reece J, Cahan C, Baharav A. Yoga for improving sleep quality and quality of life for older adults. *Altern Ther Health Med.* 2014;20(3):37–46.

37. Manjunath NK, Telles S. Influence of Yoga and Ayurveda on self-rated sleep in a geriatric population. *Indian J Med Res.* 2005;121(5):683–690.

38. Chen KM, Chen MH, Chao HC, Hung HM, Lin HS, Li CH. Sleep quality, depression state, and health status of older adults after silver yoga exercises: Cluster randomized trial. *Int J Nurs Studies.* 2009;46(2):154–163.

39. Cramer H, Lauche R, Langhorst J, Dobos G. Yoga for depression: A systematic review and meta-analysis. *Depression Anxiety.* 2013;30(11):1068–1083.

40. Kiecolt-Glaser JK, Bennett JM, Andridge R, et al. Yoga's impact on inflammation, mood, and fatigue in breast cancer survivors: A randomized controlled trial. *J Clin Oncol.* 2014;32(10):1040–1049.

41. Naveen GH, Varambally S, Thirthalli J, Rao M, Christopher R, Gangadhar BN. Serum cortisol and BDNF in patients with major depression-effect of yoga. *Int Rev Psychiatry.* 2016;28(3):273–278.

42. Tyagi A, Cohen M. Yoga and heart rate variability: A comprehensive review of the literature. *Int J Yoga.* 2016;9(2):97–113.

43. Lu WA, Kuo CD. The effect of Tai Chi Chuan on the autonomic nervous modulation in older persons. *Med Sci Sports Exerc.* 2003;35(12):1972–1976.

44. Audette JF, Jin YS, Newcomer R, Stein L, Duncan G, Frontera WR. Tai Chi versus brisk walking in elderly women. *Age Ageing.* 2006;35(4):388–393.

45. Black DS, Irwin MR, Olmstead R, Ji E, Crabb Breen E, Motivala SJ. Tai chi meditation effects on nuclear factor-kappaB signaling in lonely older adults: A randomized controlled trial. *Psychother Psychosom.* 2014;83(5):315–317.

46. Campo RA, Light KC, O'Connor K, et al. Blood pressure, salivary cortisol, and inflammatory cytokine outcomes in senior female cancer survivors enrolled in a tai chi chih randomized controlled trial. *J Cancer Survivor.* 2015;9(1):115–125.

47. Irwin MR, Olmstead R. Mitigating cellular inflammation in older adults: A randomized controlled trial of Tai Chi Chih. *Am J Geriatr Psychiatry.* 2012;20(9):764–772.

48. Ho RT, Wang CW, Ng SM, et al. The effect of t'ai chi exercise on immunity and infections: A systematic review of controlled trials. *J Altern Comp Med.* 2013;19(5):389–396.

49. Abbott R, Lavretsky H. Tai Chi and Qigong for the treatment and prevention of mental disorders. *Psychiatr Clin North Am.* 2013;36(1):109–119.

50. Wang WC, Zhang AL, Rasmussen B, et al. The effect of Tai Chi on psychosocial well-being: A systematic review of randomized controlled trials. *J Acupuncture Meridian Studies.* 2009;2(3):171–181.

51. Lavretsky H, Alstein LL, Olmstead RE, et al. Complementary use of tai chi chih augments escitalopram treatment of geriatric depression: a randomized controlled trial. *Am J Geriatric Psychiatry.* 2011;19(10):839–850.

52. Hoge EA, Bui E, Marques L, et al. Randomized controlled trial of mindfulness meditation for generalized anxiety disorder: Effects on anxiety and stress reactivity. *J Clin Psychiatry.* 2013;74(8):786–792.

53. Lumma AL, Kok BE, Singer T. Is meditation always relaxing? Investigating heart rate, heart rate variability, experienced effort and likeability during training of three types of meditation. *Int J Psychophysiol.* 2015;97(1):38–45.

54. Bottaccioli F, Carosella A, Cardone R, et al. Brief training of psychoneuroendocrinoimmunology-based meditation (PNEIMED) reduces stress symptom ratings and improves control on salivary cortisol secretion under basal and stimulated conditions. *Explore.* 2014;10(3):170–179.

55. Jindal V, Gupta S, Das R. Molecular mechanisms of meditation. *Mol Neurobiol.* 2013;48(3):808–811.

56. Creswell JD, Irwin MR, Burklund LJ, et al. Mindfulness-Based Stress Reduction training reduces loneliness and pro-inflammatory gene expression in older adults: A small randomized controlled trial. *Brain Behav Immunity.* 2012;26(7):1095–1101.

57. Whitebird RR, Kreitzer M, Crain AL, Lewis BA, Hanson LR, Enstad CJ. Mindfulness-based stress reduction for family caregivers: A randomized controlled trial. *Gerontologist.* 2013;53(4):676–686.

58. Lakhan SE, Schofield KL. Mindfulness-based therapies in the treatment of somatization disorders: A systematic review and meta-analysis. *PloS One.* 2013;8(8):e71834.

59. Wetherell J, Hershey S, Hickman S, et al. Mindfulness Based Stress Reduction for older adults with stress disorders and neurocognitive difficulties: A randomized controlled trial. *J Clin Psychiatry.* 2017 Jul;78(7):e734–e743.

60. Schutte NS, Malouff JM. A meta-analytic review of the effects of mindfulness meditation on telomerase activity. *Psychoneuroendocrinology.* 2014;42:45–48.

61. Appleton KM, Rogers PJ, Ness AR. Updated systematic review and meta-analysis of the effects of omega-3 long-chain polyunsaturated fatty acids on depressed mood. *Am J Clin Nutr.* 2010;91(3):757–770.

62. Stoll AL, Locke CA, Marangell LB, Severus WE. Omega-3 fatty acids and bipolar disorder: A review. *Prostaglandins Leukotrienes Essential Fatty Acids.* 1999;60(5-6):329–337.

63. Servan-Schreiber D. *Instinct to Heal: Curing Stress, Anxiety and Depression Without Drugs and Without Talk Therapy.* New York: Rodale Press; 2004.

64. Bountziouka V, Polychronopoulos E, Zeimbekis A, et al. Long-term fish intake is associated with less severe depressive symptoms among elderly men and women: The MEDIS (MEDiterranean ISlands Elderly) epidemiological study. *J Aging Health.* 2009;21(6):864–880.

65. Grosso G, Galvano F, Marventano S, et al. Omega-3 fatty acids and depression: Scientific evidence and biological mechanisms. *Oxidative Medicine and Cellular Longevity.* 2014;2014:313570.

66. Sublette ME, Ellis SP, Geant AL, Mann JJ. Meta-analysis of the effects of eicosapentaenoic acid (EPA) in clinical trials in depression. *J Clin Psychiatry.* 2011;72(12):1577–1584.

67. Cockayne NL, Duffy SL, Bonomally R, et al. The Beyond Ageing Project Phase 2: A double-blind, selective prevention, randomised, placebo-controlled trial of omega-3 fatty acids and sertraline in an older age cohort at risk for depression: Study protocol for a randomized controlled trial. *Trials.* 2015;16:247.

68. Lyseng-Williamson KA. Melatonin prolonged release in the treatment of insomnia in patients aged >/=55 years. *Drugs Aging.* 2012;29(11):911–923.

69. Chakraborti D, Tampi DJ, Tampi RR. Melatonin and melatonin agonist for delirium in the elderly patients. *Am J Alzheimers Dis Other Dementias.* 2015;30(2):119–129.

70. Galizia I, Oldani L, Macritchie K, et al. S-adenosyl methionine (SAMe) for depression in adults. *Cochrane Database Syst Rev.* 2016;10:Cd011286.

71. Papakostas GI, Mischoulon D, Shyu I, Alpert JE, Fava M. S-adenosyl methionine (SAMe) augmentation of serotonin reuptake inhibitors for antidepressant non-responders with major depressive disorder: A double-blind, randomized clinical trial. *Am J Psychiatry.* 2010;167(8):942–948.

72. Fux M, Levine J, Aviv A, Belmaker RH. Inositol treatment of obsessive-compulsive disorder. *Am J Psychiatry.* 1996;153(9):1219–1221.

73. Palatnik A, Frolov K, Fux M, Benjamin J. Double-blind, controlled, crossover trial of inositol versus fluvoxamine for the treatment of panic disorder. *J Clin Psychopharmacol.* 2001;21(3):335–339.

74. Kroboth PD, Salek FS, Pittenger AL, Fabian TJ, Frye RF. DHEA and DHEA-S: A review. *J Clin Pharmacol.* 1999;39(4):327–348.

75. Barrett-Connor E, von Muhlen D, Laughlin GA, Kripke A. Endogenous levels of dehydroepiandrosterone sulfate, but not other sex hormones, are associated with depressed mood in older women: The Rancho Bernardo Study. *J Am Geriatr Soc.* 1999;47(6):685–691.

76. Wolkowitz OM, Reus VI, Roberts E, et al. Dehydroepiandrosterone (DHEA) treatment of depression. *Biol Psychiatry.* 1997;41(3):311–318.

77. Schmidt PJ, Daly RC, Bloch M, et al. Dehydroepiandrosterone monotherapy in midlife-onset major and minor depression. *Arch Gen Psychiatry.* 2005;62(2):154–162.

78. Wolkowitz OM, Reus VI, Keebler A, et al. Double-blind treatment of major depression with dehydroepiandrosterone. *Am J Psychiatry.* 1999;156(4):646–649.

79. Wolkowitz OM, Reus VI, Roberts E, et al. Antidepressant and cognition-enhancing effects of DHEA in major depression. *Ann N Y Acad Sci.* 1995;774:337–339.

80. Bloch M, Schmidt PJ, Danaceau MA, Adams LF, Rubinow DR. Dehydroepiandrosterone treatment of midlife dysthymia. *Biol Psychiatry.* 1999;45(12):1533–1541.

81. Mental Health America. Complementary & Alternative Medicine for Mental Health. 2016; http://www.mentalhealthamerica.net/sites/default/files/MHA_CAM.pdf.

82. Coppen A, Bailey J. Enhancement of the antidepressant action of fluoxetine by folic acid: A randomised, placebo controlled trial. *J Affect Disord.* 2000;60(2):121130.

83. Nierenberg AA, Montana R, Kinrys G, Deckersbach T, Dufour S, Baek JH. L-methylfolate for bipolar I depressive episodes: An open trial proof-of-concept registry. *J Affect Disord.* 2017;207:429–433.

84. Fava M, Mischoulon D. Folate in depression: Efficacy, safety, differences in formulations, and clinical issues. *J Clin Psychiatry.* 2009;70(Suppl 5):12–17.

85. Papakostas GI, Shelton RC, Zajecka JM, et al. L-methylfolate as adjunctive therapy for SSRI-resistant major depression: Results of two randomized, double-blind, parallel-sequential trials. *Am J Psychiatry.* 2012;169(12):1267–1274.

86. Zajecka JM, Fava M, Shelton RC, Barrentine LW, Young P, Papakostas GI. Long-term efficacy, safety, and tolerability of L-methylfolate calcium 15 mg as adjunctive therapy with selective serotonin reuptake inhibitors: A 12-month, open-label study following a placebo-controlled acute study. *J Clin Psychiatry.* 2016;77(5):654–660.

87. Shelton RC, Pencina MJ, Barrentine LW, et al. Association of obesity and inflammatory marker levels on treatment outcome: Results from a double-blind, randomized study of adjunctive L-methylfolate calcium in patients with MDD who are inadequate responders to SSRIs. *J Clin Psychiatry.* 2015;76(12):1635–1641.

88. Wade RL, Kindermann SL, Hou Q, Thase ME. Comparative assessment of adherence measures and resource use in SSRI/SNRI-treated patients with depression using second-generation antipsychotics or L-methylfolate as adjunctive therapy. *J Manag Care Pharmacy.* 2014;20(1):76–85.

89. Klein EA, Thompson IM, Jr., Tangen CM, et al. Vitamin E and the risk of prostate cancer: The Selenium and Vitamin E Cancer Prevention Trial (SELECT). *JAMA.* 2011;306(14):1549–1556.

90. Kopecky SL, Bauer DC, Gulati M, et al. Lack of evidence linking calcium with or without vitamin D supplementation to cardiovascular disease in generally healthy adults: A clinical guideline from the National Osteoporosis Foundation and the American Society for Preventive Cardiology. *Ann Intern Med.* 2016;165(12):867–868.

91. Gariballa S, Forster S. Effects of dietary supplements on depressive symptoms in older patients: A randomised double-blind placebo-controlled trial. *Clin Nutr.* 2007;26(5):545–551.

92. Gosney MA, Hammond MF, Shenkin A, Allsup S. Effect of micronutrient supplementation on mood in nursing home residents. *Gerontology.* 2008;54(5):292–299.

93. NCCAM. *Expanding Horizons of Health Care Strategic Plan 2005–2009.* 2005.

94. McGinnis WR, Audhya T, Walsh WJ, et al. Discerning the mauve factor, part 1. *Altern Ther Health Med.* 2008;14(2):40–50.

95. Stuckey R, Walsh W, Lambert B. The effectiveness of targeted nutrient therapy in treatment of mental illness: A pilot study. *J Australian Coll Nutritional Environmental Med.* 2010;29(3):3–8.

96. Walsh WJ, Glab LB, Haakenson ML. Reduced violent behavior following biochemical therapy. *Physiol Behav.* 2004;82(5):835–839.

97. DeBusk R, Sierpina VS, Kreitzer MJ. Applying functional nutrition for chronic disease prevention and management: Bridging nutrition and functional medicine in 21st century healthcare. *Explore.* 2011;7(1):55–57.

98. Levin JS, Schiller PL. Is there a religious factor in health? *J Religion health.* 1987;26(1):9–36.

99. Koenig HG, Cohen HJ, Blazer DG, et al. Religious coping and depression among elderly, hospitalized medically ill men. *Am J Psychiatry.* 1992;149(12):1693–1700.

100. Williams DR, Larson DB, Buckler RE, Heckmann RC, Pyle CM. Religion and psychological distress in a community sample. *Social Sci Med.* 1991;32(11):1257–1262.

101. Sisask M, Varnik A, Kolves K, et al. Is religiosity a protective factor against attempted suicide: A cross-cultural case-control study. *Arch Suicide Res.* 2010;14(1):44–55.

102. Miller WR. Researching the spiritual dimensions of alcohol and other drug problems. *Addiction.* 1998;93(7):979–990.

103. Kaufman Y, Anaki D, Binns M, Freedman M. Cognitive decline in Alzheimer disease: Impact of spirituality, religiosity, and QOL. *Neurology.* 2007;68(18):1509–1514.

104. Tepper L, Rogers SA, Coleman EM, Malony HN. The prevalence of religious coping among persons with persistent mental illness. *Psychiatr Serv.* 2001;52(5):660–665.

105. Koenig HG. Religion, spirituality, and health: The research and clinical implications. *ISRN Psychiatry.* 2012;2012:278730.

106. Puchalski CM. The FICA Spiritual History Tool #274. *J Palliat Med.* 2014;17(1):105–106.

107. Koenig HG. Research on religion, spirituality, and mental health: A review. *Can J Psychiatry.* 2009;54(5):283–291.

108. Mueller PS, Plevak DJ, Rummans TA. Religious involvement, spirituality, and medicine: Implications for clinical practice. *Mayo Clin Proc.* 2001;76(12):1225–1235.

20

Neurodegenerative Diseases: Parkinson's and Alzheimer's Diseases

AVIVA ELLENSTEIN, CHRISTINA PRATHER,
AND MIKHAIL KOGAN

Parkinson's Disease

CASE STUDY

Thomas is a 72-year-old, previously healthy, retired businessman who spends his days traveling with his wife, spending time with his grandchildren, and keeping physically active by walking daily and playing tennis weekly. He visited a neurologist's office with his wife to discuss shaking that his wife initially observed in his right hand about 2 years ago and that he has also noticed for about 1 year. His wife also mentions that he's been lagging behind her on their daily walks. They have looked up his symptoms on the internet and now think he may have Parkinson's disease. They are worried about the future and confused, noting that no one in his family has ever had this problem.

A comprehensive history and examination by the neurologist reveals that his right-sided resting tremor is accompanied by the slowly progressive motor and non-motor symptoms and signs typical of Parkinson's disease. There is no evidence to suggest any of the handful of differential diagnoses that can also manifest with parkinsonism. Treatment with carbidopa/levodopa is initiated. When he returns for follow-up evaluation, he is taking carbidopa/levodopa 25/100, 1.5 tablets three times daily, and is pleased to report that his tremor is gone. He is not only moving better on the tennis court but is also faster going through his routine daily activities. His energy level has increased, and his mood is good as his worry is diminishing.

INTRODUCTION

Parkinson's disease (PD) is a slowly progressive neurodegenerative disorder. The pathophysiology, clinical subtypes, and optimal treatment of PD continue to be elucidated.[1] This chapter includes a brief scientific review of PD as well as general guidelines and selected practical recommendations for management. A comprehensive discussion of PD is beyond the scope of this manuscript.

The essential clinical features of PD are the abnormal movements of resting tremor, bradykinesia, rigidity, and postural instability, a motor symptom complex known as *parkinsonism*.[2,3] PD often includes a diverse constellation of non-motor symptoms, including but not limited to anosmia, constipation, sleep disorders, orthostatic hypotension, mood disorders, fatigue, and dementia.[4] It is increasingly appreciated that many people with PD find these symptoms among the most challenging, although they are not always evaluated clinically. Routine, comprehensive care, including individualized clinical characterization and management, is optimal.[4,5]

Given the long and varied natural history of PD, individual goals and priorities can change and should be regularly reviewed. A team of care providers is often beneficial. As research continues to advance pharmacological therapies, define nonpharmacological options, and identify effective integrative health care delivery models, individual treatment plans should reflect evidence-based guidelines.

PD is the second most common neurodegenerative disorder, following Alzheimer's disease.[1,7] PD affects approximately 1 million Americans and up to 10 million people worldwide;[6] however, its epidemiology is not completely understood. Age is the greatest risk factor for PD, with a risk of 1% to 2% above age 60 to 65 years. There is a slightly higher incidence in men than women, with a ratio of 3:2.[7] PD is a disease for which no other common environmental risk factors have been identified. Isolated populations with unusual toxic exposures (e.g., Mn and 1-methyl-4-phenyl-1,2,3,6-tetrahydropyridine [MPTP]) have manifested parkinsonian syndromes, and an association of PD with high levels of some pesticide exposure has been described; however, biased or otherwise confounded epidemiological studies provide insufficient evidence of any major toxic cause for PD.[8]

PD is pathologically characterized by the presence of Lewy bodies, intraneuronal aggregates largely composed of the protein alpha synuclein. Pathologic staging of PD is based on a stereotypical accumulation of Lewy bodies in the brain.[9] Among the neuroanatomical lesions in PD, the definitive degeneration of dopaminergic neurons in the substantia nigra renders ineffective the basal ganglia–based pathways that modulate normal movement. In association with dysfunctional cortical and cerebellar motor control networks, this degeneration leads to the slow, stiff, and tremulous symptoms typical of PD.[10,11] Non-dopaminergic pathways throughout the central and peripheral nervous system additionally contribute to the diverse array of motor and non-motor symptoms in PD.[12]

Although a discrete pathophysiological process has yet to be established, dysfunctional pathways involving α-synuclein, GBA, the ubiquitin-proteosome system, lysosomes, and mitochondria have all been implicated.[13,14] There is evidence of cell-to-cell propagated oligomerization of α-synuclein, α-synuclein-dependent mitochondrial surface protein trafficking, and cABL tyrosine kinase-mediated clearance of α-synuclein, which continue to support research aimed at rational drug design.[15–17] Microbiome changes have been implicated in the pathophysiology of PD.[18] Although it is too early to make any specific clinical recommendations, this relationship adds to a growing body of knowledge connecting the health of the brain and the gastrointestinal system. Additional studies of a broad array of biomarkers will further elucidate PD clinical subtypes and may provide novel tools to monitor both disease progression and treatment response.[19,20]

DIAGNOSIS

The diagnosis of PD is clinical. It is based on a constellation of the definitive slowly progressive motor symptoms and signs typical of PD, exclusion of alternate diagnoses, supportive non-motor symptoms, and a robust response to dopaminergic therapy.[2,3] In 2015, the International Parkinson and Movement Disorders Society (MDS) provided updated clinical diagnostic criteria.[2] The MDS criteria emphasize the value of expert clinical evaluation, particularly in assessing and re-examining features that support PD or an alternate diagnosis. Brain imaging is not required for the diagnosis of PD.[2] An abnormal dopamine transporter (DaT) SPECT scan provides evidence of dopamine deficit in the basal ganglia; however, it is not specific for PD and is also found in multiple system atrophy, progressive supranuclear palsy, and Lewy body dementia.[21]

TREATMENT

Management of PD is multifaceted, including pharmacological, physiotherapeutic, supportive, and occasionally surgical modalities. The mainstay of treatment is levodopa; however, a comprehensive discussion of standard, allopathic treatments is outside the scope of this chapter. The reader is advised to refer to current recommendations at the Movement Disorder Society (www.mds.org) and the American Academy of Neurology (www.aan.com).

Lifestyle Approaches

Exercise

It has been demonstrated that patients who exercise regularly have improved mobility, decreased disease progression, decreased cognitive decline, improved quality of life, and lessened caregiver burden.[22] Evidence suggests that programs supporting gait and balance, aerobic function, and strength are each valuable. Among the longest-studied programs, the Lee Silverman Voice Therapy LOUD (speech) and BIG (gait and balance) programs have demonstrated benefits in several studies.[23] In addition, resistance training improves not only strength but also motor symptoms and balance. Both aerobic and strength training benefit mood and cognition.[24]

Recently tai chi has been demonstrated to have sustainable benefit on balance and mobility in a number of randomized trails.[25] This low-impact, low-cost, widely available exercise can be advocated for most patients with PD.

Diet

At this point there is inconclusive evidence to recommend specific dietary modifications for PD. There is a weak association between the Mediterranean diet and a lower risk of developing PD.[26] There is weak evidence suggesting that vitamin E-rich foods, tea, coffee, and alcohol are associated with a lower risk of PD.[27] Given the lack of strong data to support dietary modification, clinicians may opt to recommend a general anti-inflammatory diet, such as the Mediterranean diet, given its overall health benefits elucidated elsewhere in this book and specifically reviewed in Chapter 2.

Specific dietary modifications may be helpful for the management of constipation. Most recently, a double-blind randomized controlled trial demonstrated that fermented milk containing pre- and probiotics improved constipation in patients with PD.[28] For patients who are dairy-free because of allergies or cultural preferences, a trial of oral probiotic supplements for constipation may be warranted. See Chapter 2 for more details on the anti-inflammatory diet and fermented foods.

Supplements and Herbs

Although supplements may provide some supportive role for patients with PD, there is no convincing data that they specifically affect PD. Since the following supplements frequently arise in discussion, familiarity with them may help clinicians provide comprehensive education for patients about their potential benefit or lack thereof. Of particular note, the use of *Mucuna pruriens*, an unregulated dopaminergic plant-based preparation, may substantially interfere with the safe and appropriate administration of the regulated dopaminergic medications, for example carbidopa/levodopa.

- *Coenzyme Q10 (CoQ10).* CoQ10 is an endogenous mitochondrial component of the electron transport chain involved in aerobic generation of ATP. Endogenous CoQ10 is depleted in most patients with PD,[29] but several trials have failed to confirm the hypothesis that repletion of CoQ10 may slow functional decline in PD by restoring low endogenous levels. Despite several early small trials with positive outcomes, a 2011 Cochrane review initially endorsing CoQ10 repletion was later withdrawn due to methodological concerns.[30] Subsequently, a large trial of high-dose CoQ10 (up to 1,200 mg/day) was stopped early due to lack of efficacy and a trend of increased side effects as compared to placebo.[31]
- *Fish oil* and other forms of supplemental omega-3 are the most commonly used supplements in the United States. Omega-3 supplements are known to have anti-inflammatory effects, and epidemiological data show that populations with high intake of omega 3-fatty acids have a lower risk of PD. While no trials have been conducted to assess effect of omega-3 on PD progression, it may be beneficial for PD-associated depression.[32]
- *N-acetylcysteine (NAC) and Glutathione (GSH).* Similar to CoQ10, brain glutathione levels are depleted in most PD patients. For years, different forms of GSH have been tried in small case series or randomized trials for PD, and there are many unsupported claims suggesting benefit of GSH for PD. Data remain too inconsistent to support the use of GSH for PD. A theoretical difficulty of using supplemental GSH is poor crossing through the blood–brain barrier.[33] Utilization of NAC as a GSH precursor is of interest since NAC readily crosses the blood–brain barrier, is available in inexpensive oral forms, and is very stable. A randomized trial evaluating 1,800 or 3,600 mg of NAC has been recently concluded, and results are expected soon.[34]
- *Mucuna pruriens.* This traditional ayurvedic leguminous plant has been used in India for the treatment of PD and other conditions for centuries. Seeds are typically used as food and contain naturally occurring levodopa in addition to a variety of flavonoids and antioxidants shown to be neuroprotective in animal models.[35] In one small double-blind randomized crossover study 30 g of *Mucuna* seeds appeared

to have a positive effect similar to 200/50 mg levodopa/carbidopa.[36] Despite its tradition of use in PD, *Mucuna* is not recommended in the United States, where it is not readily available as food and is instead formulated into supplements. Market variability and lack of standardization to allow for comparison of whole-seed preparation to extracts reasonably limits use in the United States. For important safety reasons and concern for overdosing on dopamine, *Mucuna* cannot be combined with levodopa-containing medications. In this author's experience, when patients present using or inquiring about *Mucuna*, most of the conversation circles around addressing specific fears of taking PD medications, suggesting that clinicians should remain vigilant to address underlying concerns and motivations for supplement use to provide the best personalized care.

There are a number of other supplements and herbs that are claimed to have various of benefits for patients with PD and Alzheimer's disease. See Table 20.1 for a complete list.

Acupuncture
Use of acupuncture and other traditional Chinese medicine approaches for patients with PD is very common in China. A number of Chinese and U.S. randomized trials assessed the efficacy of acupuncture for a variety of motor and non-motor symptoms.[37,38]

Pharmacological Management
Optimal pharmacological management of motor parkinsonism and non-motor symptoms includes reducing symptoms, avoiding fluctuations (periods of effective ["on"] and ineffective ["off"] responses to treatment, and minimizing side effects. Although motor symptoms such as tremor are the most immediately observable and their treatment may be the most familiar to physicians, because non-motor symptoms are often the most troubling to patients, they should be explicitly addressed. For example, a tremor in the nondominant hand that is readily observed by the clinician may not disturb the patient, while nocturia five times nightly has a negative impact on both sleep and overall function.

The mainstay of symptomatic treatment is levodopa. The biochemical precursor to dopamine, levodopa is highly effective in treating motor parkinsonism and also diminishes some non-motor symptoms. While bradykinesia and rigidity typically improve substantially with levodopa, tremor is occasionally somewhat resistant. In its most common form, oral levodopa is always given together with a peripheral dopa decarboxylase inhibitor (carbidopa or

Table 20.1. Commonly Used Supplements and Herbs for AD and PD

Name	Mechanism of action	Dosing	Side effects	Use in PD	Use in AD	Reference
Vitamin B12	As outlined in text	0.5–5 mg	Rare	Yes	Yes	See text
Methylfolate	Essential Methyl group donor, critical for Phase II detox and all methylation pathways including production of neurotransmitters	0.4–5 mg	With doses of 1 mg, irritability, nausea, anxiety in patients with COMT mutations	Yes	Yes	See text
Zinc	Outlined in text, protection against heavy metals	15–3 omg	Not reported if not overdosed	Yes	Yes	See text
Vitamin E	As outlined in text	200–400 IU	Rare	Yes	Yes	See text
Alpha-lipoic acid (ALA)	Endogenous mitochondrial molecule, antioxidant effect, Phase II detox via activation of Nrf2. Chelation effect of heavy metals in the brain.	300–1,200 mg. Not every day, in pulses	Acidic, high doses can irritate stomach and should be taken with food.	Possibly	Yes	86,87
Omega-3 fatty acids	As outlined in text	1–3 g/day of EPA/DHA Avoid >4 g	If fish oil used, fish oil aftertaste, bloating. High dose can increase risk of bleeding.	Yes	Yes	See text
Coenzyme Q10	Endogenous mitochondrial molecule, energy production, dynamic antioxidant	100–200 mg	Mild GI symptoms in doses >300 mg	Yes	Yes	29,88 and see text

(continued)

Table 20.1. Continued

Name	Mechanism of action	Dosing	Side effects	Use in PD	Use in AD	Reference
Acetyl-L-carnitine	Enhances acetylcholine production and stimulates membrane phospholipid synthesis. Conflicting data.	1.5–3.0 g	Occasional mild GI bloating and body odor. Well tolerated.	No	Yes	89,90
N-Acetylcysteine (NAC)	Strong anti-oxidant and glutathione precursor. Readily passes into brain. Positive animal models and human pilot studies.	600–1,200 mg	Occasional GI bloating and diarrhea. Well tolerated.	Yes	Yes	91 see text
Alpha-glycerylphosphorylcholine (alpha GPC), Cytidine 5′-diphosphocholine (CDP-choline)	Source of highly available choline. Low-choline diets linked to childhood brain defects and risk of AD. One randomized controlled trial showed dramatic improvement in memory in patients with mild AD.	600–1,200 mg	None reported	No	Yes	92,93
Magnesium-L-threonate	Synaptoprotective effects in the hippocampus in animal models. Randomized controlled trial under way at Stanford, CA.	1,000–2,000 mg	Not reported at recommended dose	No	Yes	NCT02210286
Nicotinamide riboside	Mitochondrial energy support, increase in SirT1 function, animal studies, randomized controlled under way	100–250 mg	None reported	No	Yes	NCT02942888

Resveratrol	Neuroprotective effect via increase in SirT1 function	0.5–2 g	Not reported. Possible interaction with Coumadin.	Possibly, no clinical data	Yes	94,95
Axona (MF) or Coconut oil	Ketogenic effect outlined in text	1–2 tablespoons	Axona often causes mild GI side effects. Coconut oil is better tolerated.	Not FDA approved	Yes	96
Cerefolin NAC (MF)	Combination of MethylB12, methylfolate, and NAC	1 tablet	As per individual nutrients	Not FDA approved	Yes	96
Bacopa monnieri	Plant used traditionally in ayurvedic medicine to improve memory. Randomized controlled trial showing improved memory in healthy elderly.	300–600 mg	None have been reported. Theoretical hormonal side effects if hypersensitization develops (not reported).	No	Yes	97
Green tea extract (EGCG)	Food-based antioxidants. Epidemiological protective data.	Food or capsules 500–1,000 mg of EGCG	High dose can cause nausea and GI upset if taken on empty stomach.	Yes	Yes	98,99
Turmeric	Small positive clinical trials for AD and animal studies for PD.	500–1000 mg of concentrated highly absorbable form	Theoretical interactions with medications, but no reports when food-based doses used.	Yes	Yes	100,101

(continued)

Table 20.1. Continued

Name	Mechanism of action	Dosing	Side effects	Use in PD	Use in AD	Reference
Ginkgo biloba	Improves microvascular circulation; conflicting data	60–120 mg	Few; theoretical increase in bleeding if combined with anticoagulation	No	Yes	102,103
Huperizine A	Plant-derived (Chinese Club moss) natural acetylcholinesterase inhibitor. Over 20 positive randomized controlled trials analyzed in recent meta-analysis. Approved for AD by Chinese FDA equivalent.	100–400 mg	Similar to Donepezil but much better tolerated. Cannot be combined with acetylcholinesterase inhibitors.	No	Yes	104
Mucuna pruriens	See text; contains naturally occurring levodopa	30 g of seeds. Use should be discouraged/	Tolerated better than levodopa-containing medications	Yes	No	36 see text
DHEA	Only if deficiency present; otherwise no evidence	5–50 mg	Few if serum level remains within normal limits	Yes	Yes	105
Pregnenolone		5–100 mg		Yes	Yes	

MF, FDA-approved medical foods for minimal cognitive impairment.

benserazide) to promote central nervous system penetration and diminish side effects. Oral carbidopa/levodopa is available in different immediate and/ or long-acting oral formulations.[4,39,40]

A variety of medications that also enhance dopamine function are commonly used independently, together, or in conjunction with levodopa to improve primary motor symptoms, mitigate fluctuations, and/or minimize levodopa-dependent side effects (e.g., choreiform movements known as dyskinesia, orthostatic hypotension). Dopamine agonists directly stimulate dopamine receptors and include oral pramipexole, oral ropinirole, transdermal rotigitone, and subcutaneous apomorphine. Two categories of enzyme inhibitors augment dopamine by slowing its biochemical degradation: the monoamine oxidase type B (MAO-B) inhibitors (oral selegiline and oral rasagiline) and the catechol-O-methyltransferase (COMT) inhibitor (oral entacapone). The dopamine agonists are manufactured individually in short- and long-acting formulations, while entacapone is available both as an individual drug and in a combined formulation with carbidopa and levodopa. Ergot dopamine agonists (e.g., pergolide, cabergoline) are not commonly used due to the risk of cardiac valvular disease, and the COMT inhibitor tolcapone is not commonly used due to a risk of liver toxicity. Some of the non-dopaminergic medications used to treat motor symptoms include an acetylcholinergic agent (trihexyphenidyl hydrochloride) and an anti-viral/NMDA receptor antagonist (amantadine). These drugs may be useful when a patient is intolerant of dopaminergic side effects or is suffering dyskinesia.[41]

Possible side effects of dopaminergic medications include but are not limited to nausea, fatigue, symptoms of orthostatic hypotension, psychosis, and compulsive reward-driven behavior (e.g., gambling, shopping, hypersexuality). Sudden-onset sleep and compulsive behaviors are more likely to be associated with dopamine agonists, and these side effects should be monitored both at initiation and with titration of these medications. Side effects are minimized overall when medications are started at low doses and slowly increased to the desired effect, which is advised; however, appropriate management of PD sometimes includes pharmacological treatment of unavoidable side effects caused by otherwise beneficial dopaminergic therapy. Alternately, as PD progresses sometimes previously effective medications may need to be decreased to minimize new side effects or symptoms of PD itself.

Surgical

The surgical treatment for PD called deep brain stimulation can be an effective option when a patient's dopaminergic benefit is robust but is accompanied by substantial dyskinesias or fluctuations. Based on current guidelines and standard practice, DBS is not the recommended treatment for most people with PD, for whom medical management is primarily advised.[51]

Alzheimer's Disease

CASE STUDY

An 89-year-old, college-educated, three-war veteran presented to an integrative clinic with a diagnosis of Alzheimer's disease (AD). The patient was very fit his entire life, spoke several languages, and was the main breadwinner for his family. At presentation his Mini-Mental Status Exam (MMSE) score was 21/30 and a second opinion obtained in a specialized memory clinic assessment confirmed the diagnosis of early AD. On detailed history, it was noted that the patient had consumed swordfish two or three times a week for over 20 years since his service in Korea. Given this information, functional mercury testing was obtained that showed a more than 100-fold elevation of total and methylmercury levels.

The patient was advised to discontinue eating swordfish completely and to minimize fish intake to only low-mercury-containing fish (this information can be obtained at Environmental Working Group website, www.ewg.org). He was also prescribed a complex detox supportive nutritional regimen that contained the following nutrients: EGCG, milk thistle, N-acetylcysteine, MethylB12 and methyl folate, zinc, omega-3 fatty acids, probiotics, Chlorella, and others. He was also encouraged to increase exercise and to regularly consume cilantro (50 g two or three times per week). Within approximately 6 months, his mercury level decreased to the level recommended by the U.S. Centers for Disease Control and Prevention and his MMSE score improved dramatically to 28/30. This case demonstrates that cognitive impairment in AD can have many confounding and possibly modifiable contributing factors.

INTRODUCTION

Major neurodegenerative disease, commonly referred to as "dementia," is typically a disease of later life, generally occurring after 65 years of age. AD, vascular dementia, and dementia with Lewy body are the most common forms of major cognitive neurodegenerative disease. An estimated 44 million people suffer from AD worldwide, including more than 5 million in the United States. According to Alzheimer's Disease International, in 2010 the annual total cost for dementia care, including medical and social care, was $600 billion worldwide.[42] The cost of dementia care in the United States alone is estimated at between $150 billion and $215 billion annually and over the last few years has exceeded the combined health care expenditure for both cancer and heart disease.[43] In addition to financial costs, the emotional burden of dementia is enormous for both patients and their families and plays a central role in dementia care as the disease evolves.

In this review, we focus on AD exclusively given that it is the most common form of dementia. Integrative treatment modalities recommended in AD are not well studied in non-Alzheimer's-type dementias, but it is hypothesized that they may have a positive effect.

AD is well recognized histologically by the development of amyloid plaques and neurofibrillary tangles in key brain regions that result in the disease's well-recognized syndrome of memory loss, language impairment, personality change, visuospatial deficits, and impaired executive functioning. Further discussion of the key proteins driving degenerative changes in AD, amyloid and tau, will be avoided in this text but may be further referenced in any allopathic neurology or dementia text or in the referenced review article.[44] In addition to the proteins amyloid and tau, it is also clear that chronic inflammation plays a key role in AD pathology. Hormonal dysregulation, vitamin deficiencies, and environmental exposure to toxins may also contribute to increased AD risk. Minimal evidence exists to support the role of environmental toxins in AD, but key suspected toxins range from aluminum, lead, mercury, and organophosphate pesticides to extremely low-frequency electromagnetic fields.[45] It is suspected that patients with specific genetic backgrounds, such as the MTHFR mutations, have an increased risk of effect. As genome sequencing moves to clinical practice, single nucleotide polymorphism (SNP) assessments are likely to become increasingly routine, permitting increased identification of genetic risk factors for AD development and subsequently opportunities for prevention and treatment.[46]

SCREENING

Due to the high prevalence of AD, regular screening is recommended for all adults over the age of 65.[47] The utility of screening is dual. The opportunity for evaluation and treatment of cognitive impairment is clear. Less well-appreciated benefits of screening include improved recognition by clinicians for the need to encourage advance care planning discussions, ensure patient safety, and provide counseling and education for care partners. Several screening tests exist to assess for cognitive function and are referenced at www.alz.org with extensive supporting information. The MMSE was formerly the most popular screening test, but due to new copyright limitations, use is now prohibited without obtaining rights from the publisher. Reliable user-friendly alternatives include the Mini-Cog and the Montreal Cognitive Assessment Test (MoCA) (Box 20.1). The Mini-Cog is a useful tool for clinicians given

Box 20.1. AD Screening Tests

Mini-Cog™©
- Use: Screening for major neurocognitive disorder
- Description: Sensitivity ranges from 76% to 99% and specificity ranges from 89% to 93% based on prevalence in the population; not validated to screen for mild cognitive impairment

http://www.alz.org/documents_custom/minicog.pdf
or https://consultgeri.org/try-this/general-assessment/issue-3.1.pdf

* Mini-Cog™© S. Borson. All rights reserved. Reprinted with permission of the author solely for clinical and educational purposes.

Montreal Cognitive Assessment (MoCA©)
- Use: Screening for minor and major neurocognitive disorder
- Description: Sensitivity ranges from 90% to 96%; sensitivity and specificity 87%; tested in 14 languages; screening assesses multiple cognitive domains
- May be used, reproduced, and distributed without permission.

http://www.mocatest.org/
or https://consultgeri.org/try-this/general-assessment/issue-3.2.pdf

ease and expediency of use while still retaining excellent sensitivity. It primarily tests memory and visuospatial capacities. Training is minimal. The MoCA tests a much broader spectrum of cognitive domains, including language, memory, attention, visuospatial, and executive functions. It is highly clinically sensitive, especially in persons with higher baseline cognitive function, but it does require brief informal training to use and daily clinical use is limited by time constraints in many practice settings. Performance on the Mini-Cog is independent of language, and the MoCA is available in most languages. An abnormal score on either test is indicative of cognitive impairment and indicates the need for further cognitive testing and evaluation for potential contributing factors.

It is imperative to remember that the diagnosis of dementia or major neurodegenerative disease is based on functional loss, specifically in regards to activities of daily living or independent activities of daily living. Cognitive deficits without functional loss may be characterized by the recognized term "minor cognitive impairment" (MCI), now referred to as minor neurodegenerative disease in the latest edition of the American Psychiatric Association's *Diagnostic and Statistical Manual of Mental Disorders*.

DIAGNOSIS

Confirmation of a suspected diagnosis of any dementia syndrome generally occurs through specialized memory clinics given the necessary complexity of obtaining a complete focused history; performing comprehensive cognitive testing; evaluating, screening for, and possibly treating factors contributing to impaired cognition; and referring for confirmatory testing when necessary. A detailed description of diagnostic algorithms is beyond the scope of this chapter; the Alzheimer's Association website at www.alz.org serves as a good initial reference. Standard evaluation includes assessment for possible contributing factors that may worsen cognition, including a comprehensive sleep evaluation, medication review, psychiatric history, sexual history, substance use history, and review for potential toxin exposure. In addition to the standard evaluation, integrative providers, including the authors, assess levels of sex hormones, cortisol, and DHEA-S, in addition to assessing functional serum or cellular levels of oxidative stress markers such as reduced glutathione (GSH), lipid peroxides, coenzyme Q10, 8-hydroxydeoxyguanosine (8-OHdG), superoxide dismutase (SOD), and several others. Total body lead or mercury load is assessed only upon clinical suspicion of toxicity from history (frequent consumption of highly contaminated fish such as tuna, swordfish, and others; occupational history), examination (multiple amalgams), or elevated oxidative stress. Routine serum heavy metal tests should be avoided as they are unable to diagnose chronic low-grade exposure, for which specialized functional tests must be done; these are beyond the scope of this review.[48]

Screening for the APOE4 gene remains controversial. Heterozygous and especially homozygous APOE4 status in healthy individuals increases the risk of developing AD later in life, but the screening is not currently part of routine AD workup nor is it recommended as standard of care. Despite a lack of evidence, lifestyle modification as a result of a positive APOE4 status most likely will lead to a decreased risk of developing AD. The www.apoe4.info community support website for and by people with a positive APOE4 status is a wonderful resource for anyone interested in learning more about this topic.

Gold standard confirmation of AD diagnosis is currently available only through brain biopsy. Recent advances in biochemical markers and functional imaging have greatly improved clinical ability to biologically confirm the diagnosis, but accessibility is limited. Functional neuroimaging to confirm amyloid deposition in the brain is now available commercially, but at the time of writing it is still not recognized by major insurance companies as standard of care, thereby leaving consumers to privately pay several thousand dollars for imaging when desired. Evaluation of cerebrospinal fluid protein biomarkers is also evolving, but routine testing is not currently used outside of research setting. Interested readers may wish to review the National Institute on Aging's "Advances in Detecting Alzheimer's Disease Progress Report" for more information.[47]

TREATMENT AND PREVENTION

To date, there are no disease-modifying treatments for AD. Despite extensive research, hundreds of experimental medications have all but failed to arrest AD progression. Emerging understanding of AD suggests that it is a complex metabolic disease that may benefit from a comprehensive metabolic protocol to address as many individual pathophysiological factors as possible, ideally before the clinical diagnosis is established or immediately following diagnosis. The first comprehensive metabolic protocol developed to address these multitudes of factors that demonstrated improvement in AD symptoms and progression was developed by Dr. Dale Bredesen and is called ReCODE (Reversal of COgnitive DEcline). This initial protocol has generated significant interest in the integrative community and promises to be a springboard for additional research.[49,50] Dr. Bredesen's book, *The End of Alzheimer's Disease*, was published in 2017 and describes in detail the research that led to, the creation of, and early clinical experience with the ReCODE protocol.

One of the key components of ReCODE is diagnostic categorization of AD according to the predominant metabolic dysregulation:

Type 1: Inflammatory
Type 1.5: Hyperglycemic
Type 2: Atrophic (hormonal deficiencies)
Type 3: Toxic

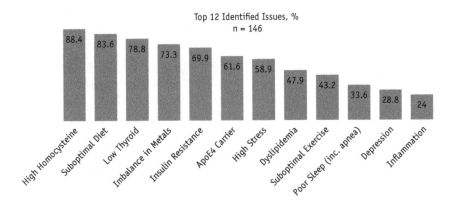

FIGURE 20.1. Top 12 identified multiple metabolic drives in patients with AD.

Treatment is structured according to the AD type; many patients have a combination of two or more types.

Lifestyle Approaches

Nutrition

Several diets, including the Mediterranean and MIND diets, have demonstrated preventive and even therapeutic AD potential in randomized prospective trials.[51,52] A detailed review of the MIND diet is provided in Chapter 2. Regardless of the specific diet chosen, adequate intake of omega-3s (essential long-chain polyunsaturated fatty acids, including alpha-linolenic acid [ALA], eicosapentaenoic acid [EPA], and docosahexaenoic acid [DHA]) is critical given their roles in cellular membrane fluidity and anti-inflammation (Box 20.2).[53] Patients who are unable to obtain adequate amounts of omega-3s from diet alone should be prescribed supplements, as discussed later in the chapter.

In addition to adequate omega-3 intake, induced episodic ketosis has become a staple of nutritional interventions for AD. Intermittent fasting that induces episodic ketosis has demonstrated benefit in animal AD models.[54] From the authors' experience, most patients comfortably tolerate about 13 or 14 hours of fasting overnight. This can be implemented from two nights a week up to every night with little to no risk, even in diabetic patients, assuming they carefully monitor their fasting sugar levels. Dr. Bredesen describes a 12-3 rule: a 12-hour fast every night with the last meal of the day being at least 3 hours before bedtime. Adding 1 tablespoon of high-grade coconut oil or purified medium-chain triglycerides (MCTs) oil to dinner further enhances ketone production and eases the intermittent fasting period. Ketogenic diets for AD are not supported by clinical studies and are difficult to sustain.

Box 20.2. Key Components of Diet for AD Prevention and Treatment

1. Low glycemic index/load diet
2. Reduction of pro-inflammatory foods such as red meat, dairy, sugar, trans fats, and all industrially processed foods
3. High amounts of fresh fruits and vegetables, including foods high in antioxidants such as berries, turmeric, and green tea
4. High amounts of foods rich in omega-3 fatty acids; nuts and seeds if unable to consume seafood
5. Overnight fasting to promote ketogenesis.

Adapted from Rakel D. *Integrative Medicine*, 4th ed. Philadelphia: Elsevier; 2017.

Exercise

Physical as well as cognitive exercises have positive effects on cognition in both MCI and AD.[55,56] Programs such as Brain HQ and Lumosity are readily available free or at a low cost and are reasonably easy to use, even for patients with early AD. When working with AD patients, exercise should be focused on strengthening, balance, and flexibility with the goal of minimizing advanced AD-related complications such as falls, sarcopenia, and contractures. Tai chi and yoga have an increasing presence in many retirement communities, senior centers, and nursing homes. These low-impact exercises combine mindfulness with movement practices and are an important component of multifaceted AD research sponsored by the National Institute of Health. Early studies show promising results.[57-59]

Mind–Body Approaches

Stress plays an essential role in many chronic illnesses. Chronic stress appears to negatively affect memory and increases neuronal damage through activation of N-methyl-D-aspartate (NMDA) receptors, leading to the damaging influx of calcium into postsynaptic neurons.[60] A number of clinical trials have shown benefits of meditation and mind–body practices for patients with early AD and MCI. Transcendental Meditation (TM), Kirtan Kriya (yogic practice of breathing combined with chanting and mudras), Tibetan sound meditation, tai chi, and yoga have all shown some positive effects. A detailed description of the neurocognitive effects of mind–body practices is provided in Chapter 4.

Sleep Optimization

Sleep apnea, or more precisely nocturnal hypoxia, has recently been shown to be a major risk factor for developing AD and should be excluded or treated if found.[61] It is important to remember that many older adults do not present with the classically taught history associated with sleep apnea, so a high index of suspicion should be maintained. Insomnia and other sleep disorders should be treated. In the authors' experience most patients with AD have some form of nocturnal hypoxia. even if they are not formally diagnosed with sleep apnea. Melatonin circadian rhythm is often disturbed in patients with AD, and supplementing with melatonin 0.5 to 10 mg at bedtime has been shown to be beneficial for sleep optimization without significant side effects.[62] Sleep evaluation should also include a comprehensive medication review to identify self-medication with supplements and over-the-counter agents as well as prescribed medications that can negatively affect cognition; when identified, these should be discontinued.

Music, Art, Pet Therapy, and Reiki

Music, art, pet-assisted therapy, and reiki (a hands-on healing touch modality) have been shown to be beneficial for dementia-associated behavioral problems such as agitation, combative behaviors, and anxiety.[63–65] Activities such as these can play a critical role in re-establishing joyful activities for both patients and their care partners, which can be critical as negative neuropsychiatric symptoms of dementia including agitation, mood lability, aggression, and anxiety evolve.[66] As AD evolves and behavioral challenges increase, the lay literature is flush with excellent resources for care partners to utilize in order to improve their knowledge and understanding about the disease in a way that is leads to improved relationships with the person suffering from AD.[67]

Supplements and Herbs

General guidelines do not recommend using any supplements for patients with AD, outside of treating obvious vitamin deficiencies such as vitamin B12 (Box 20.3). The list of supplements and herbs that patients often use for AD with at least some theoretical and/or clinical evidence is rather long. Table 20.1 summarizes the most commonly used products and provides some rationale for their use.

Frank B12 deficiency can cause pseudo-dementia or pseudo-depression and is common in the elderly. While there are no clear guidelines regarding B

Box 20.3. Recommending Multivitamins

- No additional copper and iron
- Vitamin E, mixed tocopherols, ideally containing all eight natural isomers—200–400 IU
- Methylated forms of folate—at least 400 mcg
- Non-cyanocobalamin form of B12 (methyl, hydroxy, or adeno B12)—at least 500 mcg
- Zinc—15–30 mg
- Selenium—100–200 mcg

Adapted from Rakel D. *Integrative Medicine*, 4th ed. Philadelphia: Elsevier; 2017.

vitamins and dementia, the authors advocate the use of activated forms of B12 and folate—methylcobalamin and 5-methyltetrahydrofolate (5MTHF), often called L-methylfolate— especially if the patient's methylation status is unknown. Alternatively, consider testing all AD and MCI patients for MTHFR SNPs; if positive for either A1289C or C677T, use methylfolate (1–10 mg) and avoid synthetic folic acid. In patients with MTHFR mutations, unmetabolized folic acid may cause negative consequences.[68] One strategy is to use a therapeutic B-complex or multivitamin with high doses of activated-form B12 and 5MTHF.

Vitamin E continues to have a prominent role in discussions about vitamin use in AD. Results are uniform that deficient vitamin E states are linked to AD; however, using supplemented forms of vitamin E produces conflicting results. In the past, very-high-dose vitamin E supplementation of up to 2,000 IU/day was advocated, but this approach is not supported by the research and is not recommended.[69] Ensure adequate daily intake of vitamin E through food or the use of 100 to 400 IU of supplemental mixed tocopherols.

Given accumulating evidence that low zinc and high copper levels are associated with increased risk of and more rapid AD progression, the authors recommend assessing zinc and copper levels and adjusting levels to high-normal zinc and low-normal copper.[70] One way of achieving this is by avoiding supplemental copper. Copper-rich foods contribute little to free copper serum levels, as organic forms of copper are rapidly utilized by cells, in contrast to the inorganic forms found in multivitamins and copper water pipes, which can increase serum copper levels. If needed to achieve desired levels, zinc supplementation of 15 to 30 mg is typically safe, even when used long term; regular monitoring of serum zinc levels is needed.

Despite evidence that diets low in omega-3s are associated with an increased risk of AD, supplementing with omega-3 fatty acids has not shown definitive benefits once AD develops.[53,71–73] If patients need omega-3 supplementation due to dietary restrictions, fish oil is the most easily available form. Vegan sources of omega-3 supplements are also widely available from algae or seeds. The authors typically use highly concentrated sources of fish oil that are guaranteed to be free of mercury and have a high DHA content, a DHA:EPA ratio of at least 1:1 and often 2:1. It is less clear what the target should be for the omega-6:omega-3 dietary fatty acids or supplementation ratio. One long-term strategy could be providing a 4:1 omega-6:omega-3 balanced supplement with at least 1 g of DHA/EPA.

Hormonal dysregulation is often identified in patients with AD. The relationship between hypothyroidism and cognitive impairment is elegantly presented by Dr. Yang in Chapter 14. One approach to aggressively addressing hormonal dysregulation is to routinely screen all patients with cognitive impairment for thyroid, adrenal, and sex hormone abnormalities by checking basic serum levels. Importantly, there is no evidence that hormonal treatment without the confirmed presence of a clear serological deficiency state has any clinical benefit for patients with AD. Thus, treatment should be limited to patients who are found to have low hormone levels. Specifics of hormonal treatments are discussed in Chapter 14.

Medications

The U.S. Food and Drug Administration has approved two classes of neurotransmitter-modulating agents for treatment of AD. The first class of drugs, acetylcholinesterase inhibitors, boosts available acetylcholine and is approved for use in mild (early-stage) disease. The second drug class antagonizes NMDA-dampening excitatory neurotransmitters and is approved for use in moderate (mid-stage) disease. A summary of indications, doses, and side effects for each medication is presented in Table 20.2. These medications have no role in disease modification, and their clinical impact is limited because they provide only about 12 months or less of borderline clinical improvement. Additionally, cholinesterase inhibitor use is often limited by side effects, with improved tolerance resulting from initiating the chosen medication at the lowest possible dose and titrating up slowly to level of tolerance.[74]

Initiating any medications requires careful patient and family counseling. The medications seem to have few interactions with dietary interventions, supplements, and herbs commonly used for AD, with the notable exception of Huperizine A. Another supplement to use cautiously is ginkgo, which has a theoretical interaction with acetylcholinesterase inhibitors; however, in one randomized controlled trial the combination of donepezil and ginkgo had fewer side effects than donepezil alone.[75]

Table 20.2. Medications for AD

Name	Category	Daily Dose	Approved for	Side effects
Donepezil (Aricept)	Acetylcholinesterase inhibitors	5–23 mg oral/ transdermal	All forms of AD	Bradycardia, GI bleeding, diarrhea, anorexia, nausea, syncope, headaches, hallucinations, anorexia, depression, bradycardia, nocturnal agitation (nocturnal agitation is most associated with donepezil)
Rivastigmine (Exelone)		1.5–13.3 mg oral	Mild– moderate	
Galantamine (Razadyne)		8–24 mg oral	Mild– moderate	
Memantine (Namenda)	NMDA antagonist	5–10 mg oral	Moderate– severe	Well tolerated; occasional dizziness, headaches, diarrhea

It is important to mention that in the geriatric population, prolonged use of medications with anticholinergic side effects has been linked to an increased risk of cognitive impairment, and these medications should be removed from a patient's regimen if possible.[76] As the disease progresses, many medications may be used to control the behavioral and neuropsychiatric symptoms associated with AD. Depression, irritability, and anxiety are often treated with selective serotonin reuptake inhibitors (SSRI), but use should be discontinued if a benefit is not clearly evident. Antipsychotics are often prescribed for aggressive or paranoid behaviors, but it is important to first try nonpharmacological approaches to de-escalate behaviors whenever possible. Use of antipsychotics is strongly linked to increased morbidity and mortality in patients with AD, and use in nursing homes is highly regulated.[77] Nonpharmacological methods such as frequent reorientation, music, art, touch therapy, and pet therapy should be the first-line interventions regardless of the patient's location, including acute care settings.

Use of Cannabinoids for Patients with PD and AD

As medical cannabis becomes legalized in a majority of U.S. states, use in patients with PD and AD is increasing. Cannabinoids, specifically cannabidiol (CBD), have been shown to be neuroprotective in vitro and in vivo in both PD and AD animal models.[78-80]

Heavy recreational users of cannabis have been shown to have memory and brain volume loss. This effect appears to be directly linked to a high tetrahydrocannabinol (THC) to CBD ratio found in products used for their psychotropic effects. Current data suggest that higher CBD content appears to ameliorate these negative effects.[81] The best modes for CBD delivery are sublingual, buccal, topical, or rectal in order to bypass first-pass hepatic metabolism.

Emerging evidence for cannabis use suggests efficacy for use in PD for a variety of motor and non-motor symptoms. An observational study performed in Colorado, one of first states to legalize medical cannabis in 2000, demonstrated that over 80% of patients with PD used some form of complementary and alternative medicine (CAM), reporting that massage, acupuncture, music, and cannabis were most useful. Approximately 5% of the participants surveyed reported cannabis to be the most effective intervention for a variety of motor and non-motor symptoms, including pain.[82] A small open-label study also demonstrated universal and clinically significant improvement in symptoms related to tremor, rigidity, bradykinesia, sleep, and pain.[83] While no controlled studies exist, further research is needed given these emerging data and patient interest in nonpharmacological options. At present, the U.S. Drug Enforcement Administration schedule for medical cannabis continues to dramatically limit efforts to research its effectiveness.

Multidisciplinary Approach to PD and AD

Integrative treatment involving multidisciplinary and/or palliative care approaches may be beneficial for different patients and at different stages of both PD and AD. Long-term management should include regular communication between providers—specifically, primary care physicians and neurologists when both are involved—and may be tailored when necessary to include other medical specialties (e.g., psychiatry, urology) and other health care providers (e.g., visiting nurse, physiotherapist).

Aligned with the aim of pharmacotherapy, the broad goals of nonpharmacological treatment in AD and PD are to improve immediate and long-term function, as well as safety and overall quality of life.

Eventually, most patients with PD and AD will progress toward the terminal phases of their disease. While the speed of disease progression is often hard to predict, the signs of end-stage disease are universal and well established. Early referral to a palliative care team or hospice is essential to optimize quality of life and minimize medical interventions that cannot modify disease progression and are often associated with undesirable side effects. A good and frequently encountered example is avoiding the use of feeding tubes in patients with advanced PD and AD. In this population there is no evidence that feeding tubes prolong life, and use can lead to an increased risk of infection and harm.[84,85] The recommended approach is disease education and palliative care. For a more detailed discussion of end-of-life symptoms, including management, see Chapter 31.

Key Web Resources

Alzheimer's Association (http://www.alz.org): Nonprofit organization that disseminates "information on Alzheimer's disease and dementia symptoms, diagnosis, stages, treatment, care and support resources" with a commitment to advancing research for AD and other dementias

American Parkinson Disease Association (www.apdaparkinson.org): Aims to ease the burden for Americans with PD and their families through a nationwide network of chapters, information and referral centers, and support groups. APDA pursues its efforts to find the cure by funding Centers for Advanced Research and awarding grants to fund the most promising research toward discovering the cause(s) and finding the cure for PD.

Parkinson's Disease Foundation (www.pdf.org): A leading national presence in PD research, education, and public advocacy

Michael J. Fox Foundation for Parkinson's Research (www.michaeljfox. org): Dedicated to finding a cure for PD through an aggressively funded research agenda and to ensuring the development of improved therapies for those living with PD today.

Family Caregiver Alliance: National Center on Caregiving (https://www. caregiver.org/; https://www.caregiver.org/health-issues/dementia): National agency leading the conversation about how to care for patients with cognitive impairment; includes information on caregiver education, opportunities to engage with policy and advocacy, and connecting caregivers.

ACKNOWLEDGMENTS

We thank Bianca Moiseff, medical student at George Washington University, for assistance with this chapter. Aviva Ellenstein contributed to the Parkinson's disease section of the chapter only, Christina Prather contributed to the Alzheimer's disease section only, and Mikhail Kogan contributed to both sections.

REFERENCES

1. Berg D, Postuma RB, Bloem B, et al. Time to redefine PD? Introductory statement of the MDS Task Force on the definition of Parkinson's disease. *Mov Disord.* 2014;29(4):454–462.

2. Postuma RB, Berg D, Stern M, et al. MDS clinical diagnostic criteria for Parkinson's disease. *Mov Disord.* 2015;30(12):1591–1601.

3. Rizzo G, Copetti M, Arcuti S, Martino D, Fontana A, Logroscino G. Accuracy of clinical diagnosis of Parkinson disease: A systematic review and meta-analysis. *Neurology.* 2016;86(6):566–576. doi:10.1212/WNL.0000000000002350.

4. Chaudhuri KR, Healy DG, Schapira AH. Non-motor symptoms of Parkinson's disease: diagnosis and management. *Lancet Neurol.* 2006;5(3):235–245. doi:10.1016/s1474-4422(06)70373-8.

5. Marras C, McDermott MP, Rochon PA, Tanner CM, Naglie G, Lang AE. Predictors of deterioration in health-related quality of life in Parkinson's disease: Results from the DATATOP trial. *Mov Disord.* 2008;23(5):653–659; quiz 776. http://pesquisa.bvsalud.org/portal/resource/pt/mdl-18076084.

6. Factor SA, Bennett A, Hohler AD, Wang D. Quality improvement in neurology: Parkinson disease update quality measurement set: Executive summary. *Neurology.* 2016;86:2278–2283.

7. Massano J, Bhatia KP. Clinical approach to Parkinson's disease: Features, diagnosis, and principles of management. *Cold Spring Harb Perspect Med.* 2012;2(6).

8. Bellou V, Belbasis L, Tzoulaki I, Evangelou E, Ioannidis JPA. Environmental risk factors and Parkinson's disease: An umbrella review of meta-analyses. *Parkinsonism Relat Disord.* 2015;23:1–9. doi:10.1016/j.parkreldis.2015.12.008.

9. Braak H, Del Tredici K, Rüb U, De Vos RAI, Jansen Steur ENH, Braak E. Staging of brain pathology related to sporadic Parkinson's disease. *Neurobiol Aging.* 2003;24(2):197–211.

10. Young AB, Penney JB. Neurochemical anatomy of movement disorders. *Neurol Clin.* 1984;2(3):417–433.

11. Helmich RC, Hallett M, Deuschl G, Toni I, Bloem BR. Cerebral causes and consequences of parkinsonian resting tremor: A tale of two circuits? *Brain.* 2012;135(11):3206–3226.

12. Stacy M. Nonmotor symptoms in Parkinson's disease. *Int J Neurosci.* 2011; 121(Suppl):9–17. doi:10.3109/00207454.2011.620196.

13. Singleton AB, Farrer MJ, Bonifati V. The genetics of Parkinson's disease: Progress and therapeutic implications. *Mov Disord.* 2013;28(1):14–23. doi:10.1002/mds.25249.

14. Amos D. Korczyn SH-B. Can the disease course in Parkinson's disease be slowed? *BMC Med.* 2015;13(1):295.

15. Forloni G, Artuso V, La Vitola P. Oligomeropathies and pathogenesis of Alzheimer and Parkinson's diseases. *Mov Disord.* 2016;31:771–781.

16. Di Maio R, Barrett PJ, Hoffman EK, et al. Alpha-Synuclein binds to TOM20 and inhibits mitochondrial protein import in Parkinson's disease. *Sci Transl Med.* 2016;8:342.

17. Pagan F, Hebron M, Valadez EH, et al. Nilotinib effects in Parkinson's disease and dementia with Lewy bodies. *J Parkinsons Dis.* 2016;6(3):503–517.

18. Felice VD, Quigley EM, Sullivan AM, O'Keeffe GW, O'Mahony SM. Microbiota-gut-brain signalling in Parkinson's disease: Implications for non-motor symptoms. *Parkinsons Relat Disord.* 2016;27:1–8.

19. McGhee DJ, Royle PL, Thompson PA, Wright DE, Zajicek JP. A systematic review of biomarkers for disease progression in Parkinson's disease. *BMC Neurol.* 2013;13:35.

20. Schapira AH. Recent developments in biomarkers in Parkinson disease. *Curr Opin Neurol.* 2013;26:395–400.

21. De La Fuente-Fernández R. Role of DaTSCAN and clinical diagnosis in Parkinson disease. *Neurology.* 2012;78(10):696–701.

22. Oguh O, Eisenstein A, Kwasny M, Simuni T. Back to the basics: Regular exercise matters in Parkinson's disease: Results from the National Parkinson Foundation QII registry study. *Parkinsons Relat Disord.* 2014;20(11):1221–1225.

23. Mahler L, Ramig LO, Fox C. Evidence-based treatment of voice and speech disorders in Parkinson disease. *Curr Opin Otolaryngol Head Neck Surg.* 2015;23(3):209–215.

24. Chung CL, Thilarajah S, Tan D. Effectiveness of resistance training on muscle strength and physical function in people with Parkinson's disease: A systematic review and meta-analysis. *Clin Rehabil.* 2016;30(1):11–23.

25. Ni X, Liu S, Lu F, Shi X, Guo X. Efficacy and safety of Tai Chi for Parkinson's disease: A systematic review and meta-analysis of randomized controlled trials. *PLoS One.* 2014;9(6).

26. Alcalay RN, Gu Y, Mejia-Santana H, Cote L, Marder KS, Scarmeas N. The association between Mediterranean diet adherence and Parkinson's disease. *Mov Disord.* 2012;27(6):771–774.
27. Campdelacreu J. Parkinson disease and Alzheimer disease: Environmental risk factors. *Neurol (Barcelona, Spain).* 2014;29(9):541–549. doi:10.1016/j.nrl.2012.04.001.
28. Barichella M, Pacchetti C, Bolliri C, et al. Probiotics and prebiotic fiber for constipation associated with Parkinson disease: An RCT. *Neurology.* 2016. http://www.ncbi.nlm.nih.gov/pubmed/27543643.
29. Mischley LK, Allen J, Bradley R. Coenzyme Q10 deficiency in patients with Parkinson's disease. *J Neurol Sci.* 2012;318(1-2):72–75. doi:10.1016/j.jns.2012.03.023.
30. Liu J, Wang L, Zhan SY, Xia Y. Coenzyme Q10 for Parkinson's disease. *Cochrane Database Syst Rev.* 2011;12(12):CD008150. doi:10.1002/14651858.CD008150.pub2.
31. Beal MF, Oakes D, Shoulson I, et al. A randomized clinical trial of high-dosage coenzyme Q10 in early Parkinson disease: No evidence of benefit. *JAMA Neurol.* 2014;71(5):543–552. doi:10.1001/jamaneurol.2014.131.
32. da Silva TM, Munhoz RP, Alvarez C, et al. Depression in Parkinson's disease: A double-blind, randomized, placebo-controlled pilot study of omega-3 fatty-acid supplementation. *J Affect Disord.* 2008;111(2-3):351–359.
33. Smeyne M, Smeyne RJ. Glutathione metabolism and Parkinson's disease. *Free Radic Biol Med.* 2013;62:13–25. doi:10.1016/j.freeradbiomed.2013.05.001.
34. NAC for PD RCT. https://clinicaltrials.gov/ct2/show/NCT01470027.
35. Kasture S, Mohan M, Kasture V. *Mucuna pruriens* seeds in treatment of Parkinson's disease: Pharmacological review. *Orient Pharm Exp Med.* 2013;13(3):165–174.
36. Katzenschlager R, Evans A, Manson A, et al. *Mucuna pruriens* in Parkinson's disease: A double-blind clinical and pharmacological study. *J Neurol Neurosurg Psychiatry.* 2004;75(12):1672–1677. doi:10.1136/jnnp.2003.028761.
37. Kim HJ, Jeon BS. Is acupuncture efficacious therapy in Parkinson's disease? *J Neurol Sci.* 2014;341(1-2):1–7.
38. Kluger BM, Rakowski D, Christian M, et al. Randomized, controlled trial of acupuncture for fatigue in Parkinson's disease. *Mov Disord.* 2016;31(7):1027–1032.
39. Connolly BS, Lang AE. Pharmacological treatment of Parkinson disease: A review. *JAMA.* 2014;311(16):1670–1683. doi:10.1001/jama.2014.3654.
40. Lang AE. When and how should treatment be started in Parkinson disease? *Neurology.* 2009;72(7 Supp. 2):S39–43.
41. Pahwa R, Factor SA, Lyons KE, et al. Practice parameter: Treatment of Parkinson disease with motor fluctuations and dyskinesia (an evidence-based review): Report of the Quality Standards Subcommittee of the American Academy of Neurology. *Neurology.* 2006;66(7):983–995.
42. Hurd MD, Martorell P, Delavande A, Mullen KJ, Langa KM. Monetary costs of dementia in the United States. *N Engl J Med.* 2013;368(14):1326–1334.
43. Rondeau V, Jacqmin-Gadda H, Commenges D, Helmer C, Dartigues JF. Aluminum and silica in drinking water and the risk of Alzheimer's disease or cognitive decline: Findings from 15-year follow-up of the PAQUID cohort. *Am J Epidemiol.* 2009;169(4):489–496.

44. Graham WV, Bonito-Oliva A, Sakmar TP. Update on Alzheimer's disease therapy and prevention strategies. *Annu Rev Med.* 2017;68:413–30.

45. Moorthy D, Peter I, Scott TM, et al. Status of vitamins B-12 and B-6 but not of folate, homocysteine, and the methylenetetrahydrofolate reductase C677T polymorphism are associated with impaired cognition and depression in adults. *J Nutr.* 2012;142(8):1554–1560.

46. Boustani M, Peterson B, Harris R, Lux LJ, Krasnov C, Sutton SF, Hanson L. Screening for dementia. *Agency Healthcare Res Qual.* 2003. doi:10.1037/e554782010-001.

47. Advances in Detecting Alzheimer's Disease. http://www.nia.nih.gov/alzheimers/publication/2011-2012-alzheimers-disease-progress-report/advances-detecting-alzheimers.

48. Bernhoft RA. Mercury toxicity and treatment: A review of the literature. *J Environ Public Health.* 2012;2012.

49. Bredesen DE. Reversal of cognitive decline: A novel therapeutic program. *Aging (Albany NY).* 2014;6(9):707–717.

50. Bredesen E, Amos EC, Canick J, et al. Reversal of cognitive decline in Alzheimer's disease. *Aging (Albany NY).* 2016;8(6):1–9. doi:10.18632/aging.100981.

51. Morris MC, Tangney CC, Wang Y, Sacks FM, Bennett DA, Aggarwal NT. MIND diet associated with reduced incidence of Alzheimer's disease. *Alzheimer's Dement.* 2015;11(9):1007–1014.

52. Valls-Pedret C, Sala-Vila A, Serra-Mir M, et al. Mediterranean diet and age-related cognitive decline: A randomized clinical trial. *JAMA Intern Med.* 2015;175(7):1094–1103.

53. Freemantle E, Vandal M, Tremblay-Mercier J, et al. Omega-3 fatty acids, energy substrates, and brain function during aging. *Prostaglandins Leukot Essent Fat Acids.* 2006;75(3):213–220.

54. Longo VD, Mattson MP. Fasting: Molecular mechanisms and clinical applications. *Cell Metab.* 2014;19(2):181–192.

55. Forbes D, Forbes SC, Blake CM, Thiessen EJ, Forbes S. Exercise programs for people with dementia. *Cochrane Database Syst Rev.* 2015;4:CD006489. doi:10.1002/14651858.CD006489.pub4.

56. Smith GE, Housen P, Yaffe K, et al. A cognitive training program based on principles of brain plasticity: Results from the improvement in memory with plasticity-based adaptive cognitive training (IMPACT) study. *J Am Geriatr Soc.* 2009;57(4):594–603.

57. Wayne PM, Walsh JN, Taylor-Piliae RE, et al. Effect of tai chi on cognitive performance in older adults: Systematic review and meta-analysis. *J Am Geriatr Soc.* 2014;62(1):25–39.

58. Lam LCW, Chau RCM, Wong BML, et al. A 1-year randomized controlled trial comparing mind body exercise (tai chi) with stretching and toning exercise on cognitive function in older Chinese adults at risk of cognitive decline. *J Am Med Dir Assoc.* 2012;13(6).

59. Fan J-T, Chen K-M. Using silver yoga exercises to promote physical and mental health of elders with dementia in long-term care facilities. *Int Psychogeriatr.* 2011;23(8):1222–1230.

60. Stein-Behrens B, Lin WJ, Sapolsky RM. Physiological elevations of glucocorticoids potentiate glutamate accumulation in the hippocampus. *J Neurochem.* 1994;63(2):596–602.

61. Yaffe K, Laffan AM, Harrison SL, et al. Sleep-disordered breathing, hypoxia, and risk of mild cognitive impairment and dementia in older women. *JAMA.* 2011;306(6):613. doi:10.1001/jama.2011.1115.

62. Xu J, Wang L-L, Dammer EB, et al. Melatonin for sleep disorders and cognition in dementia: A meta-analysis of randomized controlled trials. *Am J Alzheimers Dis Other Demen.* 2015;30(5):439–447.

63. Filan SL, Llewellyn-Jones RH. Animal-assisted therapy for dementia: A review of the literature. *Int Psychogeriatr.* 2006;18(4):597–611. doi:10.1017/S1041610206003322.

64. McDermott O, Crellin N, Ridder HM, Orrell M. Music therapy in dementia: A narrative synthesis systematic review. *Int J Geriatr Psychiatry.* 2013;28(8):781–794.

65. Meland B. Effects of Reiki on pain and anxiety in the elderly diagnosed with dementia: A series of case reports. *Altern Ther Heal Med.* 2009;15(4):56–57.

66. Brackey J. *Creating Moments of Joy Along the Alzheimer's Journey: A Guide for Families and Caregivers,* 5th ed. West Lafayette, IN: Purdue University Press; 2008.

67. Mace NL, Rabins P. *36 Hour Day.* 5th ed. Baltimore: Johns Hopkins University Press; 2012.

68. Smith AD, Kim YI, Refsum H. Is folic acid good for everyone? *Am J Clin Nutr.* 2008;87(3):517–533.

69. Farina N, Isaac MGEKN, Clark AR, Rusted J, Tabet N. Vitamin E for Alzheimer's dementia and mild cognitive impairment. *Cochrane Database Syst Rev.* 2012;11(11): CD002854. doi:10.1002/14651858.CD002854.pub3.

70. Brewer GJ, Kaur S. Zinc deficiency and zinc therapy efficacy with reduction of serum free copper in Alzheimer's disease. *Int J Alzheimers Dis.* 2013;2013:586365.

71. Calon F. Omega-3 polyunsaturated fatty acids in Alzheimer's disease: Key questions and partial answers. *Curr Alzheimer Res.* 2011;8(5):470–478.

72. Sydenham E, Dangour AD, Lim W-S. Omega 3 fatty acid for the prevention of cognitive decline and dementia. *Cochrane Database Syst Rev.* 2012;6:CD005379. doi:10.1002/14651858.CD005379.pub3.

73. Mazereeuw G, Lanctôt KL, Chau SA, Swardfager W, Herrmann N. Effects of omega-3 fatty acids on cognitive performance: A meta-analysis. *Neurobiol Aging.* 2012;33(7):E17–29.

74. Schneider LS, Mangialasche F, Andreasen N, et al. Clinical trials and late-stage drug development for Alzheimer's disease: An appraisal from 1984 to 2014. *J Intern Med.* 2014;275(3):251–283.

75. Yancheva S, Ihl R, Nikolova G, Panayotov P, Schlaefke S, Hoerr R. Ginkgo biloba extract EGb 761(R), donepezil or both combined in the treatment of Alzheimer's disease with neuropsychiatric features: A randomised, double-blind, exploratory trial. *Aging Ment Health.* 2009;13(2):183–190. doi:10.1080/13607860902749057.

76. Gray SL, Anderson ML, Dublin S, et al. Cumulative use of strong anticholinergics and incident dementia. *JAMA Intern Med.* 2015;175(3):401. doi:10.1001/jamainternmed.2014.7663.

77. Maust DT, Kim HM, Seyfried LS, et al. Antipsychotics, other psychotropics, and the risk of death in patients with dementia. *JAMA Psychiatry*. 2015;72(5):438–445. doi:10.1001/jamapsychiatry.2014.3018.

78. Iuvone T, Esposito G, Esposito R, Santamaria R, Di Rosa M, Izzo AA. Neuroprotective effect of cannabidiol, a non-psychoactive component from *Cannabis sativa*, on beta-amyloid-induced toxicity in PC12 cells. *J Neurochem*. 2004;89(1):134–141.

79. Esposito G, Scuderi C, Savani C, et al. Cannabidiol in vivo blunts beta-amyloid induced neuroinflammation by suppressing IL-1beta and iNOS expression. *Br J Pharmacol*. 2007;151(8):1272–1279. doi:10.1038/sj.bjp.0707337.

80. García-Arencibia M, González S, de Lago E, Ramos JA, Mechoulam R, Fernández-Ruiz J. Evaluation of the neuroprotective effect of cannabinoids in a rat model of Parkinson's disease: Importance of antioxidant and cannabinoid receptor-independent properties. *Brain Res*. 2007;1134(1):162–170.

81. Demirakca T, Sartorius A, Ende G, et al. Diminished gray matter in the hippocampus of cannabis users: Possible protective effects of cannabidiol. *Drug Alcohol Depend*. 2011;114(2-3):242–245.

82. Finseth TA, Hedeman JL, Brown RP, Johnson KI, Binder MS, Kluger BM. Self-reported efficacy of cannabis and other complementary medicine modalities by Parkinson's disease patients in Colorado. *Evidence Based Complement Altern Med*. 2015;2015:874849.

83. Lotan I, Treves T, Roditi Y, Djaldetti R. Medical marijuana (cannabis) treatment for motor and nonmotor symptoms in Parkinson's disease. An open-label observational study. *Mov Disord*. 2013;28(Suppl 1):448. doi:10.1016/S0960-9776(13)70016-X.

84. Lonnen JSM, Adler BJ. A systematic review of the evidence for percutaneous gastrostomy tube feeding or nasogastric tube feeding in patients with dysphagia due to idiopathic Parkinson's disease. *Mov Disord*. 2011;26:S170–S171.

85. Finucane TE, Christmas C, Travis K. Tube feeding in patients with advanced dementia. *JAMA*. 1999;282(14):1365. doi:10.1001/jama.282.14.1365.

86. Hager K, Kenklies M, McAfoose J, Engel J, Munch G. Alpha-lipoic acid as a new treatment option for Alzheimer's disease—a 48 months follow-up analysis. *J Neural Transm Suppl*. 2007;(72):189–193.

87. De Araújo DP, Lobato RDFG, Cavalcanti JRLDP, et al. The contributions of antioxidant activity of lipoic acid in reducing neurogenerative progression of Parkinson's disease: a review. *Int J Neurosci*. 2011;121(2):51–57.

88. Chaturvedi RK, Beal MF. Mitochondrial diseases of the brain. *Free Radic Biol Med*. 2013;63:1–29.

89. Hudson S, Tabet N. Acetyl-L-carnitine for dementia. *Cochrane Database Syst Rev*. 2003;(2):CD003158.

90. Montgomery S, Thal LJ, Amrein R. Meta-analysis of double blind randomized controlled clinical trials of acetyl-L-carnitine versus placebo in the treatment of mild cognitive impairment and mild Alzheimer's disease. *Int Clin Psychopharmacol*. 2003;18(2):61–71.

91. Adair JC, Knoefel JE, Morgan N. Controlled trial of N-acetylcysteine for patients with probable Alzheimer's disease. *Neurology*. 2001;57(8):1515–1517.

92. Fioravanti M, Yanagi M. Cytidinediphosphocholine (CDP-choline) for cognitive and behavioural disturbances associated with chronic cerebral disorders in the elderly. *Cochrane Database Syst Rev*. 2005;(2):CD000269. http://doi.wiley.com/10.1002/14651858.CD000269.pub3.

93. Moreno Moreno MDJ. Cognitive improvement in mild to moderate Alzheimer's dementia after treatment with the acetylcholine precursor choline alfoscerate: A multicenter, double-blind, randomized, placebo-controlled trial. *Clin Ther*. 2003;25(1):178–193.

94. Turner RS, Thomas RG, Craft S, et al. A randomized, double-blind, placebo-controlled trial of resveratrol for Alzheimer disease. *Neurology*. 2015;85(16):1383–1391.

95. Rocha-González HI, Ambriz-Tututi M, Granados-Soto V. Resveratrol: A natural compound with pharmacological potential in neurodegenerative diseases. *CNS Neurosci Ther*. 2008;14(3):234–247.

96. Thaipisuttikul P, Galvin JE. Use of medical foods and nutritional approaches in the treatment of Alzheimer's disease. *Clin Pract (Lond)*. 2012;9(2):199–209. doi:10.2217/cpr.12.3.

97. Calabrese C, Gregory WL, Leo M, Kraemer D, Bone K, Oken B. Effects of a standardized *Bacopa monnieri* extract on cognitive performance, anxiety, and depression in the elderly: A randomized, double-blind, placebo-controlled trial. *J Altern Complement Med*. 2008;14(6):707–713. doi:10.1089/acm.2008.0018.

98. Noguchi-Shinohara M, Yuki S, Dohmoto C, et al. Consumption of green tea, but not black tea or coffee, is associated with reduced risk of cognitive decline. *PLoS One*. 2014;9(5):e96013.

99. Mak JCW. Potential role of green tea catechins in various disease therapies: progress and promise. *Clin Exp Pharmacol Physiol*. 2012;39(3):265–273. doi:10.1111/j.1440-1681.2012.05673.x.

100. Monroy A, Lithgow GJ, Alavez S. Curcumin and neurodegenerative diseases. *BioFactors*. 2013;39(1):122–132.

101. Mythri RB, Srinivas Bharath MM. Curcumin: A potential neuroprotective Agent an Parkinson's disease. *Curr Pharm Des*. 2012;18(1):91–99.

102. Birks J, Grimley Evans J. *Ginkgo biloba* for cognitive impairment and dementia. *Cochrane Database Syst Rev*. 2009;(1):CD003120.

103. Gauthier S, Schlaefke S. Efficacy and tolerability of Ginkgo biloba extract EGb 761 in dementia: A systematic review and meta-analysis of randomized placebo-controlled trials. *Clin Interv Aging*. 2014;9:2065–2077.

104. Yang G, Wang Y, Tian J, Liu J-P. Huperzine A for Alzheimer's disease: A systematic review and meta-analysis of randomized clinical trials. *PLoS One*. 2013;8(9):e74916. doi:10.1371/journal.pone.0074916.

105. Wolkowitz OM, Kramer JH, Reus VI, et al. DHEA treatment of Alzheimer's disease: a randomized, double-blind, placebo-controlled study. *Neurology*. 2003;60(7):1071–1076.

21

Integrative Oncology

AMY LITTLEFIELD, DEIRDRE ORCEYRE,
AND STEPHANIE CHENG

Case Study

Rita M., a 67-year-old retired schoolteacher, presented in the fall of 2010 with mild bloating and digestive symptoms, including pain that was relieved with bowel movements. She was evaluated and treated with a BRAT diet for 1 month with worsening of symptoms. Within a month of her first presentation a vaginal ultrasound showed bilateral pelvic masses; her CA125 level was >4,000. Total abdominal hysterectomy with bilateral salpingo-oophorectomy was performed and the patient received treatment with intravenous and intraperitoneal chemotherapy, including Taxol, cisplatin, and carboplatin, for stage IIIC ovarian neoplasia. In addition to conventional care Rita consulted integrative oncology providers. With a broad integrative team including medical and surgical oncologists, her primary care physician, acupuncture, naturopathic physicians, nutritionists, and mental health providers she navigated multiple fistula formation and resolution. She also experienced significant fatigue, nausea and vomiting, and moderate neuropathy.

Concurrent with treatment she received intravenous vitamin C therapy, acupuncture, and evidence-based supplements targeted to the disease as well as to improving her overall metabolic functioning. Results of integrative lab assessment of markers of nutritional status, blood sugar dysregulation, inflammation, and immunity were incorporated into her treatment plan, tailored and prioritized to her needs. Without other metabolic syndrome indicators, she exhibited a tendency toward elevated blood glucose and insulin levels. The patient was highly motivated to incorporate exercise, stress management, sleep hygiene, and nutritional strategies but without hypervigilance.

Conventional treatment concluded the next spring, and her CA125 level was reduced to 11. She maintained intravenous therapies and acupuncture for 12 months. Between 2012 and 2014 she continued with integrative strategies and felt very well but began to experience recurrent and worsening bowel obstructions. She and her surgeon determined that a colostomy would provide for improved quality of life. As of January 2017, more than 6 years since diagnosis, she continues to follow an individualized lifestyle and supplement protocol that emphasizes stress management and exercise and a low-glycemic diet. Considering that the 5-year survival for a patient with distant metastases is 30%, at 6.5 years and with excellent quality of life, Rita has exceeded optimistic expectations.

Introduction

Cancer is a disease of aging, and our society is aging. People over 65 years old represented 14.5% of the population in 2014 and are expected to grow to represent 21.7% of the population by 2040.[1] In economically developed countries, 58% of all newly diagnosed cancer cases occur in patients 65 years of age and older. By 2020, the percentage of patients over 65 years old with a diagnosis of cancer is projected to exceed 70%.[2] The most common types of cancer in patients over 65 are breast, colorectal, prostate, pancreatic, lung, bladder, and stomach, and the average age of those diagnosed with all types of cancer is 70.[3] As many as 50% to 83% of adult patients with cancer in the United States report using complementary and alternative medicine (CAM) at least once after their diagnosis.[4-6] Many patients do not disclose this to their oncologist.[7]

Because the incidence of cancer is strongly associated with aging, the development and expansion of age-appropriate therapies and approaches is crucial as the population of elderly patients with cancer grows in the upcoming years. Taking into account the unique needs of this population will be of great importance. Many elderly individuals are likely to have multiple comorbidities and are subsequently likely to be taking several medications, including a high prevalence of supplement use that should be managed by a trained clinician.[8] Reduced digestive function due to aging, for example, may exacerbate digestive side effects from chemotherapy. Anemia of aging may be compounded by radiation-induced anemias. Elders may also be dealing with changes in cognition and/or functional status.

Therefore, in this population, it is especially important to look at the whole picture, taking into account the patient's other illnesses, medications, social support system, and general physical condition as all of these will impact his or her cancer care. An integrative multidisciplinary team approach can be particularly helpful when managing the complexity of health care in the elderly.[8] Additionally, some elders may be very frail, putting them at greater risk for adverse effects from cancer treatments. For these individuals, maintaining function and comfort may be more important than attempting lengthy or harsh treatments.

Geriatric patients may appreciate additional proactive integrative oncology support in the following areas:

- Support for comorbidities, which are more common in this population
- Declining hepatic and renal function and other aging-related changes lower the threshold for negative side effects and toxicities due to comorbidities
- Sarcopenia concerns and reduced nutrient absorption
- Geriatric patients have more supplement use compared to younger patients
- An integrative oncology approach will support a better quality of life for the geriatric patient.
- For "lost patients" who are dismissed due to age, integrative oncology provides closer assessment and more support
- Quality-of-life concerns may be weighted heavily over long-term survival
- Social and family support issues requiring collaboration among adult children of the patient—bring patient in, provide guidance for family members
- Palliative care and end-of-life support

Pathophysiology

The term "cancer" encompasses many diseases with widely varying natural course and treatments. While some cancers, like classic Hodgkin's lymphoma, are essentially curable, others, like glioblastoma, are rapidly fatal. Causative mutations confer neoplastic cells a growth advantage over normal cells, resulting in excessive proliferation that is independent of normal physiological growth signals. Cancers invade and destroy normal adjacent tissues and metastasize to distant sites in the body. However, some can be discovered early enough to be surgically removed or treated with systemic therapies, like chemotherapy, hormonal therapy, immunotherapy, targeted therapy, and/or radiation.[9]

Recent advances in genetics have changed how we diagnose and treat cancer. Most cancer cells have a normal cell counterpart in the body, and thus cancer has been traditionally classified based on the cell/tissue of origin. However, recent disease classifications, like those published by the World Health Organization, are frequently based on the genetic alterations in the tumor cells. More broadly, our understanding of how cancer develops, and therefore how it can be treated, has dramatically changed with the growth of genomic, proteomic, and epigenomic data. Research into the development of malignancies has led to a complex understanding of the metabolic pathways in cancer. These pathways are well organized and regulate the growth, maturity, division, metastasis, and death of cancer cells. Cell cycle mutations and dysregulated controls by the immune system fail to halt abnormal processes, leading to malignancy. The tumor microenvironment determines tumor development and regulation. Many new therapies block specific steps along various biochemical pathways essential for cancer growth. Stem cell signaling pathways are a new direction for intervention. Similarly, integrative therapies can intervene along these same pathways and influence DNA damage from environmental disturbances or chronic inflammation. Recent research has also shown that the rate of growth and spread of cancers depends not only on intrinsic cancer cell characteristics but also on the patient's immune system status, which in turn is affected by stress, nutrition, age, and chronic disease. Therefore, therapies that target cancer cells directly as well as support patients' immune systems are frequently used in combination. Many integrative therapies are emerging to have benefits in these same areas.

What Is Integrative Oncology?

The goal of integrative oncology is to reduce risk and slow or reverse existing disease processes while addressing constitutional wellness of body, mind, and spirit. The practice of integrative oncology recognizes the importance of a high quality of life and improved overall survival for patients and affords new opportunities for this beyond the conventional oncology office. Recognition of the value of lifestyle factors and social and emotional health and the emerging evidence of nutraceuticals and bodywork is pivotal to optimal integrative care. A model is emerging for collaboration among these providers, allowing for true integration. Physicians with expertise in this area receive postgraduate training from organizations such as the Society for Integrative Oncology and the Oncology Association of Naturopathic Physicians (see the list of resources at the end of the chapter). They do not necessarily administer chemotherapy but are experts in evaluating the individual, targeting evidence-based integrative care, understanding herb–drug interactions, dosing supplements, and coordinating care among a multidisciplinary integrative team.

Patients who use integrative therapies frequently report relative benefits in terms of resiliency and response. Still, most integrative oncology physicians agree that, unfortunately, there is no single "miracle cure." As much as the internet may provide encouragement about hidden treatments to cure cancer, there is no one treatment that can promise such results. Guiding and counseling patients on this fact can be an important role of the integrative practitioner.[4] With all the misinformation that abounds in this age of technology, comprehensive expertise that includes these integrative treatments is essential.

In this context of integrative oncology, we use "integrative" to mean the following:

- Integrating our approach to include the entire body—immune, nervous, digestive, endocrine systems, and so forth, each interacting with and affecting the others. This includes ongoing mindful management of comorbidities such as hypertension, obesity, and diabetes mellitus.
- Integrating the whole person—mind, body, and spirit (see Chapter 9).
- Integrating a team approach—surgery, medical oncology, radiation oncology, naturopathic oncology, reiki, acupuncture/traditional Chinese medicine, nutrition, psychotherapy, yoga, physical therapy, and so forth.

There is some confusion about the difference between integrative and alternative treatments for cancer. Generally, "integrative" refers to options offered collaboratively with conventional standards of care. "Alternative" cancer treatments include any approach that suggests a treatment to *replace* conventional approaches such as surgery, chemotherapy, radiation, hormonal therapies, or targeted therapies. Centers offering such treatments and even entire alternative cancer clinics exist worldwide, offering many treatments that are as yet unproven. Some of these treatments show potential benefit and others may cause harm. Finding an integrative oncologist for patients considering alternative treatments is essential for appropriate guidance.

The strength of scientific evidence for integrative therapies is growing but is not yet equivalent to that used to determine conventional oncology treatments. Preclinical studies abound, while clinical trials are more rare. Integrative oncology providers seek robust evidence yet strive to offer clinically relevant and safe strategies to patients. They may adopt a treatment with observed clinical benefit before it is clearly established by research, *as long as the risk profile is low*. A practice such as reiki that delivers a strong sense of wellness to the patient does not require the same level of study as that of a cytotoxic chemotherapeutic. There are therapies that can and should be adopted based on observed clinical improvements, and a double-blind placebo-controlled study is not always required.

Allied Health Providers

Oncology centers around the country are beginning to include a diversity of providers and disciplines. Many offer the services of nutritionists, mental health therapists, and physical therapists as part of standard treatment. Broadening care to include providers with expertise in the use of safe effective supplements, reiki, acupuncture, and exercise therapy, for example, is still needed. This inclusivity embraces the diversity of patients' needs and concerns.

Integrative Strategies in Prevention

In conventional medicine, prevention is understood primarily as early detection. We advocate mammography and colonoscopy, for example, as detection strategies to identify early disease processes and allow for curative treatment. Integrative oncology additionally emphasizes the nature of preventive strategies based on healthy lifestyle choices and proactive use of natural compounds that have anticancer activity. For example, for a patient who has a strong family history of breast cancer the integrative provider will certainly advocate for regular screening exams but will also offer advice on exercise, nutrition, and alcohol consumption in order to reduce risk.

Integrative Strategies in Treatment

In addition to prevention and early detection, integrative oncology supports the patient after a diagnosis has been made. Strong evidence exists for the addition of certain botanicals and nutrients into a cytotoxic regimen. With respect for and consideration of the directly cytotoxic/anticancer focus, integrative oncology physicians are trained to ease the side effects of conventional treatments, augmenting these regimens and allowing patients to tolerate them better. At the same time, the whole person is addressed. This includes lifestyle support and diet recommendations, as well as mind, body, and spirit support. Physiological function is optimized, such as the digestive and nervous systems, with particular attention paid to any comorbidities.

Integrative treatment strategies include the following:

- Lifestyle interventions
  o Exercise
  o Sleep
  o Stress management
  o Nutrition
- Supplements
  o Safety concerns
  o Constitutional support
  o Anticancer interventions
  o Side-effect management

LIFESTYLE INTERVENTIONS

Emphasis on broad lifestyle support offers tremendous value for the oncology patient. Gentle, meaningful lifestyle modifications improve quality of life without increasing mental and physiological stressors. While each lifestyle strategy is relevant independently, there is also a synergy in action that allows for patient traction and momentum, facilitating improved clinical status and a sense of well-being. In patients who sleep poorly, we observe that attention to food intake, exercise, and stress management may quickly allow for improved sleep quality. Likewise, improved sleep and optimizing food choices may allow a patient to feel sufficient energy to engage in a daily walk. Seeing the person and the wellness strategy as a whole creates a welcome momentum in the patient healing experience.

Exercise

Evidence for physical activity in cancer prevention, treatment, and survivorship is accumulating. The mechanisms vary, but we do know that the benefits of graded exercise outweigh the risks. A 2016 *JAMA* study found that exercise reduces the risk of 13 cancers independent of body size and smoking status.[10] Patients who have a history of exercise have an improved prognosis compared to their non-exercising peers. Exercise initiation during conventional treatment is associated with less fatigue, reduced cachexia and sarcopenia, and improved mood.[11] Those who continue exercise after treatment report higher quality of life and are clinically assessed with a higher functional status, and research shows improved survivorship with exercise.[12] An integrative survivorship model recognizes the benefit of exercise to comorbid conditions such as cardiac, pulmonary, and musculoskeletal disease.

Sleep

Periods of restful sleep provide opportunities for improved wellness and recuperation. Regular sleeping hours in a dark room free of disruptive artificial light is a tremendous integrative oncology strategy to improve patient wellness. This opportunity is often compromised in the geriatric population because of the physiological decline in melatonin, and the increased stress and exogenous steroid administration as part of cancer treatment. There is great value in attention to sleep hygiene. We know that disruptions of the circadian cycle increase the risk of chronic disease.[12,13] As we collaborate with the patient to improve physical activity, we are facilitating a more restful, recuperative sleep.[14] Exogenous melatonin at therapeutic doses has a role in oncology care and is discussed in the therapeutic section later in the chapter.

Stress Management

Appropriate stress interventions are imperative to an integrative oncology plan. Patients may be best supported through clergy, support groups, exercise, tai chi, meditation, and mindfulness-based stress reduction among others, including laughter. The Society for Integrative Oncology published Clinical Practice Guidelines based on a review of the literature and identified music therapy, relaxation techniques, yoga, meditation, and massage as having an evidence basis for support of stress and anxiety reduction.[15]

Mindfulness-based stress management, in particular, is currently the focus of much study. A study published in the *Journal of Clinical Oncology* found improvements in quality of life and mood among breast cancer survivors that were sustained at 3 months after this intervention.[15,16] This reinforces the expectation that stress management is optimally applied frequently and for the long term. Rather than saving stress management interventions for the end of the day as a salvage technique, short and simple interventions throughout the day are superior.

Nutrition

Patients seeking integrative oncology care have frequent misconceptions about diet or inappropriately apply strategies from internet searches. Often they place great attention on excluding "bad" foods in a manner that leads to heightened stress, malnourishment, and social isolation. Providing evidence-based guidance about what foods to include rather than emphasizing food restriction and elimination has tremendous therapeutic value. In addition to the physiological benefits of proper nutrition, this allows patients to maintain their social connection to family and meal times.

Nutritional support, especially in a geriatric oncology population, should emphasize nutrient-dense plant-dominant meals with sufficient protein to meet the high metabolic demands of oncology care. Clinically, meals with a low glycemic index that avoid simple carbohydrates and include protein, healthy fat, and fiber are useful for maintaining healthy weight, muscle mass, and energy levels. A broad intake of fruits and vegetables offer a variety of nutrients, including dietary polyphenols, with a chemopreventive benefit.[17] Polyphenols naturally occurring in the diet for which there is robust research include green tea, curcumin, garlic, and soy and are being studied for their impact on epigenetic modulation.[18] This population requires a higher protein intake to avoid catabolism and sarcopenia. Plant-based fats and fiber in legumes, avocados, nuts, and seeds are valuable to discourage insulin resistance and to facilitate fat-soluble vitamin absorption. The Mediterranean diet (see Chapter 2) or a similar diet plan incorporates many of these benefits.[17]

With regard to nutritional deficiencies in cancer, both disease progression and treatment impact, see the in-depth discussion in the 2016 review article by Gröber et al.[19]

Prior to 2009 there was concern that a diet high in soy foods may stimulate estrogen receptor-positive disease based on the demonstrated phytoestrogen activity of soy. Since then a number of human studies have actually shown an inverse relationship between dietary soy intake and cancer development and progression.[20] A 2009 *JAMA* study concluded that soy consumption in food form is "significantly associated with decreased risk of death and recurrence."[21] Many literature reviews on dietary soy use have drawn similar conclusions as well as recent clinical studies, on lung and endometrial cancers for example. Concentrated soy powders, additives, or milks used on a daily basis may have a different effect than traditional dietary use of tofu, miso paste, tempeh, edamame, and so forth. The use of soybean extracts, particularly soy isoflavones, is still controversial. However, the North American Menopause Society and the European Food Safety Authority recently concluded that isoflavones do not increase the risk of breast or endometrial cancer.[22] Similar conclusions may be drawn regarding prostate cancer.[20,23]

Patients often ask about juicing as an adjunctive treatment for cancer. Juicing fruits and vegetables concentrates valuable nutrients and provides them in an easy-to-digest form. However, many juicers remove pulp, which contains valuable fiber and helps to slow the digestion of the carbohydrates included in these foods. This leads to an unintended increase in carbohydrate ingestion and subsequent spikes in serum blood sugar and insulin levels. Some ways to address this concern are to add protein or fat to the juice, use a pulp-in or macerating juicer, split the juice into small diluted portions throughout the day, and focus on green vegetables for juicing.

The metabolism of malignant cells depends heavily on glucose. A low-glycemic diet will prevent hyperglycemia and discourage the resultant flood of growth-promoting insulin. Low-carbohydrate diets are being explored as adjunctive interventions. One such diet is the ketogenic diet, which is currently being investigated by three major U.S. medical centers for patients with glioblastoma multiforme.[24] The clinical reality, however, is that for most patients this diet is too severe and the social, mental, and emotional challenges outweigh the benefit. The target of complete sugar elimination risks weight loss and social isolation and is rarely sustainable in the long term. Generally, the best initial recommendation is to eat a low-glycemic Mediterranean-type diet.

SUPPLEMENTS

The use of supplements, often termed nutraceuticals, is a broad topic and includes the use of vitamins, minerals, botanicals, amino acids, and other nutrients in pill, powder, liquid, intravenous, intramuscular, or topical forms. Their use should be directed by a trained professional, particularly when used in conjunction with conventional treatments for cancer.[25] Nutraceuticals may be used with the goals of preventing and treating side effects, supporting the whole body, and directly intervening in the metabolic life of the malignancy. Many nutraceuticals have impact on more than one of these categories.

There is an abundance of dangerous or unreliable supplement information available to patients from family, friends, or online resources. There is a lack of providers with optimal training to guide patients through use of the supplements that are safe and for which there is evidence. Botanicals and nutraceutical supplements must be evaluated for safety and compatibility, along with interactions with function, metabolism, and excretion of conventional medical treatments. Certain chemotherapy or anesthesia drugs, for example, may be metabolized through pathways affected by particular botanicals. Integrative oncology providers are well trained in assessment of the pharmacokinetics and metabolism of natural and conventional therapies and can understand options for optimal patient care and safety. Most radiation therapies act through cell oxidation; although controversial, many agree radiation is not a time to use an abundance of antioxidant therapies.

Safety considerations for nutraceutical use include the following:

1. Will the supplement harm the patient? Certain aggressive anticancer CAM treatments may actually cause harm if used improperly.
2. Will the supplement interfere with the current conventional regimen?
   - Chemotherapy—does the supplement increase or inhibit drug metabolism? This interaction is often via hepatic metabolism pathways such as cytochrome p450. Each chemotherapy class may have different types of potential interactions. Certain supplements may augment or interfere with efficacy.
   - Radiation—does the supplement protect tissues against therapeutic radiation damage? In this case, for example, cell-protective antioxidants may work against the intentional damage caused by radiation therapy. Certain others have clear benefits.
   - Surgery—will the supplement affect anesthesia (again, via hepatic metabolism)? Will it increase bleeding or clotting?
   - Hormonal treatments and other immunotherapies must each be evaluated individually. Several professional associations and excellent books provide guidance on this.

Constitutional Support

One of the most potent strategies to improve quality of life and reduce the side effects of treatment is to identify deficiencies in a patient's nutritional status. The most clinically relevant in an oncology setting are vitamin D, omega fatty acids, B complex, and probiotics. While all have a potential role in integrative geriatrics, below is a description of their use specifically as it relates to oncology (Table 21.1).

Table 21.1. Constitutional Support

Vitamin D	45–65 ng/mL in serum or 2,000 IU daily	Bone strength, fatigue, arthralgia
Essential fatty acids in fish oil	1.5–3 g of EPA + DHA	Cachexia, depression, fatigue
B complex	1 per day, in the morning	Fatigue, depression
Probiotics	Varies	Assimilation of nutrients, immune support
Magnesium	300 mg/day	Muscle cramping, sleep, fatigue

Research about the role of *vitamin D* is expanding rapidly. The findings generally show an inverse relationship between vitamin D levels and cancer risks/progression.[19] Vitamin D levels that approximate 30 ng/ml, currently the low end of most reference ranges, are associated with a decreased risk of cancer initiation, a decreased risk of metastasis in patients with cancer, and increased survival.[26,27] In addition to risk reduction, repletion addresses quality-of-life factors relevant to this population, including mood, bone strength, arthralgias, and fatigue.[26,28] Vitamin D may also provide benefit in cachexia.[29]

Given risks among oncology patients for calcium dysregulation and bone weaknesses, it is advisable to perform formal testing rather than to provide presumptive treatment. This allows for accurate prescriptive dosing if necessary. A patient with a baseline level of 9 ng/dl will require a different strength and duration of treatment than one with a baseline of 27 ng/dl, for example; treatment of both patients with a standard daily dosage of 2,000 IU risks undertreatment of the former patient with unnecessary compromise of quality-of-life factors. Patients with hypercalcemia should be monitored closely during vitamin D repletion.

Without sufficient *essential fatty acids* in the diet, patients may experience exacerbation of neuropathy, depression, skin changes, bone loss, arthralgias, cognitive decline, and cardiac complications common in the oncology population. This role is multifactorial, including influence in eicosanoid pathways, cell signaling, and immune modulation. Marine omega fats have a role in prevention, adjuvant treatment, as well as survivorship. In 2016 *JAMA Oncology* published a study detailing the reduced risk of colorectal cancer in patients with high intake of marine omega fats.[30] In survivorship, there is evidence that symptoms of cognitive decline, arthralgias, sarcopenia, and chemotherapy-induced peripheral neuropathy show improvement in patients with higher EFA levels.[31] Given the high levels of omega-6 in the standard American diet, proactively increasing omega-3 intake with supplementation works to offset the tendency toward inflammation these patients would otherwise suffer.

One and a half grams of EPA + DHA can be obtained in a can of sardines or via a supplement. The range of concentration among fish oil products is broad and must be monitored to ensure the proper dose for the patient.[25]

With aging and the common states of hypochlorhydria in the geriatric population, *B vitamin* status decreases. Supplementation of B complex in patients with deficiency reduces the mental health symptoms and fatigue associated with oncology care. Avoidance of the synthetic folic acid in favor of a folate is preferred for cancer prevention and especially for the portion of the population with the single nucleotide polymorphism (SNP) of the MTHFR gene.[32]

Probiotics in the diet or in supplement form are an effective way to facilitate absorption of nutrients and discourage inflammatory signaling in geriatric patients. Fermented sauerkraut, kimchee, some yogurts, and kombucha
are excellent food sources of probiotics to consider. Although there is debate
among the integrative oncology community, caution is advised when considering supplemental probiotics in severely neutropenic patients. There are rare
case studies suggesting that sepsis may result from therapeutic introduction of
bacteria in pediatric populations.[25]

Magnesium levels are reduced by common acid-blocking medications, and
low magnesium states will exacerbate muscle pain, cramping, and fatigue.
Repletion allows for improved generation of ATP at the mitochondria.

Anticancer Interventions

While supporting the constitution of each patient is a fundamental part of
integrative oncology, certain cases may warrant the addition of measures to
encourage an inhospitable environment for the cancer cell (Table 21.2). One
benefit of this field is that many interventions serve a dual purpose here by
both supporting the fundamental physiology and metabolism of the patient
and providing proven benefit in fighting the disease. The goals of anticancer
supplementation are as follows:

- Support apoptosis
- Reduce angiogenesis
- Stabilize gene health
- Improve immune regulation
- Decrease inflammation
- Optimize hormonal influences

Table 21.2. Integrative Anticancer Measures

Nutrient	Dosage	Tumor type
Melatonin	20 mg	Solid tumor (breast, colon, lung, brain)
Medicinal mushrooms	1.5–3 g	Solid tumor (breast colon, lung, brain)
Curcumin	1 g liposomal form	Solid/hematological (breast, colon, non-Hodgkin's lymphoma)
Green tea EGCG extract	500–1,000 mg	Solid/hematological (breast, colon, prostate, non-Hodgkin's lymphoma)
Resveratrol	Unclear	Breast, prostate, pancreas

Medicinal mushrooms include reishi, shiitake, *Coriolus*, maitake, button mushrooms, and others. They are generally used in integrative oncology as hot-water extracts of a protein-bound polysaccharide known as beta glucan. There is evidence that these are associated with improved immune function via bone marrow modulation.[33] Overall survival improvements have also been described in multiple clinical studies. A meta-analysis in 2012 showed a 9% absolute reduction in 5-year mortality with a number needed to treat of 11. The greatest benefit found was with breast, gastric, and colon cancers.[34] A review specific to patients with curatively resected colon cancer found improved disease-free and overall survival rates in those also treated with coriolus.[35] A review of studies of *Coriolus* in lung cancer patients discussed the role of the polysaccharide in immune potentiation, reduced symptoms, and extended survival.[36] The dosage is 1.5 to 3 g/day, hot-water extract form, divided, away from food.

Curcumin is an extract from the turmeric (*Curcuma longa*) root. There is more research on this agent than any other natural anticancer therapy. Thirty years of research show that it has an effect on cell signaling pathways, reduced inflammation through reduction of NF-kB and induction of apoptosis, metastasis inhibition, and many other actions.[32,37-39] More recently, and unlike the action of conventional chemotherapy acting on mature cells, it shows promise as an agent with action against cancer stem cell lines.[39] Attention to the form and production of curcumin is important as there are limitations in bioavailability. Liposomal forms have been developed to enhance absorption.[32] The dosage is 1 g/day of curcumin standardized to liposomal curcuminoids.

Melatonin has evidence of benefit in primary prevention, adjuvant therapy, and tertiary prevention.[40] It is oncostatic, strongly antioxidant, immune-modulating, and apoptotic and acts as a hormone modulator with, for example, SERM and aromatase inhibitory activity.[40-43] As described in the lifestyle section, sleep is an important component of a wellness plan for cancer patients. In addition to potential quality-of-life benefits from improved sleep, and given the broad anticancer potential, the use of exogenous melatonin in supplement form is indicated for integrative therapy of patients with solid tumors. In meta-analyses it shows improved remission and survival rates with a decrease in treatment-related side effects.[41-43] Melatonin has been studied extensively and has shown benefit in the treatment of the side effects of cancer treatment without any compromise to efficacy.[41,42] The dosage is 20 mg at bedtime. Lower dosing may be advisable with sensitive patients, and a slow taper up starting with 3 to 5 mg can help to decrease morning drowsiness during the first weeks of treatment.

Green tea (*Camellia sinensis*) has broad anticancer properties, acting on many pathways relevant to oncology care, including antioxidant, anti-inflammatory, insulin-sensitizing, and VEGF/MMP inhibition.[44] The catechin polyphenol extracts of the tea plant, particularly epigallocatechin-3-gallate (EGCG), are linked with inhibition of many carcinogenic pathways[45] and are safe for use along with chemotherapeutic drugs.[46] In human trials benefit has been shown for cancers of the breast, digestive tract, and prostate, among others.[32,45] Notably, green tea looks exceptionally valuable with hematological malignancies, having promising evidence in patients with chronic lymphocytic leukemia. A 2013 study with 2,000 mg EGCG showed a sustained decrease in the number of absolute lymphocytes and a reduction of palpable lymphadenopathy in patients with previously untreated chronic lymphocytic leukemia.[47,48]

It is important to consider the quality and potency of a green tea product, as tea can be contaminated with pesticides and aluminum. The best option to avoid caffeine and to improve potency is to take a standardized EGCG formulation that has been tested by a third party for potency and purity. The dosage is 250 to 300 mg taken three times daily of a standardized product containing 50% EGCG, divided for optimal effect.

Resveratrol is a stilbene polyphenol found in concentrated amounts in grapes, and therefore wine. Interest in the "French paradox" has led to extensive in vitro and in vivo studies of resveratrol as an anticancer nutrient, particularly in breast and prostate malignancies. Like curcumin, resveratrol reduces oxidative stress, prevents the initiation of carcinogenesis, regulates cell cycle, inhibits metastasis, and encourages apoptosis.[32,37] It clearly activates natural killer cell activity and has an inhibitory action on cancer stem cells.[32] It is especially of value in hematological malignancies, where immune supportive therapies are controversial.[49] However, the bioavailability of resveratrol is debatable, and no clear dosage or form for ingestion has been defined at this time.[32] Many studies have used 1 to 2.5 g/day in divided doses.

Side-Effect Management

Here we discuss some of the most widely used integrative treatments to support patients during conventional treatment. A comprehensive exploration of all supportive treatments is beyond the scope of this chapter, but some key recommendations are provided. Keep in mind that many side effects are reduced or even eliminated with the constitutional support discussed earlier in the chapter. Table 21.3 provides further examples.

The family of *ginseng* plants have been used traditionally for energy, vitality, and immune tonification. Several species of ginseng have been recognized for their profound impact on cancer-related fatigue and significant

Table 21.3. Side-Effect Management

Chemotherapy-induced peripheral neuropathy	B vitamins, acupuncture, vitamin E, L-glutamine, omega-3 fatty acids
Cancer-related fatigue[15]	Ginseng, CoQ10/ubiquinol, acupuncture, qi gong, melatonin, vitamin D
Hematotoxicity	Melatonin, acupuncture, selenium, vitamin D
Chemotherapy-induced nausea and vomiting[15]	Ginger, acupuncture, acupressure, music/guided imagery therapy[83]
Mucositis	L-glutamine, zinc, honey[65]
Cognitive effects[84]	Occupational therapy, sleep support, exercise
Sleep disruption[15]	Yoga, stress management, melatonin, acupuncture
Cardiotoxicity[78]	CoQ10/ubiquinol, L-carnitine, melatonin, curcumin, resveratrol, *Ginkgo biloba*, ginseng
Stress[15,84]	Music therapy, meditation, relaxation, massage, acupuncture
Loss of appetite/ cachexia	L-carnitine, melatonin, vitamin E + omega-3 fatty acids, vitamin D, acupuncture
Alopecia	Selenium (deficient patients only)

anticancer actions.[50] An epidemiological study of Chinese cancer patients found that ginseng use before and after diagnosis was associated with a reduced risk of death and improved quality of life.[51] One recent study used 2,000 mg twice daily of *Panax quinquefolius* (American ginseng) and showed reduced cancer-related fatigue in patients undergoing treatment and after treatment.[52,53] Ginseng has been shown to be safe to use with chemotherapy in countless preclinical studies.[54,55] The dosage varies, depending on the type and preparation of ginseng.

B vitamins, particularly cobalamin (B12) and pyridoxal (B6), may prevent or reduce the onset of neuropathy from several chemotherapy drugs.[56–58] However, caution is advised as there may be interactions with high doses of B vitamins in specific situations. See the "Constitutional Support" section for general recommendations about the use of B vitamins. The dosage varies depending on the B vitamin.

Coenzyme Q10 is an essential nutrient in the production of ATP through the electron transport chain and regulates energy production in the body.[59] It is particularly concentrated in muscle tissue, and thus in the heart muscle. CoQ10 has been found to be deficient in cancer patients and may be disrupted by certain chemotherapy drugs, most notably anthracyclines.[60] Supplementation with ubiquinol, a reduced form of CoQ10, shows evidence of improving energy and reducing cardiotoxicity in patients being treated with these chemotherapy agents, with no adverse effects observed.[61,62] CoQ10 may also reduce postsurgical oxidative stress and inflammation, leading to improved recovery and outcomes after surgery, chemotherapy, radiation therapy, targeted immunotherapies, and certain hormonal therapies.[63] The dosage is 100 to 200 mg/day of ubiquinol.

The conditionally essential amino acid *L-glutamine* is a primary source of cellular energy. Using the powder in a "swish and swallow" method assists with protection and recovery of oral and gastric mucosa.[64,65] Evidence is conflicting, but several randomized controlled trials support using L-glutamine in patients with mucositis resulting from both chemotherapy and head and neck radiation.[66] Many integrative oncology experts recommend the "swish and swallow" method on days 1 through 4 following chemotherapy/radiotherapy and "swish and spit" on other days to reduce excessive action of L-glutamine on intracellular energy production. Glutamine may be used to counteract cachexia in patients with advanced solid tumor disease.[29] The dosage is 10 to 30 g/day in divided doses; the patient should mix it in water and then "swish and swallow." It can be used on an acute basis on days 1 through 4 following treatment. The patient should "swish and spit" the solution on other days to avoid concerns regarding glutamine as an undesirable intracellular energy source.

Several forms of *zinc* have been used in chemotherapy- and radiotherapy-induced mucositis with good success. A "swish and swallow" rinse of zinc L-carnosine demonstrated a reduction in mucositis, pain, and analgesic use in addition to improved recovery; other studies report similar outcomes using systemic oral zinc supplementation. Multiple randomized clinical trials clearly support this positive effect of using zinc in chemotherapy- and radiotherapy-induced mucositis.[65] The dosage is 15 to 30 mg with meals to avoid nausea. Toxicity has been reported with long-term use of doses of more than 50 mg.

Many species of *mushrooms* are used in traditional herbal medicine throughout the world; recently many have been studied and used for cancer treatment and adjunctive support. In particular, the reishi mushroom (*Ganoderma lucidum*) has extensive evidence, with an updated Cochrane review every 2 years. The most recent report states that "results showed that patients who had been given *G. lucidum* alongside with chemo/radiotherapy were more likely to respond positively compared to chemo/radiotherapy alone [and] had relatively improved quality of life in comparison to controls."[67] Reishi mushrooms have broad anti-inflammatory and immune-modulating properties. Their effects on cytokine production and circulation, most notably tumor necrosis factor-α and interleukin-6, reduce cancer-related fatigue and improve overall quality of life when used as an adjunctive treatment.[68] Studies abound on various mushroom types and extracts, including turkeytail (*Coriolus versicolor*), shiitake, maitake, chaga, *Agaricus blazei*, cordyceps, and active hexose cor-related compound (AHCC).[25,69] No serious side effects have been reported.[67] The dosage is 500 to 1,000 mg three times daily; most integrative oncology practitioners prefer a hot-water extract.

Ginger (Zingiber officinalis) has long been used for its soothing digestive properties by herbalists. Consequently, it is a first choice for chemotherapy-induced nausea/vomiting in tea, extract, and even essential oil forms. Research is demonstrating ginger's well-known efficacy in controlling this debilitating and limiting symptom of cancer treatment.[70,71] Active components gingerol and shogoal have been studied extensively and have clear beneficial effects for nausea and vomiting and inflammation in particular.[72] Several trials have demonstrated ginger's anti-nausea and antiemetic abilities.[71,73-75] Mild side effects such as heartburn or dermatitis may be observed.[73] The dosage is 1 g/day in divided doses; it best used for 10 days around the time of chemotherapy treatment.

L-carnitine is a non-essential amino acid formed in the brain, liver, and kid-neys. Acetyl-L-carnitine (ALC) is an ester form often used in dietary supple-mentation. While there was an initial indication that ALC provided protection against chemotherapy-induced peripheral neuropathy,[66] later reviews have brought that into question, particularly one double-blind randomized con-trolled trial in 2013 that showed possible worsening of taxane-induced periph-eral neuropathy with ALC use.[64,76] The mode of action of ALC may explain this difference in benefit with different chemotherapy drugs. Caution is advised at this time with therapeutic dosing of ALC for peripheral neuropathy preven-tion and treatment. However, evidence does indicate that L-carnitine may be beneficial in the treatment of cancer-related fatigue and cancer cachexia[19,62,77] as well as chemotherapy-induced cardiotoxicity.[78] The dosage is 1 to 3 g twice daily; do not use during taxane chemotherapy.

Most, but not all, studies have demonstrated a neuroprotective role of *vitamin E* in reducing chemotherapy-induced peripheral neuropathy, with no indication of negative impact.[64,66] In combination with omega-3 fatty acids, vitamin E shows promise in treating cachexia.[29,79] Use of the most potent nat-ural form, alpha-tocopherol, is generally recommended, but some clinicians prefer the more natural form of mixed tocopherols. The dosage is 200 to 400 mg alpha-tocopherol or mixed tocopherols twice daily.

Astragalus membranaceus is a botanical used extensively in Chinese medicine as a tonic. Phytochemically, it contains triterpenoid saponins and polysaccharides, for which there is extensive in vitro evidence demonstrat-ing significant immunomodulating and anticancer effects. A 2013 review by Frankel et al. thoroughly lays out the benefits of *A. membranaceus* in cancer care.[25] There is some evidence that astragalus is beneficial during chemotherapy but not during immunosuppressant treatments due to its immunomodulating effects. The dosage varies depending on the preparation.

Selenium is a trace mineral that is essential in the diet. Its role in oncology seems to be related to its formation into proteins acting with antioxidant and anti-inflammatory actions in the cell environment. Intake of selenium is inversely associated with cancer incidence, and studies of selenium supplementation indicate a role in integrative oncology, although research results are conflicting and some studies have shown a positive correlation, particularly with inorganic forms of selenium.[19,80] Use of selenium for nutritional supplementation should be limited to patients with established deficiency (with serum levels <122 mcg/l), with the optimal range being 130 to 150 mcg/l. Selenium supplementation is protective against chemotherapy-induced hepatotoxicities and nephrotoxicities and may protect against chemotherapy-induced alopecia. A reduction in radiotherapy side effects has also been noted with selenium supplementation. The dosage is 200 mcg/day selenomethionine (organic form) in patients with an established deficiency (<122 mcg/L).

The field of *Chinese medicine* includes acupuncture, acupressure, herbal medicine, and other hands-on therapies. A 2016 meta-analysis of 67 randomized controlled trials concluded that these therapies represent beneficial adjunctive therapies for adverse symptoms, including pain, fatigue, sleep disturbance, and some gastrointestinal discomfort.[81] Several studies on acupuncture, in particular, have demonstrated benefit for peripheral neuropathy, fatigue, and leukopenia, with no serious adverse events in more than 23 systemic reviews evaluated.[52,82] Please see Chapter 5 for more information about this ancient and effective system of medicine.

Survivorship

Support of quality of life and considerations for long-term sequelae of oncology treatment have greatly expanded in recent years with the increasing number of cancer survivors in the population. The goal of survivorship care is to coordinate quality of life, screening tools, and appropriate awareness of signs and symptoms of recurrence. Awareness and attention to mental health, cognitive function, fatigue, sexual function, and lifestyle health measures such as sleep, nutrition, and exercise are encouraged by both conventional and integrative providers. Integrative therapies are especially relevant in this population. Patients no longer need worry about interactions with cancer treatment and may find supportive measures for quality of life and risk reduction. The strategies already mentioned in this chapter should be utilized liberally in a survivorship support plan. Furthermore, there is conventional support available to clinicians seeking survivorship guidelines through the American Cancer Society, the American Society of Clinical Oncology, and the National Comprehensive Cancer Network. Chapter 31 provides a comprehensive discussion of the topic.

Conclusion

Oncology patients are likely to independently seek integrative intervention options throughout their cancer journey. Clinicians are encouraged to engage in meaningful dialogue with oncology patients about appropriate use of the integrative knowledge base as it relates to lifestyle medicine, supplement use, energy therapies, physical therapies, and mental health support. To do so successfully, the clinician must be aware of the safety and evidence basis of the treatments considered. The fact that patients may discover dangerous, unsubstantiated, or expensive treatments should not dilute the value of those integrative therapies that have robust evidence. The clinician is encouraged to seek options for comprehensive, effective, and integrative care from the resources provided in this chapter in order to maximize the benefits of conventional care, reduce side effects, and improve quality of life.

Further resources for integrative oncology are as follows:

Society for Integrative Oncology: https://integrativeonc.org/

Oncology Association of Naturopathic Physicians: https://oncanp.org/

"Complementary and Alternative Medicine for Health Professionals": NIH National Cancer Institute (links to multiple PDQ summary documents on integrative therapies): https://www.cancer.gov/about-cancer/treatment/cam/hp

"The Moss Report" (reports from Ralph Moss, investigative journalist, discussing integrative and alternative cancer treatments by type of cancer): http://cancerdecisions.com/

Table 21.4. Emerging Integrative Treatments

Pharmacological ascorbate (intravenous vitamin C)	https://www.cancer.gov/about-cancer/treatment/cam/hp
Mistletoe (subcutaneous injection and intravenous infusion)	https://www.cancer.gov/about-cancer/treatment/cam/hp
Cannabinoids (CBD and others) from *Cannabis sativa*	https://www.cancer.gov/about-cancer/treatment/cam/hp
Metformin use in oncology	[85,86]
Caloric restriction during chemotherapy	[87]

Table 21.5. Common Supplement Interventions by Cancer Type

Cancer Type	Treatment
Breast, colon, lung, renal, melanoma	Vitamin D, melatonin, *Coriolus*, physical activity
Hematological	CoQ10, resveratrol, green tea, quercetin
Prostate	Green tea, curcumin, I3C/DIM, melatonin, mushroom (white button, reishi, *Coriolus*, maitake), vitamin D, vitamin K

Books

- *Integrative Oncology* (Weil Integrative Medicine Library) by Donald Abrams and Andrew Weil
- *The Definitive Guide to Cancer, 3rd Edition: An Integrative Approach to Prevention, Treatment, and Healing* (Alternative Medicine Guides) by Lise Alschuler ND and Karolyn Gazella
- *Naturopathic Oncology* by Neil McKinney ND
- *Life Over Cancer: The Block Center Program for Integrative Cancer Treatment* by Keith Block MD

Table 21.4 lists some emerging integrative treatments, and Table 21.5 summarizes common supplement interventions by cancer type.

REFERENCES

1. Aging Statistics. http://www.aoa.acl.gov/aging_statistics/index.aspx. Accessed February 25, 2017.
2. Smith BD, Smith GL, Hurria A, Hortobagyi GN, Buchholz TA. Future of cancer incidence in the United States: Burdens upon an aging, changing nation. *J Clin Oncol*. 2009;27(17):2758–2765. doi:10.1200/jco.2008.20.8983.
3. Siegel RL, Miller KD, Jemal A. Cancer statistics, 2016. *CA Cancer J Clin*. 2016;66(1): 7–30. doi:10.3322/caac.21332.
4. Ebel M-D, Rudolph I, Keinki C, et al. Perception of cancer patients of their disease, self-efficacy and locus of control and usage of complementary and alternative medicine. *J Cancer Res Clin Oncol*. 2015;141(8):1449–1455. doi:10.1007/ s00432-015-1940-3.
5. Gansler T, Kaw C, Crammer C, Smith T. A population-based study of prevalence of complementary methods use by cancer survivors: A report from the American Cancer Society's studies of cancer survivors. *Cancer*. 2008;113(5):1048–1057. doi:10.1002/cncr.23659.

6. Richardson MA, Sanders T, Palmer JL, Greisinger A, Singletary SE. Complementary/alternative medicine use in a comprehensive cancer center and the implications for oncology. *J Clin Oncol.* 2000;18(13):2505–2514. doi:10.1200/JCO.2000.18.13.2505.

7. Saxe GA, Madlensky L, Kealey S, Wu DPH, Freeman KL, Pierce JP. Disclosure to physicians of CAM use by breast cancer patients: Findings from the Women's Healthy Eating and Living Study. *Integr Cancer Ther.* 2008;7(3):122–129. doi:10.1177/1534735408323081.

8. Frenkel M, Sierpina V. The use of dietary supplements in oncology. *Curr Oncol Rep.* 2014;16(11):411. doi:10.1007/s11912-014-0411-3.

9. Kumar V, Abbas AK, Aster JC. *Robbins & Cotran Pathologic Basis of Disease.* Philadelphia: Elsevier Health Sciences; 2014. https://market.android.com/details?id=book-5NbsAwAAQBAJ.

10. Moore SC, Lee I-M, Weiderpass E, et al. Association of leisure-time physical activity with risk of 26 types of cancer in 1.44 million adults. *JAMA Intern Med.* 2016;176(6):816–825. doi:10.1001/jamainternmed.2016.1548.

11. Brunet J, Burke S, Grocott MPW, West MA, Jack S. The effects of exercise on pain, fatigue, insomnia, and health perceptions in patients with operable advanced stage rectal cancer prior to surgery: A pilot trial. *BMC Cancer.* 2017;17(1):153. doi:10.1186/s12885-017-3130-y.

12. Friedenreich CM, Wang Q, Neilson HK, Kopciuk KA, McGregor SE, Courneya KS. Physical activity and survival after prostate cancer. *Eur Urol.* 2016;70(4):576–585. doi:10.1016/j.eururo.2015.12.032.

13. Reiter RJ, Tan D-X, Korkmaz A, et al. Light at night, chronodisruption, melatonin suppression, and cancer risk: A review. *Crit Rev Oncog.* 2007;13(4):303–328.

14. Cho Y, Ryu S-H, Lee BR, Kim KH, Lee E, Choi J. Effects of artificial light at night on human health: A literature review of observational and experimental studies applied to exposure assessment. *Chronobiol Int.* 2015;32(9):1294–1310. doi:10.3109/07420528.2015.1073158.

15. Greenlee H, Balneaves LG, Carlson LE, et al. Clinical practice guidelines on the use of integrative therapies as supportive care in patients treated for breast cancer. *J Natl Cancer Inst Monogr.* 2014;2014(50):346–358. doi:10.1093/jncimonographs/lgu041.

16. Hoffman CJ, Ersser SJ, Hopkinson JB, Nicholls PG, Harrington JE, Thomas PW. Effectiveness of mindfulness-based stress reduction in mood, breast- and endocrine-related quality of life, and well-being in stage 0 to III breast cancer: A randomized, controlled trial. *J Clin Oncol.* 2012;30(12):1335–1342. doi:10.1200/JCO.2010.34.0331.

17. Braakhuis AJ, Campion P, Bishop KS. Reducing breast cancer recurrence: The role of dietary polyphenolics. *Nutrients.* 2016;8(9). doi:10.3390/nu8090547.

18. Link A, Balaguer F, Goel A. Cancer chemoprevention by dietary polyphenols: Promising role for epigenetics. *Biochem Pharmacol.* 2010;80(12):1771–1792. doi:10.1016/j.bcp.2010.06.036.

19. Gröber U, Holzhauer P, Kisters K, Holick MF, Adamietz IA. Micronutrients in oncological intervention. *Nutrients.* 2016;8(3):163. doi:10.3390/nu8030163.

20. Messina M. Soy and health update: Evaluation of the clinical and epidemiologic literature. *Nutrients.* 2016;8(12). doi:10.3390/nu8120754.
21. Shu XO, Zheng Y, Cai H, et al. Soy food intake and breast cancer survival. *JAMA.* 2009;302(22):2437–2443. doi:10.1001/jama.2009.1783.
22. Zhang G-Q, Chen J-L, Liu Q, Zhang Y, Zeng H, Zhao Y. Soy intake is associated with lower endometrial cancer risk: A systematic review and meta-analysis of observational studies. *Medicine* . 2015;94(50):e2281. doi:10.1097/MD.0000000000002281.
23. Wang L-Q. Mammalian phytoestrogens: Enterodiol and enterolactone. *J Chromatogr B Analyt Technol Biomed Life Sci.* 2002;777(1-2):289–309.
24. Artzi M, Liberman G, Vaisman N, et al. Changes in cerebral metabolism during ketogenic diet in patients with primary brain tumors: (1)H-MRS study. *J Neurooncol.* 2017;132(2):267–275. doi:10.1007/s11060-016-2364-x.
25. Frenkel M, Abrams DI, Ladas EJ, et al. Integrating dietary supplements into cancer care. *Integr Cancer Ther.* 2013;12(5):369–384. doi:10.1177/1534735412473642.
26. Freedman DM, Looker AC, Abnet CC, Linet MS, Graubard BI. Serum vitamin D and cancer mortality in the NHANES III Study (1988–2006). *Ann Epidemiol.* 2010;20(9):720. doi:10.1016/j.annepidem.2010.07.085.
27. Garland CF, Gorham ED, Mohr SB, Garland FC. Vitamin D for cancer prevention: Global perspective. *Ann Epidemiol.* 2009;19(7):468–483. doi:10.1016/j.annepidem.2009.03.021.
28. Shao T, Klein P, Grossbard ML. Vitamin D and breast cancer. *Oncologist.* 2012;17(1):36–45. doi:10.1634/theoncologist.2011-0278.
29. Mochamat, Cuhls H, Marinova M, et al. A systematic review on the role of vitamins, minerals, proteins, and other supplements for the treatment of cachexia in cancer: A European Palliative Care Research Centre cachexia project. *J Cachexia Sarcopenia Muscle.* 2017;8(1):25–39. doi:10.1002/jcsm.12127.
30. Song M, Nishihara R, Cao Y, et al. Marine ω-3 polyunsaturated fatty acid intake and risk of colorectal cancer characterized by tumor-infiltrating T cells. *JAMA Oncol.* 2016;2(9):1197–1206. doi:10.1001/jamaoncol.2016.0605.
31. Fabian CJ, Kimler BF, Hursting SD. Omega-3 fatty acids for breast cancer prevention and survivorship. *Breast Cancer Res.* 2015;17:62. doi:10.1186/s13058-015-0571-6.
32. Kotecha R, Takami A, Espinoza JL. Dietary phytochemicals and cancer chemoprevention: A review of the clinical evidence. *Oncotarget.* 2016;7(32):52517–52529. doi:10.18632/oncotarget.9593.
33. Friedman M. Mushroom polysaccharides: Chemistry and antiobesity, antidiabetes, anticancer, and antibiotic properties in cells, rodents, and humans. *Foods.* 2016;5(4). doi:10.3390/foods5040080.
34. Eliza WLY, Fai CK, Chung LP. Efficacy of Yun Zhi (*Coriolus versicolor*) on survival in cancer patients: Systematic review and meta-analysis. *Recent Pat Inflamm Allergy Drug Discov.* 2012;6(1):78–87.
35. Sakamoto J, Morita S, Oba K, et al. Efficacy of adjuvant immunochemotherapy with polysaccharide K for patients with curatively resected colorectal cancer: A meta-analysis of centrally randomized controlled clinical trials. *Cancer Immunol Immunother.* 2006;55(4):404–411. doi:10.1007/s00262-005-0054-1.

36. Fritz H, Kennedy DA, Ishii M, et al. Polysaccharide K and *Coriolus versicolor* extracts for lung cancer: A systematic review. *Integr Cancer Ther.* 2015;14(3): 201–211. doi:10.1177/1534735415572883.

37. Pavan A, Silva G, Jornada D, et al. Unraveling the anticancer dffect of curcumin and resveratrol. *Nutrients.* 2016;8(11):628. doi:10.3390/nu8110628.

38. Aggarwal BB, Sung B. Pharmacological basis for the role of curcumin in chronic diseases: An age-old spice with modern targets. *Trends Pharmacol Sci.* 2009;30(2): 85–94. doi:10.1016/j.tips.2008.11.002.

39. Li Y, Zhang T. Targeting cancer stem cells by curcumin and clinical applications. *Cancer Lett.* 2014;346(2):197–205. doi:10.1016/j.canlet.2014.01.012.

40. Sánchez-Barceló EJ, Cos S, Mediavilla D, Martínez-Campa C, González A, Alonso-González C. Melatonin-estrogen interactions in breast cancer. *J Pineal Res.* 2005;38(4):217–222. doi:10.1111/j.1600-079X.2004.00207.x.

41. Seely D, Wu P, Fritz H, et al. Melatonin as adjuvant cancer care with and without chemotherapy: A systematic review and meta-analysis of randomized trials. *Integr Cancer Ther.* 2012;11(4):293–303. doi:10.1177/1534735411425484.

42. Wang Y-M, Jin B-Z, Ai F, et al. The efficacy and safety of melatonin in concurrent chemotherapy or radiotherapy for solid tumors: A meta-analysis of randomized controlled trials. *Cancer Chemother Pharmacol.* 2012;69(5):1213–1220. doi:10.1007/s00280-012-1828-8.

43. Lissoni P, Barni S, Mandalà M, et al. Decreased toxicity and increased efficacy of cancer chemotherapy using the pineal hormone melatonin in metastatic solid tumour patients with poor clinical status. *Eur J Cancer.* 1999;35(12):1688–1692.

44. Yang CS, Wang H. Cancer preventive activities of tea catechins. *Molecules.* 2016;21(12). doi:10.3390/molecules21121679.

45. Xiang L-P, Wang A, Ye J-H, et al. Suppressive effects of tea catechins on breast cancer. *Nutrients.* 2016;8(8). doi:10.3390/nu8080458.

46. Cao J, Han J, Xiao H, Qiao J, Han M. Effect of tea polyphenol compounds on anticancer drugs in terms of anti-tumor activity, toxicology, and pharmacokinetics. *Nutrients.* 2016;8(12). doi:10.3390/nu8120762.

47. Shanafelt TD, Call TG, Zent CS, et al. Phase 2 trial of daily, oral Polyphenon E in patients with asymptomatic, Rai stage 0 to II chronic lymphocytic leukemia. *Cancer.* 2013;119(2):363–370. doi:10.1002/cncr.27719.

48. D'Arena G, Simeon V, De Martino L, et al. Regulatory T-cell modulation by green tea in chronic lymphocytic leukemia. *Int J Immunopathol Pharmacol.* 2013;26(1):117–125. doi:10.1177/039463201302600111.

49. Kelkel M, Jacob C, Dicato M, Diederich M. Potential of the dietary antioxidants resveratrol and curcumin in prevention and treatment of hematologic malignancies. *Molecules.* 2010;15(10):7035–7074. doi:10.3390/molecules15107035.

50. Wang C-Z, Anderson S, Du W, He T-C, Yuan C-S. Red ginseng and cancer treatment. *Chin J Nat Med.* 2016;14(1):7–16. doi:10.3724/SP.J.1009.2016.00007.

51. Cui Y. Association of ginseng use with survival and quality of life among breast cancer patients. *Am J Epidemiol.* 2006;163(7):645–653. doi:10.1093/aje/kwj087.

52. Finnegan-John J, Molassiotis A, Richardson A, Ream E. A systematic review of complementary and alternative medicine interventions for the management of cancer-related fatigue. *Integr Cancer Ther.* 2013;12(4):276–290. doi:10.1177/1534735413485816.

53. Barton DL, Liu H, Dakhil SR, et al. Wisconsin ginseng (*Panax quinquefolius*) to improve cancer-related fatigue: a randomized, double-blind trial, N07C2. *J Natl Cancer Inst.* 2013;105(16):1230–1238. doi:10.1093/jnci/djt181.

54. He Y-S, Sun W, Wang C-Z, et al. Effects of American ginseng on pharmacokinetics of 5-fluorouracil in rats. *Biomed Chromatogr.* 2015;29(5):762–767. doi:10.1002/bmc.3354.

55. Chen S, Wang Z, Huang Y, et al. Ginseng and anticancer drug combination to improve cancer chemotherapy: A critical review. *Evid Based Complement Alternat Med.* 2014;2014:1–13. doi:10.1155/2014/168940.

56. Solomon LR. Functional vitamin B12 deficiency in advanced malignancy: Implications for the management of neuropathy and neuropathic pain. *Support Care Cancer.* 2016;24(8):3489–3494. doi:10.1007/s00520-016-3175-5.

57. Schloss JM, Colosimo M, Airey C, Masci P, Linnane AW, Vitetta L. A randomised, placebo-controlled trial assessing the efficacy of an oral B group vitamin in preventing the development of chemotherapy-induced peripheral neuropathy (CIPN). *Support Care Cancer.* 2017;25(1):195–204. doi:10.1007/s00520-016-3404-y.

58. Schloss JM, Colosimo M, Airey C, Vitetta L. Chemotherapy-induced peripheral neuropathy (CIPN) and vitamin B12 deficiency. *Support Care Cancer.* 2015;23(7):1843–1850. doi:10.1007/s00520-015-2725-6.

59. Bhagavan HN, Chopra RK. Coenzyme Q10: Absorption, tissue uptake, metabolism and pharmacokinetics. *Free Radic Res.* 2006;40(5):445–453. doi:10.1080/10715760600617843.

60. Swarnakar NK, Thanki K, Jain S. Enhanced antitumor efficacy and counterfeited cardiotoxicity of combinatorial oral therapy using doxorubicin- and coenzyme Q10-liquid crystalline nanoparticles in comparison with intravenous Adriamycin. *Nanomedicine.* 2014;10(6):1231–1241. doi:10.1016/j.nano.2014.03.003.

61. Roffe L, Schmidt K, Ernst E. Efficacy of coenzyme Q10 for improved tolerability of cancer treatments: A systematic review. *J Clin Oncol.* 2004;22(21):4418–4424. doi:10.1200/JCO.2004.02.034.

62. Iwase S, Kawaguchi T, Yotsumoto D, et al. Efficacy and safety of an amino acid jelly containing coenzyme Q10 and L-carnitine in controlling fatigue in breast cancer patients receiving chemotherapy: A multi-institutional, randomized, exploratory trial (JORTC-CAM01). *Support Care Cancer.* 2016;24(2):637–646. doi:10.1007/s00520-015-2824-4.

63. Liu H-T, Huang Y-C, Cheng S-B, Huang Y-T, Lin P-T. Effects of coenzyme Q10 supplementation on antioxidant capacity and inflammation in hepatocellular carcinoma patients after surgery: A randomized, placebo-controlled trial. *Nutr J.* 2016;15(1):85. doi:10.1186/s12937-016-0205-6.

64. Brami C, Bao T, Deng G. Natural products and complementary therapies for chemotherapy-induced peripheral neuropathy: A systematic review. *Crit Rev Oncol Hematol.* 2016;98:325–334. doi:10.1016/j.critrevonc.2015.11.014.

65. Yarom N, Ariyawardana A, Hovan A, et al. Systematic review of natural agents for the management of oral mucositis in cancer patients. *Support Care Cancer.* 2013;21(11):3209–3221. doi:10.1007/s00520-013-1869-5.

66. Schloss JM, Colosimo M, Airey C, Masci PP, Linnane AW, Vitetta L. Nutraceuticals and chemotherapy induced peripheral neuropathy (CIPN): A systematic review. *Clin Nutr.* 2013;32(6):888–893. doi:10.1016/j.clnu.2013.04.007.

67. Jin X, Ruiz Beguerie J, Sze DM-Y, Chan GCF. *Ganoderma lucidum* (Reishi mushroom) for cancer treatment. *Cochrane Database Syst Rev.* 2016;4:CD007731. doi:10.1002/14651858.CD007731.pub3.

68. Zhao H, Zhang Q, Zhao L, Huang X, Wang J, Kang X. Spore powder of *Ganoderma lucidum* improves cancer-related fatigue in breast cancer patients undergoing endocrine therapy: A pilot clinical trial. *Evid Based Complement Alternat Med.* 2012;2012:809614. doi:10.1155/2012/809614.

69. PDQ Integrative, Alternative, and Complementary Therapies Editorial Board. Medicinal Mushrooms (PDQ®): Health Professional Version. In: *PDQ Cancer Information Summaries.* Bethesda, MD: National Cancer Institute (US); 2017.

70. Sheikhi MA, Ebadi A, Talaeizadeh A, Rahmani H. Alternative methods to treat nausea and vomiting from cancer chemotherapy. *Chemother Res Pract.* 2015;2015:818759. doi:10.1155/2015/818759.

71. Bossi P, Cortinovis D, Rocca MC, et al. Searching for evidence to support the use of ginger in the prevention of chemotherapy-induced nausea and vomiting. *J Altern Complement Med.* 2016;22(6):486–488. doi:10.1089/acm.2015.0315.

72. Marx WM, Teleni L, McCarthy AL, et al. Ginger (*Zingiber officinale*) and chemotherapy-induced nausea and vomiting: A systematic literature review. *Nutr Rev.* 2013;71(4):245–254. doi:10.1111/nure.12016.

73. Ryan JL, Heckler CE, Roscoe JA, et al. Ginger (*Zingiber officinale*) reduces acute chemotherapy-induced nausea: A URCC CCOP study of 576 patients. *Support Care Cancer.* 2012;20(7):1479–1489. doi:10.1007/s00520-011-1236-3.

74. Sanaati F, Najafi S, Kashaninia Z, Sadeghi M. Effect of ginger and chamomile on nausea and vomiting caused by chemotherapy in Iranian women with breast cancer. *Asian Pac J Cancer Prev.* 2016;17(8):4125–4129.

75. Montazeri AS, Raei M, Ghanbari A, Dadgari A, Montazeri AS, Hamidzadeh A. Effect of herbal therapy to intensity chemotherapy-induced nausea and vomiting in cancer patients. *Iran Red Crescent Med J.* 2013;15(2):101–106. doi:10.5812/ircmj.4392.

76. Hershman DL, Unger JM, Crew KD, et al. Randomized double-blind placebo-controlled trial of acetyl-L-carnitine for the prevention of taxane-induced neuropathy in women undergoing adjuvant breast cancer therapy. *J Clin Oncol.* 2013;31(20):2627–2633. doi:10.1200/JCO.2012.44.8738.

77. Madeddu C, Dessì M, Panzone F, et al. Randomized phase III clinical trial of a combined treatment with carnitine celecoxib ± megestrol acetate for patients with cancer-related anorexia/cachexia syndrome. *Clin Nutr.* 2012;31(2):176–182. doi:10.1016/j.clnu.2011.10.005.

78. Lucius K, Trukova K. Integrative therapies and cardiovascular disease in the breast cancer population: A review, Part 1. *Integr Med.* 2015;14(4):22–29.

79. Gogos CA, Ginopoulos P, Salsa B, Apostolidou E, Zoumbos NC, Kalfarentzos F. Dietary omega-3 polyunsaturated fatty acids plus vitamin E restore immunodeficiency and prolong survival for severely ill patients with generalized malignancy: A randomized control trial. *Cancer*. 1998;82(2):395–402.

80. Dennert G, Zwahlen M, Brinkman M, Vinceti M, Zeegers MPA, Horneber M. Selenium for preventing cancer. *Cochrane Database Syst Rev*. 2011;(5):CD005195. doi:10.1002/14651858.CD005195.pub2.

81. Tao W-W, Jiang H, Tao X-M, Jiang P, Sha L-Y, Sun X-C. Effects of acupuncture, tuina, tai chi, qigong, and traditional Chinese medicine five-element music therapy on symptom management and quality of life for cancer patients: A meta-analysis. *J Pain Symptom Manage*. 2016;51(4):728–747. doi:10.1016/j.jpainsymman.2015.11.027.

82. Wu X, Chung VCH, Hui EP, et al. Effectiveness of acupuncture and related therapies for palliative care of cancer: Overview of systematic reviews. *Sci Rep*. 2015;5:16776. doi:10.1038/srep16776.

83. Karagozoglu S, Tekyasar F, Yilmaz FA. Effects of music therapy and guided visual imagery on chemotherapy-induced anxiety and nausea-vomiting. *J Clin Nurs*. 2013;22(1-2):39–50. doi:10.1111/jocn.12030.

84. Ernst E. Complementary therapies for supportive cancer care. *Support Care Cancer*. 2010;18(11):1365–1366. doi:10.1007/s00520-010-0991-x.

85. Coyle C, Cafferty FH, Vale C, Langley RE. Metformin as an adjuvant treatment for cancer: A systematic review and meta-analysis. *Ann Oncol*. 2016;27(12):2184–2195. doi:10.1093/annonc/mdw410.

86. Jiralerspong S, Palla SL, Giordano SH, et al. Metformin and pathologic complete responses to neoadjuvant chemotherapy in diabetic patients with breast cancer. *J Clin Oncol*. 2009;27(20):3297–3302. doi:10.1200/JCO.2009.19.6410.

87. Brandhorst S, Harputlugil E, Mitchell JR, Longo VD. Protective effects of short-term dietary restriction in surgical stress and chemotherapy. *Ageing Res Rev*. 2017;39:68–77. doi:10.1016/j.arr.2017.02.001.

22

Common Rheumatic Diseases in the Elderly

NISHA J. MANEK AND GEORGE MUÑOZ

Introduction

The scope of rheumatic diseases involves more than 150 different diagnoses, which are often chronic and carry significant morbidity and
potential disability. Given these characteristics and the lack of curative
treatments for many rheumatic disorders, the use of complementary and integrative therapies (CIM) should not be a surprise. In fact, adults with arthritis
are more likely to use CIM compared to persons with chronic conditions like
cancer, cardiovascular diseases, and diabetes.[1] Rheumatologists practicing in
the United States favor many CIM modalities for back pain and joint pain, and
there is a weakening of the perceived antagonism of conventional physicians
to CIM.[2]

In this chapter we will focus on integrative management of peripheral joint
osteoarthritis (OA), gout, and elderly onset rheumatoid arthritis (RA). Many
of the strategies of CIM for these disorders could potentially be extrapolated
to other rheumatic diseases that are commonly encountered, including poly-
myalgia rheumatica and arthritis related to calcium pyrophosphate crystals
(pseudo-gout).

Osteoarthritis

EPIDEMIOLOGY AND PATHOGENESIS

Obesity has a strong association with incident and progressive knee OA.[3,4]
By age 85 years, nearly half of the adults develop symptomatic knee OA.

The lifetime risk is highest among obese persons. underscoring the immediate need for greater use of clinical and public health interventions, especially those that address weight loss and self-management, to reduce the impact of having hip and knee OA in older adults.[5] Weight loss for obese patients with knee OA is clinically beneficial for pain reduction and improved function.[6]

Several epidemiological and experimental data support the hypothesis that diabetes could be an independent risk factor for OA in some patients, leading to the concept of a diabetes-induced OA phenotype.[7,8] If confirmed, this new paradigm will have a dramatic impact on prevention of incident OA and progression. In the experience of one of the authors (NJM), a critical analysis and better control of hyperglycemic status can lead to better joint function in elderly diabetic patients with symptomatic knee, hip, and/or hand OA.

MANAGEMENT OF PERIPHERAL OA

The need for high-quality care for OA, which has a major personal and societal impact, is recognized and several guidelines are available. The American College of Rheumatology (ACR)'s 2012 guidelines for hand, hip, and knee OA[9] and the OA guidelines from the Osteoarthritis Research Society International[10] and the National Institute for Health and Care Excellence (NICE)[11] are some of the clinical practice guidelines for the nonsurgical management of peripheral joint OA. Core elements of all guidelines are nonpharmacological management with weight management and exercise.

Integrative assessment of OA in the elderly is discussed in Chapter 12 and must address several areas, including physical and educational needs, as well as psychological and social aspects. While the effects of most CIM interventions are small to moderate in OA, they are still valuable for older patients and clinically relevant for physicians. Nearly one-third of older adults with knee OA aged 65 years and up from the Osteoarthritis Initiative reported using at least one CIM modality during the 4-year follow-up, often using conventional medicine and modalities like nutraceuticals concurrently.[12] In the case of knee OA, CIM approaches often present less potential harm to the patient compared with standard nonsteroidal anti-inflammatory medications (NSAIDs).[13]

EDUCATION AND EXERCISE

Case studies of elderly people with disabling OA who experience a remarkable turnaround in overall health are exemplified by the following report.[14]

A 71-year-old man with ankylosing spondylitis and a complex range of comorbidities presented with chronic hip OA. The patient was referred to CHAIN (Cycling against Hip PAIN), a 6-week program developed to aid self-management of hip OA through exercise, education, and advice, as defined by the NICE guidelines.[11] Significant improvements were seen in hip disability outcomes scores, sit-to-stand test, pain scores, and hip flexion. There was also a weight loss of more than 2 kg. The man reported "an amazing difference" in his affected hip and leg with improved fitness. Many clinicians would have questioned the man's suitability for the program due to his coexisting medical conditions, but this case study shows that patients are able to achieve significant improvement with exercise.[14]

In the United States, the Arthritis Self-Management Program is a community-taught, peer-led intervention in which participants attend 2-hour weekly sessions for 6 weeks.[15] These sessions are taught from an interactive model that promotes individual participation and self-management techniques that can potentially reduce pain and doctor visits.[15,16] Programs that combine intensive diet and exercise (IDEA trial) improve clinical outcomes in overweight and obese patients with knee OA and show that diet and exercise are *both* important and lead to greater weight loss than exercise alone.[18] Many other exercise programs have also been evaluated for OA, such as People with Arthritis Can Exercise (PACE),[18] and the Arthritis Foundation's Walk With Ease (WWE) program for arthritis symptoms is designed to change behavior and increase motivation and adherence in a low-intensity 6-week program.[19] The WWE is a safe, easy, and inexpensive program to promote community-based physical activity.[20,21] Patients who cannot do dry-land exercise can achieve impressive progress with pool or warm-water exercise.

Yoga and tai chi, both of which combine physical exercise with meditative components, are very popular in health clubs across the United States. To date, studies of yoga are small and the results are difficult to extrapolate to clinical scenarios.[22] Nevertheless, many patients report benefit with yoga practice, with increased joint function and better muscular strength. The low-impact nature of tai chi and qi gong make them ideal for patients who have difficulty with more traditional physical therapy (PT); indeed, tai chi is comparable in effectiveness to PT in the treatment of knee OA.[23] Patients who want to try yoga or tai chi should , it is recommended to have an individualized program under close supervision of experienced teachers. Please also refer to the sections on yoga and tai chi in Chapter 6.

Feldenkrais is a body-awareness movement therapy in which people are taught efficient ways to achieve body positions. One of the authors (NJM) has recommended Feldenkrais to many patients with OA who want to improve joint function and move with confidence. Preliminary data for Feldenkrais in OA treatment are promising.[24]

ACUPUNCTURE

Four randomized controlled trials (RCTs) that represent most of the evidence in treatment of knee OA used anywhere from 10 to 23 acupuncture sessions. The difference in the Western Ontario and McMaster Universities (WOMAC) Osteoarthritis Index for pain scale was modest but significant.[25–28] Notwithstanding this evidence, the role of acupuncture in knee OA management remains unclear, particularly if a patient is already undertaking exercise.[29–31] It is possible that acupuncture will be most beneficial in those who cannot or do not exercise. Safety considerations, cost, and choosing an acupuncture practitioner have been discussed in an excellent review.[32] The ACR 2012 guidelines recommend acupuncture for knee OA.[9]

MASSAGE

Swedish massage sessions in patients with knee OA reduced WOMAC pain scores, stiffness, and "time to walk" indices, with beneficial effects persisting for weeks following treatment cessation.[33] Further study of massage to determine optimal treatment protocols, absolute efficacy, cost-effectiveness, and generalization to other patient groups is required. A once-weekly 60-minute "dose" of massage has been suggested as a pragmatic typical real-world standard that can be a standard for future trials.[34]

MIND–BODY TECHNIQUES

In small trials or feasibility studies, other mind–body techniques such as guided imagery,[35,36] hypnosis,[37] and therapeutic touch[38–40] have been found to improve pain and level of function in patients with knee OA; however, it is unknown if the effect is sustained. In an evaluation of another "sensory" intervention, community-dwelling elderly persons with chronic OA pain perceived a reduction in pain using music therapy for 20 minutes daily.[41] In the experience of one author (NJM), for hand OA, therapy by playing on a keyboard may be tried in individual cases.[42]

DIETARY CONSIDERATIONS AND SUPPLEMENTS

There is tremendous interest in dietary polyphenols and the prevention of OA-related musculoskeletal inflammation. A diet high in fruits and vegetables, independent of lifestyle effects and body mass index, has been shown to be protective against hip OA.[43] Commonly consumed polyphenols, including curcumin, epigallocatechin gallate and green tea extract, resveratrol, nobiletin and citrus fruits, pomegranate, genistein and soy protein,[44] as well as the long-chain essential fatty acids eicosapentaenoic acid (EPA) and docosahexaenoic acid (DHA), have been suggested as preventive and treatment strategies for OA.[45]

NUTRACEUTICALS

Various clinical trials have been performed with symptomatic slow-acting drugs for knee OA (SYSADOA).[46,47] The Glucosamine/Chondroitin Arthritis Intervention Trial (GAIT) was a randomized, double-blind, placebo-controlled study comparing the efficacy and safety of glucosamine hydrochloride (GHCl), chondroitin sulfate (CS), alone and in combination, and an internal control with celecoxib for the treatment of knee OA.[48] While no statistically significant effects were observed for the combination group (GHCl + CS) in the overall study population, a significant difference was observed for the combination arm in patients with moderate to severe pain for the primary outcome, defined as a 20% decrease in the WOMAC pain score ($p = 0.002$).[48]

To confirm the effects of the GAIT trial, the Multicentre Osteoarthritis interVEntion trial with SYSADOA (MOVES) was conducted to test whether a fixed-dose combination of chondroitin sulfate (1,200 mg/day) plus glucosamine (1,500 mg/day) has comparable efficacy to celecoxib (200 mg/day) in reducing pain in patients with knee OA with moderate to severe pain after 6 months of treatment.[49] The mean ± SD age at baseline was 62.7 ± 8.9 years, and the majority of study subjects were women (83.9%). The MOVES trial found that the reduction in pain was both clinically important and statistically significant (50% reduction in both groups), as was the improvement in stiffness (46.9% reduction with the combination vs. 49.2% with celecoxib) and function (45.5% vs. 46.4%, respectively). These results confirm and extend those from the GAIT study in patients with severe knee pain.[49]

What are some takeaway messages from this research? CS and GHCl or glucosamine sulfate used alone may also be beneficial in knee OA.[46,47,50,51] Real-world efficacy is likely affected by the quality of commercially available compounds.[52] Supporting a disease modification effect, during 8 years of follow-up, glucosamine reduced the number of total knee replacements by 57%.[53] Similarly, CS may serve as a nonoperative means to protect joint cartilage and delay OA progression.[54] Overall, it seems prudent to recommend at least a 6-month trial of either compound alone or in combination. In contrast to celecoxib and acetaminophen, SYSADOAS may reduce cardiovascular mortality.[55]

AVOCADO SOYBEAN UNSAPONIFIABLES

Avocado soybean unsaponifiables (ASU) are a natural blended vegetable extract made from avocado and soybean oils that have recently been popularized as therapy for OA. ASU are formed following hydrolysis and are composed of roughly one-third avocado oil and two-thirds soybean oil. The mechanism of action of ASU is complex, and more recent work demonstrates this compound's effect on type 2 collagen synthesis.[56] Although the data are not uniform, the majority of studies suggest a beneficial effect of ASU in knee or hip OA of least 6 months duration. No serious adverse effects of ASU have been noted in any of the four trials.[57-61] Although the volume of evidence is not large, it seems reasonable to suggest a course of ASU 300 mg/day for at least 3 to 6 months in patients with moderate symptomatic OA of the hip or knee.[62,63]

S-ADENOSYLMETHIONINE

S-adenosylmethionine (SAMe), a naturally occurring compound found in living cells, participates in methylation reactions that produce cartilage proteoglycans.[64] By inference, SAMe may be important in the repair of damaged cartilage. SAMe has a serotonergic activity and has been shown to decrease depression, which is another popular use of this compound. A meta-analysis of 11 RCTs comparing SAMe with placebo or NSAIDs in almost 1,500 patients with OA (the majority had knee OA) concluded that SAMe was as effective as NSAIDs (effect size = 0.12) in reducing pain and improving function.[65] Oral doses ranging from 400 to 1,200 mg/dly were used in the studies. Furthermore, SAMe-treated patients were 58% less likely to experience adverse effects than those treated with NSAIDs. A subsequent RCT compared 1,200 mg/day SAMe with celecoxib 200 mg/day in patients with knee OA.[66] SAMe demonstrated similar efficacy as celecoxib, but SAMe had a slower onset of action, requiring nearly 1 month to achieve the same benefit as celecoxib. A safety concern is that in individuals with bipolar disorder, SAMe can trigger a manic phase.[67]

CURCUMIN

There is ample "bench" evidence for curcumin, the active component of turmeric, for its anti-inflammatory properties,[68] and encouraging data in animal models of RA were recently published.[69] There are limited data for treatment of knee OA with curcumin alone, and recent trials have used combination products of curcumin with glucosamine HCl.[70-72] The typical dose of curcumin used in clinical settings is 500 to 1,000 mg. Dietary amounts can vary from 1 teaspoon to 1 tablespoon of turmeric. Absorption of dietary turmeric is enhanced by fat and black pepper. Serious side effects have not been reported.

Additional supplements and botanicals are listed in Table 22.1.

TOPICAL THERAPIES

Capsaicin is an alkaloid derived from the seeds and membranes of the nightshade family of plants, which includes the common pepper plant. Capsaicin cream (0.025–0.075%) has been shown to be better than placebo in treating hand OA and knee OA.[84] It does have several mild drawbacks: it is somewhat inconvenient, may be irritating to eyes and mouth, and may require three or four applications per day, and improvement usually takes 3 to 4 weeks of regular use. Nevertheless, it is safe and can be used as monotherapy in patients with mild pain.

SUMMARY

Figure 22.1 illustrates a proposed schema for OA treatment with CIM approaches. Education plays a major role, with exercise, muscle strengthening, and weight management for all patients. The popular nutraceuticals glucosamine and chondroitin sulfate, alone or in combination, merit a trial in patients with symptomatic knee OA. There is some evidence for the analgesic effects of *Harpagophytum procumbens* or Devil's claw for back pain, and SAMe in the treatment of knee OA. Acupuncture has a measurable although modest benefit in treating knee OA. Exercise such as tai chi is comparable to PT in knee OA.

Table 22.1. Commonly Used Supplements and Herbs for Rheumatologic Conditions

Name	Mechanism of action	Daily dosing	Side effects	Use in RA	Use in OA	Use in gout	Reference
β-carotene	Lowers uric acid, no clear link to lowering gout risk or frequency of attacks.	10,000–25,000 IU	Increases risk of lung cancer in smokers. Avoid using in this population. Overdose is rare if used appropriately.	No	No	Yes	73
Methylfolate (L5-methyltetrahydrofolate)	See text	0.4–5 mg	With doses of 1 mg irritability, nausea, anxiety in patients with COMT mutations	Yes	Yes	Yes	See text
Vitamin D	Immune modulator; optimize level to 40–60 ng/ml	Level dependent	Not reported if not overdosed	Yes	Yes	Yes	
Vitamin B12	See text; optimize level above 500 pg/ml	1–5 mg	Rare	Yes	Yes	Yes	
Vitamin C	See text	0.5–1 gm	Rare; diarrhea if high-dose oral intake over 3g	No	No	Yes	See text
Omega-3 fatty acids, fish oil	See text	1–6 g/day of EPA/DHA	If fish oil used, fish oil aftertaste, bloating. High dose can increase risk of bleeding.	Yes	Yes	Yes	See text
Chondroitin sulfate	See text	1,200 mg	Mild GI symptoms	No	Yes	No	See text
Glucosamine sulfate	See text	1,500 mg	Mild GI symptoms	No	Yes	No	See text

(continued)

Table 22.1. Continued

Name	Mechanism of action	Daily dosing	Side effects	Use in RA	Use in OA	Use in gout	Reference
MSM	Iso-oxidized form of dimethyl-sulfoxide (DMSO). No clinical data supporting its use.	0.5–3 g	Mild GI symptoms, body odor	No	Yes	No	[74]
SAMe	See text; methyl donor involved in repair of damaged cartilage	400–1,200 mg	Can trigger manic state in bipolar patients	No	Yes	No	See text
Cherries	See text	1 cup/day or equivalent concentrate	None	No	Possibly	Yes	See text
Quercetin	Anti-inflammatory; also inhibits xanthine oxidase and lowers uric acid	0.2–2 g	Not reported	Yes	Yes	Yes	[75]
Bromelain	Extracted from pineapples; exhibits proteolytic and anti-inflammatory properties. Small positive studies with methodological problems.	0.5–2 g	Occasional mild GI symptoms	Yes?	Yes	No	[76]
ASU (avocado soybean unsaponifiables)	See text; improves type 2 collagen synthesis. Most of studies show benefit in OA.	300 mg	Not reported	No	Yes	No	See text

Boswellia serrata	Natural anti-inflammatory with broad effects. This plant produces Indian Frankincense and has been used for thousands of years. No conclusive data.	300–600 mg	Not reported	Yes	Yes	Yes	77–79
Green tea extract (EGCG)	See text	Food or capsules: 500–1,000 mg of EGCG	High dose can cause nausea and GI upset if taken on empty stomach.	Yes	Yes	Yes	See text
Curcumin		500–1,000 mg of concentrated highly absorbable form	Theoretical interactions with medications, but no reports when food-based doses used.	Yes	Yes	Yes	See text
Devil's claw	Natural COX-2 inhibitor. Typical preparations standardized to harpagoside-active ingredient.	50–100 mg of harpagoside	Theoretical risk of drug interactions with NSAIDs and anti-arrhythmics	Yes	Yes	Yes	80,81
Ginger (Zingiber officinale)	Anti-inflammatory properties similar to NSAIDs. Clinical trials show mixed results. Use of food-based ginger seems to be appropriate. No dose-specific studies done.	Not clear	Mild GI symptoms, dose-related. Possible increased risk of bleeding in patients taking anticoagulants.	Yes	Yes	Yes	82,83

(continued)

Table 22.1. Continued

Name	Mechanism of action	Daily dosing	Side effects	Use in RA	Use in OA	Use in gout	Reference
RHEUMATE	Medical Food: Combination of L-Methylfolate, Methylcobolamin 1 mg, and Curcumin 500 mg. Should be used instead of folic acid in patients with MTHFR mutations.	1 or 2 capsules	Not common, see individual ingredients	Yes	Yes	Yes	25
LIMBREL (flavocoxid)	Medical Food, flavonoid anti-inflammatory botanical compound plus zinc 20–40 mg	250–500 mg twice daily	None reported	Yes	Yes	No	26
DHEA	Only if deficiency present; otherwise no evidence	5–50 mg	Few if serum level remains within normal limits	Yes	Yes	Yes	See text

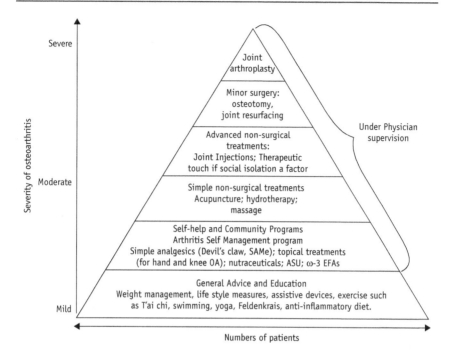

FIGURE 22.1. Proposed integrative therapies for OA
SAME, S-adenosylmethionine; ASU, Avocado Soybean Unsaponifiables; ω-3 EFA, omega-3 essential fatty acids.

Crystal-Associated Arthritis

CASE STUDY

Mr. V., a 75-year-old farmer, presented with sudden-onset left knee pain with swelling. A few days prior, he recalled consuming large amounts of beef, pork, and beer at a family wedding. The next morning, his knee was tender and rapidly progressed into significant arthritis. Mr. V. has a history of asymmetric intermittent pain and swelling in his elbows, wrists, and hand joints, such as the proximal interphalangeal joints, but his knee is involved for the first time. Joint aspiration and synovial fluid analysis confirmed intracellular monosodium urate crystals. There was no concurrent infection on synovial fluid culture. His serum urate was 10.9 mg/dl (reference range: 3.0–7.0 mg/dl) and serum creatinine was 1.7 mg/dl (reference range: 0.7–1.5 mg/dl). The glomerular filtration rate was 45 ml/min.

Mr. V.'s acute gout in his knee was treated promptly with an intra-articular corticosteroid. The physician provided him with the key information that an elevated serum acid level leads to gout. Allopurinol was started at 100 mg/day with a target serum uric acid level of less than 6 mg/dl. Colchicine 0.6 mg twice daily was also prescribed for acute gout. Mr. V. was urged to have medications "in the pocket" and was advised to start within 24 hours of onset of joint pain. His diet was changed to increase vegetables and reduce animal protein. He started vitamin C and daily cherry concentrate intake. On a return visit, his knee pain had not recurred.

INTRODUCTION

The two best-recognized and frequently encountered forms of crystal-induced joint disease in elderly patients are caused by deposition of mono-sodium urate (MSU) and calcium pyrophosphate dihydrate (CPPD) crystals. Discussion of arthritis related to CPPD is beyond the scope of this chapter. The spectrum of CPPD and its association with OA, especially destructive OA, is reviewed in a recent publication.[85] Both gout and CPPD share pathophysiological processes in the activation of NLRP3 inflammasome, and some of the anti-inflammatory strategies for gout can potentially be extrapolated to patients with acute pseudo-gout.[85,86]

FEATURES AND CLINICAL CHALLENGES IN THE ELDERLY

The clinical features of gout in elderly patients differs from gout in younger ages (Table 22.2).[87–89] Women constitute 50% to 60% of patients who have onset of gout after the age of 60, and almost all patients over the age of 80 are women. Factors like concomitant cardiac and renal disease and medications such as low-dose aspirin and diuretics contribute to chronic hyperuricemia and polyarticular disease. Heavy alcohol use seems to be less common in elderly women but may be a correctable factor in older men.

Hyperuricemia, defined as a serum urate level (SUA) greater than 6.8 mg/dl for men and 6.0 mg/dl for women, is central to the incidence and prevalence of gout but does not inevitably cause disease.[90] The accepted target for SUA is less than 6 mg/dl, well below the 6.8 mg/dl saturation point at which urate crystals precipitate from solution at body temperature.[90]

The hyperuricemia associated with diuretic therapy seen frequently in older populations results from volume depletion and consequent decreased filtered load and enhanced tubular reabsorption.[89] Diuretic use has been reported in more than 75% of patients with elderly onset gout, with a frequency of over 95% in women.[89] A retrospective cohort study documented a twofold increase

Table 22.2. Clinical Features of Gout of Typical Versus Elderly Onset

Feature	Typical gout in younger age	Elderly onset gout
Age of onset	Peak in mid-40s	Over 65 years
Gender distribution	Men >> women	Men = women
Clinical presentation	Acute monoarthritis Lower extremity (podagra 60%)	Polyarticular onset frequent Upper extremity frequent May have chronic indolent inflammatory component May mimic RA distribution in hands (pseudo-rheumatoid presentation)
Tophi	After years of attacks	Finger tophi more frequent Occurs early with or without history of prior gout attacks
Associated features and comorbidities	Elbows > fingers Chronic kidney disease of stage ≥2 Hypertension Adiposity; central obesity Hyperlipidemia Hyperglycemia Alcohol use, heavy	More common in fingers Renal insufficiency common Diuretic use, especially in women Alcohol use, less common

in risk for initiating anti-gout therapy in patients within 2 years of starting thiazide diuretics for hypertension compared with non-thiazide therapy.[89]

The ACR guidelines recommend, on a case-by-case basis, careful consideration of potential elimination of serum urate-elevating prescription medications that might be nonessential for optimal management of comorbidities (e.g., hypertension and hyperlipidemia) in a given patient. Although low-dose acetylsalicyclic acid (aspirin at a dosage of 325 mg/day or less) elevates SUA, the ACR guidelines expert panel did not recommend discontinuation as cardiovascular disease prophylaxis in patients with gout.[91]

MANAGEMENT

Acute gout should be treated promptly with pharmacological therapy within 24 hours of onset for optimal outcomes.[91,92] Pharmacologic urate-lowering therapy must be continued without interruption during an attack of gout. Conventional treatments for terminating acute gout include colchicine,

NSAIDs, selective COX-2 inhibitors, and corticosteroids. Details of pharmacological management are beyond the scope of this chapter; the reader is encouraged to refer to the ACR guidelines for the management of gout.[91] Intercritical gout is the period between attacks. For chronic gout and tophaceous gout, a xanthine oxidase (XO) inhibitor with either allopurinol or febuxostat is recommended as first-line urate-lowering therapy.[91]

LIFESTYLE AND NONPHARMACOLOGICAL APPROACHES

Lifestyle measures and dietary modifications are adjunctive to standard urate-lowering therapy and are important to implement even in the elderly, as shown in Table 22.3. Notable challenges unique to older patients are that dietary factors may not have a major impact and a strict purine-free diet has only a small effect on SUA.[93] On the other hand, older subjects (61 to over 80 years) prefer nonpharmacological interventions such as cherry extract and lifelong dietary modification to improve their gout.[94] In fact, older age was significantly associated with a high level of willingness to modify diet ($p = 0.02$).[94] It makes sense to encourage consumption of low-fat dairy products, soybeans, and other vegetable protein.

PURINE-RICH FOODS

A major advance in nutritional epidemiology relevant to gout risk was the 2004 article from the Health Professionals Follow-up Study.[95] Over 47,000 male health professionals, ages 40 to 75 years at baseline, were followed for 12 years. Members of the cohort who consumed the highest levels of meat experienced a 41% increase in risk of incident gout. In contrast, those who consumed high levels of dairy products, particularly low-fat dairy products, had a 42% *reduction* in the rate of new-onset gout.[95] These findings were informative for elucidating the relationship between dietary factors and gout incidence—that is, of a *new* (first-time) episode of gout. Avoiding or reducing the amount of purine-rich food intake, especially of animal origin, may help reduce recurrent gout.[96]

SUGAR AND FRUCTOSE

Fructose, contained in sweetened soft drinks and beverages, increases SUA and gout risk.[97,98] Eliminating sugary soft drinks from the diet of gouty patients

Table 22.3. Lifestyle Factors, Nutrition, and Supplements for Gout

Baseline recommendations for all patients with a diagnosis of gout

- Evaluate gout disease burden (tophi, frequency and severity of acute and chronic arthritis symptoms and signs).
- Patient education with initiation of lifestyle modifications
- Consider secondary causes of hyperuricemia.
- Consider elimination of nonessential prescription medications that induce hyperuricemia on a case-by-case basis.
- Consider genetic testing for HLA-B*5801 in select elderly patients if urate-lowering therapy with allopurinol is being considered, particularly in individuals of Korean ethnicity who have chronic kidney disease and Han Chinese and Thai, irrespective of renal function.
- Stay well hydrated.
- Smoking cessation
- Daily exercise, weight loss for overweight and obese patients

Food Effects on Hyperuricemia and Gout Risk

Increased Risk	Decreased or No Risk
Meats & organ meats – Liver, kidney, sweetbreads: avoid as high purine content – Limit beef, lamb, pork	Fresh cherries Unsweetened cherry juice concentrate Vitamin C supplements
Seafood – Sardines, shellfish	Low-fat dairy products, 2 servings daily Milk, yogurt, skim milk powder
Beer, spirits, wine – Avoid overuse (defined as >2 servings/day for males and 1 serving/day for females) – Avoid any alcohol during periods of acute gout or advanced gout under poor control.	Vegetables Carrots, mushrooms, peas, spinach, cauliflower Legumes such as beans & lentils Oatmeal
Fructose-containing foods & beverages – Avoid soft drinks and limit fruit juices.	Vegetable-based meat substitutes Soy-based foods
Table sugar – Avoid or limit sweets, desserts, sweetened beverages.	Coffee/decaffeinated coffee Tea: no risk
Synthetic vitamin A derivatives (retinyl esters) – Isotretinoin – Acitretin	Trend towards lower serum urate and anti-inflammatory effects for: – ß-carotene (pro-vitamin A) – Omega-3 essential fatty acids (marine fish oil) – Luteolin-rich foods (celery, green peppers)[113] – Rutin/quercetin-rich foods

Note: Promotion and maintenance of ideal health, prevention and optimal management of life-threatening comorbidities in gout patients, including coronary artery disease, obesity, metabolic syndrome, diabetes mellitus, hyperlipidemia, and hypertension emphasized.[91,95,97,98,106–108] can bring multiple health benefits. Sweet fruits (i.e., apples and oranges) have also been linked to hyperuricemia and risk of gout.[98] However, given the overall health benefits of these food items, it appears acceptable for gout patients to consume them.

CHERRIES

Cherry intake, with a serving defined as a half-cup (10–12 cherries) consumed over a 2-day period preceding a gout attack was associated with a 35% reduction in recurrent gout attacks compared to no cherry consumption, with an odds ratio of 0.65 (95% confidence interval [95% CI] 0.50–0.85). A dose-response effect was observed in that the reduction in the risk of recurrent gout attacks was successively greater in those who consumed two and three servings of cherry fruit over a 2-day period compared to those who consumed a single serving.[99] What if fresh cherries are not available? The advantage of cherry juice concentrate versus fresh fruit is that it is available throughout the year. Patients with gout experienced a significant decrease in the number of acute gout attacks within 4 months of initiating ingestion of the cherry juice concentrate ($p < 0.05$), an effect that was not seen in the control group ingesting pomegranate juice concentrate.[100] Of patients ingesting cherry juice concentrate, 55% were attack-free and stopped their regular intake of NSAIDs within 60 days of initiating consumption of cherry juice concentrate. Cherries contain anthocyanin, a naturally occurring anti-inflammatory molecule that inhibits cyclooxygenase activity and scavenges reactive nitric oxide radicals.[101] Studies demonstrated that cherries also reduce inflammation measures such as C-reactive protein and nitric oxide levels.[102,103]

VITAMIN C

In the Health Professionals Follow-up Study (n = 1,387), an inverse association was observed between intake of vitamin C and SUA.[104] In a recent meta-analysis vitamin C supplementation resulted in an aggregate reduction in SUA of 0.35 mg/dl.[105] Overall, the data suggest that a total vitamin C intake of at least 500 mg/day is associated with a reduced risk of gout, whereas the potential benefit of lower intake remains unclear. Given the general safety profile with vitamin C and its cardiovascular benefit, which is relevant among patients with gout, this nutrient may provide a useful option in the prevention of gout in older people.[106]

COFFEE AND TEA

Coffee and tea are some of the most widely consumed beverages in the world. Using data from the Third National Health and Nutrition Examination, investigators found that SUA decreased with increasing coffee intake.[107] After adjusting for age and sex, SUA associated with coffee intake of four to five and more than six cups daily was lower than that associated with no intake by 0.26 mg/dl and 0.43 mg/dl (p for trend < 0.001), respectively. A modest inverse association between decaffeinated coffee intake and SUA was also found. Tea consumption, on the hand, is not associated with lower SUA and hyperuricemia frequency.[107] Total caffeine intake was not associated with serum uric acid levels, and the inverse association appears to be via other components of coffee. Regular coffee drinking have been associated with a lower risk of gout in men.[108] It is reasonable to allow coffee drinking if a patient enjoys the beverage.

MARINE OILS

Marine-derived omega-3 polyunsaturated fatty acids such as DHA and EPA exhibit anti-inflammatory properties via inhibition of NLRP3 inflammasome activation.[109] New scientific understanding of gout pathogenesis includes insights into how MSU microcrystals activate the caspase 1–activating NLRP3 (NOD-, LRR- and pyrin domain-containing 3) inflammasome with consequent dysregulation of IL-1ß.[110] The phologistic properties of MSU crystals are clearly linked to inflammasome activation resulting in arthritis.[111,112] More research is needed, however, to determine whether omega-3 fatty acids provided as dietary intake are superior to omega-3 fatty acids provided as purified oil supplements for gout.

Table 22.1 lists other supplements and vitamins.

Rheumatoid Arthritis

EPIDEMIOLOGY

Rheumatoid arthritis (RA) affected approximately 1.5 million people in the United States in 2007, and since then that number has increased to 2.4 million. The incidence of RA is 54 per 100,000 among those age 85 and up and peaked at age 65 to 74 (89 per 100,000); there was a lower incidence in the younger population of 8.7%.[114–119] Furthermore, the prevalence of RA, at least among women, may be increasing.

TREATMENT GUIDELINES

The current strategy for treating RA in the United States is based on the ACR's revised guidelines, updated in January 2016.[120] These guidelines are self-explanatory and will not be the focus here but rather will serve as a starting point to note areas where the integrative approach has the opportunity to increase patient satisfaction, meet demand, and enhance the value of the services we provide. Nowhere in these guidelines are integrative medicine principles embedded as part of the treatment paradigm; instead, the emphasis is primarily on a pharmaceutical approach to a multisystem inflammatory condition that is now recognized to have metabolic, hormonal, neuroendocrine, environmental, and microbiome influences that are dysregulated. No single defect or cause of RA has been identified; it probably is multidimensional.[120,121] The challenge for the conventional and integrative physician will be to identify RA early to keep the disease from progressing and affecting internal organs, creating structural irreversible damage, and producing cumulative damage with comorbidities (e.g., cardiovascular disease, depression, cancer). Our challenge is to get as many people into low disease activity or if possible a remission-like state.

DEFINING LOW, MODERATE, AND HIGH DISEASE

Despite all good intentions, reaching a consensus on how to define low, moderate, and high disease remains difficult due to disparate reporting systems, differences of opinion as to which metrics are best, and the views of academics research-based criteria versus the community-based physician "in the trenches." Using metrics such as DAS 28/CDAI, Rapid-3, and perhaps serologic multiple-biomarker assays all may play a part in assessing and stratifying disease activity. This in turn tells us how much intensity and frequency may be needed to drive down the inflammatory process from high or moderate disease activity to low or remission states. Doing so may reduce comorbidities and reduce the associated care costs, which are surging into the billions as more biologics are on the launch pad. Addressing not only the primary articular issues of RA but also potential systemic comorbidities can be done through a whole-person or integrative approach.

INTEGRATING CONVENTIONAL AND WHOLE-BODY APPROACHES

Essentially, the concept is to apply the basics of an anti-inflammatory lifestyle along with appropriate nutraceutical support that makes sense in this inflamed patient population. The benefits of a plant-based diet and fasting for RA have been well delineated in the literature.[122] Elimination diets also play a role here, and strong consideration should be given to eliminating strongly antigenic foods such as cow's milk and products, along with wheat and gluten-derived foods.[123] Consideration of food sensitivities and identification in recalcitrant patients or patients exhibiting continued symptomatology such as rashes, abdominal complaints, and headaches, not associated with medication, is another strategy worth employing. In these patients, a functional approach is also worth taking, as the gut and microbiome tend to be highly dysregulated in the systemically inflamed individual. More recent data by Jose Scher et al.[124] have shown that perturbation of the microbiologic phyla may be seen not only in RA but also specific patterns associated with the other inflammatory arthropathies, including psoriatic arthritis, Reiter's, ankylosing spondylitis, and so forth. How this translates into therapeutic interventions requires more data and research, but the take-home message here is to address the microbiome, not ignore it, and attempt to define what is perturbed and attempt to eradicate pathogens, repair bowel function, and replace missing minerals (magnesium), amino acids (L-glutamine), and vitamins such as D and A, and support basic metabolic functions including methylation with adequate folate and B vitamins that are critical for immune and mitochondrial energy pathways and signaling. Some of this approach comes right out of the inflammatory bowel disease, Crohn's, and ulcerative colitis experience and literature in the use of elemental and anti-inflammatory diets, along with adequate use of omega-3 fatty acids and anti-inflammatory botanicals such as curcumin, Boswellia, and Holy Basil.[125-127] Please see Chapter 16 for a detailed functional approach to gut health.

STRESS, SLEEP, NUTRITION, SUPPLEMENTS, MICROBIOME, FUNCTIONAL APPROACHES, HORMONES, EXERCISE

The role of stress cannot be overemphasized as a major contributor and in some cases as the tipping board in causality or worsening of predisposition to RA and other inflammatory conditions. The whole-person approach in addressing stress-reduction techniques through appropriate mind–body intervention training can include mindfulness-stress based training (Jon Kabat-Zinn), breathing techniques, daily consistent meditation even if for 5 minutes, journaling, interaction with nature, and physical activity (exercise).[128] All are approaches that improve stress responses. An example for the RA patient in this regard would be to daily carry out at least one stress-reduction activity. This could be breathing exercises, starting with 1 minute per day and gradually building up to 5 minutes and if possible 15 to 30 minutes at least once daily. Powerful autonomic effects occur with this exercise, especially if practiced consistently. Low-impact cardiovascular exercises such as riding a recumbent stationary bike, using an elliptical machine, walking briskly if possible, swimming, or doing aquatic exercises are all options to consider. Rotating these activities also enhances the benefit, reduces boredom, and leverages a cross-training effect. Exercising 3 or 4 days per week, even if for 5 minutes to start, and gradually increasing to 30 to 45 minutes per session with moderate effort in individuals with well-controlled inflammation and pain would be optimal. But if deformity, moderate to severe pain, or joint biomechanical dysfunction is present, patients should do what they can consistently under the supervision of the treating physician. The general rule is to keep moving!

Sleep is another critical item in the total care of an individual, especially in RA. Quality and quantity of sleep are the two variables worth addressing—in other words, how much restful sleep occurs and how deep is the restorative level achieved for neuro-immuno-humoral benefits to occur. Generally speaking, 6 to 8 hours of total sleep are optimal for most people. Depression, pain, biorhythm disturbances, stress, and medications can perturb both quality and quantity. All the aforementioned suggestions for stress reduction can improve sleep, along with incorporating a consistent sleep ritual that involves eliminating technology, unnecessary lights, and electronics. Relaxing scents, dimmed lighting, proper temperature settings, and a pre-sleep routine all set the stage for a restful sleep experience. Botanicals such as chamomile, valerian root (*Valeriana officinales*), and hops (*Humulus lupulus*), homeopathic remedies such as Coffea cruda and Nux vomica, and nutraceuticals such as sustained-release melatonin, L-theanine, and magnesium citrate, are all beneficial in aiding sleep more naturally.[129]

Nutritionally, there is evidence that the AFMD and vegan dietary patterns reduce pain and inflammation in RA populations. Elimination diets can omit excessive pro-inflammatory sugar and high fructose-corn syrup and the numerous disguised and mislabeled equivalents that consumers must navigate to identify these potential dietary culprits and avoid their deleterious pro-inflammatory effects. Reduction and in some cases elimination (temporary or permanent) of red meat and animal-based proteins can be considered in patients with high disease activity. Similarly, marked reduction or elimination of cow's milk and its products for the highly inflamed patient is worth considering. Almond, soy, coconut, and rice milk are alternatives. Gluten has very significant gut-related pro-inflammatory effects.[130] Secondary immune responses even in the absence of detectable celiac antibodies have been noted such as rashes, abdominal pain, abdominal bloating, diarrhea, and nonspecific and even leukocytoclastic vasculitis. Rice noodles and products or other non-gluten grains should be offered as options for the gluten-sensitive or potentially sensitive individual.

Microbiome, probiotics, and dietary pattern manipulation represent another area worth discussing in the comprehensive and integrative approach to RA treatments. While the literature is exploding with data regarding these subjects, a clear consensus is missing as to cause and effect with respect to specific microbiome changes and the causality on systemic inflammation. Intervention trials modifying the microbiome exist for several rheumatic disorders, including RA. While large numbers of patients have not been studied yet, some positive results have been identified utilizing *Lactobacillus caseii* and maltodextrin. Potential causes of failures of many studies may be the few number of patients studied and a lack of understanding that manipulation of the microbiome involves more than simply adding a random probiotic.[131] A microbiome dysfunction is not merely a deficiency of one or several bacterial symbionts; rather, fixing it involves a rebalancing of the ecosystem. Hence, a functional approach makes sense to consider in approaching the complex rheumatoid inflammatory patient and to individualize each phase of the microbiome ecosystem.

Supplements that are relevant to the RA patient include omega-3 fatty acids with adequate molecularly distilled quantities of EPA/DHA. While 1 g seems adequate for general populations, for inflammatory populations higher doses seem to be more useful and tolerated. For patients with low to moderate disease activity, a dose of 2 to 3 g/day divided twice daily (BID) is appropriate as standalone treatment or with botanicals and other minerals and supportive vitamins with or without complex pharmacological regimens. Much higher doses have been advocated in the literature by some authors, especially for actively inflamed populations, in doses as high as 6 to 8 g/day of EPA/DHA; many studies in the older literature document the benefit of higher doses.[132,133]

Other supplements commonly used include folate and the L5-methyltetrahydrofolate form to bypass the fairly common MTHFR single nucleotide polymorphism (SNP) mutation (approaching 50% in incidence); this makes sense as the preferred methylation, support especially when disease-modifying therapies such as methotrexate are used for basic RA pharmacotherapy.[134] Vitamin D3 to maintain optimal serum levels and vitamins K2 and B12 are other commonly recommended vitamins in an RA protocol, along with a multivitamin/multimineral.

In addition, two Medical Foods listed in Table 22.1 deserves a mention: RHEUMATE and LIMBREL.[135,136] Purity, pharmacokinetics, and safety are advantages of this class of compounds, which may be added to the RA patient's therapeutic options of natural products in addition to classic medications as needed or other over-the-counter nutraceuticals.

Finally, hormones deserve a mention. DHEA has benefits for metabolism, reducing insulin resistance, reducing body fat, and providing anti-cancer benefits. This hormone has been most extensively studied in systemic lupus erythematosus populations and is recommended as an adjunct in therapeutic regimens for mild to moderate lupus; its ability to reduce the prednisone requirement to less than 7.5 mg/day while not causing disease flare was shown by Michelle Petri, Lahita, and others.[137,138] Its use in RA has not been as widely advocated despite its many potential metabolic benefits, including reducing insulin resistance, improving immune function, and reducing visceral fat, all of which are needed in an inflamed RA patient population.[139,140] If an individual patient has low or suboptimal DHEA sulfate levels, addition of 10 to 25 mg/day for females and 25 to 50 mg/day for males to improve energy, reduce insulin resistance, improve other quality-of-life measures, including alertness and sleep, and reduce cancer risk makes sense. Appropriate serum determination before, during, and after DHEA addition is recommended to maintain ranges of 200 to 250 (females) and 500 to 550 (males). RA patients who are overweight, who have increased body fat, who have increased insulin resistance, who are metabolically sluggish, and who have elevated leptin levels could benefit from addition of DHEA to their regimen. Optimization of other hormones is beyond the scope of this chapter, but the use of bioidentical hormones in the appropriate individual with monitoring by an experienced physician trained in such approaches is worth considering as an adjunct to the overall RA integrative management approach we have outlined thus far.

Summary

Integrative rheumatology constructs lend themselves well to the management of individuals with both inflammatory and noninflammatory arthritis. The whole-person approach makes sense and is a key construct to improving and optimizing the patient's journey while controlling costs and reducing monetary waste. All these goals are in alignment with the current mandates of the Affordable Care Act and represent a necessary evolution in the health care system whether this legislation remains in full, in part, or not at all. Patients, especially those with chronic diseases such as arthritis, share in that goal of coordinated care—that is, integrative medicine where CIM therapies become part of a whole treatment plan just as physical therapy and surgical interventions become options when the need arises.

REFERENCES

Osteoarthritis and Gout

1. Saydah SH, Eberhardt MS. Use of complementary and alternative medicine among adults with chronic diseases: United States 2002. *J Altern Complement Med.* 2006;12(8):805–812.
2. Manek NJ, Crowson CS, Ottenberg AL, Curlin FA, Kaptchuk TJ, Tilburt JC. What rheumatologists in the United States think of complementary and alternative medicine: results of a national survey. *BMC Complement Altern Med.* 2010;10:5.
3. Holmberg S, Thelin A, Thelin N. Knee osteoarthritis and body mass index: A population-based case-control study. *Scand J Rheumatol.* 2005;34(1):59–64.
4. Lee R, Kean WF. Obesity and knee osteoarthritis. *Inflammopharmacology.* 2012;20(2):53–58.
5. Murphy L, Helmick CG. The impact of osteoarthritis in the United States: A population-health perspective. *Am J Nurs.* 2012;112(3 Suppl 1):S13–S19.
6. Foy CG, Lewis CE, Hairston KG, et al. Intensive lifestyle intervention improves physical function among obese adults with knee pain: findings from the Look AHEAD trial. *Obesity (Silver Spring).* 2011;19(1):83–93.
7. Berenbaum F. Diabetes-induced osteoarthritis: From a new paradigm to a new phenotype. *Postgrad Med J.* 2012;88(1038):240–242.
8. Louati K, Vidal C, Berenbaum F, Sellam J. Association between diabetes mellitus and osteoarthritis: Systematic literature review and meta-analysis. *RMD Open.* 2015;1(1):e000077.
9. Hochberg MC, Altman RD, April KT, et al. American College of Rheumatology 2012 recommendations for the use of nonpharmacologic and pharmacologic therapies in osteoarthritis of the hand, hip, and knee. *Arthritis Care Res (Hoboken).* 2012;64(4):465–474.
10. McAlindon TE, Bannuru RR, Sullivan MC, et al. OARSI guidelines for the non-surgical management of knee osteoarthritis. *Osteoarthritis Cartilage.* 2014;22(3):363–388.
11. National Institute for Health and Care Excellence. *Osteoarthritis: Care and Management in Adults.* National Clinical Guideline Center (UK); 2014.
12. Yang S, Dube CE, Eaton CB, McAlindon TE, Lapane KL. Longitudinal use of complementary and alternative medicine among older adults with radiographic knee osteoarthritis. *Clin Ther.* 2013;35(11):1690–1702.
13. du Souich P. Comments on "OARSI guidelines for the non-surgical management of knee osteoarthritis." *Osteoarthritis Cartilage.* 2014;22(6):888–889.
14. Wainwright TW, Immins T, Middleton RG. Hip osteoarthritis: Patients with complex comorbidities can make exceptional improvements following intensive exercise and education. *BMJ Case Rep.* 2015;2015.
15. Lorig KR, Mazonson PD, Holman HR. Evidence suggesting that health education for self-management in patients with chronic arthritis has sustained health benefits while reducing health care costs. *Arthritis Rheum.* 1993;36(4):439–446.

16. *Arthritis Self-Management: What You Need to Know*. Arthritis Foundation; 2016. Accessed June 17, 2016, at http://www.arthritis.org/about-arthritis/understanding-arthritis/arthritis-self-management.php.

17. Messier SP, Mihalko SL, Legault C, et al. Effects of intensive diet and exercise on knee joint loads, inflammation, and clinical outcomes among overweight and obese adults with knee osteoarthritis: The IDEA randomized clinical trial. *JAMA*. 2013;310(12):1263–1273.

18. Callahan LF, Mielenz T, Freburger J, et al. A randomized controlled trial of the People with Arthritis Can Exercise program: symptoms, function, physical activity, and psychosocial outcomes. *Arthritis Rheum*. 2008;59(1):92–101.

19. Wyatt B, Mingo CA, Waterman MB, White P, Cleveland RJ, Callahan LF. Impact of the Arthritis Foundation's Walk With Ease Program on arthritis symptoms in African Americans. *Prev Chronic Dis*. 2014;11:E199.

20. Callahan LF, Shreffler JH, Altpeter M, et al. Evaluation of group and self-directed formats of the Arthritis Foundation's Walk With Ease Program. *Arthritis Care Res (Hoboken)*. 2011;63(8):1098–1107.

21. Walk With Ease Online Tools. Arthritis Foundation, 2016. Accessed June 17, 2016, at http://www.arthritis.org/living-with-arthritis/tools-resources/walk-with-ease/.

22. Park J, McCaffrey R, Dunn D, Goodman R. Managing osteoarthritis: Comparisons of chair yoga, Reiki, and education (pilot study). *Holist Nurs Pract*. 2011;25(6):316–326.

23. Wang C, Schmid CH, Iversen MD, et al. Comparative effectiveness of tai chi versus physical therapy for knee osteoarthritis: A randomized trial. *Ann Intern Med* 2016;165(2):77–86.

24. Webb R, Cofre Lizama LE, Galea MP. Moving with ease: Feldenkrais method classes for people with osteoarthritis. *Evid Based Complement Alternat Med*. 2013;2013:479142.

25. Berman BM, Lao L, Langenberg P, Lee WL, Gilpin AM, Hochberg MC. Effectiveness of acupuncture as adjunctive therapy in osteoarthritis of the knee: A randomized, controlled trial. *Ann Intern Med*. 2004;141(12):901–910.

26. Vas J, Mendez C, Perea-Milla E, et al. Acupuncture as a complementary therapy to the pharmacological treatment of osteoarthritis of the knee: Randomised controlled trial. *BMJ*. 2004;329(7476):1216.

27. Witt C, Brinkhaus B, Jena S, et al. Acupuncture in patients with osteoarthritis of the knee: A randomised trial. *Lancet*. 2005;366(9480):136–143.

28. White A, Foster NE, Cummings M, Barlas P. Acupuncture treatment for chronic knee pain: A systematic review. *Rheumatology (Oxford)*. 2007;46(3):384–390.

29. Manheimer E, Linde K, Lao L, Bouter LM, Berman BM. Meta-analysis: Acupuncture for osteoarthritis of the knee. *Ann Intern Med*. 2007;146(12):868–877.

30. Foster NE, Thomas E, Barlas P, et al. Acupuncture as an adjunct to exercise based physiotherapy for osteoarthritis of the knee: Randomised controlled trial. *BMJ*. 2007;335(7617):436.

31. Scharf HP, Mansmann U, Streitberger K, et al. Acupuncture and knee osteoarthritis: a three-armed randomized trial. *Ann Intern Med*. 2006;145(1):12–20.

32. Berman B. A 60-year-old woman considering acupuncture for knee pain. *JAMA.* 2007;297(15):1697–1707.
33. Perlman AI, Sabina A, Williams AL, Njike VY, Katz DL. Massage therapy for osteoarthritis of the knee: a randomized controlled trial. *Arch Intern Med.* 2006;166(22):2533–2538.
34. Perlman AI, Ali A, Njike VY, et al. Massage therapy for osteoarthritis of the knee: a randomized dose-finding trial. *PLoS One.* 2012;7(2):e30248.
35. Baird CL, Sands L. A pilot study of the effectiveness of guided imagery with progressive muscle relaxation to reduce chronic pain and mobility difficulties of osteoarthritis. *Pain Manag Nurs.* 2004;5(3):97–104.
36. Baird CL, Sands LP. Effect of guided imagery with relaxation on health-related quality of life in older women with osteoarthritis. *Res Nurs Health.* 2006;29(5):442–451.
37. Gay MC, Philippot P, Luminet O. Differential effectiveness of psychological interventions for reducing osteoarthritis pain: A comparison of Erikson [correction of Erickson] hypnosis and Jacobson relaxation. *Eur J Pain.* 2002;6(1):1–16.
38. Gordon A, Merenstein JH, D'Amico F, Hudgens D. The effects of therapeutic touch on patients with osteoarthritis of the knee. *J Fam Pract.* 1998;47(4):271–277.
39. Lu DF, Hart LK, Lutgendorf SK, Perkhounkova Y. The effect of healing touch on the pain and mobility of persons with osteoarthritis: A feasibility study. *Geriatr Nurs.* 2013;34(4):314–322.
40. Peck SD. The efficacy of therapeutic touch for improving functional ability in elders with degenerative arthritis. *Nurs Sci Q.* 1998;11(3):123–132.
41. McCaffrey R, Freeman E. Effect of music on chronic osteoarthritis pain in older people. *J Adv Nurs.* 2003;44(5):517–524.
42. Zelazny CM. Therapeutic instrumental music playing in hand rehabilitation for older adults with osteoarthritis: four case studies. *J Music Ther.* 2001;38(2):97–113.
43. Williams FM, Skinner J, Spector TD, et al. Dietary garlic and hip osteoarthritis: Evidence of a protective effect and putative mechanism of action. *BMC Musculoskelet Disord.* 2010;11:280.
44. Shen CL, Smith BJ, Lo DF, et al. Dietary polyphenols and mechanisms of osteoarthritis. *J Nutr Biochem.* 2012;23(11):1367–1377.
45. Lopez HL. Nutritional interventions to prevent and treat osteoarthritis. Part I: focus on fatty acids and macronutrients. *PM R.* 2012;4(5 Suppl):S145–S154.
46. Uebelhart D, Malaise M, Marcolongo R, et al. Intermittent treatment of knee osteoarthritis with oral chondroitin sulfate: A one-year, randomized, double-blind, multicenter study versus placebo. *Osteoarthritis Cartilage.* 2004;12(4):269–276.
47. Reginster JY, Deroisy R, Rovati LC, et al. Long-term effects of glucosamine sulphate on osteoarthritis progression: A randomised, placebo-controlled clinical trial. *Lancet.* 2001;357(9252):251–256.
48. Clegg DO, Reda DJ, Harris CL, et al. Glucosamine, chondroitin sulfate, and the two in combination for painful knee osteoarthritis. *N Engl J Med.* 2006;354(8):795–808.
49. Hochberg MC, Martel-Pelletier J, Monfort J, et al. Combined chondroitin sulfate and glucosamine for painful knee osteoarthritis: A multicentre, randomised, double-blind, non-inferiority trial versus celecoxib. *Ann Rheum Dis.* 2016;75(1):37–44.

50. Herrero-Beaumont G, Ivorra JA, Del Carmen Trabado M, et al. Glucosamine sulfate in the treatment of knee osteoarthritis symptoms: A randomized, double-blind, placebo-controlled study using acetaminophen as a side comparator. *Arthritis Rheum.* 2007;56(2):555–567.

51. Kahan A, Uebelhart D, De Vathaire F, Delmas PD, Reginster JY. Long-term effects of chondroitins 4 and 6 sulfate on knee osteoarthritis: The study on osteoarthritis progression prevention, a two-year, randomized, double-blind, placebo-controlled trial. *Arthritis Rheum.* 2009;60(2):524–533.

52. Henrotin Y, Lambert C. Chondroitin and glucosamine in the management of osteoarthritis: An update. *Curr Rheumatol Rep.* 2013;15(10):361.

53. Bruyere O, Pavelka K, Rovati LC, et al. Total joint replacement after glucosamine sulphate treatment in knee osteoarthritis: Results of a mean 8-year observation of patients from two previous 3-year, randomised, placebo-controlled trials. *Osteoarthritis Cartilage.* 2008;16(2):254–260.

54. Gallagher B, Tjoumakaris FP, Harwood MI, Good RP, Ciccotti MG, Freedman KB. Chondroprotection and the prevention of osteoarthritis progression of the knee: A systematic review of treatment agents. *Am J Sports Med.* 2015;43(3):734–744.

55. Bell GA, Kantor ED, Lampe JW, Shen DD, White E. Use of glucosamine and chondroitin in relation to mortality. *Eur J Epidemiol.* 2012;27(8):593–603.

56. Henrotin YE, Labasse AH, Jaspar JM, et al. Effects of three avocado/soybean unsaponifiable mixtures on metalloproteinases, cytokines and prostaglandin E2 production by human articular chondrocytes. *Clin Rheumatol.* 1998;17(1):31–39.

57. Blotman F, Maheu E, Wulwik A, Caspard H, Lopez A. Efficacy and safety of avocado/soybean unsaponifiables in the treatment of symptomatic osteoarthritis of the knee and hip. A prospective, multicenter, three-month, randomized, double-blind, placebo-controlled trial. *Rev Rhum Engl Ed.* 1997;64(12):825–834.

58. Maheu E, Mazieres B, Valat JP, et al. Symptomatic efficacy of avocado/soybean unsaponifiables in the treatment of osteoarthritis of the knee and hip: A prospective, randomized, double-blind, placebo-controlled, multicenter clinical trial with a six-month treatment period and a two-month followup demonstrating a persistent effect. *Arthritis Rheum.* 1998;41(1):81–91.

59. Maheu E, Cadet C, Marty M, et al. Randomised, controlled trial of avocado-soybean unsaponifiable (Piascledine) effect on structure modification in hip osteoarthritis: the ERADIAS study. *Ann Rheum Dis.* 2014;73(2):376–384.

60. Appelboom T, Schuermans J, Verbruggen G, Henrotin Y, Reginster JY. Symptoms modifying effect of avocado/soybean unsaponifiables (ASU) in knee osteoarthritis. A double blind, prospective, placebo-controlled study. *Scand J Rheumatol.* 2001;30(4):242–247.

61. Lequesne M, Maheu E, Cadet C, Dreiser RL. Structural effect of avocado/soybean unsaponifiables on joint space loss in osteoarthritis of the hip. *Arthritis Rheum.* 2002;47(1):50–58.

62. Christiansen BA, Bhatti S, Goudarzi R, Emami S. Management of osteoarthritis with avocado/soybean unsaponifiables. *Cartilage.* 2015;6(1):30–44.

63. DiNubile NA. A potential role for avocado- and soybean-based nutritional supplements in the management of osteoarthritis: a review. *Phys Sportsmed.* 2010;38(2):71–81.

64. Hosea Blewett HJ. Exploring the mechanisms behind S-adenosylmethionine (SAMe) in the treatment of osteoarthritis. *Crit Rev Food Sci Nutr.* 2008;48(5):458–463.

65. Soeken KL, Lee WL, Bausell RB, Agelli M, Berman BM. Safety and efficacy of S-adenosylmethionine (SAMe) for osteoarthritis. *J Fam Pract.* 2002;51(5):425–430.

66. Najm WI, Reinsch S, Hoehler F, Tobis JS, Harvey PW. S-adenosyl methionine (SAMe) versus celecoxib for the treatment of osteoarthritis symptoms: A double-blind cross-over trial. [ISRCTN36233495]. *BMC Musculoskelet Disord.* 2004;5:6.

67. Levkovitz Y, Alpert JE, Brintz CE, Mischoulon D, Papakostas GI. Effects of S-adenosylmethionine augmentation of serotonin-reuptake inhibitor antidepressants on cognitive symptoms of major depressive disorder. *J Affect Disord.* 2012;136(3):1174–1178.

68. Peddada KV, Shukla SK, Mishra A, Verma V. Role of curcumin in common musculoskeletal disorders: A review of current laboratory, translational, and clinical data. *Orthop Surg.* 2015;7(3):222–231.

69. Funk JL, Oyarzo JN, Frye JB, et al. Turmeric extracts containing curcuminoids prevent experimental rheumatoid arthritis. *J Nat Prod.* 2006;69(3):351–355.

70. Appelboom T, Maes N, Albert A. A new curcuma extract (Flexofytol(R)) in osteoarthritis: Results from a Belgian real-life experience. *Open Rheumatol J.* 2014;8:77–81.

71. Belcaro G, Dugall M, Luzzi R, et al. Meriva(R)+Glucosamine versus Condroitin +Glucosamine in patients with knee osteoarthritis: An observational study. *Eur Rev Med Pharmacol Sci.* 2014;18(24):3959–3963.

72. Sterzi S, Giordani L, Morrone M, et al. The efficacy and safety of using CartiJoint Forte (a combination of glucosamine hydrochloride, chondroitin sulfate and bio-curcumin) with exercise in the treatment of knee osteoarthritis: A randomized, double blind, placebo-controlled study. *Eur J Phys Rehabil Med.* 2016;52(3):321–330.

73. Ford ES, Choi HK. Associations between concentrations of uric acid with concentrations of vitamin A and beta-carotene among adults in the United States. *Nutr Res.* 2013;33(12):995–1002.

74. Brien S, Prescott P, Lewith G. Meta-analysis of the related nutritional supplements dimethyl sulfoxide and methylsulfonylmethane in the treatment of osteoarthritis of the knee. *Evid Based Complement Alternat Med.* 2011;2011:528403.

75. Takahama U, Koga Y, Hirota S, Yamauchi R. Inhibition of xanthine oxidase activity by an oxathiolanone derivative of quercetin. *Food Chem.* 2011;126(4):1808–1811.

76. Brien S, Lewith G, Walker A, Hicks SM, Middleton D. Bromelain as a treatment for osteoarthritis: A review of clinical studies. *Evid Based Complement Alternat Med.* 2004;1(3):251–257.

77. Belcaro G, Dugall M, Luzzi R, et al. Management of osteoarthritis (OA) with the pharma-standard supplement FlexiQule (Boswellia): A 12-week registry. *Minerva Gastroenterol Dietol.* 2015 Oct 22 [E-pub before print].

78. Kizhakkedath R. Clinical evaluation of a formulation containing *Curcuma longa* and *Boswellia serrata* extracts in the management of knee osteoarthritis. *Mol Med Rep.* 2013;8(5):1542–1548.

79. Sumantran VN, Joshi AK, Boddul S, et al. Antiarthritic activity of a standardized, multiherbal, Ayurvedic formulation containing *Boswellia serrata*: In vitro studies on knee cartilage from osteoarthritis patients. *Phytother Res.* 2011;25(9):1375–1380.

80. Chantre P, Cappelaere A, Leblan D, Guedon D, Vandermander J, Fournie B. Efficacy and tolerance of *Harpagophytum procumbens* versus diacerhein in treatment of osteoarthritis. *Phytomedicine.* 2000;7(3):177–183.

81. Sanders M, Grundmann O. The use of glucosamine, devil's claw (*Harpagophytum procumbens*), and acupuncture as complementary and alternative treatments for osteoarthritis. *Altern Med Rev.* 2011;16(3):228–238.

82. Grzanna R, Lindmark L, Frondoza CG. Ginger—an herbal medicinal product with broad anti-inflammatory actions. *J Med Food.* 2005;8(2):125–132.

83. Marcus DM, Suarez-Almazor ME. Is there a role for ginger in the treatment of osteoarthritis? *Arthritis Rheum.* 2001;44(11):2461–2462.

84. Cameron M, Chrubasik S. Topical herbal therapies for treating osteoarthritis. *Cochrane Database Syst Rev.* 2013;5:CD010538.

85. Rosenthal AK, Ryan LM. Calcium pyrophosphate deposition disease. *N Engl J Med.* 2016;374(26):2575–2584.

86. Mulay SR, Anders HJ. Crystallopathies. *N Engl J Med.* 2016;374(25):2465–2476.

87. Singh H, Torralba KD. Therapeutic challenges in the management of gout in the elderly. *Geriatrics.* 2008;63(7):13–18, 20.

88. ter Borg EJ, Rasker JJ. Gout in the elderly, a separate entity? *Ann Rheum Dis.* 1987;46(1):72–76.

89. Wise CM. Crystal-associated arthritis in the elderly. *Rheum Dis Clin North Am.* 2007;33(1):33–55.

90. Terkeltaub RA. Clinical practice. Gout. *N Engl J Med.* 2003;349(17):1647–1655.

91. Khanna D, Fitzgerald JD, Khanna PP, et al. 2012 American College of Rheumatology guidelines for management of gout. Part 1: Systematic nonpharmacologic and pharmacologic therapeutic approaches to hyperuricemia. *Arthritis Care Res (Hoboken).* 2012;64(10):1431–1446.

92. Khanna D, Khanna PP, Fitzgerald JD, et al. 2012 American College of Rheumatology guidelines for management of gout. Part 2: Therapy and anti-inflammatory prophylaxis of acute gouty arthritis. *Arthritis Care Res (Hoboken).* 2012;64(10):1447–1461.

93. Jordan KM, Cameron JS, Snaith M, et al. British Society for Rheumatology and British Health Professionals in Rheumatology guideline for the management of gout. *Rheumatology (Oxford).* 2007;46(8):1372–1374.

94. Singh JA, Shah N, Edwards NL. A cross-sectional internet-based patient survey of the management strategies for gout. *BMC Complement Altern Med.* 2016;16:90.

95. Choi HK, Atkinson K, Karlson EW, Willett W, Curhan G. Purine-rich foods, dairy and protein intake, and the risk of gout in men. *N Engl J Med.* 2004;350(11):1093–1103.

96. Zhang Y, Chen C, Choi H, et al. Purine-rich foods intake and recurrent gout attacks. *Ann Rheum Dis.* 2012;71(9):1448–1453.

97. Choi JW, Ford ES, Gao X, Choi HK. Sugar-sweetened soft drinks, diet soft drinks, and serum uric acid level: The Third National Health and Nutrition Examination Survey. *Arthritis Rheum.* 2008;59(1):109–116.

98. Choi HK, Curhan G. Soft drinks, fructose consumption, and the risk of gout in men: prospective cohort study. *BMJ.* 2008;336(7639):309–312.

99. Zhang Y, Neogi T, Chen C, Chaisson C, Hunter DJ, Choi HK. Cherry consumption and decreased risk of recurrent gout attacks. *Arthritis Rheum.* 2012;64(12):4004–4011.

100. Schlesinger N, Schlesinger M. Previously reported prior studies of cherry juice concentrate for gout flare prophylaxis: Comment on the article by Zhang et al. *Arthritis Rheum.* 2013;65(4):1135–1136.

101. Gelber AC, Solomon DH. If life serves up a bowl of cherries, and gout attacks are "the pits": Implications for therapy. *Arthritis Rheum.* 2012;64(12):3827–3830.

102. Jacob RA, Spinozzi GM, Simon VA, et al. Consumption of cherries lowers plasma urate in healthy women. *J Nutr.* 2003;133(6):1826–1829.

103. Kelley DS, Adkins Y, Reddy A, Woodhouse LR, Mackey BE, Erickson KL. Sweet Bing cherries lower circulating concentrations of markers for chronic inflammatory diseases in healthy humans. *J Nutr.* 2013;143(3):340–344.

104. Gao X, Curhan G, Forman JP, Ascherio A, Choi HK. Vitamin C intake and serum uric acid concentration in men. *J Rheumatol.* 2008;35(9):1853–1858.

105. Juraschek SP, Miller ER, 3rd, Gelber AC. Effect of oral vitamin C supplementation on serum uric acid: A meta-analysis of randomized controlled trials. *Arthritis Care Res (Hoboken).* 2011;63(9):1295–1306.

106. Choi HK. A prescription for lifestyle change in patients with hyperuricemia and gout. *Curr Opin Rheumatol.* 2010;22(2):165–172.

107. Choi HK, Curhan G. Coffee, tea, and caffeine consumption and serum uric acid level: The Third National Health and Nutrition Examination Survey. *Arthritis Rheum.* 2007;57(5):816–821.

108. Choi HK, Willett W, Curhan G. Coffee consumption and risk of incident gout in men: A prospective study. *Arthritis Rheum.* 2007;56(6):2049–2055.

109. Marty-Roix R, Lien E. (De-) oiling inflammasomes. *Immunity.* 2013;38(6):1088–1090.

110. Martinon F, Petrilli V, Mayor A, Tardivel A, Tschopp J. Gout-associated uric acid crystals activate the NALP3 inflammasome. *Nature.* 2006;440(7081):237–241.

111. So A, Ives A, Joosten LA, Busso N. Targeting inflammasomes in rheumatic diseases. *Nat Rev Rheumatol.* 2013;9(7):391–399.

112. So A, Busso N. The concept of the inflammasome and its rheumatologic implications. *Joint Bone Spine.* 2014;81(5):398–402.

113. Yan J, Zhang G, Hu Y, Ma Y. Effect of luteolin on xanthine oxidase: Inhibition kinetics and interaction mechanism merging with docking simulation. *Food Chem.* 2013;141(4):3766–3773.

114. Myasoedova E, Crowson CS, Kremers HM, Therneau TM, Gabriel SE. Is the incidence of rheumatoid arthritis rising? Results from Olmsted County, Minnesota, 1955–2007. *Arthritis Rheum.* 2010;62(6):1576–1582.

115. Wolfe F, Mitchell DM, Sibley JT, et al. The mortality of rheumatoid arthritis. *Arthritis Rheum.* 1994;37(4):481–494.

116. Solomon DH, Reed G, Kremer JM, et al. Disease activity in rheumatoid arthritis and the risk of cardiovascular events. *Arthritis Rheumatol.* 2015. doi: 10.1002/art.39098.

117. Yazdany J, Dudley RA, Chen R, Lin GA, Tseng C. Coverage for high-cost specialty drugs for rheumatoid arthritis in Medicare Part D. *Arthritis Rheumatol.* 2015;67(6):1474–1480.

118. "Rheumatoid Arthritis Treatment Costs." 2016. https://www.rheumatoidarthritis.org/treatment/costs/

119. Kawatkar A, et al. Direct medical expenditure associated with rheumatoid arthritis in a nationally representative sample from the Medical Expenditure Panel Survey. *Arthritis Care Res.* 2012;64(11):1649–1656.

120. Firestein GS, Ralph BC. *Kelley and Firestein's Textbook of Rheumatology,* 10th ed., vol. 1. Philadelphia: Elsevier; 2016.

121. Rakel D. *Integrative Medicine,* 3rd ed. Philadelphia: Saunders; 2012:456–463.

122. Kjeldsen-Kragh J. Rheumatoid arthritis treated with vegetarian diets. *Am J Clin Nutr.* 1999;70(3):594.

123. Hafstrom I, et al. A vegan diet free of gluten improves the signs and symptoms of rheumatoid arthritis: The effects on arthritis correlate with a reduction in antibodies to food antigens. *Rheumatology.* 2001;40(0):1175.

124. Scher JU, Littman DR, Abramson SB. Review: Microbiome in inflammatory arthritis and human rheumatic diseases. *Arthritis Rheumatol.* 2016;68(1):35–45.

125. Ahmed S, et al. Biological basis for the use of botanicals in osteoarthritis and rheumatoid arthritis: A review. *Evidence Based Compl Altern Med.* 2005;2(3):301–308.

126. Lee JY, et al. Saturated fatty acids, but not unsaturated fatty acids, induce the expression of cyclooxygenase-2 mediated through Toll-like receptor 4. *J Biol Chem.* 2001;276(20):16683.

127. Reed GW, et al. Treatment of rheumatoid arthritis with marine and botanical oils: An 18-month, randomized, and double-blind trial. *Evidence Based Compl Altern Med.* 2014;2014:857456.

128. Benson H. *The Relaxation Response.* New York: HarperCollins; 1976.

129. Rakel D. *Integrative Medicine,* 3rd ed. Philadelphia: Saunders; 2012:65–76.

130. Kohatsu W. The anti-inflammatory diet. In Rakel D, ed., *Integrative Medicine,* 3rd ed. Philadelphia: Saunders; 2012:795–802.

131. Bravo-Bias A, et al. Microbiota and arthritis: Correlations or cause? *Curr Opin Rheumatol.* 2016;28:161–167.

132. Calder PC. Omega-3 polyunsaturated fatty acids and inflammatory processes: Nutrition or pharmacology? *Br J Clin Pharmacol.* 2013;75(3):645–652.

133. Kremer J, et al. Effects of high-dose fish oil on rheumatoid arthritis after stopping nonsteroidal anti-inflammatory drugs clinical and immune correlates. *Arthritis Rheumatism.* 1995;38(8):1107.

134. Fisher MC, Cronstein BN. Meta-analysis of methylenetetrahydrofolate reductase (MTHFR) polymorphisms affecting methotrexate toxicity. *J Rheumatol.* 2009;36(3):539–545.

135. RHEUMATE. http://www.rheumaterx.com/

136. Bitto A, Squadrito F, Irrera N, et al. Flavocoxid, a nutraceutical approach to blunt inflammatory conditions. *Mediators of Inflammation*, 2014, Article ID 790851.

137. Petri M, Lahita RG, et al. Effect of prasterone on corticosteroid requirements of women with systemic lupus erythematosus. *Arthritis Rheumatism.* 2002;46(7):1820–1829.

138. Chang DM, et al. Dihydroepiandosterone treatment in women with mild to moderate systemic lupus erythematosus: A multicenter randomized, double-blind placebo-controlled trial. *Arthritis Rheumatol.* 2002;46(11):2924–2927.

139. Dhatariya K, et al. Effect of dehydroepiandrosterone replacement on insulin sensitivity and lipids in hypoadrenal women. Diabetes. 2005;54(3):765–769.

140. Watson RR. *DHEA in Human Health and Aging.* New York: CRC Press; 2012.

23

Falls

ANCA DINESCU AND MIKHAIL KOGAN

Case Study

Mr. B. is a 74-year-old art collector. He lives with his wife, a long-time advocate for integrative medicine. Four weeks prior to the visit Mr. B. sustained a fall at night while going to the bathroom. He had another nighttime fall 2 weeks later. The second fall caused severe chest pain requiring a trip to the emergency room, where a chest x-ray reveled several fractured ribs. He was prescribed Tylenol with codeine and referred to his primary care doctor for follow-up. The patient's medical problems are high blood pressure, for which he takes lisinopril and amlodipine. He also has chronic fibromyalgia, anxiety, and depression, which were managed with fish oil, duloxetine, and occasional lorazepam as needed. Over the past decade he developed insomnia, for which he was prescribed zolpidem and meditative practices, which he refused to do. His additional supplements were vitamin D 2,000 units/day and a multivitamin. Despite his medical team aggressively trying to work with him on weight loss and better management of his anxiety and depression, he refused lifestyle modifications and instead stayed on medications.

At the visit his physician learned that he had increased his lorazepam intake and at times doubled his zolpidem intake at night. On examination his vital signs were normal but he had gained 10 lbs and his body mass index (BMI) was 35. He did not have orthostatic hypotension. He had tenderness over the broken ribs. His gait and balance were normal, but he was not able to squat even with assist of his upper body, his walking was slow, and his wrist grip strength was low normal for his age. He appeared tired and anxious. Lab work of significance was a vitamin D 25-OH level of 18 ng/ml.

The patient was referred to physical therapy and tai chi classes for core strengthening and balance. His vitamin D dose was increased to 5,000 units/day with a plan to repeat the vitamin D 25-OH level in 3 months. His lorazepam was discontinued. He was also referred to a psychologist and a mindfulness-based stress reduction class (see Chapter 9), which he refused to do. However, he agreed to start working with a naturopathic doctor who specializes in weight loss programs.

At the 3-month follow-up the patient had lost 20 lbs and was very happy about his progress. He felt a lot less general pain, he slept much better, and his anxiety had improved. At the 6-month follow-up he had lost another 10 lbs and had much improved mood and sleep. His zolpidem and duloxetine doses were cut in half. The patient had not had any more near-fall or fall episodes since.

This case demonstrates importance of discontinuing medications that are associated with a high fall risk (lorazepam) and engaging the patient in core and balance strengthening exercises and further lifestyle changes, catching the moment of increased concern over his health deterioration.

Definition and Relevance

A fall represents the process in which a person comes to rest inadvertently on the ground or a lower level. Despite sharing the final outcome (i.e., the patient comes to rest on the ground), the definition of a fall does not traditionally include syncope, seizure, pseudo-seizure. or major trauma from accidents.[1] In the geriatric population falls are extremely important. At a personal level, falls are associated with a subsequent fear of falling, a decline in function, increased nursing home placement, and increased use of medical services, and complications resulting from falls represent the leading cause of death from injury in geriatric population.[1,2] At the more global level, falls in the elderly are associated with increased use of medical services and increased cost directly to the patient and also indirectly, if we add the number of hours of work lost by caregivers who will assume care of that elderly person after the fall.[3]

Falls in the elderly are very common, and their frequency increases with aging. One-third of elders over 65 years old report a fall in the previous year. In the nursing home population, 50% of residents will sustain a fall every year. In term of fall-associated injuries, most falls result in minor injuries, but 10% to 15% are associated with fracture and 5% result in major injuries such as head trauma.[1,4] Falls in the geriatric population are also associated with a stigma of weakness and are greatly under-reported. This is why it is so important to ask about falls during each encounter; indeed, this might be the only direct way to affect this issue. In the same way, the real cost of falls is hard to quantify because of the high rate of under-reporting and also because most of the falls result in minor injuries for which the patient might not seek medical attention.[1,3]

Etiology and Risk Factors

According to the most current understanding of this issue, the vast majority of falls are thought to occur as a result of interaction between intrinsic or patient risk factors (i.e., age-related decline in function), extrinsic risk factors (i.e., challenges to human erect position), and mediating/precipitating factors (i.e., situational hazards). This concept explains the observed increased frequency of falls in the elderly that matches the various age-related declines that, in the end, will make adaptation to situational hazards and environmental challenges more difficult compared to younger individuals.[1,5] Table 23.1 lists the most common intrinsic and extrinsic risk factors for falls.

Medications are by far the most correctable risk factor for falls in the elderly and unfortunately one of the most common. With the psychotropics (e.g., benzodiazepines, selective serotonin reuptake inhibitors [SSRIs], serotonin-norepinephrine reuptake inhibitors [SNRIs], and antipsychotics) and medications with anticholinergic effects at the top of the list, prescription drugs represent an important risk factor for falls. Any dose increase or

Table 23.1. Falls Risk Factors

Intrinsic	*Extrinsic*
Declining vision	Poor lighting
Gait and balance problems	Medications
Muscle weakness	Poorly fit or inappropriate use of assisting devices
Postural hypotension	Tripping obstacles (commonly rugs)
Vitamin D deficiency[6]	Uneven or slippery surfaces
Chronic medical problems such as Parkinson's disease	Poor building design • Lack of stair handrails • Lack of bathroom grab bars • Poor stair design
Previous falls and fear of future falls	
Advanced age	

Modified from CDC website: https://www.cdc.gov/steadi/pdf/risk_factors_for_falls-a.pdf

decrease or starting or stopping of medications represents a possible hazard for falls, as well as taking more than three or four medications in general. Alcohol and illicit/recreational drugs are other well-known risk factors for falls but are frequently not asked about during the interview of the geriatric patient.[7]

Evaluation and Management

From a general, practical approach, falls management has three arms.

The first is **ongoing screening** of geriatric patients for identification and correction (when possible) of risk factors to prevent a first fall. Screening for the occurrence of a first fall is recommended at every office visit by simply asking patients if they have fallen since the previous visit. If no fall has occurred, screening for the known risk factors in the elderly might seem easy, but it is at times a lengthy list and requires a systematic approach including the known risk factors mentioned earlier.[8]

Immediate post-fall management depends on the presence or absence of injury. Beyond the care for visible wounds, minor or major, attention should be focused on assessing for less visible injuries (hip fracture, subdural hematoma, intracerebral hemorrhage), assessing for the presence of delirium, and providing supportive care.

Prevention of subsequent falls follows the same principles used in the assessment and correction of risk factors prior to the first fall, possibly with more insight derived from the lessons learned from the recent event.

Assessment of Risk Factors

A detailed history of the index fall, if known or if witnessed, represents an excellent starting point. Particular attention should be paid to the social history, with a focus on environmental hazards and use of alcohol and illicit drugs. A thorough review of medications, including dose adjustments, is crucial as this is the most modifiable risk factor for preventing future falls.

The Comprehensive Geriatrics Assessment is one of the best approaches in assessing geriatric syndromes, including falls. The physical examination should start with assessment of vision changes, hearing changes (at times associated with balance changes), proprioception testing, gait and balance testing, pain assessment, focused neurological examination, orthostatic hypotension check, and vital signs.[9] Laboratory and other diagnostic tests are not routinely recommended; the decision should be informed by the previous history and physical examination findings.

Correcting the Identified Risk Factors

The following interventions have variable degrees of evidence in decreasing the risk of falling among elderly adults:

Minimizing medications
Initiating a tailored exercise program including strengthening, balance, and gait training
Treating vision impairment
Correcting foot problems
Treating postural hypotension and arrhythmias
Adding vitamin D supplementation
Making home/environment modifications.[6,10,11]

Integrative Approaches for Falls

MOVEMENT AND EXERCISE

Tai chi has gained popularity as a falls prevention strategy given that it is reasonably easy to learn, does not require complex equipment, and is inexpensive. There are a lot more tai chi teachers even in remote areas than comprehensive falls prevention exercise programs, and evidence supporting use of tai chi for falls prevention is robust.[12] Surprisingly, yoga does not appear to be effective at falls prevention.[13]

NUTRITION AND SUPPLEMENTS

The anti-inflammatory, Mediterranean diet has been shown to reduce the risk of frailty and falls in the elderly.[14] Adequate protein intake of 1.0 to 1.2 g per kilogram of body weight per day is important as part of frailty prevention and is discussed in detail in Chapter 2.[15]

Vitamin D optimization has strong evidence for falls prevention. Minimum recommended intake for all elders is 800 to 1,000 IU/day.[6] The authors recommend maintaining the vitamin D level at at least 30 and ideally in the range of 40 to 60 ng/ml.

Table 23.2. Summary of Integrative Program for Falls Prevention

Diet	Mediterranean, anti-inflammatory diet including increased fatty fish intake and anti-inflammatory herbs such as turmeric
Exercise	Promote mobility, walking, resistance training, tai chi
Supplements	Vitamin D, increased protein intake
Hormones	Not recommended for routine use. Treat deficiency states on individualized basis.

ANDROGEN REPLACEMENT

Routine hormonal treatments as part of falls prevention is not recommended, but low levels of dehydroepiandosterone (DHEA) and testosterone are associated with frailty and falls.[16,17] Given the growing body of evidence supporting the clinical use of carefully monitored DHEA supplementation to maintain a normal DHEA-S level, the authors recommend individualized assessment and treatment.[18] The typical daily DHEA dose is 25 to 50 mg for men and 5 to 25 mg for women. Initiating testosterone treatment is much more challenging and should not be based on the risk of falls alone. While a number of safety concerns of using testosterone replacement have been raised, some concerns may be overstated, and avoiding any replacement in all patients seems to be unwarranted.[19] For a more detailed review of testosterone replacement see Chapter 10.

Table 23.2 summarizes some integrative programs for preventing falls.

REFERENCES

1. Przybelski RJ, Shea TA. Falls in the geriatric patient. *WMJ.* 2001;100(2):53–56.
2. Aschkenasy MT, Rothenhaus TC. Trauma and falls in the elderly. *Emerg Med Clin North Am.* 2006;24(2):413–432. doi:10.1016/j.emc.2006.01.005.
3. Heinrich S, Rapp K, Rissmann U, Becker C, König HH. Cost of falls in old age: A systematic review. *Osteoporos Int.* 2010;21(6):891–902. doi:10.1007/s00198-009-1100-1.
4. Sterling DA, O'Connor JA, Bonadies J. Geriatric falls: Injury severity is high and disproportionate to mechanism. *J Trauma.* 2001;50(1):116–119. doi:10.1097/00005373-200101000-00021.
5. Bueno-Cavanillas A, Padilla-Ruiz F, Jiménez-Moleón JJ, Peinado-Alonso CA, Gálvez-Vargas R. Risk factors in falls among the elderly according to extrinsic and intrinsic precipitating causes. *Eur J Epidemiol.* 2000;16(9):849–859. doi:10.1023/A:1007636531965.
6. Lappe JM, Binkley N. Vitamin D and sarcopenia/falls. *J Clin Densitom.* 2015;18(4):478–482. doi:10.1016/j.jocd.2015.04.015.

7. Zia A, Kamaruzzaman SB, Tan MP, et al. Polypharmacy and falls in older people: Balancing evidence-based medicine against falls risk. *Postgrad Med.* 2015;127(3): 330–337. doi:10.1080/00325481.2014.996112.

8. Ambrose AF, Cruz L, Paul G. Falls and fractures: A systematic approach to screening and prevention. *Maturitas.* 2015;82(1):85–93. doi:10.1016/j.maturitas.2015.06.035.

9. Stuck AE, Siu AL, Wieland GD, Adams J, Rubenstein LZ. Comprehensive geriatric assessment: A meta-analysis of controlled trials. *Lancet.* 1993;342(8878):1032–1036. doi:10.1016/0140-6736(93)92884-V.

10. Kenny RA, Romero-Ortuno R, Cogan L. Falls. *Medicine (Baltimore).* 2013;41(1): 24–28. doi:10.1016/j.mpmed.2012.10.010.

11. Drootin M. Summary of the updated American Geriatrics Society/British Geriatrics Society clinical practice guideline for prevention of falls in older persons. *J Am Geriatr Soc.* 2011;59(1):148–157. doi:10.1111/j.1532-5415.2010.03234.x.

12. Schleicher MM, Wedam L, Wu G. Review of tai chi as an effective exercise on falls prevention in elderly. *Res Sport Med.* 2012;20(1):37–58. doi:10.1080/15438627.2012.634697.

13. Cramer H, Sibbritt D, Adams J, Lauche R. The association between regular yoga and meditation practice and falls and injuries: Results of a national cross-sectional survey among Australian women. *Maturitas.* 2016;84:38–41. doi:10.1016/j.maturitas.2015.10.010.

14. León-Muñoz LM, Guallar-Castillón P, López-García E, Rodríguez-Artalejo F. Mediterranean diet and risk of frailty in community-dwelling older adults. *J Am Med Dir Assoc.* 2014;15(12):899–903. doi:10.1016/j.jamda.2014.06.013.

15. Landi F, Calvani R, Tosato M, et al. Anorexia of aging: Risk factors, consequences, and potential treatments. *Nutrients.* 2016;8(2). doi:10.3390/nu8020069.

16. Voznesensky M, Walsh S, Dauser D, Brindisi J, Kenny AM. The association between dehydroepiandrosterone and frailty in older men and women. *Age Ageing.* 2009;38(4):401–406. doi:10.1093/ageing/afp015.

17. Kurita N, Horie S, Yamazaki S, et al. Low testosterone levels, depressive symptoms, and falls in older men: A cross-sectional study. *J Am Med Dir Assoc.* 2014;15(1): 30–35. doi:10.1016/j.jamda.2013.11.003.

18. Rutkowski K, Sowa P, Rutkowska-Talipska J, Kuryliszyn-Moskal A, Rutkowski R. Dehydroepiandrosterone (DHEA): Hypes and hopes. *Drugs.* 2014;74(11):1195–1207. doi:10.1007/s40265-014-0259-8.

19. Schwartz E, Morelli V, Holtorf K. Hormone replacement therapy in the geriatric patient: Current state of the evidence and questions for the future: Estrogen, progesterone, testosterone, and thyroid hormone augmentation in geriatric clinical practice: Part 2. *Clin Geriatr Med.* 2011;27(4):561–575. doi:10.1016/j.cger.2011.07.004.

24

Skin, Vision, and Hearing

ILANA SEIDEL AND JUSTIN SEVIER

As you delve into this chapter you will learn about skin cancers, xerosis, pressure ulcers, vision changes, and hearing loss in the geriatric population. These subjects are placed together due to the fact that skin and the epithelia of the eyes and ears stem are from the same embryonic layer, the ectoderm.[1] Over time, organs lose their ability to adapt to the oxidative stressors from internal and external environments, though exercise and other lifestyle factors may alleviate the effects of aging. We will further delineate the effects of the physical transformations later in this chapter. The aging process brings on not only physical changes, but also changes that can affect an individual emotionally.

Cells, including skin cells, lose their capacity to repair DNA and overcome oxidative stress with age. Increased cancer risk, decreased elasticity, and an increased propensity toward bruising[2] can lead to depression over subjective loss of beauty and anxiety over changes in skin color or texture. The incidence of pressure ulcers increases with age, resulting in not only an increase in the risk of infection but also an increase in pain and discomfort, resulting in a higher level of distress[3] and possibly leading to a more depressed mental state.

Vision can be affected by a loss of lens flexibility[4] and an increased risk of cataract formation due to protein misfolding caused by exposure to ultraviolet light.[5] The resulting presbyopia and decreased visual acuity may lead to decreased driving for affected individuals, so they will require more aid while shopping or reaching social centers.[6] Hearing changes and loss bring their own difficulties, but when accompanied by vision loss, also known as dual sensory loss, the patient experiences a decreased ability to communicate, social isolation, depression, and difficulty with daily activities such as transportation.[6] This chapter provide some alternative recommendations for prevention or delaying age-related skin conditions, eye diseases, and hearing loss, along with mock case studies to help explain risk factors.

Skin and Aging

Researching skin aging is complex because anatomical and histological skin layers age independently and respond differently to the same stressors.[7] Extrinsic factors such as ultraviolet radiation and tobacco smoking cause skin aging in sun-exposed areas.[8] The skin develops deep wrinkles that do not disappear upon stretching, epidermal thickening, roughness, and mottled discoloration.[9,10] Intrinsic factors such as genetic predisposition[11] and endocrine milieu[12] are major players in skin aging for covered areas. In this instance, the skin develops a thin and atrophic appearance, fine wrinkles that disappear with stretching, loss of underlying fat, reduced elasticity and prominent dryness with pruritus.[7]

MELANOMA

Jon is a 67-year-old blond green-eyed white male with a childhood history of blistering sunburns while sailing, a current recent unplanned weight loss, and a 7-mm asymmetrical brown and black lesion with border irregularity, diagnosed as malignant melanoma on biopsy.

Prevention for Jon's melanoma would have included avoiding bursts of sun exposure and receiving annual skin examinations. His blond hair, green eyes, pale skin, and inability to tan predisposed Jon to melanoma.[13] Evans et al. reported additional predisposing factors such as a personal history of keratinocyte cancer (previously categorized as non-melanoma skin cancers), melanoma cutaneous cancer, actinic keratosis, higher socioeconomic status, and increased neocytic nevi.[13]

Nutrients, botanicals, and supplements have been shown to be beneficial for both prevention and treatment of skin cancers. Serini found that the omega-3 DHA in food enhances MITF expression and PKA-dependent nuclear B catenin phosphorylation, which suppresses melanoma progression to invasive malignancy.[14] In vivo and in vitro studies indicate that curcumin has a cytotoxic, antiproliferative,[15] and apoptotic[16] effect on melanoma cells.[17,18] Recommended dosages range from 500 to 1,000 mg three times a day for its anti-inflammatory effects.[17] Green tea polyphenols inhibit melanoma cell growth through class I histone deacetylases inhibition.[19] Fortes found that consuming nutrients from the Mediterranean diet exhibited a protective effect for melanoma.[20]

In addition to supporting health via food choices, certain probiotic species have preliminarily been found to confer anti-melanoma activity. Though additional research is needed, Gueniche indicated that a change in skin homeostasis caused by ultraviolet exposure could be decreased by *Lactobacillus johnsonii* NCC 533.[21]

KERATINOCYTE CANCER

Amy is a 66-year-old female CEO with a history of tanning bed usage presenting with a pearly pink papule with telangiectatic vessels on her back. William is an 82-year-old fair-skinned, blue-eyed male with difficulty tanning who presents with an ulcerated red plaque on his forehead. Workup of the lesions indicated keratinocyte cancer (KC), Amy with basal cell carcinoma and William with squamous cell carcinoma.

KC is the most common type of cancer among Americans.[22] At least 3 million individuals in the United States are diagnosed with KC annually.[23] Prevention of KC includes minimizing sunburns, including from tanning beds. Katta et al. reported a "promising trend [of reducing the risk of KC] when dietary antioxidants (vitamin C, vitamin E, beta carotene, selenium) were provided via eating whole foods rather than via taking supplements."[22] Although natural ingestion of antioxidants through food is often preferred due to the antioxidants' synergistic mechanism of action in foods, supplementation can sometimes be beneficial. Chen et al. reported that 500 mg of nicotinamide twice a day significantly decreased the rate of new KC and new-onset actinic keratosis at 12-month follow-up appointments. Of note, there were no adverse effects, but the positive effects lasted only while actively taking the nicotinamide.[24] Treatment for KC includes Mohs micrographic surgery as first-line treatment, cryotherapy for tumors less than 3 mm deep, and topical imiquimod or fluorouracil for low-risk tumors.[25] Mohs surgery involves injection of a local anesthetic, removal of the thinnest possible layer of visible cancerous tissue, having the patient wait in the waiting room while the dermatologist examines the tissue, and then having the patient return to surgery if an additional layer needs to be removed. Cryotherapy uses low temperatures to freeze lesions.[25]

SUN EXPOSURE

As previously mentioned, predisposition to skin cancers includes a history of sunburns. A Cochrane review[26] of sun protection for preventing basal cell and squamous cell skin cancers that included physical barriers in the search terms found one randomized controlled study that was suitable for inclusion. This study ended up not demonstrating whether sunscreens are effective in preventing KC; in fact, there seemed to be no difference in the risk of developing KC between those applying sunscreen daily and those who did not. Some experts have indicated alternative avenues for protection. Wearing protective clothing may minimize sunburns; polyester has the highest ultraviolet light absorption and cotton has the lowest.[27] Hats protect the head and neck and sunglasses protect the periorbital region.[28] It is important to remember that minimizing sunlight exposure may lead to vitamin D deficiency and depression.[29] Therefore, one general approach is to avoid exposure during high-intensity sunlight to minimize the risk of sunburns.

XEROSIS

George is a relatively healthy 82-year-old African American man who comes to his primary care physician complaining of rough, tight, flaky and ashen skin with an itchy sensation. This had started about 6 months after he had omitted most fats from his diet because he was told that fats were unhealthy. This presentation of xerosis is not inevitable, but it is multifactorial.[30,31] It turns out that fat is an important key to healthy skin. In fact, intrinsic factors affecting the development of xerosis include changes in keratinization and lipid content. Brosche reports that borage oil consumption induces a statistically significant improvement of cutaneous barrier function and less dry skin in elderly people.[32] De Spirt et al found that a dose of 2.2 g of total fatty acids with either flax seed or borage oil caused significantly increased skin hydration after 12 weeks of treatment.[33]

Dehydration is a major external factor associated with the development of xerosis. It can be induced by the use of diuretics and comparable medications, low fluid intake, and use of heaters and air conditioners.[30,31] Allman reminds us that there is an increased risk of dehydration in the geriatric population due to the altered physiological control systems associated with thirst and satiety.[34] Levi recommends at least nine 8-ounce cups of fluid daily.[35] Serving high-fluid meals such as soups, casseroles, and gelatin in addition to increasing fluid intake with medication may aid in increasing overall water content.[35] Another method of improving skin hydration is via moisturizing with glycerol.[36] In fact, Fluhr linked distal extremity xerosis to decreased sebaceous gland activity causing glycerol depletion in mice.[37] Coderch et al. reported that a mixture of three lipids (cholesterol, free fatty acids, and ceramides) in an equimolar ratio repaired a skin barrier faster than applying one lipid or a mixture of two lipids.[38]

PRESSURE ULCERS

The topic of pressure ulcers is beyond the scope of this book and would require a full chapter in itself, but here we will list a few nutritional factors that are important, such as vitamin C, selenium, zinc, propolis, protein, and fatty acids, all of which form the general prevention of malnutrition.

There are many factors that can cause and contribute to the formation of pressure ulcers, such as age, uncontrolled diabetes, vascular disease, malnutrition, trauma, and immunosuppressive drugs.[39] In regards to malnutrition, currently there is much controversy over the effectiveness of vitamin C, selenium, and zinc on the reduction and prevention of pressure ulcers, but clinical research has presented promising results showing reduced healing time of the skin,[39] leading to less severity of infection and fewer occurrences.

The use of propolis has shown great promise in the treatment of pressure ulcers, with results similar to those of vitamin C, selenium, and zinc: reduced healing time, an increase in wound contraction, and accelerated tissue repair.[40] Though very limited, the analysis of Stan Scheller's study showed that the use of propolis was associated with complete healing of pressure ulcers in 9 of 10 patients.[40] This was due to the antimicrobial properties of propolis, which resulted in reduced infection that permitted the ulcer to heal.

While these topical and cofactors have not been sufficiently tested, the primary method of pressure ulcer prevention is proper nutritional support. Along with adequate hydration and tissue viability, tissue repair processes can be preserved, reducing the occurrence and healing time of pressure wounds.[41] In addition, a balanced diet comprising protein and fatty acids will ensure that the skin has a high level of health. By using these methods in combination, it is probable that many cases of pressure ulcers could be prevented and healed.

Vision

From sun damage, exposure to chemicals, polluted rain, chlorine in pool water, dirt particles in the wind, or simply just age, our eyes naturally take quite a beating throughout our lives. While deterioration or degeneration is not guaranteed as we age, the chances of developing one of the most common degenerative diseases (cataracts, macular degeneration, and glaucoma) increase exponentially.[42–44]

CATARACTS

There seems to be a lack of preventive care for the eyes and an over-reliance on surgery for handling degenerative eye diseases.[45] Within the traditional medical community, it is common to wait for surgical intervention, and while modern eye technology and surgical techniques have proven to be effective at removing cataracts and restoring vision, there can be negative side effects.[45] Also, not everyone has access to proper medical and surgical facilities, especially in the developing world. This necessitates the implementation of more accessible alternative methods for preventing and slowing cataract growth.[46] Since age-related cataracts are the cause of blindness for over 50% of the world's blind people,[47] it is important to spread the information about preventive techniques so that more patients could utilize them before experiencing issues.

Keith, a 64-year-old overweight male, complains of diminished and cloudy vision. He says his eyes feel very dry or he feels like there is something in his eye. He has a history of hypertension, arthritis, and type 2 diabetes, all diagnosed at around 40 years of age, but all have been controlled with medication. Keith started smoking at age 16 but has been smoke-free for the past 10 years. After being seen by an ophthalmologist, Keith is told he has an early cataract. The cause is said to be age-related, and it is determined that Keith will undergo surgery when the cataract progresses.

Cataracts have been linked to low concentrations of antioxidants in the lens, including coenzyme Q10[48] and glutathione.[45] With the reduction of key components of detoxification, the eye cannot control the presence of free radicals as effectively, and this may increase the chances of cataract formation.[45] It is thought that a low antioxidant content in the lens can increase the chances of cataract formation; thus, by increasing glutathione levels prolonged protection can be provided from oxidative stress and the onset of cataracts can be delayed.[45] Research has also shown that diabetes can increase the probability of developing cataracts due to the oxidative stress brought on by the excess of sugars in the system.[49,50] By maintaining an appropriate and healthy weight, people can reduce their chances of developing type 2 diabetes[51] and help to equip the immune system to handle stress. Methods such as quitting smoking[46] and using coping mechanisms such as meditation or other types of stress reduction will provide additional benefits[49,50,52]

Proper nutrition and hydration, along with numerous vitamins and supplements, could provide supportive care as an antioxidant and/or as a support for the liver. The consumption of flavonoid-containing foods, such as berries and leafy greens,[53] may strengthen and improve capillary flow, and the consumption of DHA and other free fatty acids may also slow growth.[54]

For Keith, surgery is the most definitive form of treatment, but measures can be taken to slow the growth of the cataract and prepare him for lifestyle changes to decrease the chances of another cataract forming once this one is removed. Keith should be started on a lutein and zeaxanthin supplement at 10 mg/day for the first month followed by 6 mg/day as a routine dose. Olmedilla et al. have shown that supplementation with these can reduce the rate of growth of early cataracts and even improve vision function altogether, including visual acuity and glare sensitivity, due to the antioxidant and protective nature of lutein.[55] A supportive study has indicated that soluble propolis may reduce oxidative stress and thus diminish the growth and formation of cataracts related to sugars in the body.[56] Concurrently, Keith should follow a diet and exercise plan to reduce stress and weight, and begin to include supplementation for detoxification, antioxidant support, and liver support, reducing his chances of developing another cataract.

MACULAR DEGENERATION

Sam is an 84-year-old male complaining of sudden diminishment of vision that he cannot explain. A detailed medical history shows that he has been a pack-a-day smoker since the age of 17, has a history of alcoholism and currently drinks six to eight beers each night, has a generally inactive lifestyle, and believes that nutrition has no effect on his health. Upon ophthalmic examination he is found to have early age-related macular degeneration (AMD).

AMD affects 10% of people over 65 years of age, and that percentage rises to 30% after the age of 75.[57] Research shows that the risk factors and preventive care for AMD are similar to those for cataracts—that is, negative environmental factors and the addition of positive nutritional and lifestyle changes.[58]

Early detection through screening is paramount in order to have more options for alternative therapies due to the slow, sometimes unnoticed progression of the disease. Almost identical to the preventive methods for cataracts and resulting in the same benefits, patients should use proper stress management techniques, exercise regularly and maintain an active lifestyle, maintain adequate hydration, get plenty of sleep, and optimize whole-body health with proper nutrition.[59,60]

The Age-Related Eye Disease Study Research Group indicates that the combination of vitamins C and E, beta-carotene, and zinc slowed the progression of macular degeneration, possibly due to the supportive and antioxidant nature of these vitamins and minerals.[61] In addition, people who consume DHA via cold-water fish at least once per week were half as likely to experience macular degeneration as those consuming DHA less frequently.[62,63]

GLAUCOMA

Lauren is a 70-year-old woman who has been diagnosed with non-acute chronic glaucoma. She presents with a family history of glaucoma and through regular screening, due to a likely genetic component, discovered the degeneration of the optic nerve early. Commonly with open-angle chronic glaucoma, most patients will not experience any symptoms until sight loss has already taken effect and the degeneration has already progressed.[64] Her ophthalmologist has prescribed some of the typical medications for maintaining a healthy intraocular pressure (IOP), but she has not been able to tolerate them. Due to this intolerance, Lauren's ophthalmologist has recommended alternative means for controlling the IOP elevation and, if need be, surgery to resolve the problem.

It is not largely understood the exact mechanisms that cause and contribute to glaucoma, but it is believed that IOP is associated with the degeneration of nerve cells, reduced ocular blood flow, and increased oxidative stress.[65] Many factors can link glaucoma with other neurodegenerative disorders, including issues related to the immune and central nervous system, proper blood flow to the eye, and oxidative stress.[66] By focusing on what can contribute to the progression of disease, one can apply numerous alternative methods to improve IOP and ocular blood flow and reduce oxidative stress.

Similar to alternative methods for cataracts, vitamin C given at 0.5 g/kg, as well as flavonoids such as bilberry and pine bark extract and fish oil, has shown a reduction in IOP.[67] Intravenous delivery of vitamin C resulted in an even greater drop of IOP, with some patients responding to just 2 g/day while others need higher doses such as 35 g/day. Vitamin C can also increase blood osmolarity and improve outflow of aqueous fluid, thus reducing IOP with a significant increase in ocular blood flow.[67] Also, exercise has shown promise in lowering IOP within 1 hour of moderate to heavy exercise; effects could last up to 3 weeks in some patients.[64] While exercise has not been shown to reduce IOP in all patients, increased physical activity brings a host of other benefits, such as increased blood flow, better sleep, better stress management, and a stronger immune system.[64]

Each day Lauren should take vitamin C 0.1 to 0.5 g/kg; bioflavonoids 1,000 mg; magnesium 300 mg due to its ability to improve visual fields in glaucoma patients;[68] and chromium 100 mcg, as the mineral has shown to improve focusing power within the eye and research has shown a direct link between glaucoma, chromium, and vitamin C deficiency leading to IOP.[69]

For prevention and treatment of chronic glaucoma patients can take a combination of bilberry (160–240 mg/day) and pine bark extract (150–300 mg/day); mostly for normotensive glaucoma, patients can take 120 to 320 mg of *Ginkgo biloba* each day as research has shown that it increases ocular blood flow while not affecting heart rate or IOP[70] and significantly increases visual field indices.[64,71]

To optimize the effectiveness of these methods, patients should limit their caffeine intake and maintain control of allergies, as both caffeine and allergies have been proven to increase IOP. Corticosteroids should be avoided for their inhibiting effect on collagen.[64] Another alternative method that needs to be addressed is the use of cannabis for the reduction of IOP. While inhaled marijuana has been proven to reduce IOP, its effectiveness lasts only up to 4 hours. This limited amount of time, coupled with the mental and physical effects and high cost, limit its use.[72] The study by Jampel et al. has shown that there are known cannabinoid receptors in the eye, but there is difficulty providing an effective local dose as these specific chemicals are not readily water-soluble. However, the development of ophthalmic cannabinoid preparations is under way, and they may provide an interesting alternative to glaucoma medications.

Table 24.1 provides a summary of vitamins and supplements for preventing and treating cataracts, glaucoma, and macular degeneration.

Table 24.1. Vitamins and Supplements for Ophthalmic Use

Vitamins/Supplements	Cataracts	Glaucoma	Macular Degeneration
Alpha-lipoic acid			x
Arginine			x
Astragalus	x		
Beta-carotene	x		x
Choline (B4)			x
Chromium		x	
Cobalamin (B12)			
Copper			x
Curcumin	x		
DHA	x	x	x
Fish oil	x	x	x
Flavonoids	x	x	x
Folate (B9)			x
Garlic	x		
Gingko biloba		x	x

(continued)

Table 24.1. Continued

Vitamins/Supplements	Cataracts	Glaucoma	Macular Degeneration
Glutathione	x	x	x
Lutein	x		x
Magnesium		x	x
Melatonin		x	
Milk thistle	x		
Niacin (B3)	x		
Propolis	x		
Pyridoxine (B6)			x
Riboflavin (B2)	x		
Oleander	x		
Omega-3	x·		x
Sage			x
SAMe	x		
Selenium			x
Taurine			x
Thiamine (B1)	x		
Tocopherols			x
Turmeric root	x		
Vitamin A	x		x
Vitamin C	x	x	x
Vitamin E	x		x
Wheat sprouts	x		
Zeaxanthin	x		x
Zinc			x

Hearing

Lily is an 80-year-old woman who says that it is becoming difficult to hear her family and friends when they are talking to her. A specialist determined that there is nothing structurally wrong with her ear and that her hearing loss is just the result of old age. She was prescribed hearing aids and encouraged to utilize other methods to slow the rate of hearing loss, such as a regimen of vitamins and minerals and a diet rich in key nutrients found to be beneficial to presbycusis.

Forty percent of people over the age of 75 suffer from presbycusis (age-related hearing loss), making it the leading cause of deafness in the world. Studies continue to show that, much like every other bodily system, diet and nutrition play a role in prevention and maintenance of deficiencies, with presbycusis being no different. It is thought that the frequent exposure to loud sounds in our daily lives, such as listening to music through headphones, traffic and construction noise, and simply just changes in the internal structure of our ears, can cause hearing loss.[73]

Research has shown that many alternative methods, from simply proper nutrition to regulation of homocysteine and an adequate level of vitamins (e.g., B12 and folate) and minerals, may reduce the likelihood of developing presbycusis.[74] Oxidative stress is thought to play a significant role in gradual hearing loss, leading practitioners and researchers to look to "free-radical scavengers" as possible ways to deter or prevent presbycusis.[74]

Use of some vitamins and minerals may improve, or at a minimum decrease, one's chances of developing presbycusis. For example, vitamin C and rebamipide, scavengers of free radicals, improved hearing in 23 patients for all tested fields of sound except for 1,000, 2,000, and 4,000 Hz.[75] CoQ10 supplementation has shown improvements in all the fields not improved upon listed in the previous sentence.[76] However, more thorough studies are needed to verify these findings and the combination of these two methods of prevention and reduction, as some studies determined that these findings are insignificant.[77]

For Lily, by combining many of the studies about nutritional deficiencies in the elderly and alternative methods of protection, we can design a health plan to support her auditory system and delay more invasive measures. Because of their studied benefit in improving the quality of hearing, she should take a combination of vitamins A, E, and D and magnesium. In addition, vitamin B12 and folate can help to regulate her homocysteine levels. Finally, she should begin to add supportive foods into her diet to improve blood flow and microcirculation, such as oily fish, berries, *Ginkgo biloba*, copper-containing foods, and fresh fruits and vegetables. It is also thought that allergies can cause an issue in which a viscous fluid fills the ear instead of air, resulting in a dampening of sound vibrations. This can cause hearing loss, making it important for proper maintenance by ruling out any allergies along with the supplements and nutritious diet.[73]

Summary

As we age many deficiencies can develop, but the belief that there is nothing we can do to prevent damage to or support the skin, vision, and hearing in the elderly is a dangerous state of mind. Many of the supportive methods listed above are relatively cheap, are generally safe under professional guidance, and are very accessible to much of the population. They will not only have the potential to protect body systems but will likely have a systemic benefit for the patient beyond what the treatments are specifically prescribed for. By supporting more thorough studies of these vitamins and supplements, clinicians could reduce the amount of age-related deficiencies and ultimately help save or lengthen the elderly population's ability to see, hear, and live.

REFERENCES

1. Germ layers and their derivatives. Chapter 25 in *Review of Medical Embryology*, LifeMap Discovery. http://discovery.lifemapsc.com/library/review-of-medical-embryology/chapter-25-germ-layers-and-their-derivatives. Accessed January 12, 2017.
2. Physical changes with aging—geriatrics. *Merck Manuals Professional Edition*. http://www.merckmanuals.com/professional/geriatrics/approach-to-the-geriatric-patient/physical-changes-with-aging. Accessed January 12, 2017.
3. Payne D. Strategies to support prevention, identification and management of pressure ulcers in the community. *Br J Community Nurs*. 2016;21(Sup6). doi:10.12968/bjcn.2016.21.sup6.S10.
4. Heys KR, Friedrich MG, Truscott RJW. Presbyopia and heat: Changes associated with aging of the human lens suggest a functional role for the small heat shock protein, α-crystallin, in maintaining lens flexibility. *Aging Cell*. 2007;6(6):807–815. doi:10.1111/j.1474-9726.2007.00342.x.
5. Chauss D, Brennan LA, Bakina O, Kantorow M. Integrin αVβ5-mediated removal of apoptotic cell debris by the eye lens and its inhibition by UV-light exposure. *J Biol Chem*. 2015;290(51):30253–30266. doi:10.1074/jbc.m115.688390.
6. McDonnall M, Crudden A, LeJeune B, Steverson A, O'Donnell N. Needs and challenges of seniors with combined hearing and vision loss. *J Vis Impairment Blindness*. 2016;110(6):399–411. Accessed January 12, 2017.
7. Kanaki T, Makrantonaki E, Zouboulis CC. Biomarkers of skin aging. *Rev Endocr Metab Disord*. 2016;17(3):433–442. doi:10.1007/s11154-016-9392-x.
8. Makrantonaki E, Bekou V, Zouboulis CC. Genetics and skin aging. *Dermatol Endocrinol*. 2011;4:280–284.
9. Makrantonaki E, Zouboulis CC. Molecular mechanisms of skin aging: State of the art. *Ann N Y Acad Sci*. 2007;1119(1):40–50. doi:10.1196/annals.1404.027.
10. Nikolakis G, Makrantonaki E, Zouboulis CC. Skin mirrors human aging. *Hormone Mol Biol Clin Invest*. 2013;16(1). doi:10.1515/hmbci-2013-0018.
11. Makrantonaki E, Zouboulis CC. The skin as a mirror of the aging process in the human organism: State of the art and results of the aging research in the German National Genome Research Network 2 (NGFN-2). *Exp Gerontol*. 2007;42(9):879–886. doi:10.1016/j.exger.2007.07.002.

12. Makrantonaki E, Schönknecht P, Hossini AM, et al. Skin and brain age together: The role of hormones in the ageing process. *Exp Gerontol.* 2010;45(10):801–813. doi:10.1016/j.exger.2010.08.005.

13. Evans RD, Kopf AW, Lew RA, et al. Risk factors for the development of malignant melanoma—I: Review of case-control studies. *J Dermatol Surg Oncol.* 1988;14(4):393–408. doi:10.1111/j.1524-4725.1988.tb03373.x.

14. Serini S, Zinzi A, Vasconcelos RO, et al. Role of β-catenin signaling in the antiinvasive effect of the omega-3 fatty acid DHA in human melanoma cells. *J Dermatol Sci.* 2016;84(2):149–159. doi:10.1016/j.jdermsci.2016.06.010.

15. Abusnina A, Keravis T, Yougbaré I, Bronner C, Lugnier C. Anti-proliferative effect of curcumin on melanoma cells is mediated by PDE1A inhibition that regulates the epigenetic integrator UHRF1. *Mol Nutr Food Res.* 2011;55(11):1677–1689. doi:10.1002/mnfr.201100307.

16. Bush JA, Cheung K-JJ, Li G. Curcumin induces apoptosis in human melanoma cells through a Fas receptor/caspase-8 pathway independent of p53. *Exp Cell Res.* 2001;271(2):305–314. doi:10.1006/excr.2001.5381.

17. Odot J, Albert P, Carlier A, Tarpin M, Devy JRM, Madoulet C. In vitro and in vivo anti-tumoral effect of curcumin against melanoma cells. *Int J Cancer.* 2004;111(3):381–387. doi:10.1002/ijc.20160

18. Qiu Y, Yu T, Wang W, Pan K, Shi D, Sun H. Curcumin-induced melanoma cell death is associated with mitochondrial permeability transition pore (mPTP) opening. *Biochem Biophys Res Comm.* 2014;448(1):15–21. doi:10.1016/j.bbrc.2014.04.024.

19. Prasad R, Katiyar S. Polyphenols from green tea inhibit the growth of melanoma cells through inhibition of class I histone deacetylases and induction of DNA damage. *Genes Cancer.* 2015;6(1-2):49–61. doi:10.18632/genesandcancer.52.

20. Fortes C, Mastroeni S, Melchi F, et al. A protective effect of the Mediterranean diet for cutaneous melanoma. *Int J Epidemiol.* 2008;37(5):1018–1029. doi:10.1093/ije/dyn132.

21. Guéniche A, David P, Philippe B, Stephanie B, Elif B, Isabelle C-H. Probiotics for photoprotection. *Dermato-Endocrinology.* 2009;1(5):275–279. doi:10.4161/derm.1.5.9849.

22. Katta R, Brown DN. Diet and skin cancer: The potential role of dietary antioxidants in nonmelanoma skin cancer prevention. *J Skin Cancer.* 2015;2015:1–10. doi:10.1155/2015/893149.

23. Skin cancer (non-melanoma): Statistics. Cancer.Net. http://www.cancer.net/cancer-types/skin-cancer-non-melanoma/statistics. Published March 8, 2016. Accessed January 7, 2017.

24. Chen A, Martin A, Choy B, et al. A phase 3 randomized trial of nicotinamide for skin-cancer chemoprevention. *N Engl J Med.* 2015;373:1618–1626. doi:10.1056/NEJMoa1506197.

25. Firnhaber J. Diagnosis and treatment of basal cell and squamous cell carcinoma. *Am Fam Physician.* 2012;86(2):161–168.

26. Sanchez G, Nova J, Rodriguez-Hernandez A, et al. Sun protection (including sunscreens) to prevent basal cell carcinoma and cutaneous squamous cell carcinoma of the skin. *Cochrane Database System Rev.* 2016;(7). doi:10.1002/14651858.CD011161.pub2.

27. Diaz JH, Nesbitt LT. Sun exposure behavior and protection: Recommendations for travelers. *J Travel Med.* 2013;20(2):108–118. doi:10.1111/j.1708-8305.2012.00667.x.

28. Klostermann S, Bolte G. Determinants of inadequate parental sun protection behaviour in their children: Results of a cross-sectional study in Germany. *Int J Hygiene Envir Health.* 2014;217(2-3):363–369.

29. Maslin DL. Do suncreens protect us? *Int J Dermatol.* 2014;53(11):1319–1323. doi:10.1111/ijd.12606.

30. Hurlow J, Bliss DZ. Dry skin in older adults. *Geriatr Nurs.* 2011;32(4):257–262. doi:10.1016/j.gerinurse.2011.03.003.

31. White-Chu EF, Reddy M. Dry skin in the elderly: Complexities of a common problem. *Clin Dermatol.* 2011;29(1):37–42. doi:10.1016/j.clindermatol.2010.07.005.

32. Brosche T, Platt D. Effect of borage oil consumption on fatty acid metabolism, transepidermal water loss and skin parameters in elderly people. *Arch Gerontol Geriatr.* 2000;30(2):139–150. doi:10.1016/s0167-4943(00)00046-7.

33. Spirt SD, Stahl W, Tronnier H, et al. Intervention with flaxseed and borage oil supplements modulates skin condition in women. *Br J Nutr.* 2008;101(03):440–445. doi:10.1017/s0007114508020321.

34. Desforges JF, Allman RM. Pressure ulcers among the elderly. *N Engl J Med.* 1989;320(13):850–853. doi:10.1056/nejm198903303201307.

35. Levi R. Nursing care to prevent dehydration in older adults. *Aust Nurs J.* 2005;13:21–23.

36. Breternitz M, Kowatzki D, Langenauer M, Elsner P, Fluhr J. Placebo-controlled, double-blind, randomized, prospective study of a blycerol-based emollient on eczematous skin in atopic dermatitis: Biophysical and clinical evaluation. *Skin Pharmacol Physiol.* 2008;21(1):39–45. doi:10.1159/000111134.

37. Fluhr JW, Mao-Qiang M, Brown BE, et al. Glycerol regulates stratum corneum hydration in sebaceous gland deficient (Asebia) mice. *J Invest Dermatol.* 2003;120(5):728–737. doi:10.1046/j.1523-1747.2003.12134.x.

38. Coderch L, Pera MD, Fonollosa J, Maza ADL, Parra J. Efficacy of stratum corneum lipid supplementation on human skin. *Contact Dermatitis.* 2002;47(3):139–146. doi:10.1034/j.1600-0536.2002.470303.x.

39. Vega A. A review of the efficacy of zinc, selenium, and vitamin C in the treatment of pressure ulcers. *Topics Clin Nutr.* 2011;26(2):115–125. doi:10.1097/tin.0b013e31821931be.

40. Kucharzewski M, Kubacka S, Urbanek T, Wilemska-Kucharzewska K, Morawiec T. Stan Scheller: The forerunner of clinical studies on using propolis for poor and chronic nonhealing wounds. *Evidence Based Compl Altern Med.* 2013;2013:1–5. doi:10.1155/2013/456859.

41. Posthauer ME, Banks M, Dorner B, Schols JMGA. The role of nutrition for pressure ulcer management. *Advances Skin Wound Care.* 2015;28(4):175–188. doi:10.1097/01.asw.0000461911.31139.62.

42. Babalola OE, Murdoch IE, Cousens S. Blindness: How to assess numbers and causes? *Br J Ophthalmol.* 2003;87:282–284.

43. Friedman DS, O'Colmain BJ, Muñoz B. Prevalence of age-related macular degeneration in the United States. *Arch Ophthalmol.* 2004;122:564–572.

44. Baisakhiya S. Correlation between age, gender, waist-hip ratio and intra-ocular pressure in adult North Indian population. *J Clin Diag Res*. 2016;10(12): CC05–CC08. doi:10.7860/jcdr/2016/21487.8991.

45. Thiagarajan R, Manikandan R. Antioxidants and cataract. *Free Radical Res*. 2013;47(5):337–345. doi:10.3109/10715762.2013.777155.

46. Langford-Smith A, Tilakaratna V, Lythgoe PR, Clark SJ, Bishop PN, Day AJ. Age- and smoking-related changes in metal ion levels in human lens: Implications for cataract formation. *PLoS One*. 2016;11(1). doi:10.1371/journal.pone.0147576.

47. Pascolini D, Mariotti SP. Global estimates of visual impairment: 2010. *Br J Ophthalmol*. 2011;96(5):614–618. doi:10.1136/bjophthalmol-2011-300539.

48. Kernt M, Hirneiss C, Neubauer AS, Ulbig MW, Kampik A. Coenzyme Q10 pre-vents human lens epithelial cells from light-induced apoptotic cell death by reduc-ing oxidative stress and stabilizing BAX/Bcl-2 ratio. *Acta Ophthalmol*. 2010;88(3). doi:10.1111/j.1755-3768.2010.01875.x.

49. Bunce G. Animal studies on cataract. In Taylor A (ed), *Nutritional and Environmental Influences on the Eye*. Boca Raton, FL: CRC Press, 1999:105–115.

50. Janghorbani M, Amini M. Cataract in type 2 diabetes mellitus in Isfahan, Iran: Incidence and risk factors. *Ophthalmic Epidemiol*. 2004;11:347–358.

51. Sá CD, Heizen PG, Corralo V, Santos GGD, Soares NM. Chronic effect of aero-bic exercise on anthropometric, biochemical and hemodynamic variables in indi-viduals with type 2 diabetes mellitus: A systematic review. *Revista Andaluza de Medicina del Deporte*. 2016;9(4):173–179. doi:10.1016/j.ramd.2015.09.005.

52. Passo MS, Goldberg L, Elliot DL, Van Buskirk EM. Exercise training reduces intra-ocular pressure among subjects suspected of having glaucoma. *Arch Ophthalmol*. 1991;109:1096–1098.

53. Meyer CH, Sekundo W. Nutritional supplementation to prevent cataract forma-tion. *Dev Ophthalmol*. 2005;38:103–119.

54. Chang D, Rong S, Zhang Y, et al. Serum free fatty acids level in senile cataract. *J Am Coll Nutr*. 2014;33(5):406–411. doi:10.1080/07315724.2013.875420.

55. Olmedilla B, Granado F, Blanco I, Vaquero M. Lutein, but not alpha-tocopherol, supplementation improves visual function in patients with age-related cataracts: A 2-y double-blind, placebo-controlled pilot study. *Nutrition*. 2003;19:21–24.

56. Shibata T, Shibata S, Shibata N, et al. Propolis, a constituent of honey, inhibits the development of sugar cataracts and high-glucose-induced reactive oxygen species in rat lenses. *J Ophthalmology* 2016;2016:1917093.

57. Friedman DS, O'Colmain BJ, Muñoz B. Prevalence of age-related macular degen-eration in the United States. *Arch Ophthalmol*. 2004;122:564–572.

58. Seddon JM. Multivitamin multimineral supplements and eye disease: Age-related macular degeneration and cataract. *Am J Clin Nutr*. 2007;85:304S–307S.

59. Cho E, Seddon JM, Rosner B. Prospective study of intake of fruits, vegetables, vitamins, and carotenoids and risk of age-related maculopathy. *Arch Ophthalmol*. 2004;122:883–892.

60. Parekh N, Voland RP, Moeller SM. Association between dietary fat intake and age-related macular degeneration in the Carotenoids in Age-Related Eye Disease Study

(CAREDS): An ancillary study of the Women's Health Initiative. *Arch Ophthalmol.* 2009;127:1483–1493.

61. Age-Related Eye Disease Study Research Group. A randomized placebo-controlled clinical trial of high dose supplementation with vitamins C and E, beta-carotene and zinc for age-related macular degeneration and vision loss. AREDS report No. 8. *Arch Ophthalmol.* 2001;119:1417–1436.

62. Smith W, Mitchell P, Leeder S. Dietary fat and fish intake and age-related maculopathy. *Arch Ophthalmol.* 2000;118:401–404.

63. Augood C, Chakravarthy U, Young I. Oily fish consumption, dietary docosahexaenoic acid and eicosapentaenoic acid intakes, and associations with neovascular age-related macular degeneration. *Am J Clin Nutr.* 2008;88:398–406.

64. Pizzorno JE, Murray MT. *Textbook of Natural Medicine.* Edinburgh: Churchill Livingstone; 1999.

65. Mozaffarieh M, Flammer J. Ocular blood flow and glaucomatous optic neuropathy. Springer-Verlag Berlin Heidelberg, 2009. doi:10.1007/978-3-540-69443-4.

66. Schwartz M. Lessons for glaucoma from other neurodegenerative diseases: Can one treatment suit them all? *J Glaucoma.* 2005;14(4):321–323. doi:10.1097/01.ijg.0000169412.86387.ad.

67. Steigerwalt RD, Gianni B, Paolo M, et al. Effects of Mirtogenol on ocular blood flow and intraocular hypertension in asymptomatic subjects. *Mol Vis.* 2008 Jul 10;14:1288–1292.

68. Gaspar AZ, Gasser P, Flammer J. The influence of magnesium on visual field and peripheral vasospasm in glaucoma. *Ophthalmologica.* 1995;209:11–13.

69. Lane BC. Diet and glaucomas. *J Am Coll Nutr.* 1991;10:536.

70. Chung HS, Harris A, Kristinsson JK, et al. Ginkgo biloba extract increases ocular blood flow velocity. *J Ocul Pharmacol Ther.* 1999 Jun;15:233–240.

71. Quaranta L, Bettelli S, Uva MG, et al. Effect of Ginkgo biloba extract on preexisting visual field damage in normal tension glaucoma. *Ophthalmology.* 2003 Feb;110:359–362.

72. Jampel H. American Glaucoma Society Position Statement: Marijuana and the treatment of glaucoma. *J Glaucoma* 2010;19(2):75–76.

73. Lazarides L. Nutrition and age-related hearing loss. www.positivehealth.com/. http://www.positivehealth.com/article/nutrition/nutrition-and-age-related-hearing-loss. Published December 2002. Accessed July 2016.

74. Gopinath B, Flood VM, Rochtchina E, Mcmahon CM, Mitchell P. Serum homocysteine and folate concentrations are associated with prevalent age-related hearing loss. *J Nutr.* 2010;140(8):1469–1474. doi:10.3945/jn.110.122010.

75. Takumida M, Anniko M. Radical scavengers: A remedy for presbyacusis. A pilot study. *Acta Oto-Laryngol.* 2005;125(12):1290–1295. doi:10.1080/00016480510037032.

76. Guastini L, Mora R, Dellepiane M, Santomauro V, Giorgio M, Salami A. Water-soluble coenzyme Q10 formulation in presbycusis: Long-term effects. *Acta Oto-Laryngol.* 2010;131(5):512–517. doi:10.3109/00016489.2010.539261.

77. Polanski JF, Cruz OL. Evaluation of antioxidant treatment in presbyacusis: Prospective, placebo-controlled, double-blind, randomised trial. *J Laryngol Otol.* 2013;127(02):134–141. doi:10.1017/s0022215112003118.

25

Functional Laboratory Studies

DEIRDRE ORCEYRE, RONAK MEHTA, AND MIKHAIL KOGAN

Each day millions of laboratory tests are done in the United States. For example, in 2009 the Centers for Medicare & Medicaid Services Medicare Part B clinical laboratory claims processed 26.1 million basic metabolic profiles.[1] Clearly, laboratory studies are an important part of clinical care in all fields, and geriatrics is no exception.

While most tests are ordered to diagnose a specific condition or disease, in this chapter we describe less commonly used but no less valuable functional laboratory testing. The term "functional laboratory testing" comes from the field of functional medicine and deserves a short explanation. The field is the brainchild of Dr. Jeffrey Bland, a nutritional biochemist who began using individualized evidence-based biochemical nutritional and nutraceutical approaches over 25 years ago. This pioneering work is summarized in his *Textbook of Functional Medicine.*[2,3]

The Institute of Functional Medicine (IFM), a teaching organization, is dedicated to educating clinical providers on practical applications of functional medicine in practice and is the main resource for this new field of medicine.[4] The IFM defines functional medicine as follows: "It addresses the underlying causes of disease, using a systems-oriented approach and engaging both patient and practitioner in a therapeutic partnership." The IFM provides a variety of resources such as a comprehensive certification program in functional medicine and a number of useful online and paper resources and publications.

Functional medicine laboratory tests are often ordered not to diagnose any specific medical problems but instead to identify the patient's unique biochemical states. For example, instead of testing stool for the presence of parasites or pathological bacteria, the functional medicine provider may opt to look into

Table 25.1. Functional Laboratory Companies

	ALCAT	Genova	Quick Silver	Diagnostechs	Doctors Data	Spectracell	Cyrex	23andme	ZRT
GI stool	X	X		X	X				
Food sensitivity	X	X		X	X		X		
Heavy metals		X partial	X		X		X		
Adrenal stress index	X	X		X	X				X
Nutritional: Minerals/ vitamins		X	X			X			
Organic acids		X			X				
Fatty acids		X			X				
Oxidative stress		X			X	X			
Toxicities		X			X		X		
Intestinal permeability		X					X		
Non-food allergy	X	X							
Methylation	X	X				X			
Genetic		X						X	
Cardiovascular		X							
Hormones: male/female				X					X
SIBO		X							
Immune							X		
Insurance coverage:									
Medicare	no	yes	no	yes	no	yes	no	no	partial*
Medicaid	no	no	no	No	no	partial*	no	no	partial*
Tri-Care	no	yes	no	yes	no	yes	no	no	partial*
Commercial	no	partial	no	No	no	varies*	no	no	partial*

* Insurance coverage changes all the time, and this table's accuracy may be compromised by ongoing fluctuations in the health care market.

Labrix	Pharmasan	Salveo Diagnostics	Diagnostic Solution Labs	Analytical Research Lab	European Lab Nutrients/ HDRI	IGeneX	US Biotek	Breathtrackers/ Quin Tron	NCNM Clinic Laboratory
		X	X		X				
	X	X			X		X		
					X				
X	X	X							
	X			X	X		X		
					X		X		
	X								
							X		
		X			X		X		
					X				
X	X								
	X	X							
X	X	X							
								X	X
	X	X			X	X			
*varies	*varies	partial*	*varies	no	no	yes	no	no	No
no	no	partial*	no	no	no	no	no	no	p
*varies	*varies	partial*	yes	no	no	yes	no	no	partial*
partial*	*varies	partial*	partial	no	no	*varies	no	*varies	partial*

the global functioning of the patient's digestion by simultaneously assessing a variety of different markers such as pancreatic function, presence of normal healthy flora, level of total intestinal IgA, and a number of other biochemical markers.

Many functional medicine tests have some or all parts that are hard to distinguish from traditional laboratory tests. For example, Spectracell tests levels of vitamins, minerals, antioxidants, fatty acids, and others through a blood sample.[5] At first glance, it appears to be a routine methodology. However, instead of analyzing serum levels, this company analyzes intra-lymphocyte levels, thereby assessing the intracellular compartment and understanding intracellular metabolism.[5]

To continue this comparison, let's use magnesium testing. Checking serum magnesium levels rarely leads to correctly identifying patients with magnesium deficiency. Serum levels of magnesium are under tight control, often at the expense of intracellular magnesium stores. While serum magnesium plays an important role, it represents a very small amount of the total body magnesium, with most magnesium being in the intracellular form. This intracellular magnesium has many critical functions, and deficiency can contribute to clinical problems such as headaches, asthma, muscle cramps, and others. Intracellular magnesium depletion often coexists with normal serum magnesium, making intracellular level assessment quite important, particularly if a magnesium-related metabolism disturbance is suspected.[6]

Detailed training in functional medicine and functional medicine laboratory testing is beyond the scope of this chapter. Many trainings are available in this topic. The goal of this chapter is to provide a basic understanding of what is available in terms of functional lab techniques and companies. There are multiple types of functional labs, broken down by category here. Table 25.1 lists some of the most widely recognized functional lab companies.

Categories

The most commonly used categories of specialty testing are endocrine, digestive, food sensitivities, nutritional status, immune, and toxicity.

ENDOCRINE

Endocrine lab testing looks at several different systems—adrenal, thyroid, female hormone, androgen, endocrine pancreas, and pituitary. In particular, thyroid, androgen, pituitary, and endocrine pancreas are well evaluated with conventional bloodwork. However, adrenal and female hormone levels in the blood do not reflect optimal intracellular levels. For this reason, salivary and/or urine testing may be used instead of blood.[7]

Cortisol hormone testing is best evaluated via salivary methods. Scientific communities have been using this method for decades. Chronic stress can disrupt metabolism and ultimately contribute to neurological conditions, gastrointestinal symptoms, skin issues, disruption of thyroid hormone production and balance, and other complications.[8,9] Cortisol increases gut permeability, thereby contributing to food sensitivities, resulting in more symptoms and increased stress.[10] Using a one-day serial salivary collection, the circadian rhythm of cortisol excretion by the adrenal gland may be evaluated. For a detailed review of diurnal cortisol testing please refer to Chapter 14.

Female hormones may be evaluated in the blood, saliva, or urine. Blood levels reflect what is produced and circulating in the blood; salivary levels reflect what has been absorbed into the cell and excreted into the saliva, the argument being this will better reflect intracellular levels; urine levels reflect what is filtered through the kidney, broken down, and excreted as urinary metabolite.[7] There is great debate within the functional lab world as to which method is preferable. Additionally, what is preferable for a woman being treated with hormones may be different than for an untreated woman. Determining the right test for a given patient requires an educated medical opinion after evaluating the case thoroughly (Table 25.2).

DIGESTIVE

The typical digestive analysis in a primary care office is the ova and parasite test. This test does not evaluate digestive function, microbiome balance, digestive tract inflammation, or bacteria and yeast growth. Several functional lab companies provide digestive stool analyses to look for these various functions integral to digestive health and well-being. These companies analyze specific stool and salivary markers for gastrointestinal

Table 25.2. Hormones Tested and Best Method(s)

• Ovarian: saliva (direct)/urine (metabolites)	• Pancreas (insulin): blood
• Androgen: blood	• Thyroid: blood
• Adrenal: saliva (cortisol)/blood (DHEA)	• Pituitary: blood

function. This may include digestive enzyme breakdown products, inflammatory markers, short-chain fatty acids, DNA-identified or cultured bacteria, cultured yeast, ova and parasite microscopy, pH, occult blood, and more.

An emerging technology that should be mentioned is the use of PCR-DNA analysis to identify bacteria making up the individual microbiome of each patient. There is still debate over whether this new technology is superior to the traditional bacterial identification using culture growth. Arguments as to which method best identifies *living* bacteria abound.

Several labs offer testing for a functional condition called intestinal permeability (also known as leaky gut syndrome), a laxity of the gap junctions between enterocytes. Permeable gap junctions weaken the normal intestinal barrier, leading to absorption into the bloodstream and subsequent recognition by the immune system of foreign compounds such as incompletely digested foods, bacterial antigens, and toxins. Intestinal permeability is associated with increased sensitivities to foods, hyperreactivity of the immune system, and systemic symptoms and conditions associated with gastrointestinal inflammation.[11]

In certain disease states of the small intestine, such as gluten-sensitive enteropathy, permeability to large molecules may increase while permeability to small molecules decreases—a result of damage to the microvilli. In this way, a person may have malnutrition concurrent with hyperreactivity of the immune system secondary to intestinal permeability.[12]

A special category arising within the functional digestion arena is testing for a condition known as *small intestinal bowel overgrowth* (SIBO). SIBO is a complex condition of microbiome imbalance within the small intestine, leading to intestinal symptoms such as gas, bloating, constipation, and diarrhea. As with any digestive compromise, SIBO may also lead to systemic symptoms stemming from nutritional deficiency and/or inflammation. The gold standard for SIBO testing is a hydrogen/methane breath test. Discussion is ongoing as to the best technology and procedure for this testing; for example, companies may offer a 2-hour, 3-hour, or 4+-hour breath collection (Table 25.3).[13]

Table 25.3. Two- and Three-Hour Tests

2-hour test: Genova Diagnostics	*3-hour test:* Biohealth Laboratory; Breath Trackers/Quin Tron; NCNM Clinic SIBO Lab

Conditions that may benefit from the use of functional digestive lab testing include the following:

- Irritable bowel syndrome (IBS)
- Inflammatory bowel disease
- Diabetes
- Chronic loose stools or diarrhea
- Chronic constipation
- Excessive eating or anorexia
- Obesity
- Cardiovascular disease
- Celiac and other malabsorption disorders
- Suspected or known malabsorption issues
- Chronic abdominal discomfort or pain
- Chronic skin conditions
- Mood disorders
- Autoimmune
- Autism
- Sudden changes in bowel habits
- Gas and bloating
- Chronic fatigue
- Acute loose stools or diarrhea, particularly after travel or camping

FOOD SENSITIVITIES

Food sensitivity testing is worthy of a textbook all on its own. Simply stated, there is no one best way to test food sensitivities, and many options exist for evaluation. Other than type 1 IgE hypersensitivity (the only true *allergy)*, other methods are not well evidenced but are widely used and considered useful by many practitioners.

IgE tests are the most commonly used, traditional food allergy tests, such as the RAST/blood test or the skin prick test. They look for type 1 acute hypersensitivity reactions.

IgG (blood) and IgA (blood, stool, or saliva) tests are widely used by many of the larger companies along with lymphocyte reactivity assays or other non-antibody-mediated cytotoxicity tests. These are type 2 hypersensitivity reactions.

The most difficult type of reaction to evaluate are the types 3 and 4 hypersensitivities, as these use many different reactive processes within the complex

Table 25.4. Companies and Techniques

Skin prick	IgE dermal test
RAST	IgE blood test
US Biotek	IgG/E/A blood test
Genova	IgG/IgE blood test
ELISA/ACT	Lymphocyte reactive assay
ALCAT	Cellular reactions
VEGA test	Electrodermal/acupuncture point
Applied kinesiology/muscle testing and pulse testing	

immune system. Neutrophils, complement, IgG, T-cell-mediated reactions, and more may be involved. Some companies evaluate lymphocyte reactivity or calculate cytokine activity. Some techniques use acupuncture points, pulse rate, or muscle strength to assess food sensitivities (Table 25.4).[14]

Conditions that may benefit from the use of food sensitivity testing are as follows:

- Gastrointestinal disorders (e.g., diarrhea/constipation, bloating, IBS, gastritis, reflux, colitis, associated malabsorption [nutritional deficiencies])
- Neurological symptoms (e.g., migraines, headaches, memory problems, chronic fatigue, mood swings, depression [neuroendocrine immune system], attention-deficit/hyperactivity disorder, neuropathy, cognitive impairment)
- Respiratory disease (e.g., chronic cough, wheezing/bronchoconstriction, sinusitis, asthma)
- Metabolic/endocrine disorders (e.g., obesity, diabetes, metabolic syndrome)
- Inability to lose weight, weight loss, thyroid illness and diseases, infertility history
- Skin symptoms (e.g., eczema, psoriasis, rashes, keratosis pilaris, urticaria, acne)
- Muscular/skeletal disorders (e.g., stiff or sore joints, arthritis, tendinitis)
- Immune system and other comorbidities (e.g., reduced immunity against infections, allergies, autoimmune diseases, heart problems, progression of tumors, other symptoms related to chronic activation of the immune system)
- Insomnia
- Fatigue
- Ear infections

- Weight loss
- Anemia
- Blood clotting abnormalities

The gold standard in food sensitivity testing is still considered to be the elimination and reintroduction diet, either eliminating one food at a time or using a broad elimination diet. As the half-life of reactive immune factors may be many weeks (e.g., 21 days for IgG), it is often recommended to avoid the food(s) for a minimum of 3 to 6 weeks to determine reactivity. Patients keep a symptom journal during the diet and as foods are carefully reintroduced. The reintroduction process is key in identifying food triggers. Unfortunately, because this method is tedious, many patients are unable to do it.

When discussing food sensitivities, *gluten sensitivity* deserves particular attention. Traditionally, celiac disease has been recognized as an autoimmune gluten enteropathy, with particular changes to the villi of the small intestine, leading to inflammation of the intestines and malabsorption, with subsequent deficiency conditions such as vitamin B12 deficiency, anemia, dermatitis herpetiformis, fat malabsorption, diarrhea, and fatigue. The gold standard for celiac disease diagnosis was a positive biopsy of the small intestine showing loss of villi. Additionally, certain blood tests were used for diagnosis, such as anti-gliadin antibody (IgG/IgA), tissue transglutaminase antibodies (IgG/IgA), anti-reticulin antibodies, and/or anti-endomysial antibodies. Finally, certain genes were identified predisposing for celiac disease, known as the HLA-DQ proteins.[15]

Many clinicians have recognized that this method for diagnosing frank celiac disease misses many cases of *gluten sensitivity*, or a reaction of the immune system to the ingestion of gluten proteins.[16] Gluten sensitivity may not include the significant changes to the villi of the small intestine that are diagnostic of celiac disease but may trigger inflammatory attacks on other systems, including the nervous, endocrine, and rheumatologic systems. It is widely recognized that certain autoimmune conditions have a direct correlation to gluten sensitivity.[17] Clinically, learning to identify risk factors for non-celiac gluten sensitivity and to differentiate among celiac disease, non-celiac gluten sensitivity, and other grain-related conditions such as SIBO is critically important.[18,19]

NUTRITIONAL STATUS

Functional lab evaluation of nutritional status generally refers to intracellular nutrients or metabolites via blood cells and plasma, but it may include urine and hair analysis. Certain tests use data analytics algorithms to identify patterns of functional nutritional deficiency or insufficiency.

For example, quantities of certain intracellular biomarkers give an indication of essential fatty acid absorption and utilization, helping to guide supplementation with omega 3-6-9 fatty acids and other types of dietary fats. Science has moved quickly, and such data analysis can give information about the actual functional availability of vitamins and minerals, along with indicators of the intestinal microbiome, neurotransmitter metabolism, energy production and mitochondrial function, vitamin and mineral metabolism, detoxification, and much more using blood and urine samples. A unique feature of these complex tests is their inclusion of assessment of oxidative stress. For example, NutrEval includes glutathione and CoQ10 levels; if low, these could indicate increased oxidative stress.[20,21]

Conditions that may benefit from the use of functional nutritional lab testing include the following:

- Behavioral disorders
- Chronic fatigue or fibromyalgia
- Mood disorder
- Anxiety
- Depression
- Mental and behavioral disorders such as depression and attention-deficit/hyperactivity disorder
- Headache
- Weight issues
- Sleep abnormalities
- Immune dysfunction
- Insomnia
- IBS
- Joint pain
- Chemical sensitivities
- Cardiovascular disease
- Senile neurological degeneration
- Hormonal disorders
- Autoimmune disorders
- Arthritides
- Learning disorders
- Nutritional deficiencies
- Food allergies
- Inflammatory disorders
- Hair and skin conditions, such as dermatitis, alopecia, acne, brittle nails coarse dry hair, and frequent infections

TOXICITY

Some chronic health conditions do not respond as expected to treatment. Sometimes patients experience a constellation of symptoms that do not clearly stem from one disease or diagnosed condition. In these complex and chronic illnesses, it may be helpful to evaluate whether there is an accumulation of toxic chemicals and elements to which we are exposed through our food, air, and environment. This accumulation is not without consequences: toxins may cause damage to organ systems, disrupt normal metabolism, and interfere with the balance of essential nutrients. Chronic health conditions like autoimmune and neurodegenerative diseases, as well as cancer and even diabetes, have been associated with ongoing exposure to environmental toxins.[22]

Functional lab evaluations attempt to measure the body burden of or the immune system's reactivity to toxic chemicals within the body. This may include heavy metals such as mercury, lead, and arsenic as well as environmental chemicals known as persistent organic pollutants (POPs). POPs are emerging as important factors in chronic health conditions.[23] These include PCBs, pthalates, parabens, organophosphates, bisphenol A (BPA), volatile solvents, chlorinated pesticides, and many others:

> Approximately 2,300 new chemicals are annually submitted for review to the U.S. Environmental Protection Agency (EPA); less than half of the high-volume chemicals have been tested for toxic risk to humans and only 7 percent have been assessed for developmental effects in children. Unknown to many, the effects of multiple chemical exposures, or synergistic effects are rarely evaluated—researchers are only now beginning to learn of the serious and far-reaching consequences.[24]

Review Chapter 4 for additional resources on this topic.

To clear these toxins, the body has natural detoxification functions, primarily through the liver. Certain functional lab tests can help to identify how well these detoxification systems work, as they may be impacted by metabolic nutritional deficiencies and even genetic predisposition.

GENETICS

Mapping of the human genome has allowed investigation into the genetics of health and wellness. Many small genetic changes (single nucleotide polymorphisms [SNPs]) have been identified that impact metabolic pathways within the body. The most famous of these may be the MTHFR pathway, which has wide effects on the nervous system, cardiovascular system, and more. Some functional physicians are specializing in this type of testing as a way of individualizing care. SNP testing is available for assessing the cardiovascular system, endocrine/estrogen levels, gluten/food sensitivities, detoxification, and more. While this type of testing is rapidly growing, the lack of clinical studies and standardization makes it hard to utilize it in clinical practice.

ACKNOWLEDGMENT

The authors thank Jenna Abdelhadi, 2017 B.S. Candidate, Exercise and Nutrition Science, Pre-Medical Concentration, The George Washington University.

REFERENCES

1. Passiment E, Meisel JL, Fontanesi J, Fritsma G, Aleryani S, Marques M. Decoding laboratory test names: A major challenge to appropriate patient care. *J Gen Intern Med*. 2013;28(3):453–458. doi:10.1007/s11606-012-2253-8.
2. Jones D, ed. *Textbook of Functional Medicine*. Gig Harbor, WA: Institute of Functional Medicine; 2005.
3. Leyton E. Functional Medicine. *Can Fam Physician*. 2006;52(12):1540.
4. Institute for Functional Medicine website. https://www.functionalmedicine.org/. Published 2016.
5. Nutritional Status and Health. SpectraCell Laboratories website. https://www.spectracell.com/clinicians/products/mnt/. Published 2016.
6. de Baaij JHF, Hoenderop JGJ, Bindels RJM. Magnesium in man: Implications for health and disease. *Physiol Rev*. 2015;95(1):1–46. doi:10.1152/physrev.00012.2014.
7. Aardal-Eriksson E, Karlberg BE, Holm AC. Salivary cortisol—an alternative to serum cortisol determinations in dynamic function tests. *Clin Chem Lab Med*. 1998;36(4):215–222. doi:10.1515/CCLM.1998.037.
8. Olson KL, Marc DT, Mcmanus CJ. The hypothalamic-pituitary-adrenal axis: The actions of the central nervous system and potential biomarkers. In: Klatz R, Goldman R, eds. *Anti-Aging Therapeutics Volume XIII*. Chicago, IL: American Academy of Anti-Aging Medicine; 2012:91–100.
9. Fall DJ, Kellermann S-A. Addressing adrenal imbalance: The future of adrenal health. *Neurosci Inc*. 2012.
10. Yang P-C, Jury J, Söderholm JD, Sherman PM, McKay DM, Perdue MH. Chronic psychological stress in rats induces intestinal sensitization to luminal antigens. *Am J Pathol*. 2006;168(1):104–114; quiz 363. doi:10.2353/ajpath.2006.050575.

11. Buret AG. How stress induces intestinal hypersensitivity. *Am J Pathol.* 2006; 168(1):3–5.

12. Vojdani A. Molecular mimicry as a mechanism for food immune reactivities and autoimmunity. *Altern Ther Health Med.* 2015;21:34–45.

13. Siebecker A. SIBO breath testing resources. siboinfo.com.

14. Marc D, Olson K. Hypersensitivity reactions and methods of detection. *Townsend Lett.* January 2011:69–71.

15. Sollid LM, Thorsby E. HLA susceptibility genes in celiac disease: Genetic mapping and role in pathogenesis. *Gastroenterology.* 1993;105(3):910–922.

16. Sapone A, Bai JC, Ciacci C, et al. Spectrum of gluten-related disorders: consensus on new nomenclature and classification. *BMC Med.* 2012;10(1):13. doi:10.1186/1741-7015-10-13.

17. Fasano A, Sapone A, Zevallos V, Schuppan D. Nonceliac gluten sensitivity. *Gastroenterology.* 2015;148(6):1195–1204. doi:10.1053/j.gastro.2014.12.049.

18. Elli L, Branchi F, Tomba C, et al. Diagnosis of gluten related disorders: Celiac disease, wheat allergy and non-celiac gluten sensitivity. *World J Gastroenterol.* 2015;21(23):7110–7119. doi:10.3748/wjg.v21.i23.7110.

19. Elli L, Roncoroni L, Bardella MT. Non-celiac gluten sensitivity: Time for sifting the grain. *World J Gastroenterol.* 2015;21(2127):8221–8226. doi:10.3748/wjg.v21.i27.8221.

20. Mytilineou C, Kramer BC, Yabut JA. Glutathione depletion and oxidative stress. *Parkinsonism Relat Disord.* 2002;8(6):385–387. doi:10.1016/S1353-8020(02)00018-4.

21. Sohal RS, Forster MJ. Coenzyme Q, oxidative stress and aging. *Mitochondrion.* 2007;7(Suppl.):S103–111. doi:10.1016/j.mito.2007.03.006.

22. Sears ME, Genuis SJ. Environmental determinants of chronic disease and medical approaches: Recognition, avoidance, supportive therapy, and detoxification. *J Environ Public Health.* 2012;2012:356798. doi:10.1155/2012/356798.

23. Li QQ, Loganath A, Chong YS, Tan J, Obbard JP. Persistent organic pollutants and adverse health effects in humans. *J Toxicol Environ Health A.* 2006;69(21): 1987–2005. doi:10.1080/15287390600751447.

24. Landrigan PJ, Schechter CB, Lipton JM, Fahs MC, Schwartz J. Environmental pollutants and disease in American children: Estimates of morbidity, mortality, and costs for lead poisoning, asthma, cancer, and developmental disabilities. *Environ Health Perspect.* 2002;110(7):721–728. doi:10.1289/ehp.02110721.

26

Primary Care for Homebound Patients

ROBERT L. JAYES AND ROBERT M. KAISER

ome-based primary care, once a nearly universal practice, declined markedly in the mid-20th century but has experienced a recent resurgence.[1] It is now on the rise for several reasons: an aging population for which office-based care is less convenient, favorable changes in Medicare fee-for-service reimbursement, and a greater recognition that the care of sick homebound adults may be better done in their home.[2,3]

Medicare is the primary payer for most home-based primary care in the United States, as most patients who require this care are elderly. Medicare has two requirements for patients receiving home visits: (1) patients receiving home care must be homebound, and going out to see the doctor would be a burdensome, taxing effort requiring the assistance of another person, and (2) the visit is medically necessary.[4] Most other payers (e.g., private insurance and Medicaid) have adopted similar requirements. In addition to fee-for-service Medicare, Medicare Advantage plans have played an increasing role in the management of homebound patients. In the public sector, the U.S. Veterans Health Administration (VHA) has had a home-based primary care program for over four decades—since the 1970s—and now serves approximately 25,000 veterans daily.[5]

There are a growing number of home care providers and a steadily increasing number of home visits annually in the United States. Practices range in size from primarily office-based practitioners seeing a few patients at home each week to large provider groups who see hundreds of homebound patients daily. Most practices accept available insurance, but there are a small but growing number of "concierge" practices who do not.[6] Most larger home care practices have evolved into multidisciplinary teams, where the skills of coordinators, social workers, and other disciplines augment the services of the direct care providers.[3] Nurse practitioners and physician assistants play a large role as care providers in most practices.

Although most home care practices focus on primary care, there have been intriguing experiments in providing specialty care and even "hospital at home" care for some illnesses. The management of selected patients with congestive heart failure and pneumonia who would otherwise have been admitted to the hospital has been studied[7–9] as well as treatment for many psychiatric conditions.[10] Most of these experiments have shown better outcomes for patients[9] but have not been adopted widely because they have not been supported by existing fee-for-service reimbursements. Alternative payment models, such as in accountable care organizations, are experimenting with the use of house calls as a way to reduce readmissions and other aspects of overutilization.[11,12]

In the future, virtual visits over the telephone or video conferencing will play an increasing role in extending medical care into the home. The safety, efficacy, and funding of these efforts are being explored.[13,14] Managed care organizations like Kaiser Permanente have embarked on such efforts, which include homebound as well as ambulatory patients.[15]

Potential Economic Impact of Home Care Practice

There is growing evidence that home care practices can care for homebound patients with multiple comorbidities more efficiently, with lower costs and equivalent or superior outcomes.[16–19] VHA has reduced hospital days by 63%, nursing home days by 83%, and total cost of care by 24%.[19] De Jonge et al. have demonstrated a similar reduction in total Medicare costs (17%) for sick homebound elders while measuring high patient and family satisfaction.[17] The Affordable Care Act funded the Independence at Home (IAH) demonstration project to assess the feasibility of incentivizing health care teams to reduce expenditures for homebound patients with three or more chronic conditions. Initial results have shown a promising reduction in expenses, and Congress has extended the IAH demonstration project. It is possible that a similar reimbursement scheme could soon be approved for national dissemination, which would provide a strong incentive for provider groups to organize similar efforts to provide home-based care for the Medicare population. If IAH becomes more widely available to Medicare recipients, some authors suggest that there could be billions of dollars in savings in the nation's Medicare budget.[20]

Components of a Home Visit

Home care is invaluable for individuals who may not be able to travel easily to a clinician's office: (1) those with disability (medical, functional, or cognitive) and multiple chronic medical conditions, who require ongoing home-based primary care; (2) those recovering from illness after a hospitalization, who need close follow-up for several weeks; and (3) those needing short-term care for a specific need, such as skilled wound care.

Primary care home visits include the initial comprehensive assessment, the continuity visit, the urgent visit, and the post-hospital visit. The home visit must address both the patient's and the clinician's agendas, which may be separate and sometimes divergent. The clinician must perform several important tasks: (1) asking the patient and caregiver about their foremost concerns; (2) checking vital signs; (3) assessing pain; (4) reviewing medications; (5) taking a history; (6) doing a physical examination; and (7) checking to see if the caregiver is overburdened. The home visit allows the clinician to find out firsthand if an individual is safe, feeling well medically and psychologically, eating normally, taking medications regularly, performing activities of daily living and instrumental activities of daily living, and receiving adequate social support.[21]

Other Programs Supporting Homebound Patients

Clinicians may often draw on governmental and nongovernmental resources in the community to assist patients at home:

- State and local Offices on Aging may provide information or referrals to useful programs, including delivery of meals, adult day care, transportation, home health aides, and caregiver support.[22]
- For those patients who are Medicaid-eligible, Medicaid Waiver Programs can offer extensive services in the home, such as home health aide services, in lieu of placement in a skilled nursing facility.[23]
- Medicare- or Medicaid-eligible patients may be referred for skilled services, such as wound care or physical or occupational therapy in the home, if clinically indicated.[24]
- Medicare patients with terminal illness may be referred to a community hospice program, which can provide home visits by a nurse and other members of the hospice team (physician, social worker, chaplain, and other disciplines) and can also provide home health aide support.[25]

- VHA has a nationwide Home-Based Primary Care Program through which eligible veterans may receive regularly scheduled visits from an interdisciplinary team at home.[26]

Integrative Health Practitioners' Current and Future Roles

Integrative medicine may provide helpful treatment modalities for individuals being cared for at home—in particular, complementary treatments for common conditions such as chronic pain, falls, depression, anxiety, and insomnia. Acupuncture[27] and massage[28] may be useful for those with pain that has not responded to traditional therapies. Patients with gait instability and a history of falling may benefit from tai chi.[29] Mindfulness training, relaxation exercises, and meditation[30] are additional practical interventions for patients with depression, anxiety, and insomnia. Integrative practitioners are not yet widely available for home care patients, but they have the potential to yield certain benefits, such as better pain control, a reduction in medication use, and increased patient satisfaction.

Teaching Students and Trainees in the Home

The home is an important educational setting in which learners can readily acquire the knowledge, skills, and attitudes that are essential in providing optimal care for complex, frail patients.[31] The home provides a rich context for acquiring fundamental clinical knowledge about patients—many of them older—with common chronic conditions. These conditions include the geriatric syndromes of falls, delirium, dementia, incontinence, polypharmacy, pressure ulcers, and depression. They also include chronic illnesses such as osteoarthritis, coronary artery disease, cerebrovascular disease, congestive heart failure, chronic obstructive pulmonary disease, hypertension, and neurological diseases such as stroke, multiple sclerosis, and amyotrophic lateral sclerosis. The home also provides the proper context for learning how to successfully integrate palliative and hospice care principles into patients' daily lives. Furthermore, the home is a setting where trainees can develop and hone essential clinical skills such as communication, history-taking, eliciting goals of care, medication review, physical examination, safety assessment, caregiver assessment, and inter-professional collaboration. Furthermore, seeing patients in the home can help trainees to cultivate positive attitudes such as respect for individual autonomy, empathy for individuals with chronic illness and disability, and professionalism toward patients and members of the interdisciplinary team.

The home is an ideal environment for students and trainees to learn about primary care for frail, complicated patients and their families. In the home, one can obtain a comprehensive picture of the patient's medical condition, mobility, function, nutritional status, medication adherence, psychological state, economic stability, family relationships, and social support system. It is a place where the patient may feel more comfortable and in control, compared with a traditional encounter in an office, where the clinician is in charge and may be a more formidable and imposing presence. This sense of comfort that the patient and family may feel in their own home can make it easier to carry on conversations, gather information, gain understanding of how a patient is doing day to day, and build effective and mutually beneficial clinical partnerships that will allow the patient to remain in the community and avoid emergency room visits, hospitalization, and institutionalization.[32]

The following are useful online resources:

American Academy of Home Care Medicine: http://www.aahcm.org
Area Agencies on Aging: https://caring.com/local/area-agency-on-aging
Medicaid Waiver Program: https://www.medicaid.gov/medicaid-chip-program-information/by-topics/waivers/home-and-community-based-1915-c-waivers.html
VA Home-Based Primary Care: http://www.va.gov/GERIATRICS/Guide/LongTermCare/Home_Based_Primary_Care.asp

REFERENCES

1. Peterson LE, Landers SH, Bazemore A. Trends in physician house calls to Medicare beneficiaries. *J Am Board Family Med.* 2012 November/December;25(6):862–868.
2. Landers SH. Why health care is going home. *N Engl J Med.* 2010 Oct 28;363(18):1690–1691.
3. DeCherrie LV, Soriano T, Hayashi J. Home-based primary care: A needed primary-care model for vulnerable populations. *Mt Sinai J Med.* 2012 Jul-Aug;79(4):425–432.
4. https://www.cms.gov/Regulations-and-guidance/Guidance/Transmittals/Downloads/R172BP.pdf Accessed May 1, 2016.
5. Edes T, Kinosian B, Vuckovic NH, et al. Better access, quality, and cost for clinically complex veterans with home-based primary care. *J Am Geriatr Soc.* 2014 Oct;62(10):1954–1961.
6. Leff B, Weston CM, Garrigues S, et al. Home-based primary care practices in the United States: Current state and quality improvement approaches. *J Am Geriatr Soc.* 2015 May;63(5):963–969.

7. Leff B, Burton L, Mader SL. et al. Hospital at home: Feasibility and outcomes of a program to provide hospital-level care at home for acutely ill older patients. *Ann Intern Med.* 2005;143:798–808.

8. Cryer L, Shannon SB, Van AM. et al. Costs for "hospital at home" patients were 19 percent lower, with equal or better outcomes compared to similar inpatients. *Health Aff (Millwood).* 2012; 31:1237–1243.

9. Caplan GA, Sulaiman NS, Mangin DA, et al. A meta-analysis of "hospital in the home". *Med J Austral.* 2012;197:512–519

10. Reckrey JM, DeCherrie LV, Dugue M, et al. Meeting the mental health needs of the homebound: A psychiatric consult service within a home-based primary care program. *Care Manag J.* 2015;16(3):122–128.

11. Wong FKY, Chow SKY, Chan TMF, Tam SKF. Comparison of effects between home visits with telephone calls and telephone calls only for transitional discharge support: A randomised controlled trial. *Age Ageing.* 2014 Jan;43(1):91–97.

12. Wong FKY, So C, Chau J, Law AKP, Tam SKF, McGhee S. Economic evaluation of the differential benefits of home visits with telephone calls and telephone calls only in transitional discharge support. *Age Ageing.* 2015 Jan;44(1):143–147.

13. Husebo AML, Storm M. Virtual visits in home health care for older adults. *Scientific World Journal.* 2014;2014:689873.

14. Van Offenbeek MAG, Boonstra A. Does tele-home consultation lead to substitution of home visits? Analysis and implications of a tele-home care program. *Stud Health Technol Inform.* 2010;157:148–153.

15. https://www.washingtonpost.com/business/capitalbusiness/innovators-at-kaiser-permanente-technology-brings-the-doctors-office-to-your-living-room/2014/02/28/ef6ae39c-9e56-11e3-a050-dc3322a94fa7_story.html Accessed May 1, 2016.

16. Stall N, Nowaczynski M, Sinha SK. Systematic review of outcomes from home-based primary care programs for homebound older adults. *J Am Geriatr Soc.* 2014 Dec;62(12):2243–2251.

17. De Jonge KE, Jamshed N, Gilden D, Kubisiak J, Bruce SR, Taler G. Effects of home-based primary care on Medicare costs in high-risk elders. *J Am Geriatr Soc.* 2014 Oct;62(10):1825.

18. Wajnberg A, Wang KH, Aniff M, Kunins HV. Hospitalizations and skilled nursing facility admissions before and after the implementation of a home-based primary care program. *J Am Geriatr Soc.* 2010 Jun;58(6):1144–1147.

19. Chang C, Jackson SS, Bullman TA, Cobbs EL. Impact of a home-based primary care program in an urban Veterans Affairs medical center. *J Am Med Dir Assoc.* 2009 Feb;10(2):133–137.

20. Boling PA, Leff B. Comprehensive longitudinal health care in the home for high-cost beneficiaries: A critical strategy for population health management. *J Am Geriatr Soc.* 2014 October;62(10):1974–1976.

21. Unwin BK, Tatum PE. House calls. *Am Fam Physician.* 2011 Apr 15;83(8):925–931.

22. Caring.com. AAAs Explained. 207-2016. Accessed on May 24, 2016, at: https://caring.com/local/area-agency-on-aging

23. Medicaid.gov. 1915(c) Home & Community-Based Waivers. Accessed on May 24, 2016, at: https://www.medicaid.gov/medicaid-chip-program-information/by-topics/waivers/home-and-community-based-1915-c-waivers.html

24. LongTermCare.gov. Medicare, Medicaid, and More. Accessed on May 24, 2016, at http://longtermcare.gov/medicare-medicaid-more/

25. CMS.gov. Hospice. Accessed on May 24, 2016, at: https://www.cms.gov/Medicare/Medicare-Fee-for-Service-Payment/Hospice/index.html

26. VA.gov. Home Based Primary Care. Accessed on May 24, 2016, at: http://www.va.gov/GERIATRICS/Guide/LongTermCare/Home_Based_Primary_Care.asp

27. Vickers, AJ, Cronin AM, Maschino AC, et al. Acupuncture for chronic pain. *Arch Intern Med.* 2012 Oct;172(19):1444–1453.

28. Crawford C, Boyd C, Paat CF, et al. The impact of massage therapy on function in pain populations—A systematic review and meta-analysis of randomized controlled trials: Part I, Patients experiencing pain in the general population. *Pain Medicine.* 2016 [E-pub ahead of print].

29. Hempel S, Shekelle PG, Taylor SL, et al. Evidence map of tai ihi. QUERI Evidence Based Synthesis Program. September 2014. Accessed on June 3, 2016, at: www.hsrd.research.va.gov/publications/esp/taichi-REPORT.pdf

30. Goyal M, Singh S, Sibinga EMS, et al. Meditation programs for psychological stress and well-being: A systematic review and meta-analysis. *JAMA Intern Med.* 2014 Jan;174(3):357–368.

31. Yuen JK, Breckman R, Adelman RD, Capello CF, LoFaso V, Reid MC. Reflections of medical students on visiting chronically ill older patients in the home. *J Am Geriatr Soc.* 2006 Nov 54(11):1778–1783. DOI: 10.1111/j.1532-5415.2006.00918.x

32. Kao H, Conant R, Soriano T, McCormick W. The past, present, and future of house calls. *Clin Ger Med.* 2009;25(1):19–34.

27

Person-Directed Health Care Across the Lifespan: The Veterans Affairs Health Care System

ELIZABETH L. COBBS, AMANDA HULL,
AND ALYSSA ADAMS

T he VA is the largest and most comprehensive health care system in the United States today and aims to provide an integrated, seamless continuum of person-directed care blending healing approaches across the lifespan (Table 27.1). The VA system has been recognized as being a highly evidence-based and cost-effective approach to serving the nation's veterans[1] and is especially important for older persons or those living with serious illness because it incorporates the idea of *becoming whole* even in the face of incurable illness or death.

The VA system has a number of elements that support this highly sophisticated and effective system. A well-established electronic comprehensive patient record system (CPRS) facilitates access to clinical patient information. Everything from the immunization history to the cardiac catheterization video is immediately visible to providers. A consultant seeing a 90-year-old gentleman for the first time can view discharge summaries from every VA hospital stay, primary care notes, other consultant notes, lab values, and test results in a few moments. Documentation of an advance care planning discussion is easily found and updated, allowing providers to offer nuanced advice that is compatible with each individual's values and goals.

Primary care is a key component of the VA health system, with every patient assigned to a designated primary care provider with a patient-aligned care team. Pharmacists are active in optimizing medication management and reconciliation. Social workers link patients and families to VA and community resources. All team members engage in telephone management to support patients and families between visits. Telehealth management tools for

Table 27.1. VA Continuum of Health Care Across the Lifespan

Ambulatory Care	Hospital	Nursing Home	Home
Primary care teams	Inpatient hospitalist teams	Primary care teams	Home-based primary care teams
Mental health	Mental health	Mental health	Mental health
Specialty care	Specialty care	Specialty care	Specialty care
Geriatrics care	Geriatrics care	Geriatrics care	Geriatrics care
Palliative care	Palliative care	Palliative care	Palliative care
		Hospice care	Hospice care
Integrative care	Integrative care	Integrative care	
			Home health aides
Caregiver support			Caregiver support
Women's health care			
Homeless outreach and support			

hypertension, diabetes mellitus, and other chronic conditions are widely integrated into the care. Specialized women's health services are widely available. Longstanding commitments to measuring important health processes and outcomes (e.g., blood pressure, hemoglobin A1C, patient satisfaction, pain relief, hospital and emergency department utilization, colon cancer screening, immunizations) have contributed to a robust culture of safety, reliability, and evidence-based treatment (http://www.hsrd.research.va.gov/publications/esp/quality.pdf).

Mental health care is provided by a spectrum of providers, including physicians, psychologists, social workers, and other counselors. Evidence-based psychotherapy and care coordination are key elements of mental health services, and CPRS is well utilized to identify patients at risk for suicide and violent behavior. Specialized programs exist for substance abuse recovery and homelessness, among others. No other health system offers this degree of access and depth of services. Measurement of important outcomes (e.g., homelessness, suicide, access) drives improvement and accountability.

Geriatrics, extended care, and palliative care support the VA's commitment to meet the needs of older veterans and those living with serious illness. Emphasis on advance care planning discussions ("Honoring Veterans Preferences") is central to the person-directed practice. Services range from hospital consultations for geriatrics and palliative care, to outpatient consultations and primary care, to home-based primary care, to home hospice, to nursing home care for rehabilitation, long-term living, or hospice/palliative care. Functionally dependent veterans are entitled to VA-paid home health aide services that support them to remain in their own homes in the community as their need for personal assistance grows. Only Medicaid programs in selected states provide similar services to homebound persons living with functional dependency. Caregiver support programs assist caregivers to effectively care for their loved ones at home. VA Home Based Primary Care (HBPC) is delivered by inter-professional teams including physicians, nurse practitioners, nurses, social workers, physical therapists, psychologists, and pharmacists. HBPC has led the nation in demonstrating outcomes of reduced hospital and emergency department use by homebound veterans, improved care, and reduced overall costs.[2] Access to home hospice services has increased care at home near the end of life, with evidence of reduced deaths in the hospital.

Integrative health approaches have become more widely available in the VA to better meet the needs of persons living with chronic conditions. Education in self-care techniques such as mindfulness, meditation, yoga, and other practices has expanded. Resources to promote healthy weight attainment, regular exercise programs, and reduction of inflammatory influences are made available through programs across the VA. The field of healing and creative arts is increasingly recognized as an important domain of healthful environments of care serving older persons and those living with serious illness or nearing the end of life. The VA Centers for Community Living (residential programs for persons needing nursing home care) incorporate creative pursuits to help residents engage in meaningful activity and help resolve many of the post-traumatic stress symptoms that plague veterans (http://www.creativeaging.org/programs-people/healing-creativity-washington-dc-va-medical-center). Additionally, self-care continues to emerge as a major theme to build resiliency and compassion among the VA health care workforce.

Education remains a major theme in the VA. The VA fosters education for health professionals through the Office of Academic Affairs supporting graduate medical education as well as training for psychologists, dentists, therapists, and nurses. The delivery of clinical education in the inter-professional programs of the VA promotes improved collaboration of health care professionals needed to improve the value of health care services. Additionally, the Office of Patient Centered Care and Cultural

Transformation (OPCC&CT) has developed the Whole Health Education Program, which is designed to educate VA employees in providing a proactive, whole-person approach. This includes learning how to effectively implement integrative health approaches. This is an inter-professional training that includes VA physicians, nurses, dietitians, social workers, psychologists, peer support specialists, chaplains, and other staff.

Innovation and scholarly activity have been central to the VA's strategy to achieve excellence in service delivery. World-class research on topics important to veterans has been steadily produced utilizing the VA's vast patient population and database. VA research has produced major bodies of evidence to guide treatment of cardiovascular conditions, cancer, mental health, and quality improvement. Geriatric Research and Education and Clinical Centers have been in existence since the 1980s and have been major contributors to the field of geriatric medicine and the training of geriatricians and other aging experts (http://www.va.gov/grecc/).

The VA health system is outperforming every other U.S. system in comprehensiveness, incorporation of multidimensional approaches (from disease-modifying medical treatments, to integrative health approaches, to prevention and personal care), using a shared electronic medical record that integrates the efforts of multiple professional providers over time, and commitment to caring for persons across the lifespan.

Although the VA is a large and comprehensive health care system, VA leadership recognizes the need for transformation of health care to better promote health and well-being. Not just the VA but all health care systems across the United States fail to effectively address the increasing epidemic of preventable chronic diseases resulting in great human and financial burdens. Failure to prevent disease, not to mention improve health, is the result of systems that are reactively focused on disease events, with limited success engaging people in improving their health and well-being. Thus, within VA, there is a philosophical transformation occurring where disease care and disease management is shifting to a personalized, proactive, patient-centered approach to health care, where the veteran, not the disease, is at the center of care.[3] OPCC&CT within the VA Central Office was established in 2011 to drive this paradigm shift (http://www.va.gov/patientcenteredcare/about.asp).

The call for health care transformation is outlined in current VA strategic documents, including the VA's strategic priorities and the VA's current operational guide (http://www.va.gov/health/docs/VHA_Blueprint_for_Excellence.pdf), which calls for a transition "from 'sick care' to '*health* care' in the broadest sense."[4] If the VA is to move from a model of sick care to a provider of health care, it must move from a reactive, disease-based model to a whole-health approach focused on proactive health partnerships. Thus, the personalized, proactive, patient-driven approach, coined "whole health," is at the heart of the health care transformation within the VA. Personalized care means putting veterans needs first and partnering with them to create a customized health plan based on their goals, personal history, and lifestyle. Proactive care means that the veteran's care team actively works with the veteran to find preventive, rather than reactive, options that strengthen his or her individual, innate capacity for health and healing. Patient-driven care puts veterans at the head of their personal health care team so that clinicians can give veterans the skills, resources, and support to drive their own care. In its full form, the whole-health approach promotes a reorientation of the veteran's experience with the VA and combines "state of the art" conventional medicine with personalized health planning, integrative health services, and innovative self-care approaches. The VA's Undersecretary of Health has identified whole health as the way forward for VA health care, explaining that "Our 'whole health' model of care is a key component of the VA's proposed future delivery system. This model incorporates physical care with psychosocial care focused on the veteran's personal health and life goals, aiming to provide personalized, proactive, patient-driven care through multidisciplinary teams of health professionals."[5]

The VA has begun to design a whole-health implementation strategy, the Whole Health Partnership, which is a systematic approach to providing whole-health care early in the relationship between the VA and the veteran, emphasizing self-care in the larger context of well-being, and incorporating a full range of conventional and integrative health approaches. The Whole Health Partnership model promotes a more continuous engagement of the health system and the veteran across the lifespan.

The Whole Health Partnership design includes three central components: the Pathway, Wellbeing Centers, and Clinical Care (Fig. 27.1). The Pathway partners with veterans at the point of enrollment and creates an overarching personal health plan that integrates VA and non-VA care. Wellbeing Centers will be easily accessible to veterans throughout the nation within VA or non-VA settings and will focus on providing an integrative health approach to optimize health and well-being. Clinical Care represents the conventional clinical care with an enhanced emphasis on healing environments, healing relationships, and the integration of integrative health and personal health planning practices into treatment plans. A number of VA medical centers have been early innovators in this work, capitalizing on both leadership investment and grassroots movements to establish the components of the Whole Health Partnership. In fiscal year 2016, seven VA medical centers were funded by OPCC&CT to design the Pathway, and many are also implementing the other

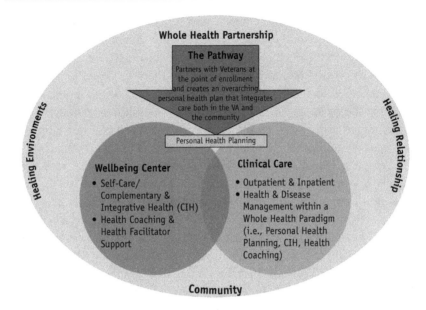

FIGURE 27.1. Whole Health Partnership Model.

components of the Whole Health Partnership, including Washington DC VA Medical Center, Jesse Brown VA Medical Center, VA Boston Healthcare System, W. G. Hefner VA Medical Center, Harry S. Truman Memorial Veterans' Hospital, Gulf Coast Veterans Health Care System, and VA North Texas Health Care System.

The Washington DC Veterans Affairs Medical Center (DCVA) exemplifies the Whole Health Partnership model. DC was one of the first VA medical centers to create a Wellbeing Center, entitled the Integrative Health and Wellness (IHW) program, which is a patient-centered, integrative health program for veterans served by the DCVA. This program was established in 2012 and currently resides within the Patient Centered Care Service. The program's mission is to promote comprehensive whole-health programming for veterans and staff by providing integrative health services to support personalized, proactive, patient-driven care and resilient staff that empowers veterans to design their own care and to live to their fullest potential.

The IHW program operates in a dedicated space in the DCVA and offers integrative health programming 5 days per week. Veterans are referred by a provider and after completing a program orientation session they are able to attend various integrative health services at the frequency of their choosing.

In fiscal year 2015, providers from over 50 different departments at the DCVA referred veterans to the IHW program. Regardless of referral source, pain or mental health symptoms were the primary health concern of veterans participating in the program. The total number of newly enrolled veterans has increased every year since consult inception, with the majority of referrals coming from primary care. During fiscal year 2015, 16% of IHW referrals were for veterans older than 65, with 55% of veterans over age 65 referred to IHW enrolling in the program. Of those veterans over the age of 65 referred to the IHW program during fiscal year 2015, 7% served during the Korean War, 6% served during the Persian Gulf War, 78% served during the Vietnam War, 3% served between the Korean and Vietnam Wars, and 5% were post-Vietnam. A considerable number of older veterans engaged in integrative health services, and over half of those offered enrollment in an integrative health clinic accepted.

The IHW program organizes itself along two tracks: an integrative medicine track, which includes an integrative medicine physician and energetic wellness services; and a well-being and education track, which includes group-based integrative health services. Within the integrative medicine track, an integrative medicine physician provides consultation services 1 day per week for outpatient veterans at the DCVA. Veterans with fibromyalgia, chronic pain, chronic fatigue, and gastrointestinal issues are referred to this consult service by a medical provider. In fiscal year 2015, 50% of veterans receiving care in the integrative medicine clinic were over age 65. Additionally, 25% of veterans receiving energetic wellness services within the IHW program were over age 65. It is clear that integrative health services are accepted and well utilized by older veterans, and these services may offer a unique benefit in an older population with various chronic conditions.

Within the well-being track, integrative health programming includes wellness massage, auricular acupuncture, yoga, meditation, iRest Yoga Nidra, biofeedback, qi gong, tai chi, nutrition workshops, an integrative nutrition group, Mindfulness Based Stress Reduction, and a Whole Health education group. Please see http://www.washingtondc.va.gov/Wellness/index.asp for additional resources. During fiscal year 2015, within the IHW program, 28% of veterans engaging in auricular acupuncture and 24% of veterans participating in health education groups (i.e., Whole Health education and integrative nutrition education) were over the age of 65. Additionally, meditative practices were well attended by older adults: 31% of veterans engaging in iRest Yoga Nidra and 37% of veterans attending meditation groups were over the age of 65. Further, movement-based groups, such as gentle yoga, qi gong, and tai chi, were popular with older adults: 76% of veterans engaging in movement-based groups were over the age of 65. Older Veterans are accepting of and benefiting from engaging in integrative health approaches. Movement-based practices and meditation were the best-attended integrative health groups by older veterans.

In sum, integrative health approaches are well received by older veterans, and inclusion of these approaches may support the psychological, physical, and spiritual health of our older veteran population.

National VA leadership continues to support the development of whole health and integrative health, as evidenced by supporting OPCC&CT to develop the Integrative Health Coordinating Center and the Whole Health Partnership model. The VA has the opportunity to become the national leader in whole health care delivery, and the Whole Health Partnership model is a roadmap to this paradigm shift.

REFERENCES

1. Longman P. Before the State of VA Health Care Hearings, U.S. Senate Committee on Veterans' Affairs, May 14, 2014.
2. Edwards ST, Prentice JC, Simon SR, Pizer SD, Home-based primary care and the risk of ambulatory care–sensitive condition hospitalization among older veterans with diabetes mellitus. *JAMA Intern Med.* 2014;174(11):1796–1803. doi:10.1001/jamainternmed.2014.4327
3. Krejci LP, Carter K, Gaudet T. Whole health: The vision and implementation of personalized, proactive, patient-driven health care for Veterans. *Medical Care.* 2014;52:S5–S8.
4. Department of Veterans Affairs Blueprint for Excellence: Veterans Health Administration. 2014.
5. Shulkin DJ. Beyond the VA crisis—becoming a high-performance network. *N Engl J Med.* 2016;374:1003–1005.

28

Long-Term Care/Residential Care

TAHIRA I. LODHI AND TANIA ALCHALABI

According to the latest World Health Organization (WHO) statistics,[1] between 2015 and 2050, the proportion of the world's population who are over 60 years old will nearly double, from 12% to 22%. This change is occurring across nations, from Asia Pacific to North America and from the Middle East to Europe. By 2050, 80% of older people will be living in low- and middle-income countries. Accordingly, the norms of long-term care systems will be forced to change in societies all over the world.

In the United States, the long-term care system has evolved considerably. Before the Industrial Revolution of the 1820s through 1870, long-term care meant multigenerational families living under one roof. The younger members of the family helped take care of the old. With the economic change, an inevitable sociocultural change ensued, rendering this arrangement nonviable for future generations. Thereafter, older Americans with resources hired help, while those without resources had to move to almshouses.

With the establishment of the Centers of Medicare and Medicaid Services[2] in 1965, the face of long-term care changed again. Most of the almshouses of prior years were converted to nursing homes. Under the Omnibus Budget Reconciliation Act of 1987,[3] the federal government converted these nursing homes into one of the most regulated bodies in the country. The basic objective of this reform act was to ensure that residents of nursing homes receive quality care in order to achieve and maintain their best possible physical, mental, and psychosocial health. It made provision of certain basic services to each resident mandatory and established a Nursing Home Residents' Bill of Rights.

In the mid-1970s, the dissatisfaction with nursing homes led to the introduction of the "assisted living facilities" concept. The idea was to maintain independence in the elderly while supporting "aging in place" in a non-medical, home-like environment. Today, these facilities are regulated by the individual states[4] and provide various levels of care, endeavoring to support independence in activities of daily living (ADLs; eating, bathing, dressing, toileting, transferring [walking], and continence) as well as instrumental activities of daily living (IADLs; food preparation, laundry, telephone use, medication management, finances, and transportation).

In addition to the above, there are several other short- and long-term care options available to elders and patients with disabilities depending on the need and circumstance. To understand these, we will consider a clinical real-life situation so the reader can walk through the maze of various care facilities and hopefully learn to navigate the system better.

It is important for health care providers to understand the social support systems and living situations of their patients because adherence to medication, follow-up on multiple medical problems, and care transitions depend on these support systems. A patient who has a disability because of cognitive impairment and ADL dependence may not be able to adhere to a regimen requiring medication administration three times daily. His or her family or a visiting nurse may be an option, or placement in an assisted living facility may be the answer. Similarly, a patient with abnormal weight loss may not be able to live independently because of medical conditions such as debilitating arthritis that may limit his or her access to proper nutrition.

In addition, for patients residing in long-term care facilities, it is important for the health care providers to know the roles of providers at the facilities and their limitations in providing care for the patients. For example, certified nursing assistants can provide ADL support but cannot dispense medications; a registered nurse or a licensed practical nurse can dispense medications. While nursing homes are required to have a medical director, assisted living facilities are not required by local health departments to have a medical director on site. When a patient is sent to such a facility, the nursing staff there would need orders for all medications, including over-the-counter medications; otherwise, they would not be able to administer them.

Role of Complementary and Alternative Medicine

Complementary and integrative health care can have a significant impact on quality of life, pain control, and several other outcomes in different long-term care settings. Integrating acupuncture, reiki, pet therapy, and music and massage therapies are evidence-based modalities to help improve pain and functional status for the elderly.[5] These modalities exist in different long-term care facilities to different extents based on patient and family interest, level of functioning, and comorbidities. It is easier to incorporate them in assisted living and senior living facilities because usually the patients' level of functioning is higher and they are not as tightly regulated by state or federal regulations. More work is needed to establish a safe way to implement integrative modalities in long-term care settings.[6]

Case Study

Mr. and Mrs. Smith, an elderly couple, decided to retire after 45 years of service in the local government. They had three children, two of whom lived in the area. The children were regularly in contact with their parents and the oldest daughter was identified as the medical power of attorney. They made their advance directive clearly known to the children and had their wills drawn up. Their primary care physician, a local geriatrician, had known them since they turned 65 years of age and saw them regularly every 3 months. They were physically active, belonged to the local senior center, and accompanied their grandchildren to soccer practice every week. They lived in a three-level single-family home and were independent in ADLs and IADLs.

Mr. Smith was 80 years old. He had a history of 20 pack-years of tobacco use, although he quit smoking about 15 years ago. He also had mild chronic obstructive pulmonary disease, hypertension, hyperlipidemia, diabetes, and mild dementia, but no behavioral disturbances. He had several falls and his memory was constantly declining. He missed payments on several bills so that his daughter had to intervene and help with financial management. She also had to start transporting her parents to various appointments because Mr. Smith got lost while driving in his own neighborhood, so the daughter had to take away his car. All of his medical problems were otherwise well controlled on six medications.

Mrs. Smith was 82 years of age. She was a lifelong non-smoker. She had a history of osteoporosis, osteoarthritis, and hypertension. She also had mild cognitive impairment, but no dementia. She had been stable medically and took five medications on a regular basis. She helped her husband with his medications too. While doing some chores around the house, Mrs. Smith had a fall that resulted in a right hip intertrochanteric fracture. She was hospitalized and had an open reduction/internal fixation surgery done. The hospitalization was complicated by delirium. Because of her delirium, she was not able to ambulate soon after surgery and developed a stage 2 sacral decubitus ulcer. She needed help with bathing, dressing, and medication management. Her surgical wound needed dressing. The hospital rehab team helped her exercise regularly, but she was not able to tolerate the 3 to 4 hours of intensive rehab in the hospital. Instead, it was recommended that she go to a sub-acute rehab facility[2] based on the fact that:

1. She required more skilled services under the supervision of licensed clinicians including skilled nursing and 2 to 3 hours of rehabilitation services per day, at least 6 days per week.
2. She needed frequent on-site evaluation by a physician, nurse practitioner, or physician assistant to manage her medications, delirium, and pain associated with surgery.
3. Medically necessary services could only be safely provided in an inpatient sub-acute care facility and could not be safely provided in a less restrictive clinical setting (e.g., at home with skilled home health services, or an outpatient setting).

Mrs. Smith and her family were told that sub-acute rehab might be a stand-alone facility or part of a nursing facility (NF) or skilled nursing facility (SNF). Although "nursing facility" and "skilled nursing facility" are terms often used interchangeably, there are some technical differences between the two. They are both long-term care facilities certified by the state survey agency. NFs provide long-term care and rehabilitative services to Medicaid beneficiaries following hospital discharge. SNFs, on the other hand, provide the same services to Medicare beneficiaries. Facilities can have both "NF beds" and "SNF beds"; they are said to be "dually certified." Medicaid beneficiaries occupy NF beds, while Medicare beneficiaries occupy SNF beds. Individuals can be "dual beneficiaries," eligible both for Medicare and for Medicaid. Such individuals can move from the SNF portion of a facility to the NF portion (in the event that long-term care is needed).

The following services could be provided to Mrs. Smith by the interdisciplinary team at sub-acute rehab:

- *Rehabilitative care*: At least 2 hours of direct therapy per day, at least 6 days per week (i.e., at least 12 hours of direct therapy per week). This required her to be physically and cognitively willing and able to participate in the rehab program and show that she was benefitting from it.
- *Pain management*: Monitoring and adjustment of a complex pain management treatment plan including frequent dose adjustment, changes in the route of medication administration, or skilled intervention for uncontrolled pain and/or an unstable medical condition

- *Parenteral fluids and/or medications*: Administration of two or more different oral, intramuscular, or intravenous medications on a daily basis (may include dosage adjustments and/or lab monitoring)
- *Wound care*: Complex wound care requiring aseptic technique, packing, debridement, irrigation, and/or frequent assessment for complications such as infection or vascular compromise. If needed, a wound vacuum device requiring multiple setting changes could be provided. Surgical wounds, burns, or stage 3 or 4 decubiti could also be managed.

Although Mrs. Smith did not require them, following services could also be provided by the facilities if needed:

- *Catheter*: Nursing management of indwelling urinary bladder catheter, nephrostomy tube, or supra-pubic tube during the early post-insertion period (not routine care), or in case of catheter complications. Insertion, sterile irrigation, and/or replacement of supra-pubic catheters.
- *Central line*: Administration of parenteral nutrition, medications, or fluids via a central line (e.g., Hickman catheter, Port-a-Cath). Central lines that are in place but not in active use will not be maintained.
- *Enteral tube feedings*: Skilled management of enteral feeding regimen for a newly inserted nasogastric tube, J-tube, or G-tube when a patient is functionally incapable of sufficient oral intake to sustain life
- *Diabetic care*: Daily monitoring of unstable blood sugar levels and administration of sliding-scale insulin. A physician's order for sliding-scale insulin does not constitute SNF level of care if insulin is not being administered daily.
- *Ostomy care*: Management and/or teaching about new colostomy or ileostomy (no routine care for old ostomies) during the early postoperative period
- *Respiratory care*: Skilled nursing observation and assessment to evaluate the patient's need for modifications of treatment, including chest physical therapy and/or aerosol delivery of medication (to mobilize secretions) at least three times a day. New respiratory treatments including initial phases of a regimen involving administration of medical gases (e.g., oxygen, bronchodilator).

Mrs. Smith had Medicare Part A, B, and D, so she could go to an SNF for sub-acute rehab. She decided to go to one that was close to her house. For the first 20 days, Medicare covered her room and board and rehab services 100%.

After that, up to 80 days, she had a 20% co-pay. After a 4-week stay, part of which she had to pay out of pocket, she was overjoyed when she was ready to be discharged. She was not particularly happy with the low-salt diet she was given at the rehab nor did she like to be around other people who were sicker. She confided to her husband that she would like to stay in her own house as long as possible, and if she had to move, she would want to go to a place where they could both be together. The social worker in the sub-acute rehab facility arranged for home physical and occupational therapy by orders of the rehab physician. She also arranged for a home health aide because at this point Mrs. Smith still needed help with bathing and food preparation, although she could dress herself independently. These outpatient home health services were provided by a home health agency and covered by Medicare Part A and/or B, depending on the needs.[7]

Once at home, Mrs. Smith's occupational therapist visited and made recommendations for grab bars to be installed in her bathroom. Her physical therapist did a visit for home safety evaluation and recommended that some area rugs be removed from her bedroom because they were a potential fall hazard. Mrs. Smith was not happy to have her cherished Oriental rugs be taken away, but agreed to comply.

After 8 weeks of therapy at home, she was not making much progress. She was able to ambulate with a cane, could dress herself, and needed standby assistance with bathing. This was deemed to be her new baseline. She continued to do her exercises on her own. Medicare paid for home health aides to help her 4 hours a day 2 days a week. Mr. Smith, while trying to take care of his wife, did his best to maintain his health but missed taking his medications frequently. As a result, his blood sugar levels and blood pressures were erratically controlled. Mrs. Smith was unable to resume the caregiving role she had before her fall. This required their adult children to play a more active caregiving role on a daily basis.

Over the following year, the couple continued to decline functionally. They were more sedentary than before. The daughter paid out of pocket to extend home health aide hours for her parents 5 hours a day 6 days a week.

On one occasion, the couple's daughter went out of the country for a month. Upon her return, she found signs of significant decline. Mr. and Mrs. Smith ate less, maybe one full meal a day, and took frequent naps. Both had falls intermittently without any serious injury. This time, the daughter used up their savings to pay for home health aides to stay with Mr. and Mrs. Smith 24 hours a day 7 days a week.

A month into this new arrangement, the daughter received a call from one of her parents' aides that her father was more agitated than usual and was intermittently disoriented. Alarmed, she decided to take him to the emergency room. He was found to be in ketoacidosis secondary to a urinary tract infection and dehydration. He was admitted to the intensive care unit. After 48 hours he was stable enough to be shifted to the regular medical floor. His mental status slowly improved to baseline during the hospital stay. Functionally, he was very unsteady on his feet, with some delirium superimposed on his dementia. The rehab team in the hospital recommended sub-acute rehab, but he insisted on going home with visits from physical and occupational therapists. He received therapy services for 2 weeks but then refused to participate.

Over the next few months at home, Mr. and Mrs. Smith continued to decline and became almost completely dependent for ADLs. They needed help with bathing and dressing. They could feed themselves but needed food to be prepared for them. The biggest challenge was Mr. Smith's worsening dementia and associated behavioral issues, anger and "sundowning." He needed frequent reorientation. He had multiple falls when he refused to accept the caregivers' help for ADL care.

During a regular visit with the primary care geriatrician, the daughter expressed significant caregiver burden. She was very concerned about her parents living by themselves. Not only were resources dwindling for 24-hour caregiving, but also their caregiving needs could not be met at their multilevel house. A family meeting was arranged with the geriatrician, her outpatient social worker, Mr. and Mrs. Smith, and their daughter. Everybody agreed that it was no longer safe for the couple to continue living in their house, but the couple was depressed and tearful at the idea of having to leave it. The social worker provided them with options of community-based services[8] as listed in Table 28.1.

The options that did not require moving from the residence were rejected because Mr. and Mrs. Smith had already tried most of these resources. They were mostly looking to move to a facility where they could age in place. They realized at this point that depending on their functional level at any given time and their underlying medical issues, they would need more and more ADL support going forward. After much consideration, they decided to move into an independent apartment at a CCRC after selling their house. The major upside to the move was that there would be more activities on the premises. In addition to having a Medicare-paid caregiver 2 hours a day 4 days a week, the daughter combined her parents' social security income and contributed out of pocket to pay for home health aides to stay with her parents 24/7. They were provided with meals at the facility.

Three months later, the primary care physician met with the couple and their daughter. Mr. Smith's memory had declined further. There were days when he forgot his children's names or became agitated with Mrs. Smith in the evenings and had multiple more falls because he wouldn't allow the caregivers

Table 28.1. Community-Based Programs

No Change in Residence	Requires Change in Residence
Adult Day Care - Social supports in congregate setting - Services range from non-skilled custodial care to advanced skilled services. - Available staff on site includes registered nurse providing clinical assessment and monitoring and assistance with medications. - Used as respite for ADL assistance and supervision while primary caregivers work - Not covered by Medicare; some costs covered by Medicaid or other insurers **Day Hospitals** - Provide skilled nursing care usually in rehabilitation centers or chronic care hospitals - Can provide parenteral antibiotics, chemotherapy, and intensive rehabilitation - Patients requiring multidisciplinary rehab or psychiatric illness benefit from these. - Services are covered under Medicare with similar requirements as home health care. **Program of All-Inclusive Care for the Elderly (PACE)** - Care provided to Medicare- and Medicaid-eligible patients who are living in the community but require a nursing home level of care by an interdisciplinary team in an adult day care setting	**Assisted Living** - Based on social not medical model of care; provides varying levels of care within and between stages - Also called personal care homes, residential care homes, domiciliary care, and sheltered care and community residences - Considered to be transition between home and nursing; average length of stay 2 years - Run by states and local health departments. Regulations vary throughout the country. Only requirement that is uniform to all is an individualized service plan (ISP). - Most frequent citation across the country is medication administration. Depending on the state licensing requirements, medication administration and management can be directed by skilled, nonskilled, or fully licensed nursing staff. - Cost of care varies greatly across the country. Care in assisted living is cheaper than nursing homes. - Services are not covered by Medicare. - Health Insurance Association of America reports that all 11 of the companies selling long-term care insurance offer assisted living coverage, but most Americans do not have long-term care insurance. - Certain services are paid under Supplementary Security Income and Social Services Block Grant programs. - Thirty-eight states reimburse or plan to reimburse for assisted living as a Medicaid service. **Group Homes** - Including domiciliary care, single-room-occupancy residences, board-and-care homes, and some congregate living situations - Often serve patients with chronic mental illness or dementia - Residents have their own bedrooms but shared living room, dining room, and kitchen. - Low cost; opportunities for isolation; higher staff-to-patient ratios

Table 28.1. Continued

No Change in Residence	Requires Change in Residence

– Interdisciplinary team consists of a geriatrician, nurse practitioner, social worker, pharmacist, dietitian, physical and occupational therapists, and transportation workers.
– Services vary; can include hearing aids, eyeglasses, and other benefits at discretion of PACE team (e.g., paying patient's electricity and gas bills).
– Permanent program under Medicare but optional under Medicaid; very few other insurance plans cover it
Managed Long-Term Care Programs (MLTCs)
– An effort by different states to start programs to avoid nursing home placement or hospital admission
– For Medicare and Medicaid or dually eligible candidates who have chronic conditions that have impaired their ability to live independently
Home Hospital
– A more intensive form of home health care providing more complex care at home that otherwise may have required hospitalization
– Patients have access to an on-call system of nurses and physicians on regular basis and for episodic care.
– High satisfaction rates
Technological Innovations at Home
– Personal emergency response systems worn around neck or arm
– Newer devices can provide medication administration and management, transmit vital signs, and connect to telemedicine.
– Home robotics under development to help with ADLs and IADLs
– Computers and smartphones may also be used.
	– Mostly for-profit and may require state licensure
	Adult Foster Care
	– A family sponsors the elderly person under state regulations, sometimes requiring licensure.
	– More family-like atmosphere, with ADL support
	– Longest experience with this is in Oregon.
	– Some states cover services through Medicaid.
	Sheltered Housing
	– Funded through Older Americans Act and offered as Section 8 housing, Housing and Urban Development programs for seniors and disabled persons
	– Services include personal care assistance, housekeeping services and meals, social work services, and activities coordinators.
	– Clients are charged on a sliding scale; fees may be up to 30% of their income.
	Continuing-Care Retirement Communities (CCRCs)
	– Chosen by most affluent seniors
	– Variety of living options such as apartments or condominiums, assisted living, skilled nursing home care, so residents can shift through levels of care while aging in place
	– Three financial models are common:
	  • All-inclusive: provides total health care coverage, including long-term care
	  • Fee-for-service: payments match level of care
	  • Modified coverage: covers long-term care to a predetermined maximum
	– Additional fees may include a nonrefundable entry fee plus a monthly fee for supportive services.
	– Largely private funding. Some may have Medicare- or Medicaid-funded beds for skilled

to help him. He refused to take medications frequently and was found chok-ing on his food. At the physician's suggestion, the couple was moved into the assisted living part of the CCRC. The nurses there managed their medications. This was a very expensive option, however, and they were fast running out of their limited resources.

About 3 months into this arrangement, per the daughter's request, an inter-disciplinary team meeting was held with Mr. and Mrs. Smith, their daughter, the social worker, the administrator, and the director of nursing at the assisted living facility. Mr. Smith's dementia had progressed further. He did not recog-nize Mrs. Smith or the rest of the family members and he was losing weight. The family decided to move Mr. Smith into the locked-down dementia unit, where his behavior could be managed more closely, he could be fed by the onsite caregivers, and Mrs. Smith could spend time with him during the entire day. Mrs. Smith decided to remain in the assisted living facility but moved into a smaller unit to save her dwindling resources. It was also decided that going forward, Mr. and Mrs. Smith wanted to remain as comfortable as possible. In accordance with their advance directive, their emergency care was changed to "Do Not Resuscitate/Do Not Intubate" (DNR/DNI). They wanted to be kept comfortable and pain-free and have hospice services as needed. They did not want to be hospitalized but agreed to be treated conservatively by onsite physi-cians for any reversible medical issues.

Over the next 2 months, Mr. Smith declined further. After a fall with hip fracture, he became bedbound. Mrs. Smith also started having more issues with memory and depression as Mr. Smith transitioned to the dementia unit. At this point, the family agreed to transfer them both to the nursing home[9] portion of the CCRC. Hospice services (service by Medicare Part A) were started for him. He died peacefully, pain-free, and surrounded by his family members 2 months later. Because she had hospice services, Mrs. Smith was able to receive bereavement care by the hospice providers over the next year.

Mrs. Smith had a visit with her primary care physician and expressed inter-est in pursuing non-medical, integrative modalities to help with her pain asso-ciated with osteoarthritis, depression, and developing urinary incontinence. She discussed acupuncture, reiki, yoga, massage therapy, and tai chi. She started doing acupuncture and yoga and over some weeks expressed that she was happy with the results.

Future of Long-Term Care

As health care becomes integrated with technology elsewhere, advance ana-lytics and telehealth can be used to fine-tune patient- and family-centered options. "The Internet of things" (IoT) includes the idea of augmenting medical services, such as shower mats with sensors that can detect falls, bed overlays that can detect limb movements during the night, and glucometers that can transmit data to health care personnel for closer blood sugar monitoring. According to the "Key Findings from a National Survey of Older Americans" carried out by the Kaiser Family Foundation, 70% of Americans age 50 to 64 years have gone online; of these, 51% are online every day.[10] The obvious future direction is the provision of a ubiquitous long-term health care environment for the elderly. This environment is triggered not only by the cost-effectiveness but also by the ease of use of the e-health or telemedicine applications. The seamlessness allows for an environment where the elderly can be independent while maintaining safety.

REFERENCES

1. http://www.who.int/mediacentre/factsheets/fs404/en/
2. www.cms.gov
3. http://www.ncmust.com/doclib/OBRA87summary.pdf
4. https://aspe.hhs.gov/basic-report/compendium-residential-care-and-assisted-living-regulations-and-policy-2015-edition
5. Evans R, Vihstadt C, Westrom K, Baldwin L. Complementary and integrative healthcare in a long-term care facility: A pilot project. Complementary and Integrative Healthcare in a Long-term Care Facility: A Pilot Project. *Glob Adv Health Med.* 2015 Jan; 4(1):18–27. doi:10.7453/gahmj.2014.072
6. Bauer M, Rayner J. Use of complementary and alternative medicine in residential aged care. *J Altern Complement Med.* 2012 Nov;18(11):989–993. doi:10.1089/acm.2011.0582.
7. https://www.medicare.gov/coverage/home-health-services.html
8. Medina-Walpole A, Pacala J. Geriatrics Review Syllabus, *American Geriatric Society*, 2016, 9th ed. www.americangeriatrics.org
9. https://www.cms.gov/Medicare/Provider-Enrollment-and-Certification/GuidanceforLawsAndRegulations/Nursing-Homes.html
10. https://kaiserfamilyfoundation.files.wordpress.com/2013/01/e-health-and-the-elderly-how-seniors-use-the-internet-for-health-information-key-findings-from-a-national-survey-of-older-americans-survey-report.pdf

ADDITIONAL READINGS

AMDA. White Paper on Determination and Documentation of Medical Necessity in Long Term Care Facilities. 2001. http://www.amda.com/library/whitepapers/mednecwhitepaper.htm. Accessed April 30, 2016.

AMDA. Role of Attending Physician in the Nursing Home, 2003. http://www.amda.com/governance/resolutions/e03.cfm. Accessed April 30, 2016.

Bonner AF. Falling into place: A practical approach to interdisciplinary education on falls prevention in long-term care. *Ann Long-Term Care.* 2006; 4(6):21–29.

Carlson BL, Foster L, Dale SB, et al. Effects of cash and counseling on personal care and well-being. *Health Serv Res.* 2007;42:467–487.

29

Interprofessional Team-Based Care

BEVERLY LUNSFORD AND TERRY A. MIKOVICH

Introduction

Longevity has increased substantially in the past 50 years, and the fastest-growing segment of the population is people over 85 years of age. Along with increased longevity is an increase in chronic illness. In 2012, about 50% of Medicare beneficiaries (older adults and disabled) in the United States had at least one chronic condition,[1] 25% had more than one chronic illness, and 20% had five or more chronic health conditions.[2]

Chronic illnesses are associated with intermittent and/or progressive functional decline, requiring regular monitoring, disease management, and coordination of care. Multiple providers across settings help prevent, delay, or minimize decline in health and maintain quality of life. Older adults with functional limitations need personal assistance for activities of daily living (eating, bathing, dressing, toileting, and walking) as well as instrumental activities of daily living (shopping, medication, financial management, and housekeeping). These services can enable people with functional disabilities to live safely in their homes as long as possible.[3]

Health care systems are being redesigned to address the unique needs of older adults and individuals with chronic illness. The current health care system was developed in the early 1900s for short-term illness (e.g., acute infection, heart attack, trauma). Now the most common illnesses are noncommunicable diseases, such as coronary artery disease, cancer, diabetes, and dementia, which are chronic and long-term illnesses that may cause progressive loss of functioning and cognitive capacity over many years. In addition, people over 60 experience disability from age-related hearing loss, visual loss, frailty, and movement difficulties.[4] These conditions require a different care system that includes primary care, acute care, specialty care, rehabilitative and long-term care, and community resources and supportive services.

Realigned systems of care for older adults require many health care professionals from different specialties and disciplines, such as cardiology, nephrology, endocrinology, ophthalmology, and social work. Older adults traverse several levels of care, from primary to acute and rehabilitative care and community-based services, requiring timely and effective communication to achieve optimal outcomes. Each provider, individual, and family needs comprehensive information about other conditions, hospitalizations, and specialty care for making immediate health care decisions. Practitioners cannot provide care for just a select condition(s), as it may not be independent of other issues/problems. This could result in increased costs from duplication of services and prescriptions, unnecessary hospitalization, and/or longer periods of illness.[5] In addition, many people utilize complementary and alternative therapies, so practitioners need a greater awareness of their value.

Seamless and accurate flow of information throughout the system of care, including the individual and family, ensures the integration of all relevant components and informed decision making to optimize outcomes. A primary health provider who knows the older adult well can facilitate addressing mind, body, and spiritual needs and coordinating care with a team of practitioners. This approach is person-centered and enables the team to gain a greater knowledge of the social determinants of health that may impact the individual's health and well-being.

Interprofessional or Interdisciplinary Teams?

The terms *interdisciplinary* and *interprofessional* are frequently used interchangeably when referring to teams, but there is an important distinction in function. Interdisciplinary team members work within the roles and abilities of their discipline, and clinicians run the risk of being isolated to their own professional standards of care. The complex needs of older adults with chronic health conditions require the different disciplines to work and communicate more effectively. Interprofessional care means that each member utilizes knowledge, skills, and attitudes to augment and support the contributions of other members of the team.[6] Each health care team member seeks knowledge about the role of other professions involved to provide integrated, continuous care for the older adult and his or her family, while promoting a person-centered approach that decreases duplication and fragmentation, reduces costs, and results in better outcomes. Team members are held equally accountable, and they work cohesively to share information from their unique perspectives with peers without fear of criticism or dismissiveness.[7]

Team-based care may be difficult to define because it occurs within different settings, as well as across settings.[8] There are primary care and home-based teams, acute care or hospital teams, emergency response teams, and so forth. Teams may include different constellations of team members, and they may interact through different modes, such as face-to-face or via medical records, phone, or email. In addition, teams can be geographically dispersed.

Teams function more effectively if they have a common goal focused on the individual and his or her family, including optimal physical functioning and quality of life. Team members should address their individual and organizational needs so they do not distract the team from the individual as the primary focus of the team's collaboration. Professionals on the team should be experienced in the clinical fields pertaining to the client's diagnosis, and during team development, time must be spent on learning about the other professions involved. Many professionals do not learn about other professions' knowledge, skills, and roles in client care during their educational process, so they may lack fundamental knowledge of how other professions contribute along the health care continuum.

While decisions are made as a team, there may be an identified leader who facilitates communication and engages team members regularly to promote a smooth process for collaboration, or at critical times for problem-solving. A leader creates an atmosphere of trust to achieve the primary goal. However, when teams are widely dispersed across several settings, the "leader" may change depending on the current site of care or critical problems being addressed. A formal leader also facilitates team formation by establishing mission, policies, and procedures.

A new role of care coordinator or geriatric case manager is emerging to coordinate care within and across settings. The Agency for Healthcare Research and Quality (AHRQ) defines care coordination as "deliberate organization of patient care activities between two or more participants (including patient) involved in a patient's care to facilitate the appropriate delivery of healthcare services. Organizing care involves marshaling personnel and other resources needed to carry out all required patient care activities."[9] These may include negotiating responsibilities, facilitating transitions, assessing needs/goals, creating a proactive plan of care, monitoring, following up, responding to change, supporting self-management, and linking the patient and family to community resources.

In the United States, financial incentives have been implemented for care coordination and interprofessional collaboration for individuals with complex health needs to improve health outcomes, prevent hospitalization, and reduce the cost of care for older adults.[10] As of January 2015, U.S. physicians are able to bill monthly to provide care coordination for individuals with two or more chronic conditions.[11] This includes non–face-to-face chronic-care management services, such as consulting with other providers who care for the same patients, coordinating care with home and community-based clinical providers, and communicating with caregivers/decision makers (i.e., family members) to ensure that the right care is being given, at the right time, and in the right setting.[12]

The Dartmouth Report has observed patterns that indicate that it may be more difficult to achieve goals of coordination in some regions than others.[13] An example is that the volume of services required based on contact days and inpatient days presents a higher level of difficulty in care coordination. In the Chicago region the average number of inpatient days is 5.3 to 7.6 per Medicare beneficiary compared to the Wyoming region, with 3.8 to 4.3 days.[13 P29] New payment models like primary medical homes and comprehensive primary care require care coordination, but in some regions the specialists may play a more prominent role, whether they are aware of it or not. Older adults or family members may need to discuss this with the care providers to determine who will be responsible for helping them coordinate care as they age.

For older adults utilizing long-term care services (e.g., nursing homes, assisted living, or home care), the health care team may include physicians, advanced practice nurses, nurses, physician assistants, physical therapists, occupational therapists, social workers, dietitians, art therapists, and activities coordinators. For optimal care, each service provider needs to be aware of the core clinical skills of other providers and how their services align with team goals and expectations to provide person-centered care. This is exemplified by the case of an older adult who experienced a stroke for the first time and receives services from a neurology team, a physician, an advanced practice nurse, nurses, physical therapists, occupational therapists, speech therapists, a dietitian, massage therapists, and expressive arts therapists with recommendations for medications, food intake, activity therapies, and arts engagement (for meaningful activity and stress reduction). If changes in levels of activity, medication, food tolerance, and the individual's and family goals are not communicated among the team members, this could result in negative clinical outcomes, such as inadequate management of blood pressure, duplication of services, depression, and lack of client and family ability to follow through (participate) with care.[14]

Transitions between care settings (i.e., home, nursing home, assisted living, and acute care) are particularly vulnerable times for older adults, and they can benefit from interprofessional collaboration. Transitions may involve different systems of care (transfer to emergency room from long-term care), different health care providers and teams (outpatient clinical services and long-term care facility), and changes in treatment protocols and needs (e.g., stroke precautions) when moving to different units in the hospital or discharge back home. Some of the common barriers and problems include lack of a person-centered focus, lack of feedback or information between specialists and primary care providers,[15,16] difficulty obtaining medical records and laboratory results on the part of providers,[17,18] and lack of hospital follow-up with home discharge,[19] which is commonly referred to as a "Swiss cheese" model. Collaboration and communication that allows smooth transfer of information is needed among all levels of the team while maintaining a focus on the individual's needs, fears, and preferences.

Two evidence-based models for integrating systems of care are the transitional coaching model (TCM)[20] and the care transitions program.[21,22] For older adults who are transitioning from hospital to home, the TCM is a good example of interprofessional collaboration for safe transitions. This model focuses on hospital discharge of people with chronic illness. Advanced practice nurses make inpatient visits and then post-discharge home visits with additional phone consultation. The nurse forms a partnership with the individual and his or her caregiver and coordinates care with physicians, nurses, pharmacists, and social workers. This model has demonstrated significantly lower rates of repeat hospital admissions, deaths, and total costs for the intervention group versus the usual care group.

The care transitions program proposes two opportunities for improving care coordination: patient activation and a coach to manage care coordination. In this model, the coach (an advanced practice nurse) works with the patient and family members so they can coordinate their own care. The coach teaches the individual and family members, which promotes independence and a greater competence in self-care skills. This model was associated with reduced hospital admissions for the same condition and reduced costs of care at 6 months after discharge.

Interprofessional Team Models

There are several emerging models of team-based care reflecting the unique needs of older adults for maintaining well-being, managing multiple chronic illnesses, and/or frailty.

HEALTH-ORIENTED TEAMS

The first two examples in integrative geriatric care are the health promotion model and the disease-oriented team.[23] The health promotion model may include a health-oriented team that works with individuals who may seek to reduce stress, maintain optimal weight, or manage pain. The interprofessional team for weight management may include the primary care provider, a nutritionist, an exercise physiologist, a mindfulness eating instructor, an acupuncturist, and a spiritual guide.

In contrast to the health promotion team is the disease-oriented team, in which the focus of care is for the person experiencing major health problems, such as cancer or renal failure. The team for renal disease, for example, may include a nephrologist, a dialysis technician, a surgeon, a pharmacist, a renal nurse, a mind–body coach, and a spiritual director. This provides an integrated approach using traditional disease management with holistic mind, body, and spirit care that is person-centered and promotes quality of life.

In the 1990s, integrative medical clinics began opening in academic medical centers (e.g., University of Arizona, University of California at San Francisco, and University of Maryland) to provide integrative care.[23] Integrative medicine centers have since added complementary and alternative medicine (CAM) centers.[24] During this time, other integrative medicine clinics have evolved outside of academic centers, such as at Scripps and the Beth Israel Continuum Center.

Integrative medicine teams are also established in acute care settings. A 2010 study of U.S. hospitals found that 42% offer one or more CAM therapies.[24] This is in comparison to 37% in 2008 and 26.5% in 2005. Hospitals attribute this rise in offering alternative therapies to patient demand (84%) and clinical effectiveness (67%) These services can significantly increase the number of disciplines represented in team-based care, as the services may include art therapy, yoga, tai chi, meditation, acupuncture, chiropractic, and so forth. It is imperative that CAM providers gain a good understanding of the other disciplines, including defining terminology, sharing medical system theories, and patient communication. Similar to other team-based care, this requires a cultural shift for physicians to move from a traditional model of "all-knowing" to a "shared knowledge" model for team care.[25]

HOME AND COMMUNITY-BASED SERVICES

Home and community-based services, a subset of long-term services and supports, provide care and service coordination outside of institutional settings. They include supports for individuals, their families, and other unpaid caregivers to maximize the person's independence in the community. For the first time, home and community-based services accounted for a majority of Medicaid expenditures for long-term services and supports in fiscal year 2013, and given the need for promoting independence and well-being for older adults outside of institutional settings, this expenditure is expected to grow.[26]

HOME-BASED PRIMARY CARE

Home-based primary care is an interprofessional team-based model of care that focuses on the 5% of older adults who are most ill and who represent almost 50% of Medicare expenditures.[26-29] These patients are more likely to be older, with multiple chronic conditions, and they enter skilled nursing facilities at a higher rate.[30] Home-based primary care includes medical and social services for seniors who are unable to or find it difficult to get to an office for medical care. There are more than 150 home-based primary care sites in the Department of Veterans Affairs (VA), and they are reported to reduce hospital and nursing home usage, with 24% lower total VA costs and 11% lower Medicare costs.[30,31] The VA home-based primary care teams include physicians, nurses, social workers, dietitians, psychologists, pharmacists, rehabilitative therapists, and other professionals who provide integrated care. The team coordinates care with each other, the patient, and family caregivers (if available) and provides referrals to other needed services and resources outside of the VA.[31]

To test the effects of this model in the Medicare fee-for-service area, a case-controlled concurrent study of 722 home-based primary care cases and 2,161 controls matched for sex, age bands, race, and Medicare buy-in status, long-term nursing home status, cognitive impairment, and frailty examined Medicare costs, utilization events, and mortality.[32] The mean age was 83.7 years for cases and 82 years for controls, and a majority of both groups were female (77%) and African American (90%). After 2 years of follow-up the cases had lower Medicare and hospital costs ($44,455 vs. $50,977 in controls and $17,805 vs. $22,096 in cases), lower skilled nursing facility costs ($4,821 vs. $4,098), higher home health costs ($6,579 vs. $4,169), and higher hospice costs ($3,144 vs. $1,505). The cases had 23% fewer subspecialist visits and 105% more generalist visits. Overall, the cases had 17% lower Medicare costs over 2 years with no difference in mortality or time to death between cases and controls. Thus, home-based primary care results in lower Medicare costs with similar survival outcomes.

An additional advantage of home-based primary care in the VA is that there is no end date for the care. Consequently, at times the patient will transition to hospice. When a need for the hospice level of care becomes evident, the provider, nurse, and social worker will meet with patient and family/caregiver to discuss hospice. If needed, the psychologist can participate in the meeting. If the patient agrees, a referral is made to hospice. The home-based primary care team continues to provide primary care and collaborates with the hospice staff.

ACUTE CARE FOR ELDERS

An Acute Care for Elders (ACE) unit provides an interdisciplinary model of care in acute care settings that includes the proactive identification and management of geriatric syndromes with teams that focus on person-centered care. The teams may consist of geriatricians, nurse practitioners, nurses, rehabilitation therapists, pharmacists, dietitians, care managers, and social workers who work collaboratively to develop patient-centered care plans. Care transitions are planned from the day of admission with communication of care plans to the caregivers, including physicians, nurses, family members, and the patient. Care includes consideration of environmental modifications that enhance safety, mobility, and cognitive stimulation and provide a more home-like atmosphere.

The ACE unit may include the use of contrasting colors for individuals with low vision, handrails in rooms and hallways, furniture adapted for easier transfer, and a central gathering place for group activities. A randomized controlled study of 1,632 older adults indicated that individuals in ACE units had a significantly shorter length of stay (6.7 days per person vs. 7.3 days in usual care). This reduced the total inpatient costs from $10,451 per patient receiving usual care to $9,477 per patient in an ACE unit. In addition, patients were able to maintain their functional abilities, and hospital readmission rates were not increased.[33]

COMPREHENSIVE GERIATRIC ASSESSMENT IN ACUTE CARE

Another model of care for older adults in acute care settings is a dedicated team of geriatric specialists who provide consultative services across the institution instead of a dedicated geriatric ward. The effectiveness of these multidisciplinary specialist wards versus specialist teams in acute care hospital wards was shown in a meta-analysis of 22 randomized controlled trials with a total of 10,315 patients across six countries, in which older adults who received comprehensive geriatric assessment (specialist teams on dedicated hospital unit) were more likely to be alive and in their own homes up to a year after admission, compared to older adults who received general medical care.[34] In addition, older adults who received comprehensive geriatric assessment were less likely to be institutionalized, less likely to die or experience deterioration, and more likely to benefit from improved cognition.

PROGRAM OF ALL-INCLUSIVE CARE FOR THE ELDERLY

The Program of All-Inclusive Care for the Elderly (PACE) provides comprehensive medical and social services for frail individuals so that they can live safely in the community. PACE includes integrated preventive, acute care, and long-term care services that address the frequent complex medical, functional, and social needs of frail older adults. PACE provides flexibility for clients, family members, caregivers, and health care professionals to meet the person's health care needs. Patients over age 55 who are eligible for nursing home care may join this comprehensive service program to remain in the community.[35]

Most participants are dually eligible for Medicare and Medicaid benefits. PACE provides an interdisciplinary team of health professionals with the sole source of financing from Medicaid and Medicare benefits. It enables practitioners to provide participants with all needed services rather than only services reimbursed by Medicare and Medicaid fee-for-service plans.

It has been difficult to conduct experimental studies to measure the effectiveness of PACE due to the limitations of finding an appropriate comparison group. A review of research for PACE programs indicate that there is no significant effect on reducing Medicare costs, and PACE programs may increase Medicaid costs.[36] While enrollees may have fewer hospital admissions, they may have higher rates of nursing home admission. There may be improvement in quality of care for older adults, indicated by lower rates of pain and lower mortality rates. PACE enrollees express satisfaction with medical and personal care.

PALLIATIVE CARE TEAMS

Palliative care teams address pain and symptom management for individuals with acute or chronic medical conditions and their families. A dedicated palliative care team offers medical, nursing, social services, and chaplaincy, in addition to coordinating other therapies (CAM, physical, occupational, and speech therapy) that address specific needs. Similarly, hospice provides an interdisciplinary team that includes doctors, nurses, therapists (speech, occupational, and physical therapists), home health aides, social workers, chaplains, counselors, and trained volunteers. Integrative and complementary medicine specialists may be part of both palliative and hospice care teams to provide pain and symptom management, support and education for the family and caregivers, as well as an opportunity for the dying individual to find a sense of transcendence and peace with dying.

Interprofessional Team Training

The Partnership for Health in Aging (PHA), a coalition of more than 30 organizations representing health care professionals who care for older adults, developed a position statement to inspire the development and expansion of academic and continuing education to provide interprofessional team training.[37–40] The education must include attitudes, beliefs and experiences about providing team care; the differing commitment of faculty and students from different disciplines to the training; the value of education by matching the level of student education and interprofessional experiences in the clinical setting; less hierarchical clinical settings with shared leadership among health professions for more effective student education; and institutional and financial support for education and practice settings for meaningful interprofessional training.

The Agency for Healthcare Research and Quality (AHRQ), in collaboration with the Department of Defense's Patient Safety Program, has developed a comprehensive curriculum for teaching team care, TeamSTEPPS.[41] It is designed to improve the culture of safety in medical teams that is rooted in 20 years of research and lessons learned in applying the principles of team care. The curriculum is designed for different settings of care and aims to increase the awareness of team functioning, clarifying roles and responsibilities, resolving conflicts, improving information sharing, and eliminating barriers to quality and safety. AHRQ engages groups of professionals within organizations in the training to improve patient safety by building more effective teamwork across their organization.

The Interprofessional Education Collaborative fosters opportunities for health professions students from different disciplines to learn about, from, and with each other.[42] This collaborative has developed core competencies to guide health professions education in team-based practice to foster greater collaboration and better health outcomes.

REFERENCES

1. Ward BW, Schiller JS, Goodman RA. Multiple chronic conditions Among US adults: A 2012 update. *Prev Chronic Dis.* 2014;11:130389. doi:http://dx.doi.org/10.5888/pcd11.130389.
2. Warshaw G. Introduction: Advances and challenges in care of older people with chronic illness. *Generations.* 2006;30:5–10.
3. Kassner E. Home and community-based long-term services and supports for older people fact sheet. Washington, DC: AARP Public Policy Institute, 2011. http://assets.aarp.org/rgcenter/ppi/ltc/fs222-health.pdf Accessed April, 15, 2016.
4. World Report on Ageing and Health. Geneva: World Health Organization, 2015. http://apps.who.int/iris/bitstream/10665/186463/1/9789240694811_eng.pdf?ua=1/.
5. AHRQ Innovations Exchange Team. Chronic disease management can reduce readmissions. AHRQ Healthcare Innovations Exchange, https://innovations.ahrq.gov/perspectives/chronic-disease-management-can-reduce-readmissions. Last updated March 26, 2014.
6. Hall P, Weaver L. Interdisciplinary education and teamwork: A long and winding road. *Medical Education.* 2001;35:867–875.
7. Inter-professional collaboration and education. *Am J Nurs.* 2015;115(3):47–64.
8. Mitchell P, Wynia M, Golden R, et al. Core principles and values of effective team-based health care. Discussion Paper, Institute of Medicine, Washington, DC; 2012. www.iom.edu/tbc.

9. Care Coordination, Quality Improvement. Agency for Healthcare Research and Quality, Rockville, MD. http://www.ahrq.gov/research/findings/evidence-based-reports/caregaptp.html.

10. New York Academy of Medicare, Policy, Research, and Practice. Issue Brief Volume 1, page 1: Issue 2, October 2013.

11. Centers for Medicare and Medicaid Systems (CMS). The Center for Consumer Information & Insurance Oversight Regulations and Guidance. October 31. Baltimore, MD: CMS. https://www.cms.gov/cciio/resources/regulations-and-guidance/.

12. https://www.medicare.gov/manage-your-health/coordinating-your-care/coordinating-your-care.html

13. Bynum J, Meara E, Chang C, Rhoads J. Our Parents, Ourselves: Health Care for an Aging Population. February 17, 2016. A Report of the Dartmouth Atlas Project, The Dartmouth Institute for Health Policy & Clinical Practice. http://www.dartmouthatlas.org/downloads/reports/Our_Parents_Ourselves_021716.pdf.

14. Geriatric Interdisciplinary Team Training Workbook. VISN 3 Geriatric Research, Education, and Clinical Center (GRECC). Geriatrics, Palliative Care, and Interdisciplinary Teamwork Curriculum Module #2.

15. Forrest CB, Glade GB, Baker AE, Bocian A, von Schrader S, Starfield B. Coordination of specialty referrals and physician satisfaction with referral care. *Arch Pediatr Adolesc Med.* 2000;154:499–506.

16. Gandhi TK, Sittig DF, Franklin M, Sussman AJ, Fairchild DG, Bates DW. Communication breakdown in the outpatient referral process. *J Gen Intern Med.* 2000;15:626–631.

17. Gandhi TK. Fumbled handoffs: One dropped ball after another. *Ann Intern Med.* 2005;142:352–358.

18. Schoen C, Osborn R, Huynh PT, et al. Primary care and health system performance: Adults' experiences in five countries. *Health Aff.* 2004;Suppl Web Exclusives:W4-487–W4-503.

19. Schoen C, Osborn R, Huynh PT, et al. Taking the pulse of health care systems: Experiences of patients with health problems in six countries. *Health Aff.* 2005;Suppl Web Exclusives:W5-509–W5-525.

20. Naylor MD, Brooten DA, Campbell RL, Maislin G, McCauley KM, Schwartz JS. Transitional care of older adults hospitalized with heart failure: A randomized, controlled trial. *J Am Geriatr Soc.* 2004;52:675–684. [Erratum, *J Am Geriatr Soc.* 2004;52:1228.]

21. Coleman EA, Parry C, Chalmers S, Min S. The care transitions intervention: Results of a randomized controlled trial. *Arch Intern Med.* 2006;166:1822–1828.

22. Coleman EA, Smith JD, Frank JC, Min S, Parry C, Kramer AM. Preparing patients and caregivers to participate in care delivery across settings: The care transitions intervention. *J Am Geriatr Soc.* 2004;52:1817–1825.

23. Mitchell P, Wynia M, Golden R, et al. Core principles and values of effective team-based health care. Discussion Paper, Institute of Medicine, Washington, DC, 2012. www.iom.edu/tbc.

24. American Hospital Association. 3rd Biannual Complementary and Alternative Medicine (CAM) Survey of Hospitals. 2008. http://www.aha.org/aha/pressrelease/2008/080915-pr-cam.html Accessed April 15, 2016.

25. Hansson A, Friberg F, Segesten K, et al. Two sides of the coin: General practitioners' experience of working in multidisciplinary teams. *J Interprofessional Care.* 2008;22(1):5–16. doi:10.1080/13561820701722808.

26. Holtz-Bakin D. High-cost Medicare beneficiaries. Health and Human Services (HHS), May 2005. https://www.cbo.gov/publication/16487.

27. MEDPAC. The Medicare Modernization Act and Chronic Care Improvement. Report to the Congress. New Approaches in Medicare. MEDPAC Report, 2004.3.

28. Liu K, Wall S, Wissoker D. Disability and Medicare costs of elderly persons. *Milbank Q.* 1997;75:461–493.

29. Manton KG, Stallard E. Analysis of underwriting factors for AAPCC (adjusted average per capita cost). *Health Care Financ Rev.* 1992;14:117–132.

30. Holtz-Bakin D. High-cost Medicare beneficiaries. Health and Human Services (HHS), May 2005. https://www.cbo.gov/publication/16487.

31. Beales JL, Edes T. Veterans Affairs home-based primary care. *Clin Geriatr Med.* 2009;25:149x–154x.

32. DeJonge KE, Jamshed N, Gilden D, et al. Effects of home-based primary care on Medicare costs in high-risk elders. *J Am Geriatr Soc.* 2014;62:1825–1831.

33. Barnes ED, Palmer RM, Kresevic DM, et al. Acute care for elders units produced shorter hospital stays at lower cost while maintaining patients' functional status. *Health Aff.* 2012;31(6):1227–1236.

34. Ellis G, Whitehead M, Robinson D, et al. Comprehensive geriatric assessment for older adults admitted to hospital. *Cochrane Database Syst Rev.* 2011;7:CD006211. doi:10.1002/14651858.CD006211. pub2.

35. PACE. https://www.medicare.gov/your-medicare-costs/help-paying-costs/pace/pace.html

36. Assistant Secretary for Planning and Evaluation. Evaluating PACE: A review of the literature—executive summary January 2014. Washington, DC: U.S. Department of Health and Human Services. https://aspe.hhs.gov/execsum/evaluating-pace-review-literature-executive-summary.

37. Partnership for Health in Aging Workgroup on Interdisciplinary Team Training in Geriatrics. Position statement on interdisciplinary team training in geriatrics: An essential component of quality health care for older adults. *J Am Geriatr Soc.* 2014;62:961–965. http://dx.doi.org/10.1111/jgs.12822.

38. MEDPAC. The Medicare Modernization Act and Chronic Care Improvement. Report to the Congress. New Approaches in Medicare. MEDPAC Report, 2004.

39. Liu K, Wall S, Wissoker D. Disability and Medicare costs of elderly persons. *Milbank Q.* 1997;75:461–493.

40. Manton KG, Stallard E. Analysis of underwriting factors for AAPCC (adjusted average per capita cost). *Health Care Financ Rev* 1992; 14:117–132.

41. About TeamSTEPPS®. Agency for Healthcare Research and Quality, Rockville, MD. http://www.ahrq.gov/teamstepps/about-teamstepps/index.html.

42. Interprofessional Education Collaborative. https://www.ipecollaborative.org/about-ipec.html.

30

Bioethical Issues in Integrative Geriatrics

KATALIN ROTH

Ethical issues in integrative geriatrics include those specific to geriatrics and those specific to the use of complementary and alternative medicine (CAM). Older persons and their doctors are faced with complex ethical issues in medical decision making. Older persons bring to their medical decision making a lifetime of values and choices and, for many, a more nuanced appreciation of loss and death. Of importance are considerations of safety versus independence, life-extending therapies versus quality of life, the burdens of caregiving, and the influence of advanced age on the risks and benefits of various medical interventions.

Many older persons have used some forms of CAM. Studies show that baby boomers have a high acceptance of chiropractic, acupuncture, massage, and nutritional and other integrative therapies.[1,2] Immigrants in particular, depending on their countries of origin, may have more experience with therapies used in integrative medicine. However, many are reluctant to disclose their use of these therapies for fear of physician disapproval.[3] Also, physicians often fail to ask about patients' use of herbal or nutritional supplements or other CAM modalities when they interview patients.[3-5]

Geriatrics has been described by some as "slow medicine," and an integrative approach is very consistent with the more holistic model of geriatric care.[6] Slow medicine refers to the delicate balancing of important goals to preserve function. Of course this does not mean that older patients should not be treated promptly and aggressively in an emergency or when good treatment options exist; rather, when considering interventions, weight should be given to the patient's current economic and psychosocial circumstances, functional status, and long-term goals. A conventional disease-oriented model of medical treatment fails to account for the complexity of medical conditions confronting older adults as well as maximizing their quality of life.

The relationship between CAM and conventional allopathic medicine continues to evolve, but it is fair to say that among allopathic providers there is a growing acceptance of many aspects of integrative medicine.[5] Since 1991 the National Center for Complementary and Alternative Medicine (now the National Center for Complementary and Integrative Health) at the National Institute of Health has funded studies of CAM therapies. The Institute of Medicine has recognized that CAM therapies are part of the established medical landscape.[7] The Cochrane Collaboration now tracks and evaluates the evidence base of CAM therapies. Furthermore, doctors now routinely accept and promote such aspects of health as vitamins, exercise, and nutrition, which were not so long ago regarded as "complementary." Nonetheless, the relationship of integrative therapies to conventional geriatric medical practice raises potential ethical issues.

The first ethical challenge for any geriatric integrative provider of health care to older adults is to understand the patient's values and goals of care. Active listening and empathy is critical to delivering good integrative medical care, and history taking should include an assessment of the patient's history of CAM use and openness to CAM. Open, free communication underlies all of the ethical principles discussed below.

Modern medical ethics draws upon four essential principles: beneficence, nonmaleficence, autonomy, and justice.[8]

Beneficence, or acting on behalf of the patient's best interests, considers beneficial therapeutic options in the context of the specific goals and values of the patient. Maintaining independence, respecting family obligations, preserving function, and maintaining quality of life are integral aspects of the decision as to whether a proposed treatment may be beneficial. Providing scientific evidence for recommended treatments is part of the obligation of beneficence.

Nonmaleficence, or "do no harm," requires that the doctor avoid treatments that may be ineffective, that are likely to cause distressing side effects, or that may provide survival without honoring the patient's values. Treatments with marginal benefit or with a poor evidence base waste time and money and may cause suffering. "Slow medicine" can be seen as a way of expressing the ethical value of nonmaleficence.

Advanced age and functional status are prognostic factors for treatment complications in the older patient. The routine incorporation of prognostic factors into the design of appropriate treatment plans can be viewed as an ethical imperative consistent with beneficence and nonmaleficence.

Beneficence and nonmaleficence require that the doctor should endeavor to act in the patient's best interest rather than the doctor's self-interest. Conflicts of interest should be avoided, or if unavoidable, should always be disclosed. Adherence to evidence-based practice ensures that the patient's best interests are uppermost.

Palliative medicine is consistent with the values of beneficence and non-maleficence. A patient-centered integrative approach to care at the end of life requires a strong knowledge base in palliative medicine.

It can be argued that the use of restraints, physical or chemical, subverts beneficence and nonmaleficence. While providing nutrition to patients with advanced dementia via a feeding tube might be consistent with values of nurturance, restraining the elderly patient who refuses to eat or who repeatedly pulls out a feeding tube is an assault on the person.

Autonomy, or respect for persons, requires that the clinician offer medical treatment choices that are consistent with the patient's value system. The corollary is that the doctor must respect the patient's value choices. The doctor should not abandon a patient who does not follow his or her advice but rather chooses alternative options (non-abandonment).

Autonomy is the underlying justification for the doctrine of informed consent. The use of CAM therapies requires that full information be provided to the patient. It can be argued that there should be a higher standard for informed consent when CAM treatments are offered, somewhat analogous to that required in research and experimental therapies.

Autonomy requires autonomous decision-making capacity. The high prevalence of dementia in the geriatric population implies that all geriatric patients should be screened for cognitive impairment. However, many persons with mild cognitive impairment can express preferences even if they cannot weigh complex medical decisions. Informed consent is a pretense when patients have advanced dementia, and physicians should not confuse acquiescence with truly informed decision making.

The final ethical principle is *justice*. Physicians have an obligation to strive to ensure that health resources are allocated justly. Ideally, all patients should receive similar treatment for similar conditions. In the individual clinical situation, physicians should act as patient advocates and provide the best possible available care at the bedside. Rationing decisions for the health system as a whole should not influence the practitioner in the clinical encounter.

Nonetheless, the investment of expensive health resources at the end of life is a policy question for society. Some ethicists have argued that expenditures should be more limited in the very old so that health care resources are fairly distributed to young and old alike. Bioethicist Daniel Callahan, for instance, proposes that there is such a thing as a natural lifespan, a full life, and that it may not always be wise to keep "elderly people with chronic diseases expensively alive."[9,10]

Ability to pay is a criterion that directly or indirectly affects many health care decisions. There may not be a just distribution of the benefits of CAM. Many CAM therapies are not covered by Medicare and other insurance plans in the United States. On the other hand, some European countries cover many CAM therapies. Despite these differences in insurance coverage, integrative providers should always endeavor to provide the best possible treatments for their patients.

Advance Care Planning

Geriatricians routinely integrate advance care planning into their practice. Advance care planning should be undertaken in the care of all older persons and all persons who face life-limiting serious illness. An important part of advance care planning is the patient's identification of surrogate decision makers. It is always prudent to anticipate a future need for surrogate decision makers. Capable patients should be encouraged to identify family or friends who can be included in health care discussions and decisions. Older patients should designate a health care proxy decision maker to make health care decisions for them should they become incapacitated.

Many older persons do not want heroic or high-tech therapies at the end of their lives and do not wish to spend their remaining time in a state of dependency. For instance, it is well known that prolonged debility, usually irreversible, often ensues after cardiopulmonary resuscitation in the elderly.[11] If these preferences are not discussed with family members prior to a health emergency, or prior to the onset of dementia, surrogate decision makers who are unaware of their relative's preferences may choose more aggressive care. When persons cannot make informed decisions, because of dementia or severe illness, the value of autonomy may be less important than making decisions based on the best interest of the patient (beneficence). This best interest test should still take into account the patient's preferences and values insofar as they are known.

There is a high burden on surrogate decision makers to make choices based on well-established standards of care. Surrogates should take care, if choosing CAM therapies, that the patient's values are respected and that more conventional therapies have not been sufficient.

Integrative interventions such as exercise and nutrition may be regarded as enhancing patient autonomy. However, integrative practitioners should discourage the use of treatments that have not been shown to benefit older patients. Complementary therapies should not be offered as first-line therapy when conventional treatments have demonstrated benefit. For older patients whose treatment choices may include observation, patients need to be informed that many complementary therapies, while they may enhance a sense of well-being, have not been shown to affect the course of the illness.

Patients and their families should be encouraged to make use of available resources for advance care planning—many tools are now free and available online.[12,13]

Confidentiality

Respect for patient autonomy requires physicians to maintain patient confidentiality. When patients do not wish their family members or neighbors to know of their condition, their confidentiality should be respected. However, confidentiality may conflict with other important considerations, such as patient safety. For example, if the doctor believes that the patient's infirmity precludes safe driving, yet despite counseling the patient will not stop driving, then the safety of the patient and the safety of the public are jeopardized. In this case the doctor has an affirmative obligation to report the patient to the department of motor vehicles and to inform family members of his concern.

Truth Telling

Physicians have an obligation to be truthful with patients. Physicians must be honest with patients about their illness, treatment options, and prognosis, so that they might best be able to make informed choices. The use of complementary therapies may make sense when the goal is to support the autonomy and dignity of the older person. Integrative physicians have an obligation to ensure that patients are well informed. Care must be taken to ensure that therapies without a strong evidence base are not used in place of well-established treatments without giving extensive disclosure to patients. This is another way of saying that proper informed consent must be obtained.

Patient Preferences

Respect for patient autonomy obligates the doctor to learn about the reasons underlying the patient's choices. For example, nonadherence to prescribed medications might be because the patient must choose between an expensive medication or paying the rent; missed doctors' visits may be due to lack of transportation. Failure to inquire more deeply into a patient's life circumstances can create profound misunderstanding in the doctor–patient relationship. Many older adults have responsibilities as caregivers to spouses and other relatives, and they may choose to avoid recommended treatments because such treatments might interfere with their responsibilities. Patients may make choices to avoid hospitalization, fearing the loss of independence, and whenever possible such choices should be respected and supported.

Case Study

Mr. D., a 76-year-old African-American married man with mild hypertension, is diagnosed with localized prostate cancer. His urologist recommends surgery, but Mr. D. is reluctant. Dr. M., his primary care geriatrician, discusses the variable course of prostate cancer in the older patient and offers the option of observation. She tells Mr. D., "Beware, there are a lot of quack therapies out there" and does not inquire about his attitudes toward or personal use of CAM. Mr. D. has heard from friends and from reading on the internet that prostate cancer can be an indolent disease in the elderly. He also has heard that vitamins and cleansing therapies may be of benefit, and he buys various remedies on the internet. Mr. D has been scheduled to see Dr. M. every 6 months but he does not return for 2 years. In the interim he has been receiving acupuncture, taking herbs, and using other CAM therapies. He has also stopped drinking alcohol and has become a vegetarian. Recently he developed back pain, for which he consulted a chiropractor. The chiropractor evaluated him, elicited the history of prostate cancer, and referred him back to his primary care provider. On exam Dr. M. finds that Mr. D.'s legs are weak and he has significant tenderness over his thoracic spine. His prostate-specific antigen level is markedly elevated, and plain spine films show metastatic erosion of several vertebral bodies. A computed tomography scan shows tumor impingement on the spinal cord, and Dr. M. recommends hospital admission, emergency radiation therapy, and steroids to avert imminent cord compression. Mr. D. agrees to hospital management of his metastatic prostate cancer.

Mr. D. was clearly upset and frightened by his cancer diagnosis. Observation was an option that he did not realize was available to him, and in his decision to delay surgery, he was likely harmed by his long absence from medical care. Perhaps he would have returned sooner had Dr. M. not made disparaging remarks about CAM. His relationship with his physician suffered as a result of the doctor's skepticism about his interest in CAM.

Perhaps at the outset Dr. M. and the urologist might have offered less invasive treatments (such as radiation or hormone treatments), as surgery was not acceptable to Mr. D. Going forward, Dr. M. should support Mr. D.'s need to take some control of his care, by understanding and helping him navigate through available CAM therapies. She might support his healthful dietary improvements and work with him and his family to better understand his choices now that his disease has advanced. For his pain, Dr. M. should include CAM modalities in her treatment plan. Dr. M. should assist Mr. D. with advance care planning, identifying a surrogate decision maker and clarifying his wishes regarding resuscitation and comfort measures at the end of life.

Professional Responsibilities of Integrative Geriatricians

The relationship between traditional allopathic medicine and integrative medicine is a troubled one, and providers need to be honest with their patients and with themselves about CAM. As part of continuing medical education and maintenance of skills, integrative providers need to update their understanding of CAM therapies. Traditional medical thinking included skepticism and even prohibition of association with CAM practitioners and osteopaths. Doctors of osteopathy are now trained and accredited according to similar standards as allopaths, and there is now broad acceptance of osteopathic-trained physicians in allopathic residency and fellowship training programs. Osteopaths and allopaths enjoy equal status before state licensing boards. The American Medical Association's code of ethics now concedes that chiropractors might provide acceptable care in certain respects and allows for professional association between allopaths and chiropractors.[14–17] CAM professional organizations have codes of ethics that are consistent with conventional bioethics, and CAM providers need to become familiar with them.

LICENSING

Protection of the public requires that CAM providers should be subject to licensing and regulation. It is beyond the scope of this chapter to discuss training and licensing, but CAM providers should investigate the applicable regulations in their jurisdictions. Acupuncturists, massage therapists, and chiropractors have established training curricula, accredited teaching institutions, and institutional standards that review and validate credentials. Integrative physicians should encourage their patients to seek care from practitioners who are qualified and credentialed. Licensure is an important professional standard for CAM providers, and allopathic physicians should be familiar with the licensing requirements in their area. Chiropractors are licensed in every state, massage therapists and acupuncturists are licensed in more than half of the states, and naturopaths are licensed in about 12 states.[18]

For allopathic physicians who offer CAM to their patients, the Federation of State Medical Boards has issued Model Guidelines for the Use of Complementary and Alternative Therapies in Medical Practice.[19] These guidelines give state medical boards guidance in regulating physicians who incorporate CAM and recognize that patients have a right to seek CAM. The guidelines stress the safety and also the efficacy of CAM treatments and stress that CAM therapies (1) must be compared with established treatment models for the same condition; (2) should have a favorable risk/benefit ratio compared to other treatments for the same condition; (3) should be based on a reasonable expectation of favorable outcome, including prevention practices; and (4) should be based on the expectation that a greater benefit will be achieved than that expected with no treatment.

MALPRACTICE

Physicians offering CAM therapies are liable to malpractice for CAM as well as for other therapies, and in this regard patient participation in decision making, full disclosure to patients, and informed consent are critical. Failure to treat with conventional care and failure to offer proven conventional therapies leave the physician open to a claim of malpractice. Malpractice generally requires findings that (1) the physician violated a duty to provide a standard of care; (2) the care provided was below professional standards; (3) harm was caused to the patient because the provider failed to meet the professional standard; and (4) the patient's injury can be compensated with damages.[20]

Research Questions in CAM for Integrative Geriatricians

Studies undertaken to assess CAM therapies should conform to ethical standards for biomedical research. Studies conducted under the auspices of the National Center for Complementary and Alternative Medicine conform to the standards set by the National Institute of Health.[21] In its 2005 report on CAM, the Institute of Medicine outlined an ethical framework for CAM research. The report proposed five components: a social commitment to public welfare; a commitment to protect patients; respect for patient autonomy; recognition of medical pluralism; and public accountability.

Summary

Ethical practice of integrative geriatrics requires a strong knowledge base in geriatrics and an understanding of the special challenges faced by seniors nearing the end of life. In considering whether to offer CAM therapies, the provider should consider the severity and acuteness of illness, the curability with conventional treatment, and the invasiveness and toxicities of conventional treatment. The quality of evidence and safety of CAM therapies should be discussed with the patient. Excellent, open communication between patient and doctor is essential. This includes an exploration of the patient's views and intention regarding CAM. The principles of beneficence, nonmaleficence, autonomy, and justice help guide clinicians.

Informed consent is an essential component of ethical practice. In the case of CAM therapies, informed consent must include discussion of the conventional treatment alternatives and the curability with conventional treatment as well as the quality of evidence of safety and efficacy of CAM. The patient's capacity should be assessed and consent cannot be presumed. Advance care planning provides an opportunity to explore the patient's values and goals and helps to tailor therapy to the individual patient and family.

Integrative physicians should strive to refer patients to well-trained, licensed, and credentialed CAM providers. CAM research should follow established guidelines.

Useful online resources include the following:

- www.theconversationproject.org: "The Project is dedicated to helping people talk about their wishes for end-of-life care."
- www.acpdecisions.org
- https://nccih.nih.gov/research/statistics: detailed review of CAM statistics including National Health Interview Survey (CDC and NCCIH)

REFERENCES

1. https://nccih.nih.gov/research/statistics.
2. Kaptchuk TJ, Eisenberg DM. The persuasive appeal of alternative medicine. *Ann Intern Med.* 1998;129:1061–1065.
3. Astin J. Why patients use alternative medicine. *JAMA.* 1998;279(19):1548–1553.
4. Ryder PT, Wolpert B. Complementary and alternative medicine use among older African-Americans. *Arch Intern Med.* 1998;158(20):2200–2211.
5. Eisenberg DM. Advising patients who seek alternative medical therapies. *Ann Intern Med.* 1997;127:61–69.

6. Zuger A. Review of "My Mother Your Mother" by Dennis McCullough. *New York Times*, Feb. 26, 2008.

7. Institute of Medicine Committee on the Use of Complementary and Alternative Medicine by the American Public. Washington DC: The National Academies Press; 2005.

8. Beauchamp T, Childress J. *Principles of Biomedical Ethics*, 5th ed. New York: Oxford University Press, 2001.

9. Callahan D. On dying after your time. *New York Times*, Nov. 13, 2013.

10. Callahan D. *Setting Limits: Medical Goals in an Aging Society*. Washington DC: Georgetown University Press; 1995.

11. Ehlenbach WJ, Barnato AE, Curtis JR, et al. Epidemiologic study of in-hospital cardiopulmonary resuscitation in the elderly. *N Engl J Med*. 2009;361(1):22–31.

12. www.theconversationproject.org

13. www.acpdecisions.org/

14. AMA Code of Medical Ethics Opinion 3.04, April 1977.

15. AMA Code of Medical Ethics Opinion 3.041, March 1992.

16. http://journalofethics.ama-assn.org/2011/06/pfor1-1106.html

17. http://journalofethics.ama-assn.org/2011/06/coet1-1106.html

18. Cohen M. Legal and risk management issues in complementary and alternative medicine. In Snyder L, ed., *Complementary and Alternative Medicine: Ethics, the Patient and the Physician*. Totowa, NJ: Humana Press; 2007.

19. FSMB Report on Professional Conduct and Ethics, April 2000. http://www.fsmb.org/Media/Default/PDF/FSMB/Advocacy/2000_grpol_Professional_Conducts_and_Ethics.pdf

20. Cohen MH, Eisenberg DM. Potential physician malpractice liability associated with complementary and integrative therapies. *Ann Intern Med*. 2002;136:596–603.

21. Emanuel E, Wendler D, Grady C. What makes research ethical? *JAMA*. 2000:283(20):2701–2711.

31

Integrative Palliative Care

ANGELA LEE, STEPHANIE CHENG, AND DALE LUPU

This chapter provides an overview of hospice and palliative care. We discuss integrative approaches to the most common symptoms encountered in palliative care, palliative approaches to communication and advance care planning, and considerations in providing care at the end of life. Integrative medicine and palliative medicine are philosophical cousins. Many of the basic tenets of palliative medicine—interdisciplinary care, person-centered care, care of the whole person and of the family, careful communication and goal setting[1]—are also foundational to integrative medicine. As the World Health Organization states:

> Palliative care is an approach that improves the quality of life of patients and their families facing the problem associated with life-threatening illness, through the prevention and relief of suffering by means of early identification and impeccable assessment and treatment of pain and other problems, physical, psychosocial and spiritual.[2]

The National Consensus Project for Quality Palliative Care enumerates the following features of palliative care philosophy and delivery:

- Care is provided and services are coordinated by an interdisciplinary team.
- Patients, family, and palliative and non-palliative health care providers collaborate and communicate about care needs.

- Services are available concurrently with or independent of curative or life-prolonging care.
- Patient and family hopes for peace and dignity are supported through the course of illness, during the dying process, and after death.[3]

With the exception of special support during the dying process and bereavement period, all these features are also part of integrative medicine. Both integrative and palliative medicine emphasize the patient's experience, including quality of life as defined by the patient and functional status related to the patient's own goals. Both treat the patient in the context of his or her family and social setting. Both pay careful attention to the mind–body continuum. Both are best delivered by transdisciplinary teams. And both cultivate the healer's skill in listening, communicating, and embodying a compassionate presence.

In contrast to palliative medicine, integrative medicine may deploy strategies to cure an underlying condition as well as to alleviate the symptoms. Palliative medicine focuses on the relief of suffering, leaving attempts at cure of the underlying disease to other parts of medicine. However, it is a common mistake to assume that palliative medicine can ONLY be used when curative efforts have ceased. "Upstream" palliative care working in concert with the curative health care system has shown the biggest impact on both quality of life and length of life.[4,5] In sum, while integrative medicine includes ameliorating and curing underlying conditions and palliative medicine includes a special (but not exclusive) focus on the end of life, both specialties embrace a holistic approach to enhancing quality of life, optimizing function, and relieving suffering.

Given that integrative medicine and palliative medicine share a philosophical approach, this chapter will cover two major topics: (1) integrative medicine approaches that may be useful in treating the most common and troublesome problems encountered by palliative medicine practitioners and (2) key palliative medicine skills and expertise that may be useful to the integrative practitioner.

Integrative Approaches to Palliative Symptom Management

While symptoms vary from patient to patient depending on the disease process, there are some commonly experienced symptoms toward the end of life and in those who are seriously ill. This section discusses integrative approaches to the most common symptoms encountered in palliative care.

PAIN

Pain is a symptom that receives much attention in palliative care. Chapter 12 discusses integrative pain management. Special considerations about treating pain at the end of life are discussed in this section.

It can be helpful to think of pain in terms of somatic and neuropathic pain. For somatic pain, opioids, nonsteroidal anti-inflammatories (NSAIDs), and acetaminophen (Tylenol) are commonly used. As always, benefits and risks must be weighed for each medication as these pain medications are not without risks/side effects (e.g., constipation and altered level of consciousness with opioids, bleeding and abdominal discomfort with NSAIDs, and liver damage with excessive amounts of Tylenol). For patients with neuropathic pain, common treatments include gabapentin; pregabalin; tricyclic antidepressants like amitriptyline, nortriptyline, and desipramine; carbamazepine; selective serotonin reuptake inhibitors like fluoxetine and paroxetine; mixed reuptake inhibitors like venlafaxine and duloxetine; topical lidocaine patches; intravenous or oral ketamine (limited data in older adults); and methadone and other opioids.

A systematic review looked at the evidence of integrative modalities for treating pain toward the end of life and found that acupuncture, massage, aromatherapy, psychological therapies, music therapy, and hypnosis may ease pain sensation and suffering.[6] However, use of integrative modalities at the end of life should be determined on a case-by-case basis.[7]

NAUSEA AND VOMITING

Nausea and vomiting are frequent complaints associated with cancer and its therapies, as well as other disease processes, especially toward the end of life. A thorough history and physical exam are essential as the etiology and therefore treatment can vary significantly. Nausea is mediated through the gastrointestinal lining, the vestibular system, the cerebral cortex, and the chemoreceptor trigger zone in the medulla oblongata. Common causes of nausea are dysmotility, obstruction, medication side effects, brain metastases, and vestibular apparatus irritation. Often overlooked, constipation is a common cause of nausea and vomiting and can be easily addressed.

Nutrition/Botanicals

Ginger has been shown to help with nausea in a variety of settings, including postoperative nausea,[9] HIV/antiretroviral-induced nausea,[10] and motion sickness. Ginger may also reduce chemotherapy-induced nausea, but data thus far have been conflicting, which may be explained by the nonstandard-ized preparations of ginger used.[11] Marx et al. performed a systematic litera-ture review and found that five of seven included studies reported favorable results; they suggested that the mixed results may be due to the varying dos-ages used in different studies.[12] Results from mixed-model analyses showed that all concentrations of ginger significantly reduced the incidence of acute, but not delayed, nausea, with 0.5 and 1.0 g being the most effective.[13] Bioactive compounds within the rhizome of ginger interact with several pathways that

> are directly implicated in chemotherapy induced nausea in addition to pathways that could play secondary roles by exacerbating symptoms. These properties include 5-HT$_3$, substance P, and acetylcholine receptor antagonism; anti-inflammatory properties; and modulation of cellular redox signaling, vasopressin release, gastrointestinal motility, and gastric emptying rate.[14]

The dosage is 500 to 1,000 mg ginger root extract every 4 to 6 hours as needed, or 1 teaspoon or 5 g of crystallized ginger every 2 to 3 hours, as needed. The patient can also drink ginger tea. Ginger should be avoided in patients with thrombocytopenia given its anticoagulant effects. Excessive doses can cause heartburn.

Medical marijuana (cannabis) has been shown to help alleviate nausea and vomiting. A recent Cochrane review analyzed 23 randomized controlled tri-als of cannabinoids compared with placebo or with other antiemetic drugs. Patients were more likely to report a complete absence of nausea and vom-iting with cannabis than with placebo, and there was little discernable dif-ference between the effectiveness of cannabinoids and of prochlorperazine, metoclopramide, domperidone, and chlorpromazine. Of note, however, none of the trials involved the agents now most widely used—the serotonin 5-HT3 antagonists.[15] Cannabis contains several potentially therapeutic cannabinoids, including delta-9-tetrahydrocannabinol (THC), the most psychoactive can-nabinoid in the plant, and cannabidiol (CBD).

The dosage of Marinol (dronabinol) (THC only) is 2.5 to 10 mg three or four times daily. Cannabis is also available as a tincture, edible, transdermal patch, salve, and other forms (and of variable THC:CBD ratios) from individual dis-pensaries. Dosing should be discussed with the dispensary staff. Dry mouth, fatigue, dizziness, agitation, and poor memory are potential side effects. Side effects are significantly more common and more severe with high-dose, pure THC products, both botanicals or medical. Severe delirium has been reported from both nabilone and dronabinol. Most patients prefer the botanical form of cannabis for a variety of reasons, mostly due to the lowest chances of side effects and easiest control of the dosage.

Acupuncture/Acupressure

Several studies have been performed showing the benefit of acupuncture and acupressure for nausea and vomiting.[16] Acupressure in the form of a wristband (popularly found under the name "Sea-Band") has been used for chemotherapy-related nausea with good effect (and other causes of nausea).[17,18] Acu-stimulation bands like "ReliefBand" are also available.

Pharmaceuticals

Pharmacological antiemetic agents abound and target a variety of receptors (including serotonin, dopamine, histamine, acetylcholine, and neurokinin). Tables 31.1 and 31.2 list typical first-line antiemetics for various common clinical scenarios.

CONSTIPATION

Constipation is a common and distressing symptom in seriously ill patients, and fecal impaction is more common in older adults (and can lead to urinary retention).[19] Additionally, constipation is prevalent toward the end of life and involves a complex interaction of anatomical, neurological, and iatrogenic factors.[20] Palliative medicine patients are at especially high risk due to the following factors:

- Low intake of food, fluid, and fiber
- Impaired mobility
- Opioid analgesics and other drugs that impair gut motility
- Complicating medical conditions, such as bowel obstruction or hemorrhoids

Dehydration can lead to constipation, so taking in adequate fluid is important. Drinking 8 to 12 glasses of water daily is recommended if possible. In addition, flaxseed meal or oil (1 tablespoon on cereal or mixed in water, juice, or a smoothie three times a day) can help with bowel function.[21,22] There are no data to support the use of one laxative over another. In the palliative population,

Table 31.1. Common Clinical Scenarios Associated with Nausea and Vomiting at the End of Life

Clinical Scenario	Mechanism of Nausea and Vomiting	Typical First-line Antiemetics
Opioid-induced nausea and vomiting	Stimulation of CTZ (D2) Gastroparesis (D2) Constipation (H1, muscarinic acetylcholine receptor) Sensitization of labyrinth (H1, muscarinic acetylcholine receptor)	Metoclopramide, haloperidol, prochlorperazine
Chemotherapy-induced nausea and vomiting	5HT3 released in gut, stimulating peripheral pathways Stimulation of CTZ (D2, 5HT3, NK1) Anxiety	5Ht3 antagonists (such as ondansetron), dexamethasone, and aprepitant
Malignant bowel obstruction	Stimulation of CTZ (D2) Stimulation of peripheral pathways (H1, muscarinic acetylcholine receptor)	Metoclopramide (if incomplete obstruction), haloperidol, and dexamethasone or hyoscyamine, nasogastric tube, venting gastrostomy tube
Impaired gastrointestinal tract mobility of advanced cancer	Gastroparesis (D2)	Metoclopramide
Radiation-associated nausea and vomiting	Stimulation of peripheral pathways via 5HT3 released from enterochromaffin cells in gastrointestinal tract	5HT3 antagonists
Brain tumor	Increased intracranial pressure or meningeal irritation activates meningeal mechanoreceptors, which stimulate the vomiting center.	Dexamethasone
Motion-associated nausea and vomiting	Stimulation via vestibulocochlear nerve (muscarinic acetylcholine receptor, H1)	Scopolamine, diphenhydramine, promethazine

Abbreviations: CTZ, chemoreceptor trigger zone; D2, dopamine type 2 receptor; H1, histamine type 1 receptor; NK1, neurokinin type 1 receptor; 5HT3, 5-hydroxytryptamine type 3 receptor.

Adapted from Table 2 in Wood GJ, et al. Management of intractable nausea and vomiting in patients at the end of life: "I was feeling nauseous all of the time . . . nothing was working." *JAMA.* 2007;298(10):1196–1207.[8]

Table 31.2. Antiemetics

Antiemetic (trade name)	Presumed Primary Receptor Site of Action	Dosage/Route	Major Adverse Effects
Metoclopramide (Reglan)	D2 (primarily in GI tract) or 5HT3 (only at high doses)	5–20 mg orally or subcutaneously or intravenously before every meal and before bed	Dystonia, akathisia, esophageal spasm, and colic in gastrointestinal tract and obstruction
Haloperidol (Haldol)	D2 (primarily in CTZ)	0.5–4 mg orally or subcutaneously or intravenously every 6 hours	Dystonia and akathisia
Prochlorperazine (Compazine)	D2 (primarily in CTZ)	5–10 mg orally or intravenously every 6 hours or 25 mg rectally every 6 hours	Dystonia, akathisia, and sedation
Promethazine (Phenergan)	H1, muscarinic acetylcholine receptor or D2 (primarily in CTZ)	12.5–25 mg orally or intravenously every 6 hours or 25 mg rectally every 6 hours	Dystonia, akathisia, and sedation
Diphenhydramine (Benadryl)	H1	25–50 mg orally, intravenously, or subcutaneously every 6 hours	Sedation, dry mouth, and urinary retention
Scopolamine (Transderm scop)	Muscarinic acetylcholine receptor	1.5-mg transdermal patch every 3 days	Dry mouth, blurred vision, ileus, urinary retention, and confusion
Hyoscyamine (Levsin)	Muscarinic acetylcholine receptor	0.125–0.25 mg sublingually or orally every 4 hours or 0.25–0.5 mg subcutaneously or intravenously every 4 hours	Dry mouth, blurred vision, ileus, urinary retention, and confusion
Ondansetron (Zofran)*	5HT3	4–8 mg orally by pill or dissolvable tablet or intravenously every 4–8 hours	Headache, fatigue, and constipation

(continued)

Table 31.2. Continued

Antiemetic (trade name)	Presumed Primary Receptor Site of Action	Dosage/Route	Major Adverse Effects
Mirtazapine (Remeron)	5HT3	15–45 mg orally every night	Somnolence at low dose, dry mouth, and increased appetite

Abbreviations: CTZ, chemoreceptor trigger zone; D2, dopamine type 2 receptor; H1, histamine type 1 receptor; 5HT3, 5-hydroxytryptamine type 3 receptor.

*Ondansetron is included as an example of 5HT3 antagonists because it was the first agent of this class and was adopted in many hospital formularies. Its inclusion is not meant to indicate superiority over other members of the class, such as dolasetron, granisetron, and palonosetron.

Adapted from Table 3 in Wood GJ, et al. Management of intractable nausea and vomiting in patients at the end of life: "I was feeling nauseous all of the time . . . nothing was working." *JAMA.* 2007;298(10):1196–1207.[8]

the mainstay of constipation treatment is to start with a bowel stimulant (e.g., senna) and escalate doses as needed. An osmotic agent (e.g., polyethylene glycol, milk of magnesia) may be added if needed. Suppositories, enemas, or manual disimpaction may also be required. A rectal exam should be performed to rule out fecal impaction and a kidney, ureter, and bladder x-ray (KUB) should be considered to rule out obstruction. Of note, a stool softener and/or laxative should be started prophylactically (and given regularly) with the start of any opioid. In general, bulk-forming fiber agents (e.g., psyllium, methylcellulose) have little role in palliative care because of their tendency to form impactions when patients stop taking in adequate amounts of fluids. There are limited data supporting the use of newer agents like the small intestinal secretagogues lubiprostone and linaclotide at the end of life. Various therapies are summarized in Table 31.3.

DYSPNEA

Dyspnea is a symptom experienced by almost all terminally ill patients at some point in their disease course. Dyspnea is defined by the Thoracic Society of America as "a subjective feeling of breathing discomfort."[19] There are several possible etiologies, and dyspnea is often multifactorial. Common causes of dyspnea include infection, fluid overload, malignancy, muscle weakness, chronic obstructive pulmonary disease, and anxiety. If possible, any underlying (and potentially reversible) causes should be addressed first. If dyspnea

Table 31.3. Prevention and Treatment of Constipation

Medication	Dosage and Frequency	Comments
Stool Softener (Detergent Laxative)		
Docusate sodium (capsules/tablets or liquid) (Colace)	Starting dose: 100 mg orally twice daily or 200 mg; titrate dose up to two or three times daily. Max. 600 mg/day.	Generally well tolerated and safe; generally insufficient if used alone
Stimulants		
Senna (Sennokot)	1 tablet orally daily; titrate up to 4 tablets orally twice daily	Useful when added to docusate; can cause cramping, can worsen colic in bowel obstruction; also available as tea
Bisacodyl (Dulcolax)	Start with 1 (5-mg) tablet orally daily; titrate to 3 tablets twice daily. Suppository 10 mg per rectum daily as needed.	Can worsen colic in bowel obstruction; bisacodyl suppository causes more cramping than glycerin suppository; bisacodyl tablets can cause more cramping than senna tablets
Osmotic Agents		
Glycerin suppository	1 per rectum daily prn	Acts as both lubricant and osmotic agent; generally well tolerated, but rarely adequate alone
Sorbitol	15–60 ml orally two to four times daily	Sweet taste can be unpleasant; can cause bloating
Lactulose (10 g/15 ml)	15–60 ml orally two or three times daily	More expensive than sorbitol but with similar efficacy and side effects
Polyethylene glycol (Miralax)	17 g powder dissolved in liquid taken orally one to three times daily	Tasteless; often well tolerated; available over the counter
Magnesium hydroxide (milk of magnesia)	15–30 ml daily as needed	Can cause cramping; high magnesium load with renal failure
Magnesium citrate	200–400 mg powder daily in divided doses; 195–300 ml oral solution given once or in divided doses	Can cause cramping; high magnesium load with renal failure
Enemas		
Warm tap water	One administration per rectum, can repeat daily or twice daily	Rectal administration can soften stool before manual disimpaction.

(continued)

Table 31.3. Continued

Medication	Dosage and Frequency	Comments
Mineral oil	One administration per rectum	Oral dosing should be avoided; risk of severe pneumonitis if aspirated; rectal administration can soften stools before manual disimpaction.
Milk and molasses (or corn syrup)	Added to a liter of water; per rectum administration	Combines both osmotic and colonic stimulant; traditional use has been when all else fails
Soap suds	One administration per rectum	Not recommended: colon irritant, risk of bowel-wall damage with large dose or repeated use
Other Agents		
Prune juice	120–240 ml orally one or two times daily	Combines both soluble fiber and stimulant; a recognized traditional approach; good adjuvant
Metoclopramide	10–20 mg orally every 6 hours	Pro-motility agent; may be helpful for some patients; contraindicated in complete bowel obstruction, potential for tardive dyskinesia (U.S. Food & Drug Administration black box warning); avoid prolonged use
Methylnaltrexone	0.15 mg/kg of body weight (up to 12 mg) subcutaneous injection every other day	Need to rule out bowel obstruction prior to use; requires subcutaneous injection; usually produces bowel movement within 30 minutes; peripheral mu-opioid receptor antagonist; effectively treats opioid-induced constipation without reversing analgesia or precipitating withdrawal; expensive, generally used as rescue therapy in refractory cases
Lubiprostone	8–24 mcg orally twice daily with food	Chloride channel activator; approved by U.S. Food & Drug Administration for constipation-predominant irritable bowel syndrome and chronic idiopathic constipation; may cause nausea

Adapted from Quill TE et al. *Primer of Palliative Care*, 6th ed. American Academy of Hospice and Palliative Medicine; 2014:82–83.[19]

remains after disease-focused treatment, the focus should be on treating dyspnea as a symptom.

Behavioral

Positioning can impact a patient's sensation of breathing comfort, and many patients find that sitting up can bring greater ease. In addition, increasing air movement by opening a window or placing a fan in front of the patient's face can ease dyspnea. Adjusting humidity by using a humidifier or air conditioner can be helpful. Breathing exercises, guided imagery, and hypnotherapy can also help dyspnea. Discontinuing intravenous fluids in imminently dying patients is appropriate.

Pharmaceuticals

Opiates have been the mainstay of treatment of dyspnea at the end of life as well as in dyspnea refractory to disease-focused treatments.[23] However, a recent Cochrane review found that there is only some low-quality evidence showing benefit for the use of oral or parenteral opioids to relieve breathlessness. They suggest that more research is needed with larger numbers of participants, using standardized protocols and with quality of life measures included[23] (Table 31.4).

Treatment with other medications can be helpful, such as anticholinergics (e.g., scopolamine transdermal patch, atropine drops, glycopyrrolate IV/SQ, or hyoscyamine tablets) for secretions; benzodiazepines (e.g., lorazepam) for anxiety (which can be a large component of dyspnea); and bronchodilators, corticosteroids, and diuretics for their disease-modifying effects.

Supplemental Oxygen

Widespread use of oxygen is not recommended for relief of dyspnea, even in the dying phase.[25] However, a therapeutic trial of oxygen supplementation to relieve dyspnea in hypoxemic patients can be helpful. For non-hypoxemic patients, there are not data supporting use of supplemental oxygen for dyspnea, though some patients may report some relief. Use of oxygen in hypoxemic and non-hypoxemic patients should be based on symptom relief, not pulse oximetry, when used in dying patients. Patients generally prefer a nasal cannula, but masks or face-tents can also be used.

Table 31.4. Opioid Dosing for Management of Dyspnea

Opioid Tolerance	Dosage
Opioid naïve	5 mg oral morphine equivalent as single dose; if tolerated, can administer every 4 hours around the clock, hold for sedation; an additional dose every hour in between scheduled doses can be made available as needed for severe dyspnea
Older adults, CO_2 retainers, or patients with renal impairment	Consider reducing starting dose by half. Avoid use of morphine in patients with renal disease.
If current opioid dosage is inadequate	Titrate by increments of 25% to 50% to effect.
Dyspnea with exertion or movement	Give 30 minutes prior to activity.
If acutely dyspneic or actively dying	Use intravenous morphine bolus (2–5 mg or 10% of daily dosage) every 5–10 minutes as needed, titrate to effect (decline of self-reported dyspnea on 10-point scale); consider starting a continuous infusion based on the dosage needed to improve the patient's symptoms. For patients who cannot self-report, an improvement of nonverbal signs of distress or a decline in elevated respiratory rate toward the normal range may be used as surrogate markers of dyspnea.
If on stable opioid dosage	Consider a trial of scheduled short-acting opioid or long-acting opioid as baseline, with immediate-release opioid as needed in between.

Adapted from Quill TE, et al. *Primer of Palliative Care,* 6th ed. American Academy of Hospice and Palliative Medicine; 2014:51,[19] who adapted table from Brown DJ. Palliation of breathlessness. *Clin Med.* 2006;6:133–136.[24]

FATIGUE

Fatigue is one of the most common end-of-life symptom across all disease states. Prevalence estimates of fatigue range from 48% to 97%.[19] Reported prevalence rates are highest among those with cancer; however, patients with chronic or end-stage renal, hepatic, pulmonary, or cardiac disease, HIV, or neurological disease also frequently experience fatigue, which has been associated with poorer quality of life.[26,27] Fatigue has been defined as "a subjective feeling of tiredness, weakness, or lack of energy" and may have both physical and cognitive dimensions.[19] Fatigue is frequently multifactorial, and as always, a thorough history and physical are essential to diagnosing underlying factors. In many cases, patients experience primary fatigue (related directly to disease mechanism) in addition to secondary fatigue (related to non-disease-specific factors that are often reversible, such as medications, untreated pain, infection, sleep apnea). In cases of primary fatigue, the following treatment modalities may be helpful. Of note, there are limited data to guide treatment of fatigue, and most research to date has focused on stimulants, but results have been mixed.

Sleep Hygiene

Educating patients about sleep hygiene can help improve sleep quality and decrease daytime fatigue.

Exercise and Yoga

Meta-analyses evaluating the effect of various exercise programs on fatigue in cancer patients have found that physical exercise improved fatigue.[28] However, the optimal exercise intensity and duration are unclear. Given this, and given the fact that the patient's functional status may be limited, an individualized exercise plan is recommended based on each individual's capabilities. There is evidence that yoga can improve symptoms of fatigue in patients with cancer[29,30] and end-stage renal disease.[31]

Massage, Acupuncture, and Reiki

Studies suggest that massage, acupuncture, and reiki may play a beneficial role in reducing fatigue in cancer patients.[32-34]

Meditation and Hypnosis

Several studies have found that meditation can improve fatigue in a number of conditions, including heart failure and cancer.[35-37]

Hypnosis in combination with cognitive-behavioral therapy has been shown to ease fatigue in patients with breast cancer and may ease fatigue in other patient populations.[38]

IMPORTANT CAVEATS

When recommending natural products for a palliative care population, the clinician should be aware of the following:[39]

1. The potential harm of natural products in patients with limited renal or hepatic function
2. The potential harm of interactions between natural products and drugs
3. The potential harm of natural products due to poor manufacturing quality.

Because there are relatively few studies of complementary and integrative approaches in the palliative care population, further research is needed to guide care.

Palliative Care Approaches to Communication and Advance Care Planning

Fundamental to both integrative and palliative medicine are interdisciplinary care, whole-person care, and person-centered care through communication and goal setting. Both focus on the intersection of "healing" and care of the whole person: body, mind, spirit, patient, and family. Patients initially seek care with an initial hope that they can be restored to their former state of health and functioning. Should that goal become unlikely to be realized, the clinician should then guide patients through a process of formulating new goals for their health and well-being. Excellent communication skills facilitate this process.

Although many guidelines call for more communication about care planning, shared decision making, and advance care planning, the evidence shows that these functions are performed too little, and often too late. Common barriers to implementing better care planning include cultural barriers; psychological barriers; fears on the part of the patient, family, and physician; listening barriers; organizational barriers; language barriers; and medical terminology. A barrier that may particularly impact integrative medicine practitioners is uncertainty over roles. Patients expect their physicians to initiative these discussions, but there is ambiguity about whether the primary care physician or the specialist should take the lead.[40] Integrative medicine clinicians may assume that someone else—internist, cardiologist, oncologist—is taking the lead, but those practitioners may be too busy or may not have a systematic way to address the task, leaving the issues unaddressed. Because integrative medicine practitioners expressly concern themselves with holistic care, a systematic

Table 31.5. Reasons to Initiative Palliative Care Planning Conversations

Reasons for Palliative Conversations
– Shift in focus from cure to managing disease/disease symptoms
– Shift from quantity of life to quality of life
– Shift from managing disease to preparing for death
– Discussing prognosis when time is short
– Shifting goals when patient's initial goals are not achievable
– Discussing patient's desire to return home but patient cannot
– Discussing patient's desire to live to see a particular event but unlikely given life expectancy

Source: Goldstein NE, Morrison RS, et al. *Evidence-Based Practice of Palliative Medicine.* Philadelphia, PA: Elsevier Saunders; 2013:244.[41]

approach to care planning and advance care planning should be part of the care of any patient with serious illness seen by the integrative medicine team. Table 31.5 shows common reasons, or "triggers," that should prompt the integrative team to talk more fully about care planning for the impact of serious illness.

As shown in Figure 31.1, care planning, advance care planning, and shared decision making are all related process, but there is much confusion over the use of the terms. We use "care planning" as the broadest term covering all aspects of helping patients and families to articulate their goals and to develop realistic plans to address them. Shared decision making applies when several courses of action are open to the patient and selection of the appropriate one is best done through a collaborative process that allows patients and their providers to make health care decisions together, taking into account the best clinical evidence available as well as the patient's values and preferences.[42]

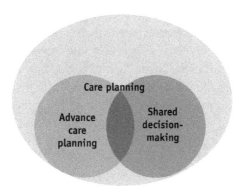

FIGURE 31.1. Care planning, advance care planning, and shared-decision-making.

Advance care planning is the process of having patients state what they would want in the future if they become unable to communicate or make decisions for themselves. Advance care planning also includes appointing someone to be the designated health care decision maker (or "proxy") in the future.

The communication skills that the practitioner needs to apply when unable to meet the goal of restoring a person to health include the following:

- Establishing rapport
- Helping patients articulate their goals and values as applicable to their health state
- Delivering "bad news," including prognostic information
- Providing medical information and information about treatment options (including probable efficacy and burdens)
- Guiding the advance care planning process

As practitioners, we are trained in the art and science of medicine and our role is to apply our knowledge to best assist patients in their health and well-being goals. These goals can vary significantly from person to person. We must develop excellent communication skills so that we treat the whole person rather than an isolated aspect of himself or herself. Our goal in these conversations is to establish what is important for the patient as a whole person, not assuming that all patients place equal weight on length of life or weigh the burdens of treatment in the same way. An additional task is to provide information about conditions and treatments such that the patient can grasp essential information, filter it through his or her values and preferences, and arrive at a decision. Finally, care planning is a process that takes place over time, is iterative, and responds to changes in the patient's health, function, and goals.

ESTABLISHING RAPPORT

Effective communication decreases patient distress, increases adherence to treatments, and results in higher satisfaction with care.[43] These skills take time and practice. Two sources for obtaining online guidance on skill building are VitalTalk (www.vitaltalk.org)[44] and E-prognosis (http://eprognosis.ucsf.edu/communication/).[45] VitalTalk is also helpful for becoming more effective in teaching these skills to others.[44] Highly effective techniques include asking broad-based, open-ended questions such as, "Tell me about yourself."

One important aspect of the initial communication approach is to establish how patients prefer to communicate, especially when difficult topics are discussed. Some patients may prefer to have family members with them; indeed, some may prefer to delegate decisions to family members. Establishing the patient's preferences for the communication process is an early step in most communication frameworks.

CLARIFYING PATIENT VALUES AND PREFERENCES

After establishing how patients wish to communicate, the next step is to explore what gives their life meaning. We work with them to identify concerns and to assess their unique cultural and spiritual values. When assessing spirituality, we assess their faith and beliefs, the importance they place on their faith and their faith community, and how it influences their medical care.[46] Gathering a sense of a patient's values contributes greatly to making medical treatment recommendations.

DELIVERING "BAD NEWS"

Several protocols have been developed to remind physicians of the steps in sensitive communication when sharing difficult news. All involve the following: arrange the physical and emotional atmosphere, find out how much the patient knows, find out how much the patient wants to know, share the information, respond to the patient's feelings, make a plan, and follow through. The simplest protocol to remember is "Ask-Tell-Ask," which counsels the physician to do just that.[47] SPIKES is a more detailed protocol. Both are summarized in Table 31.6.

PROVIDING INFORMATION ABOUT PROGNOSIS

Almost all patients consider it "very important" to receive information about what to expect in their illness.[48,49] The American College of Physicians' High Value Care Task Force recommends two steps. The first is to explore a patient's understanding of the prognosis in order to understand the patient's awareness and acceptance of the illness. This allows communication to be titrated to the patient's level of understanding. The second step is to provide prognostic information to the degree desired by the patient (and within the limits knowable to the physician) to enable the patient to factor this information into his or her decisions.[40]

Table 31.6. Two Protocols for Communicating Difficult News

Ask-Tell-Ask[47]	SPIKES

STEPS AND EXAMPLE
 	
Ask: Begin by **asking** an open-ended question about the patient's/family members' understanding of the medical illness, as well as their needs and concerns.
 	
Tell: Next, **tell** the patient/family members information based on the the patient's level of understanding discovered in the first "ask" (i.e., addressing issues that do not seem clear to the patient/family, discussing any areas of misunderstanding). Use non-technical words—for instance, "spread" instead of "metastasized."
 	
Ask: Lastly, either **ask** what the patient understood using a "teach-back" technique and whether this information has changed his or her own views of the illness or prognosis.
	S: Setup: set up interview
	• Learn about patient's medical condition.
	• Before the interview, meet with other providers to determine goals, establish roles during the meeting, discuss treatment options and prognostic information.
	• Invite patient, family, friends.
	• Identify surrogate decision maker if appropriate.
	• Sit down.
	• Introduce meeting participants.
	P: Perception
	• Ask the patient what he or she knows about his or her medical condition.
	  • "Tell me what you understand."
	  • "What have the doctors told you?"
	I: Invitation
	• Find out how much the patient wants to know about his or her condition.
	K: Knowledge
	• Explain the medical facts.
	• Explain gradually using language patient will understand.
	• Give a warning shot:
	  ▪ I have some bad news.
	  ▪ The news is not what we hoped for.
	• Confirm patient information.
	• If asked about prognosis:
	  ▪ Check if everyone present wishes to know.
	• Ensure patient and family members understand that prognosis is not a fixed time period. Prognosis changes with changing medical condition. "Based upon what we know so far and your present medical condition, it is likely . . ."
	• Provide general timeframes; do NOT give specific time/dates: hours to days, days to weeks, weeks to months, many months.
	E: Emotions, Empathize
	• Acknowledge emotions for patient and practitioner.
	  ▪ "I find it difficult to tell you."
	  ▪ "I wish things were different."
	S: Strategy or Summary
	• Support realistic hope.
	• Reframe hope: "We always have hope, but what we hope for may change."
	• Briefly review meeting.[1]
	• Establish next step.

Source: Buckman R. Communication skills in palliative care: A practical guide. *Neurol Clin.* 2001;19:4.[58]

ADVANCE CARE PLANNING

Given that many patients with serious illness will reach a point when they are unable to make decisions for themselves, it is helpful for physicians to guide patients through the process. Table 31.7 shows the basic types of documents used to record a patient's instructions and preferences.

SUPPORTING HOPE

There is a widespread misperception that disclosing a poor prognosis will "take away hope."[50] In reality, sensitive communication of the prognosis in the context of broader discussions about a person's goals and values can help in reframing so that hope is maintained.[51,52] Strategies for helping patients develop realistic goals that are part of a general sense of hopefulness include the following:

- Assess goals
- Address hope

Table 31.7. **Advance Care Planning Documents and Resources**

Types of Advanced Care Planning Documents	
Substantive Directive	Allows a patient to specify wishes for future care; may also allow designation of proxy decision maker
- Living Will	
- Five Wishes	
- Personal Wishes Statement	
Process Directives	Designates a surrogate decision maker; does not specify wishes for care
- Health care power of attorney	
- Health care proxy	
- Durable power of attorney for health care	
Physician Order for Life-Sustaining Treatment	- Physician's orders regarding cardiopulmonary resuscitation, medical interventions such as antibiotics, artificial nutrition and hydration - Travels with patient across care sites - Legally valid as order for transit
Code status	Order or document at a specific institution on cardiopulmonary resuscitation in the event of clinical decompensation

(continued)

Table 31.7. Continued

Advance Care Planning Resources

Resource	Description	Web Address
Massachusetts Medical Society: End-of-Life Care	Instructional website for patients; discusses advance care planning with focus on designation of health care proxy	www.healthcareproxy.org
Better Ending	Guides for patients in Massachusetts about how to do advance care planning; includes videos and guides in multiple languages	www.betterending.org
Aging with Dignity	Distribution site for: – Five Wishes – Next Steps how to discuss five wishes	www.agingwithdignity.org
Americans for Better Care of the Dying	National non-profit that advocates for better end-of-life care via policy change – Excerpts from "Handbook for Mortals"	www.abcd-caring.org
The POLST paradigm	Physician Order for Life-Sustaining Treatment (POLST), how to use it and access it in each state	www.polst.org
American Bar Association: Consumer's Toolkit for Health Care Advance Planning	Toolkit covering all aspects of advance care planning; includes resources, books	www.abanet.org/aging (under Resources)
Caring Connections	Guide from National Hospice and Palliative Care Organization; has link to state-specific advance directives	www.caringinfo.org
Respecting Choices	National online and onsite courses for medical professionals in advance care planning; from group at Gunderson Lutheran Medical Foundation	www.respectingchoices.org

Source: Goldstein NE, Morrison RS, et al. Evidence-Based Practice of Palliative Medicine. Philadelphia, PA. Elsevier Saunders; 2013:259.

- Hope for the best but prepare for the worse
- Reframe hope
- Focus on the positive

End of Life

As an individual's functional status declines, it is appropriate to revisit goals regarding medical interventions to support the patient's values, goals, and preference. To fully assess goals, it is necessary to address the whole person, body, mind, spirit, for the patient and family. Too often, the approach focuses on what *not* to do, but emphasizing avoiding resuscitation or other procedures misses the need to actively do many things to support the patient and family through the end of life. Involving family members can alleviate some of the loneliness dying patients experience. Dying patients have many fears, and open and direct conversations may relieve some of them: the fear of pain, of indignity, of abandonment, of loneliness, and of the unknown.[53-55] Balaban provides examples of appropriate questions to guide conversations regarding planning for the end of life.[56] Table 31.8 summarizes the issues that should be addressed when life expectancy is weeks to days.

Table 31.8. Issues to Be Addressed in the Last Weeks and Days of Life

End of Life
Prepare the family; educate family on ways of interacting with their dying loved ones:
– Talk to them; hearing is the last sense to be lost
– Respect dying loved one's dignity
– Reminisce, or be a quiet supportive presence
Prepare family when end of life is near
Provide knowledge of what to expect
Determine how much families wish to know
Signs of Approaching Death
Weeks to Months:
– Withdrawal
– Focus more internally
– Loss of interest in outside activities
– Increased sleep
– Touch and wordless companionship are valuable.
– Decreased need for food and fluid
– Variable interest in food/drink
– Taste changes
– This is NORMAL and EXPECTED.

(continued)

Table 31.8. Continued

Days to Weeks
– Disorientation
– Confusion is common
– Hearing, seeing, or having conversations with deceased loved ones becomes more common.
– Terminal delirium/agitation
  – Restlessness, agitation
  – May require medication and is often upsetting
  – Treat with antipsychotics, benzodiazepines; address pain issues

Hours to Days
– Physical changes
  – Change in complexion
  – Hypotension, tachycardia, thready pulse
  – Labile temperatures; treat with cool cloths, acetaminophen suppositories
  – Changes in breathing
  – Periods of apnea
  – Cheyne-Stokes breathing (long pause followed by rapid breathing)
  – Kussmaul breathing (deep, rapid breathing)
  – Agonal breathing (shallow rapid breathing)
  – Mottling
  – Respiratory secretions (formerly known as terminal secretions/death rattle); treat with repositioning, anticholinergics
  – Glazed eyes
– Nonresponsiveness
– Pre-death rally: hours to days before death patient may have period of lucidity, increased activity, may ask for favorite food or interact with family/friends; may give families a false sense of patient's recovery

Current Challenges in Providing Integrative Palliative Care

LACK OF EVIDENCE BASE

Even when the evidence for a complementary therapy is solid in a general population, there is usually very little evidence to guide its application to the palliative care population—people who are likely older and frailer and with many more comorbidities than the population in which the therapy was originally tested. Therefore, abundant caution needs to be used when considering how the evidence generalizes to people using palliative care.

UNCERTAINTY ABOUT BEST PRACTICE MODELS

While complementary or integrative therapies are sometimes used by palliative care or hospice teams, the actual integration of the two services is rare and there is no published evidence we are aware of to guide practice. There are two different approaches available. In the first approach, an embedded model, the integrative medicine practitioner becomes a regular part of the hospice or palliative care team, or a palliative care practitioner could be embedded within an integrative practice. The second approach keeps the services separate but encourages referral and active consultation between them.

ACCEPTANCE BY AND COLLABORATION WITH OTHER PROVIDERS

Both palliative care and integrative medicine face barriers in gaining the trust of other practitioners. Palliative care is sometimes seen derisively as just "hand holding and Band-Aids" and the same, or worse, is sometimes said about integrative medicine. Consulting etiquette is needed to build effective collaborations with initially skeptical colleagues.[57] Demonstrating a willingness to be helpful, to solve problems, and to put patient needs first can eventually win over colleagues and convert them into allies. Helping colleagues to manage difficult cases (such as families in conflict or patients with refractory symptoms) teaches them skills to use in similar cases and wins the consultant a steady stream of future referrals. Palliative care practitioners have found it useful to use "trigger lists" to screen for appropriate cases so that referrals are not left until too late.

LACK OF FUNDING MECHANISM AND DISPARITIES

Hospice is well covered in the United States for Medicare beneficiaries and for most privately insured patients. Hospices are able to, and are expected to, cover any appropriate treatments in the care plan for the terminal illness, and many routinely cover less expensive modalities such as massage and music therapy. But early (non-hospice) palliative care has no separate funding mechanism other than physician billing. Thus, coverage for integrative approaches that may not typically be covered by insurance may create an out-of-pocket burden for patients. For patients with fewer financial resources, lack of insurance coverage may make integrative approaches effectively out of reach.

QUALITY MEASUREMENT AND IMPROVEMENT

Quality measurement for palliative care is in its infancy; quality measurement for integrative care may still be prenatal. Measures that focus on functional

---

Box 31.1. Selected Educational Resources for Palliative Care Skills

Comprehensive information on all topics in short, one-page "bites": Palliative Care
Fast Facts and Concepts, http://www.mypcnow.org/fast-facts
    Comprehensive training programs online:
    EPEC-O: https://www.cancer.gov/resources-for/hp/education/epeco
    Stanford Palliative Care Training Portal: https://palliative.stanford.edu/
    Communication: Vitaltalk www.vitaltalk.org
    Prognosis calculators: E-prognosis http://eprognosis.ucsf.edu/calculators/#/

---

improvement, quality of life, and attainment of patient goals are promising
but nascent in these areas. Much more work is needed both to bolster the evidence base for effectiveness and to ensure that patients receive the best care.

Box 31.1 lists selected education resources for palliative care skills.

REFERENCES

1. Institute of Medicine. *Dying in America: Improving Quality and Honoring Individual Preferences near the End of Life*. Washington, DC: National Academies Press; 2014.
2. World Health Organization. NCDs/Palliative Care. 2015.
3. National Consensus Project for Quality Palliative Care. *Clinical Practice Guidelines for Quality Palliative Care*, 3rd ed. 2013.
4. Temel JS, Greer J, Muzikansky A, et al. Early palliative care for patients with met-astatic non-small-cell lung cancer. *N Engl J Med*. 2010;363(8):733–742. doi:10.1056/NEJMoa1000678.
5. Parikh RB, Kirch RA, Smith TJ, Temel JS. Early specialty palliative care—translating data in oncology into practice. *N Engl J Med*. 2013;369(24):2347–2351. doi:10.1056/NEJMsb1305469.
6. Pan CX, Morrison RS, Ness J, et al. Complementary and alternative medicine in the management of pain, dyspnea, and nausea and vomiting near the end of life. A systematic review. *J Pain Symptom Manage*. 2000;20(5):374–387. doi:10.1016/S0885-3924(00)00190-1.
7. Lafferty WE, Downey L, McCarty RL, Standish LJ, Patrick DL. Evaluating CAM treatment at the end of life: A review of clinical trials for massage and meditation. *Complement Ther Med*. 2006;14(2):100–112. doi:10.1016/j.ctim.2006.01.009.
8. Wood GJ, Shega JW, Lynch B, Von Roenn JH. Management of intractable nausea and vomiting in patients at the end of life. *JAMA*. 2007;298(10):1196. doi:10.1001/jama.298.10.1196.
9. Mandal P, Das A, Majumdar S, Bhattacharyya T, Mitra T, Kundu R. The effi-cacy of ginger added to ondansetron for preventing postoperative nausea and

vomiting in ambulatory surgery. *Pharmacognosy Res.* 2014;6(1):52–57. doi:10.4103/0974-8490.122918.

10. Dabaghzadeh F, Khalili H, Dashti-Khavidaki S, Abbasian L, Moeinifard A. Ginger for prevention of antiretroviral-induced nausea and vomiting: A randomized clinical trial. *Expert Opin Drug Saf.* 2014;13(7):859–866. doi:10.1517/14740338.2014.914170.

11. Marx W, McCarthy AL, Ried K, et al. Can ginger ameliorate chemotherapy-induced nausea? Protocol of a randomized double blind, placebo-controlled trial. *BMC Complement Altern Med.* 2014;14(1):134. doi:10.1186/1472-6882-14-134.

12. Marx WM, Teleni L, McCarthy AL, et al. Ginger (*Zingiber officinale*) and chemotherapy-induced nausea and vomiting: A systematic literature review. *Nutr Rev.* 2013;71(4):245–254. doi:10.1111/nure.12016.

13. Ryan JL, Heckler CE, Roscoe JA, et al. Ginger (*Zingiber officinale*) reduces acute chemotherapy-induced nausea: A URCC CCOP study of 576 patients. *Support Care Cancer.* 2012;20(7):1479–1489. doi:10.1007/s00520-011-1236-3.

14. Marx W, Ried K, McCarthy AL, et al. Ginger: Mechanism of action in chemotherapy-induced nausea and vomiting: A review. *Crit Rev Food Sci Nutr.* 2017;57(1):141–146. doi:10.1080/10408398.2013.865590.

15. Smith LA, Azariah F, Lavender VTC, Stoner NS, Bettiol S. Cannabinoids for nausea and vomiting in adults with cancer receiving chemotherapy. *Cochrane Database Syst Rev.* 2015;11(11):CD009464. doi:10.1002/14651858.CD009464.pub2.

16. Rithirangsriroj K, Manchana T, Akkayagorn L. Efficacy of acupuncture in prevention of delayed chemotherapy-induced nausea and vomiting in gynecologic cancer patients. *Gynecol Oncol.* 2015;136(1):82–86. doi:10.1016/j.ygyno.2014.10.025.

17. Molassiotis A, Helin AM, Dabbour R, Hummerston S. The effects of P6 acupressure in the prophylaxis of chemotherapy-related nausea and vomiting in breast cancer patients. *Complement Ther Med.* 2007;15(1):3–12. doi:10.1016/j.ctim.2006.07.005.

18. Taspinar A, Sirin A. Effect of acupressure on chemotherapy-induced nausea and vomiting in gynecologic cancer patients in Turkey. *Eur J Oncol Nurs.* 2010;14(1):49–54. doi:10.1016/j.ejon.2009.07.006.

19. Quill T, Bower K, Holloway R, et al. *Primer of Palliative Care*, 6th ed. AAHPM; 2014.

20. Sykes NP. The pathogenesis of constipation. *J Support Oncol.* 2006;4(5):213–218.

21. Aliasghari F, Homayouni Rad A, Motayagheni N, Homayouni Rad H, Sahhaf F. Application of laxative foods in prevention and treatment of constipation. *MOJ Food Process Technol.* 2016;2(4):45. doi:10.15406/mojfpt.2016.02.00045.

22. Ramos CI, Andrade de Lima AF, Grilli DG, Cuppari L. The short-term effects of olive oil and flaxseed oil for the treatment of constipation in hemodialysis patients. *J Ren Nutr.* 2015;25(1):50–56. doi:10.1053/j.jrn.2014.07.009.

23. Barnes H, McDonald J, Smallwood N, Manser R. Opioids for the palliation of refractory breathlessness in adults with advanced disease and terminal illness. *Cochrane Database Syst Rev.* 2016;3:CD011008. doi:10.1002/14651858.CD011008.pub2.

24. Brown DJF. Palliation of breathlessness. *Clin Med.* 6(2):133–136.

25. Campbell ML, Yarandi H, Dove-Medows E. Oxygen is nonbeneficial for most patients who are near death. *J Pain Symptom Manage.* 2013;45(3):517–523. doi:10.1016/j.jpainsymman.2012.02.012.

26. Walke LM, Gallo WT, Tinetti ME, Fried TR. The burden of symptoms among community-dwelling older persons with advanced chronic disease. *Arch Intern Med.* 2004;164(21):2321–2324.

27. Horigan AE. Fatigue in hemodialysis patients: A review of current knowledge. *J Pain Symptom Manage.* 2012;44(5):715–724. doi:10.1016/j.jpainsymman.2011.10.015.

28. Tomlinson D, Diorio C, Beyene J, Sung L. Effect of exercise on cancer-related fatigue. *Am J Phys Med Rehabil.* 2014;93(8):675–686. doi:10.1097/PHM.0000000000000083.

29. Pachman DR, Barton DL, Swetz KM, Loprinzi CL. Troublesome symptoms in cancer survivors: Fatigue, insomnia, neuropathy, and pain. *J Clin Oncol.* 2012;30(30):3687–3696. doi:10.1200/JCO.2012.41.7238.

30. Buffart LM, van Uffelen JGZ, Riphagen II, et al. Physical and psychosocial benefits of yoga in cancer patients and survivors, a systematic review and meta-analysis of randomized controlled trials. *BMC Cancer.* 2012;12(1):559. doi:10.1186/1471-2407-12-559.

31. Yurtkuran M, Alp A, Yurtkuran M, Dilek K. A modified yoga-based exercise program in hemodialysis patients: A randomized controlled study. *Complement Ther Med.* 2007;15(3):164–171. doi:10.1016/j.ctim.2006.06.008.

32. Fleisher KA, Mackenzie ER, Frankel ES, Seluzicki C, Casarett D, Mao JJ. Integrative reiki for cancer patients: A program evaluation. *Integr Cancer Ther.* 2014;13(1):62–67. doi:10.1177/1534735413503547.

33. Boyd C, Crawford C, Paat CF, et al. The impact of massage therapy on function in pain populations: A systematic review and meta-analysis of randomized controlled trials: Part II, Cancer pain populations. *Pain Med.* 2016;17(8):1553–1568. doi:10.1093/pm/pnw100.

34. Lau CHY, Wu X, Chung VCH, et al. Acupuncture and related therapies for symptom management in palliative cancer care. *Medicine (Balt).* 2016;95(9):e2901. doi:10.1097/MD.0000000000002901.

35. Kim YH, Kim HJ, Ahn S Do, Seo YJ, Kim SH. Effects of meditation on anxiety, depression, fatigue, and quality of life of women undergoing radiation therapy for breast cancer. *Complement Ther Med.* 2013;21(4):379–387. doi:10.1016/j.ctim.2013.06.005.

36. Kwekkeboom KL, Bratzke LC. A systematic review of relaxation, meditation, and guided imagery strategies for symptom management in heart failure. *J Cardiovasc Nurs.* 2016;31(5):457–468. doi:10.1097/JCN.0000000000000274.

37. Carlson LE, Garland SN. Impact of mindfulness-based stress reduction (MBSR) on sleep, mood, stress and fatigue symptoms in cancer outpatients. *Int J Behav Med.* 2005;12(4):278–285. doi:10.1207/s15327558ijbm1204_9.

38. Witt CM, Cardoso MJ. Complementary and integrative medicine for breast cancer patients: Evidence-based practical recommendations. *Breast.* 2016;28:37–44. doi:10.1016/j.breast.2016.04.012.

39. Leong M, Smith TJ, Rowland-Seymour A. Complementary and integrative medicine for older adults in palliative care. *Clin Geriatr Med*. 2015;31(2):177–191. doi:10.1016/j.cger.2015.01.004.

40. Bernacki RE, Block SD. Communication about serious illness care goals: A review and synthesis of best practices. *JAMA Intern Med*. 2014;174(12):1994–2003. doi:10.1001/jamainternmed.2014.5271.

41. Goldstein NE, Morrison RS (Rolfe S. *Evidence-Based Practice of Palliative Medicine*. Philadelphia, PA: Elsevier Saunders; 2013.

42. Informed Medical Decisions Foundation. Why shared decision making? http://www.informedmedicaldecisions.org/shareddecisionmaking.aspx. Accessed December 8, 2016.

43. Griffin SJ, Kinmonth A-L, Veltman MWM, Gillard S, Grant J, Stewart M. Effect on health-related outcomes of interventions to alter the interaction between patients and practitioners: A systematic review of trials. *Ann Fam Med*. 2004;2(6):595–608. doi:10.1370/afm.142.

44. Vital Talk. http://www.vitaltalk.org/.

45. ePrognosis: Communication. http://eprognosis.ucsf.edu/communication/.

46. Puchalski CM. The role of spirituality in health care. *Proc Bayl Univ Med Cent*. 2001;14(4):352–357.

47. ePrognosis: Communication Skills: Ask Tell Ask. http://eprognosis.ucsf.edu/communication/video-ask-tell-ask.php.

48. Clayton JM, Butow PN, Arnold RM, Tattersall MHN. Discussing life expectancy with terminally ill cancer patients and their carers: A qualitative study. *Support Care Cancer*. 2005;13(9):733–742. doi:10.1007/s00520-005-0789-4.

49. Steinhauser KE, Christakis NA, Clipp EC, McNeilly M, McIntyre L, Tulsky JA. Factors considered important at the end of life by patients, family, physicians, and other care providers. *JAMA*. 2000;284(19):2476–2482.

50. Warm E, Weissman DE. Fast Fact #21: Hope and Truth Telling. Palliative Care Network of Wisconsin Fast Facts. http://www.mypcnow.org/blank-ficho. Published 2015. Accessed December 8, 2016.

51. Evans W, Tulsky J, Back A, Arnold R. Communication at times of transitions: How to help patients cope with loss and re-define hope. *Cancer J*. 2006;12(5):417–424.

52. Coulourides Kogan A, Penido M, Enguidanos S. Does disclosure of terminal prognosis mean losing hope? Insights from exploring patient perspectives on their experience of palliative care consultations. *J Palliat Med*. 2015;18(12):1019–1025. doi:10.1089/jpm.2015.0038.

53. Lynn J, Teno JM, Phillips RS, et al. Perceptions by family members of the dying experience of older and seriously ill patients. SUPPORT Investigators. Study to Understand Prognoses and Preferences for Outcomes and Risks of Treatments. *Ann Intern Med*. 1997;126(2):97–106.

54. Lynn J. An 88-year-old woman facing the end of life. *JAMA*. 1997;277(20):1633. doi:10.1001/jama.1997.03540440067034.

55. Callahan D. Pursuing a peaceful death. *Hastings Cent Rep.* 23(4):32–38.

56. Balaban RB. A physician's guide to talking about end-of-life care. *J Gen Intern Med.* 2000;15(3):195–200.

57. von Gunten C, Weissman D. Fast Fact #266: Consultation etiquette in palliative care. Palliative Fast Facts and Concepts. http://www.mypcnow.org/blank-j2555. Published 2013. Accessed December 8, 2016.

58. Buckman R. Communication skills in palliative care: A practical guide. *Neurol Clin.* 2001;19(4):989–1004.

32

Positive Aging

MICHELLE SIERPINA AND BEVERLY LUNSFORD

Case Study

At age 81, Bob, a former military pilot, oil industry executive, and entrepreneur, happened upon and joined a community-based organization offering college-level academic courses, fitness activities, and opportunities for social interactions for those over 55. He reports that at the time he was suffering from neuropathies and other physical ailments, tiring easily, and experiencing muscle aches that impaired his mobility, so he lacked any regular physical activity. He experienced diminishing interest in leaving the house as he noticed what he perceived as his declining state. After a series of lifestyle changes offered in this new group, he discovered improved quality of life and better physical and mental status in his eighth decade. As a result of incorporating increased socialization, moderate group fitness activities, walking, group practice of life review, a literature discussion group, and other similar activities, Bob reported, at age 86, that his neuropathies were disappearing and his mental and psychological outlook had reversed. After a fall in a bathroom, he was able to get up by himself, a feat he attributed to his functional fitness training at his senior community program.

In the life story group, he wrote vignettes that brought back long-forgotten memories that he enjoys sharing with family and friends. One study found that the protocol his group used decreased depressive symptoms in older adults.[1] Another literature appreciation group he joined has supplied joy and laughter he seldom experienced in any other settings and at any other time in his life. The friends he has made have truly proven the meaning and value of "community."

Bob's story represents numerous others like himself who demonstrate that progressive decline and deterioration can at least be slowed, and in his case were actually reversed. In this chapter, we share a variety of tools to achieve such results.

Introduction

People gather every day in the Osher Lifelong Learning Institute—OLLI at UTMB Health with friends, and others who will become friends, as they expand their social, intellectual, physical, and spiritual dimensions. Ages 55 to 105, these folks represent a new archetype of aging where the final years of life are filled with meaning, fulfillment, hope, and opportunities for generativity. As a group, they offer living confirmation that while certain aspects of the aging process alter physical, mental, and social capabilities, new coping mechanisms and new perspectives encourage a more dynamic view of longevity and the tools to achieve that.

In this chapter, we share case histories that allow you to meet individuals whose stories will equip you with options and resources to share with your patients and clients. Marsha, for instance, heard her geriatrician warn that she had to make major lifestyle changes or suffer serious health consequences. She started with a modest indoor walking practice, added seated fitness, then was ready for yoga, and finally completed a 5K fun run/walk, resulting in improved clinical lab markers. She achieved a remarkable improvement in self-esteem and outlook, developing a group of new friends who provided support and encouragement for her healthy lifestyle choices. Those choices and activities served as a springboard to improving Marsha's social, intellectual, and creative pursuits.

Larry's wife suffered a protracted illness that required his devoted attentiveness for years. After her death, he was an adrift and inconsolable widower. His daughter encouraged participation in community activities but he resisted. After some months, he succumbed to her persistence and began enjoying ballroom dance classes with a new-found friend, which led to his involvement in yoga, nutrition, and healthy eating classes, followed by numerous other experiences luring him to join his new community of friends for one learning and living experience or another every day, filling his life with joy and meaning. He transformed a hopeless future into a vital new reality by making new choices and opening himself to new experiences and people.

Harold's perspective on dating after 80 will bring you to the heart of longing and late-life love. A former health care provider himself, he understood the physiological and psychological components of how one might experience emptiness after decades in a committed relationship to find oneself alone and lonely.

Let us then meet the new aging cohort, the face of aging in the future. Here, later life becomes an adventure in creativity, the arts, humanities, and artistic expression, whether in music, dance, art, poetry, creative writing, or personal reflection. Yoga, tai chi, walking, ballroom dance, and water aerobics offer possibilities for vibrant growth rather than the stereotype of inevitable decline in the later years of life. Most of the individuals we introduce participate in an Osher Lifelong Learning Institute on a barrier island off the Texas Gulf Coast. At this writing there are 119 OLLIs across the nation. In the United States and beyond, thousands of other academies for lifelong learning, institutes for learning in retirement, and senior centers offer an endless array of opportunities for socialization, physical activity, volunteering, and self-improvement.

Get a Move On!

"The motion is the lotion" summarizes a sound theory in rehabilitation. Those committed to healthy lifestyles at any age must develop enjoyable, sustainable forms of physical activity. Sometimes favored sports or physical activity from earlier stages in life can be continued as one grows older. Those fortunate enough to continue lifelong practices, such as the 92-year-old competitive ballroom dancer, likely represent the minority.

Often, realities of an aging body or other factors may preclude pick-up basketball, hours on the golf course, touch football, or daily jogging. However, options for age-appropriate movement activities abound for aging individuals. Walking, a universal pastime, can be done almost anywhere, at any time, and by most people. One study explored the value of walking compared to ballroom dance for effectiveness in preventing cognitive decline. The authors concluded, "A physically active lifestyle has the potential to prevent cognitive decline and dementia, yet the optimal type of physical activity/exercise remains unclear."[2] Like many other studies, the message is to keep in motion. Walking can be done safely in most places, but indoor walking tracks or even the neighborhood shopping mall may provide a climate-controlled environment, making walking possible in any weather.

Ballroom dance continues to prove an effective (and fun) method for enhancing both physical and mental capacity. Some studies have examined the value of tai chi for falls prevention, balance, and gait issues. One study found that ballroom dance and tai chi both had benefits.[3]

Yoga has been shown to have positive health benefits in a multitude of ways, including memory enhancement training;[4] it also provides an effective motivational attraction for those who participate.[5] According to that study, only activities that bring pleasure and personal satisfaction will become a regular, sustainable practice.

Whether science supports tai chi over yoga or ballroom dance over walking or whatever the comparison, here is a crucial point: "Providing diversity in exercise programs targeting seniors recognises the heterogeneity of multicultural populations and may further increase the number of taking part in exercise."[2] In other words, by providing numerous options and thus encouragement for fitness activities, participants can find the style of activity that best suits their needs, interests, and lifestyle. One review article covers a variety of suggestions.[6] As mobility declines, some activities like yoga and tai chi can even be adapted by using chairs. Water therapy is another example of a positive physiotherapy and exercise that allows those with painful joints to move in the buoyancy and support of water.

Creative Expression, Play, Dance, Art, Theater

The National Center for Creative Aging (NCCA) challenges us to "Envision a world where all individuals flourish across their lifespan through creative expression." The center is "dedicated to fostering an understanding of the vital relationship between creative expression and healthy aging, and to developing programs that build upon this understanding in a world where all individuals flourish across their lifespan through creative expression."[7]

Consider incorporating art, music, dance, exercise, poetry/literature, theater, life reflection, and coupling and sexuality in prognosis and treatment plans for your clients/patients. Take cues and advice from NCCA, then look to your own community for options and opportunities. Check out your local YMCA, YWCA, county extension service, community college, faith-based organization, or some other group that provides opportunities for art, music, dance, or other creative outlets for older adults. Refer patients to these resources as part of their treatment plan for lifestyle choices.

Meaning, Generativity, and Sexuality in Aging

Eric Erikson,[8] George Vaillant,[9] and others commonly accept generativity as promoting growth in others who are younger. Meaning in life, quality of life, and generativity have expanded to include promoting growth in others of any age. Great power results when older adults share their wisdom and life experiences with younger generations to educate, encourage, and empower. In later years, though, any of the categories discussed in this chapter, creative expression, life reflection, meditation, gratitude, even physical activity, can provide opportunities for mentoring, inspiring, and challenging others. A grandmother who practices yoga or Pilates three times a week or an uncle who blogs regularly might motivate someone from a younger generation. Those practices can be equally motivating to a friend, neighbor, or sibling of a similar or even older age. Whether going to a fitness session, attending a lecture, or painting a watercolor, aging individuals challenge their peers by simply showing up and continuing the practice, thus setting an example.

Elders might fulfill the longing for generativity by sharing their artistic and creative skills mentoring local schoolchildren of any age. In our community, partnerships with local school districts and art organizations welcome older adults with time and talent to give and wisdom to impart. While mentoring others, older adults can also fulfill their personal needs for creativity. A local arts and environmental group offers a course on sustaining wetlands. The experience culminates in enhanced environmental awareness and leads to opportunities to participate in environmental projects while mentoring others. Boys and Girls Clubs seek "grandparents" for children. One man satisfies his longing for theatrical performance by playing Santa Claus, generativity and creativity intersecting in his life.

Older adults sometimes have formalized roles in generativity through educating future health care providers. Medical students, resident physicians, nurses, and other health care professionals who rotate through community-based programs for older adults gain a rich perspective on the possibilities and tools available to achieve healthy aging. In one study, "Preliminary results using descriptive analysis revealed an increase in positive images of aging and a decrease in negative images of aging among the five student participants."[10]

Sexuality and the need for intimacy continue after a loved one passes away. One man wrote about this in his life story group, describing "dating" as complicated and confusing. "At 80, I had the advantage that the female-to-male ratio of singles over 70 seemed about 50 to 1. I soon found dating in high school and college is quite different from dating by the aged. The biggest problem was 'intimacy'. If I/we were to go on a cruise around the world, the expense of two cabins would be prohibitive. Also I did not know my own capabilities and, having the medical knowledge of aged women's difficulties, I had trouble approaching the subject." One study in Spain reported, "Residential Aging Care Facilities staff should have an opportunity to receive training on residents' sexuality, as sexual interest and behavior is a key dimension of residents' lives."[11]

Conclusions

The Alzheimer's Association believes that "The public should know what the science concludes: certain healthy behaviors known to be effective for diabetes, cardiovascular disease, and cancer are also good for brain health and for reducing the risk of cognitive decline."[12] They have launched a new brain health education program, *Healthy Habits for a Healthier You*. Like Stanford's Sightlines Project, the aim is to provide a combination of current research and useful information about ways that consumers "can take care of their bodies and brains to age as well as possible."[12] Healthy lifestyle choices can and must become a norm for positive aging. In *Seven Strategies for Positive Aging*, Robert D. Hill asserts "the characteristics of positive aging come from practicing strategies that promote optimal adjustment in old age."[13]

The following is a list of key online resources, but please consider expanding your horizon to many others. Investigate each website with caution as you assess evidence-based criteria. Aging services must offer evidence in order for you to devote resources to those you serve.

- *The Creativity and Aging Study*Landmark study on the effects of arts participation on an aging population (https://cahh.gwu.edu/arts-aging-study). This study, the first controlled study to assess whether participation in the creative arts, apart from traditional medical care, can promote healthier aging was led by Gene D. Cohen, MD.
- *Think Positive about Aging and Live Longer*, by Mark Stibich, PhD (http://longevity.about.com/od/mentalfitness/p/positive_aging.htm). Research shows that how you perceive aging affects how long you will live. In a study of 660 people, those with more positive perceptions of their own aging lived an average of 7.5 years longer. This effect remained after other factors such as age, gender, income, loneliness, and health status were controlled.
- *Program for Positive Aging*—a place for everyone's brighter future (http://www.programforpositiveaging.org/). Positive aging involves more than just maintaining good health for as long as possible. Physical wellness is vital and valuable, but it isn't the whole solution. Positive aging is also about quality of life and enjoyment of living. Overall wellness depends upon attitude, spirit, resilience, and adaptability to the new opportunities and challenges of later life.
- *Positive Aging Newsletter* from the Taos Institute (http://www.taosinstitute.net/positive-aging-newsletter): The newsletter brings to light resources—from scientific research on aging, gerontology practices,

and daily life—that contribute to an appreciation of the aging process. Challenging the longstanding view of aging as decline, the newsletter provides resources for understanding aging as an unprecedented period of human development.

- *The Sightlines Project* at Stanford University (http://longevity3.stanford. edu/wp-content/uploads/2016/05/Sightlines-Project.pdf): Seeing our way to living long and living well in 21st-century America.

REFERENCES

1. Chippendale T, Bear-Lehman J. Effect of life review writing on depressive symptoms in older adults: A randomized control trial. *Am J Occup Ther.* 2012 Jul-Aug;66(4):438–446.
2. Merom D, et al. Cognitive benefits of social dancing and walking in old age: The dancing mind randomized controlled trial. *Front Aging Neurosci.* 2016 Feb 22;8:26. doi: 10.3389/fnagi.2016.00026.
3. Rahal MA, et al. Analysis of static and dynamic balance in healthy elderly practitioners of Tai Chi Chuan versus ballroom dancing. *Clinics (Sao Paulo).* 2015 Mar;70(3):157–161.
4. Eyre HA, et al. Changes in neural connectivity and memory following a yoga intervention for older adults: A pilot study. *J Alzheimers Dis.* 2016;52(2):673–684. doi:10.3233/JAD-150653.
5. Wertman A, Wister AV, Mitchell BA. On and off the mat: Yoga experiences of middle-aged and older adults. *Can J Aging.* 2016 Jun;35(2):190–205. DOI: 10.1017/S0714980816000155.
6. Bamidis PD, et al. A review of physical and cognitive interventions in aging. Applied Neuroscience: Models, methods, theories, reviews. A Society of Applied Neuroscience (SAN) special issue. *Neurosci Biobehav Rev.* 2014;44:206–220.
7. http://www.creativeaging.org/about-ncca Accessed June 8, 2016.
8. Erikson EH, Erickson JM, Kivnick HQ. *Vital Involvement in Old Age.* New York: W.W. Norton; 1986.
9. Vaillant GE. *Aging Well: Surprising Guideposts to a Happier Life.* Boston: Little Brown; 2002.
10. Chippendale T. Elders' life stories: Impact on the next generation of health professionals. *Curr Gerontol Geriatr Res.* 2013;2013:493728. doiI:10.1155/2013/493728.
11. Villar F, Celdrán M, Fabà J, Serrat R. Staff members' perceived training needs regarding sexuality in residential aged care facilities. *Gerontol Geriatr Educ.* 2016 Feb. 17 [E-pub before print]. doi:10.1080/02701960.2015.1127811
12. Baumgart M, et al. Summary of the evidence on modifiable risk factors for cognitive decline and dementia: A population-based perspective. *Alzheimers Dementia.* 2015;11(6):718–726.
13. Hill RD. *Seven Strategies for Positive Aging.* New York: W.W. Norton; 2008.

INDEX

women's health, 171–83. *See also* menopause
  breast health, 177–78
  genitourinary problems, 178–81
  hormone replacement therapy, 182–83
  life expectancy data, 171
  post-menopause skin changes, 176–77
  sexual response, 182
  vasomotor symptoms, 174–76
  white women, decreasing life
    expectancy, 1
Women's Health Initiative (WHI), 174,
    178, 182
World Federation of Chiropractic, 95
World Health Organization (WHO)
  disease classifications, 423–24
  on ischemic heart disease, 215
  magnesium recommendation, 220
  palliative care, defined, 565
wound healing, 118, 176
WP Thyroid, 246

xanthine oxidase (XO) inhibitor,
    for gout, 462

Yin and Yang (in TCM), 77
yoga
  Alzheimer's disease and, 408
  cognitive function benefits, 111, 595
  colon cancer and, 304
  components of, 108
  COPD and, 348
  delivery methods, 109
  in exercise prescription, 50, 59
  fatigue and, 577
  for fibromyalgia, 208
  flexibility and, 158

gene expression and, 61
historical background, 108
for HPA axis dysfunctions, 258
immune system and, 320
for irritable bowel syndrome, 310
for myofascial pain syndrome, 204
osteoarthritis and, 450
osteoporosis-related fractures and, 110
as positive aging activity, 595
positive aging and, 595
postural control and mobility and, 110
principles of, 108
psychiatric disorders and, 373
research studies, findings, 110
sleep, depression, and, 110
teacher accreditation, 109
Therapeutic Yoga for Seniors program, 109
at VA centers, 529
yoga therapy vs., 108–9
Yoga for Healthy Aging blog, 109
YOGA My Heart Study, 225
Yoga Nidra, 529

Zhang Sanfeng, 104
zinc
  Alzheimer's disease and, 410
  in cancer side effect management, 437
  deficiency symptoms, 34
  ejection fraction/micronutrient study
    findings, 223
  gastrointestinal issues and, 35
  for irritable bowel syndrome,
    inflammatory bowel disease, 311
  macular degeneration and, 493
  osteoporosis and, 275
  respiratory infections and, 331